Impact of Digital Solutions for Improved Healthcare Delivery

Nilmini Wickramasinghe
La Trobe University, Australia

IGI Global
Publishing Tomorrow's Research Today

Published in the United States of America by
    IGI Global
    701 E. Chocolate Avenue
    Hershey PA, USA 17033
    Tel: 717-533-8845
    Fax: 717-533-8661
    E-mail: cust@igi-global.com
    Web site: https://www.igi-global.com

Library of Congress Cataloging-in-Publication Data

CIP PENDING

ISBN13: 9798369352373
Isbn13Softcover: 9798369352380
EISBN13: 9798369352397

Vice President of Editorial: Melissa Wagner
Managing Editor of Acquisitions: Mikaela Felty
Managing Editor of Book Development: Jocelynn Hessler
Production Manager: Mike Brehm
Cover Design: Phillip Shickler

British Cataloguing in Publication Data
A Cataloguing in Publication record for this book is available from the British Library.

This book is dedicated to the 3Gs in my life who have always guided me and grounded me so I can always do my best, aim for excellence and never settle for less and my 2 Ms and last but definitely not least J whose support and encouragement is not only valued and appreciated but without which it would not be possible to have the clarity of thought to embark upon let alone complete such an opus.

Editorial Advisory Board

Table of Contents

Detailed Table of Contents

Chapter 1

Yordanka Karayaneva, Teesside University, UK
Sara Sharifzadeh, Swansea University, UK
Ala Szczepura, Coventry University, UK
Yanguo Jing, Leeds Trinity University, UK
Bo Tan, Tampere University, Finland

Many countries world-wide are facing the public health challenge of caring for an aging population. Meanwhile, there is a belief that in care settings unobtrusive sensors and physical robots will eventually address this challenge. However, research into factors influencing older users' acceptance of such technology in these environments has received little attention. This paper describes a study undertaken in a UK care home 'living lab' environment exploring older people's preferences for sensors and robots. An in-depth qualitative study examined the preferences of a cross-section of 21 older adults (aged 81-99) in the care home setting. In addition to two dimensions (usefulness and ease-of-use) included in the Technology Acceptance Model (TAM) framework, the importance of other elements such as physical appearance, functionality, cost, trust and control were investigated. The resulting framework is presented to support future co-design of sensors and robots with older adults.

    Omar F. El-Gayar, Dakota State University, USA
    Giridhar Reddy Bojja, Michigan Tech, USA
    Loknath Sai Ambati, Oklahoma City University, USA
    James Boit, Grand Valley State University, USA
    Nevine Nawar, Alexandria University, Egypt

The increasing demand for efficient healthcare has spurred the adoption of IoT technologies, promising reduced costs and improved outcomes. This study addresses the integration of IoT in healthcare, focusing on patient-centered applications across prevention, diagnosis, and treatment. We explore three research questions concerning the main IoT applications, their drivers and challenges, and their impact on healthcare delivery. This systematic literature review synthesizes evidence from the literature to identify trends and mappings in IoT applications. The review includes a comprehensive framework for IoT in healthcare, enhancing patient engagement and care delivery. The study is structured first to define IoT paradigms and technologies, followed by proposing a healthcare framework, describing our methodology, and discussing the implications of our findings on future healthcare innovations.

    William Alberto Cruz Castañeda, Universidade Tecnológica Federal do
        Paraná, Brazil

Healthcare is facing challenges, such as the rising cost of care, an increase in the elderly population, and the prevalence of chronic diseases. To address these challenges, there is a need to transform healthcare from a hospital-centered to a patient-centered model focused on disease management to improve well-being. To achieve this, decentralized healthcare services are integrated with the Internet of Things and cloud technologies. As a result, cost-effective digital healthcare services have emerged. These digital services use body sensor networks and wearable devices for health monitoring, ensuring access to health data. Nevertheless, data from several digital services is difficult to handle using conventional analysis procedures. Thus, this chapter proposes small-scale and large-scale digital smart healthcare service architectures to allow autonomy and decision-making founded on artificial intelligence, multiple criteria decisions, sixth-generation communication, cloud technologies, and wearable Internet of Things for point-of-care and chronic disease management.

Artificial Intelligence encompasses a range of technologies which includes machine learning, natural language processing and predictive analytics and all of which are being integrated into healthcare systems. These applications are optimizing clinical workflows, aiding in more accurate diagnoses and providing data-driven insights that enhance decision-making for healthcare professionals. The diagnostic tools powered by AI are proving instrumental in early detection of diseases ultimately leading to improved treatment plans and outcomes. With accelerating outcomes, improving patient experiences and transforming traditional approaches, AI is reshaping the healthcare industry in profound ways. This chapter provides in-depth exploration into the transformative impact of Artificial Intelligence on healthcare outcomes, specifically focusing on enhancing the patient experience in the digital era. It also explores the multifaceted ways in which AI is accelerating healthcare outcomes and reshaping patient experiences which contributing to the overall transformation of the healthcare industry.

In the age of multi-resistant bacteria and viruses, sterilizing surgical instruments effectively and efficiently impacts hospital-acquired infections. In a hospital sterilization and decontamination unit (HSDU), contaminated equipment arrives after their use in the operating theatre, intensive care unit, diagnostics facilities, and wards. Items are unpacked, checked, inventoried, washed, dried and packed. Each activity requires resources and inefficient management can lead to increasing lead times for items to be processed and, thus, poses an increased risk of hospital-acquired infections. A simulation model was developed for the National Health Service in the U.K. Data relating to staffing levels and machine availability has been collected and the arrival patterns of items are considered. A heuristic simulation-optimization approach was employed to produce an improved staffing pattern that meets the required service level. Furthermore, the output ensures that instruments are processed within a 5-hour target time and is developed and applied to real-world scenarios.

A frequent cancer worldwide is skin cancer. Non-melanoma exists. Melanoma kills more than non-melanoma skin malignancies. Successful treatment and early diagnosis improve skin cancer survival. Cancer burden and prognosis vary depending on the diagnosis type and stage. The biopsy method used to diagnose skin cancer is imprecise. To diagnose and treat skin cancer early, onco-dermatologists must enhance diagnostic accuracy. Doctors use several tools to diagnose skin lesions. Through image processing, AI has enhanced early skin cancer diagnosis. Radiology adopted artificial intelligence (AI) sooner than dermatology. AI is now more accessible because of technology, AI-powered expert systems can detect skin cancer early. This chapter examines early skin cancer diagnosis using machine learning (ML) models and the problem of automating skin cancer diagnosis with AI algorithms. This study sheds light on past and future efforts to diagnose early skin cancer and other concerns.

This chapter explores Applications of smartphone technology in cancer diagnosis make it a game-changing part of healthcare, especially in terms of better early diagnosis and empowering patients. This abstract synthesizes some recent developments of the application of smartphones in detecting cancer, focusing on skin and cervical cancers. Recent studies have reported that AI algorithms developed on smartphones could accurately estimate skin lesions for malignancy. For instance, a clinical validation study assessed two neural network algorithms that attained sensitivities of 96.4% and 95.35% in detecting malignant skin lesions, hence establishing the potential of the smartphone as a diagnostic tool in dermatology. Widespread use of smartphones enables access to methods of early detection, mainly in underserved regions of a country, reducing the healthcare burden from late-stage cancer diagnoses.

Several important challenges come to the forefront when it comes to mobile solutions for clinical decision support systems (CDSS) that focus on comorbidities, particularly in the context of type 2 diabetes. To protect patient information, mobile CDSSs handling sensitive medical data must provide strong encryption, safe data transmission, and adherence to laws like the Health Insurance Portability and Accountability Act. For smooth data interchange and care coordination, integration with current electronic health record (EHR) systems and other healthcare IT infrastructure is essential. Interoperability is facilitated by standards such as FHIR (Fast Healthcare Interoperability Resources) and HL7 (Health Level Seven International). On the basis of current clinical data and evidence-based guidelines, the CDSS ought to offer precise and trustworthy suggestions. Sufficient validation and updates are important to guarantee pertinence and efficacy.

Hypertension is a major risk factor worldwide for early death. Well-established interventions like the Dash diet on average have modest results (5 mmHg systolic and 3 mmHg diastolic pressure improvement). We compare three employee eHealth intervention pilots with results that are three to six times larger, analysing them for eSupport design lessons. In these pilots, various tools and daily microlearning strategies have been used. Small-scale Self-Management Support (SMS) groups for hypertension control foster high degrees of learning, interaction, and personalization. Average blood pressure improvements in the pilots were 161/112 to 129/90 mmHg, resp. 145/92 to 126/86 mmHg, and 155/95 to 139/85 mmHg. User evaluation (n=20) showed the importance of core SMS components: information transfer, daily monitoring, promoting health competences and follow-up. A cross-case finding is that more daily social learning and ICT-enabled microlearning feedback increases success: for competence building and for blood pressure results.

Smart living, healthcare, cognitive smart cities, and social systems are impartial a rare of the areas in which technology related to health is being applied these days. A component of the rapidly evolving modern technology that deserves more attention is the intelligent, dependable, and pervasive healthcare system. Predicting, preventing, and treating illnesses is made possible for doctors by data collecting methods such as sensors aided by the Internet of Things (IoT). In order to assist doctors in monitoring the importance of symptoms and the course of therapy, machine learning (ML) algorithms have the latent to progress the accurateness of medical diagnosis and prognosis based on sensing data. A neurodegenerative condition affecting the neurological system is Parkinson's disease.

A lot of works exist in the literature that compares regression algorithms on different datasets. This chapter presents a model that uses best subset selection approach for the predictors and performs an exhaustive empirical comparison of eight regression algorithms Linear Regression, Multi-Linear Regression, Polynomial Regression, K-Nearest Neighbors, Lasso, Ridge, Decision Tree, Gradient Boost Tree, and Random Forest Regression algorithms on various predictors from Covid-19 dataset. The model is evaluated for train accuracy on metrics R2, Root Mean Square Error, and Mean Absolute Error. The test R2 and adjusted-R2 metrics evaluate the model on cross-validation prediction test errors. The predicted values of dependent variables are checked for similarity and validation using statistical z-test.

The use and design of digital technologies for the self-management of chronic diseases are increasing. Self-management systems designed without theoretically driven design principles are ineffective and inconsistent. This chapter proposes design principles based on the characteristics of the digital technologies: (1) re-programmability, (2) homogenization of data, and (3) self-referential nature. The design principles are instantiated in a diabetes mobile app and illustrated in use case diagrams. The proposed principles increase the projectability of system design principles and simplify the complexity of the problem space for ICT-enabled self-management systems.

Addressing the pervasive issue of mental illnesses in the U.S. necessitates innovative approaches. This study explores the potential of social media platforms as valuable sources for detecting mental health issues, leveraging the spontaneous and open expression of users' thoughts and feelings. Previous research has applied machine learning techniques to social media data to predict mental health states, which this study aims to expand by providing a holistic view of the strategies used for identifying mental health concerns through social media analysis. Our research questions focus on the strategies for utilizing social media data, the efficacy of these strategies, the challenges faced, and the broader implications for healthcare delivery. Employing a tertiary investigation approach, we review secondary studies to identify trends and synthesize findings, aiming to offer comprehensive insights and guide future research in mental health service delivery through social media engagement.

This chapter explores the potential of digital health technologies in preventive cardiology, including telemedicine, wearables, sensors, artificial intelligence, and mobile health platforms. These technologies have shown effectiveness in reducing cardiovascular risk factors and improving patient outcomes. However, barriers to widespread adoption include digital literacy gaps, limited internet access, data privacy concerns, and technical complexities. To overcome these, this chapter proposes strategies like national e-Health guidelines, stakeholder engagement, improved regulatory standards, human-centered design principles, integration with existing healthcare systems, technology infrastructure investments, and fair pricing models. Addressing data security, accessibility, and ethical considerations is crucial for a future of personalized, proactive, and accessible cardiovascular care. The chapter concludes by highlighting the challenges of digital health technologies in preventive cardiology.

Recent advancements in healthcare technologies, particularly wearable devices, have significantly enhanced the delivery and efficiency of healthcare. Wearable devices integration with mobile apps provides many functionalities to users including but not limited to vital sign monitoring and physical activity tracking. This chapter is a survey of current trends in wearable design with a particular focus on the impact on improved healthcare delivery. The chapter provides a foundation for the design features of wearable devices, focusing on users' experience, acceptance, adoption, and continuous use of such devices.

This study examines the effectiveness of conventional and spatial augmented reality in assisting individuals with amnestic mild cognitive impairment, which is characterized by memory loss and cognitive challenges. As neurodegenerative diseases become more prevalent in the aging population, AR solutions can improve daily functioning and independence. This study compares the usability and user perceptions of wearable AR and projection-based SAR in augmented living spaces. Results show that SAR significantly reduces cognitive load and anxiety compared to traditional wearable systems. Its intuitive interface and seamless environmental integration lead to improved user satisfaction and higher adoption rates. Participants consistently rated spatial augmented reality higher on all usability metrics, suggesting its suitability as a digital health intervention for individuals with aMCI. Adding to the theoretical discourse on the cognitive adoption of innovative digital health solutions, these findings highlight the need for user-centered AR technologies that improve health outcomes.

Valerianus Hashiyana, University of Namibia, Namibia
Fosia Shavuka, University of Namibia, Namibia
Willbard Kamati, University of Namibia, Namibia

Breast cancer is a leading cause of cancer-related deaths globally, particularly affecting developing countries. In Namibia, it is the most prevalent cancer type, highlighting the need for enhanced awareness and early detection strategies, especially in rural areas. This study evaluated the knowledge and awareness of breast cancer among Namibian women, identifying gaps and exploring the development of an online support group. The research collected qualitative data from randomly selected participants in the Khomas region through questionnaires, as well as secondary data from online archives, which included a comprehensive literature review and observation of the existing structures and systems in place. The study employed interpretive phenomenological analysis and qualitative content analysis to interpret the collected data. It emphasized the importance of psychosocial support for patients and caregivers, suggesting the establishment of an online support group platform to facilitate emotional and moral support, ultimately enhancing the fight against breast cancer in Namibia.

Chapter 18
The Impact and Significance of Diabetes Mellitus as a Global Health
Ayesha Thanthrige, La Trobe University, Australia
Nilmini Wickramasinghe, La Trobe University, Australia

Diabetes mellitus is a critical global health problem affecting millions of individuals and imposing a significant economic burden worldwide. A RLR across multiple selected databases was conducted to provide a detailed analysis regarding the significance of diabetes as a disease, with a particular focus on the evolving role of digital health interventions in diabetes management. Key areas discussed include global prevalence and projections, economic costs, complications and comorbidities, psychological factors, and history of diabetes understanding. The review includes studies conducted both before and after the COVID-19 pandemic to provide a comprehensive understanding of how digital health technologies, such as mobile health applications, telemedicine have evolved and been adapted in response to the pandemic's challenges. The paper also discusses the advancement and features of self-management methods. By examining this evolution, the study provides new insights into the effectiveness, challenges, and future potential of these technologies in enhancing diabetes care.

Preface

Impact of Digital Solutions for Improved Healthcare Delivery sets out to highlight the breadth of possibilities today's digital technological advances can bring to healthcare delivery. Digital solutions for healthcare are revolutionising care delivery much like automation and the assembly line had such a significant impact in the Industrial Age or antibiotics was such a game changer for Medicine over 100 years ago. Specifically, armed with technology, we have for the first time the potential to deliver to a healthcare value proposition of better access, quality and value for all, anytime, anywhere. Moreover, this care is highly personalised and precise at scale; thereby, ensuring optimal clinical resources, timely as well as effective, efficient and efficacious care, happier patients, a smarter and supported clinical workforce and a healthier community.

This book serves to build on past books that have introduced the potential of e-health or IS/IT for healthcare and lays out a clear road map and vision around what high quality, high value care for all is and can be if our digital solutions are harnessed and maximised. In short, it serves to describe the digital transformation taking place in healthcare delivery today. The target audience includes students and researchers of digital health and related fields, clinicians and allied health workers, management and senior management in healthcare as well as other areas within the web of healthcare such as regulators and/or payers and even those individuals in industry sectors like pharma and med tech and last but not least for the everyday citizen. This is because healthcare is an industry that affects us all, we all interact with healthcare; in short it is not a spectator sport; we must all actively participate in making our healthcare delivery the best it can be.

The book consists of 18 chapters which taken together highlight the breadth and possibilities for digital health solutions as follows:

Chapter 1: AI-Enhanced Healthcare and Eldercare Delivery using Non-Intrusive Sensors and Physical Robots: An Exploratory Study by Karayaneva et al. describes a study undertaken in a UK care home 'living lab' environment exploring older people's preferences for sensors and robots.

Chapter 2: The Impact of Internet of Things in Healthcare Delivery: A Tertiary Study by El-Gayar et al., unpacks key issues around the adoption of various Internet of Things devices for supporting superior healthcare delivery.

Chapter 3: Artificial Intelligence, Decision-Making, 6G, and Wearable IoT: The Next Generation´s Backbone for Digital Smart Healthcare Services by Castañeda proposes small-scale and large-scale digital smart healthcare service architectures to allow autonomy and decision-making founded on artificial intelligence, multiple criteria decisions, sixth-generation communication, cloud technologies, and wearable Internet of Things for point-of-care and chronic disease management.

Chapter 4: Accelerating Healthcare Outcomes Uplifting Patients Experience Pairing Artificial intelligence (AI): Transforming Healthcare Industry in Digital Arena by Singh et al., provides in-depth exploration into the transformative impact of Artificial Intelligence on healthcare outcomes, specifically focusing on enhancing the patient experience in the digital era.

Chapter 5: Modelling and Optimizing the Decontamination Process of Surgical Instruments by England et al. examines in a hospital sterilization and decontamination unit (HSDU), contaminated equipment arrives after their use in the operating theatre, intensive care unit, diagnostics facilities, and wards

Chapter 6: Revolutionizing Skin Cancer Diagnosis with Artificial Intelligence: Insights into Machine Learning Techniques by Shafik outlines unique approaches empowered with artificial intelligence for better and effective diagnosis of skin cancer.

Chapter 7: Empowering Early Cancer Detection: The Role of Smartphone Technology in Diagnosing Skin and Cervical Cancers by Babu et al. describes the role of smartphone technology in specific tumour streams.

Chapter 8: Important Concerns with Comorbidities and Type 2 Diabetes in Clinical Decision Support Systems Based on Mobile Solutions by Ruban et al. discusses mobile solutions for clinical decision support systems (CDSS) that focus on comorbidities, particularly in the context of type 2 diabetes.

Chapter 9: Beyond Average Results in Hypertension e-Support & Self-Management: 3 Pilot Studies with Social Learning by Simons et al. serves to compare three employee eHealth intervention pilots with results that are three to six times larger, analysing them for eSupport design lessons.

Chapter 10: IoT and Machine Learning for Early Prediction of Neurological Disorder by Shobana et al discussed opportunities for IoT and machine learning techniques to assist with early prediction of various neurological disorders so that treatment can be started sooner.

Chapter 11: A Predictive Analysis of the Covid-19 Pandemic for Traditional and Tree-Based Regression Algorithms by Singh et al. outlines the use of analytics and machine learning techniques to predict the COVID-19 pandemic and lessons from this.

Chapter 12: Design Principles for Chronic Disease Self-Management Systems: A Technical Investigation Based on the Characteristics of Digital Technologies by Dagar et al. examines key design principles for the development of suitable digital technologies for better chronic disease self-management.

Chapter 13: Using Social Media Data to Predict Mental Health Issues: A Tertiary Study by Haldar et al. examines how digital health, and social media can better assist with mental health diagnosis

Chapter 14: Digital Health Technologies for Preventive Cardiology by Mala et al. presents opportunities for digital health solutions to better support cardiac prevention and wellness management.

Chapter 15: Designing Wearables for Improved Healthcare: A Survey of Current Trends and Future Directions by Wahbeh et al. explores the opportunities and trends for wearable devices for self-management and prevention.

Chapter 16: Bridging the Gap between Augmentation and Cognition: A Comparative Analysis of Wearable and Spatial Augmented Reality for People with aMCI by Böhmer et al. explores the gap between wearables and special augmented reality and how this might be bridged.

Chapter 17: Enhancing the Fight of Breast Cancer in Namibia through Awareness and Online Social Network Support by Hashiyana et al. assess the knowledge and awareness of breast cancer in Namibia, focusing on both patients and caregivers.

Chapter 18: The Impact and Significance of Diabetes Mellitus as a Global Health Challenge by Thanthrige et al discusses the advancement and features of self-management methods with digital health interventions in the context of type 2 diabetes.

Taken together, this miscellany of chapters serves to introduce all readers to the power and potential of digital health solutions. Moreover, it illustrates the possibilities for personalised and precise care delivery every time for everyone and everywhere enabled through the digital transformation of healthcare that is only made possible through embracing our digital health solutions. This is indeed a brave new world, and it is my hope that all who read this book are inspired to delve further either by embracing such solutions in practice or facilitating their adoption or researching further so we can push the envelope. It should be clear after reading this book that the future for healthcare delivery is both bright and challenging and let us all work together to realise the full potential of our digital solutions for better healthcare delivery.

Nilmini Wickramasinghe
La Trobe University, Australia
September 10, 2024.

Acknowledgement

This book would not have been possible without the efforts of so many people. First and foremost, a big thank you to all the contributing authors, your chapters are what have made this book so unique and provided the breadth and depth of content in the following pages. In addition, I want to acknowledge the work of those who reviewed chapters; without your diligence and dedication the caliber and quality of this final product could not have been achieved. I am most grateful to my colleagues for all their suggestions, coffee catch up discussions and feedback which have helped to keep this project on track and to point. Further, I am indebted to my organization for affording me the time to work on this project. I greatly appreciated and valued the support the team at IGI provided. Last but not least, a special thank you to my family whose support and encouragement is greatly valued and appreicated.

Chapter 1
AI-Enhanced Healthcare and Eldercare Delivery Using Non-Intrusive Sensors and Physical Robots:
An Exploratory Study

Yordanka Karayaneva
Teesside University, UK

Sara Sharifzadeh
https://orcid.org/0000-0003-4621-2917
Swansea University, UK

Ala Szczepura
https://orcid.org/0000-0001-6244-9872
Coventry University, UK

Yanguo Jing
https://orcid.org/0000-0001-9581-4215
Leeds Trinity University, UK

Bo Tan
https://orcid.org/0000-0002-6855-6270
Tampere University, Finland

DOI: 10.4018/979-8-3693-5237-3.ch001

ABSTRACT

Many countries world-wide are facing the public health challenge of caring for an aging population. Meanwhile, there is a belief that in care settings unobtrusive sensors and physical robots will eventually address this challenge. However, research into factors influencing older users' acceptance of such technology in these environments has received little attention. This paper describes a study undertaken in a UK care home 'living lab' environment exploring older people's preferences for sensors and robots. An in-depth qualitative study examined the preferences of a cross-section of 21 older adults (aged 81-99) in the care home setting. In addition to two dimensions (usefulness and ease-of-use) included in the Technology Acceptance Model (TAM) framework, the importance of other elements such as physical appearance, functionality, cost, trust and control were investigated. The resulting framework is presented to support future co-design of sensors and robots with older adults.

1. INTRODUCTION

The need to support the older population is an ongoing challenge world-wide which has led to numerous scientific discoveries and breakthroughs. According to a recent report by the United Nations, the number of adults aged 65 or over is expected to increase from 771 million in 2022 to 1.6 billion in 2050 (United Nations, 2022). At the same time, a declining birthrate is leading to reductions in the workforce available to provide care (Ince Yenilmez, 2015). The older population is commonly affected by specific neurocognitive conditions such as dementia, which is an umbrella term for a number of conditions leading to significant care needs due to cognitive decline. Specifically in the United Kingdom (UK), the number of adults living with dementia is currently estimated to be 982,000, while this number is projected to double to 1.4 million in 2040 (Alzheimer's Society, 2024). As stated earlier, within this context the need for innovations to support the older population is becoming even more crucial and necessary.

There exists a number of devices for smart monitoring of the older population. Such devices include depth-vision cameras, wearable technologies, infrared sensors, Doppler radars, among others. Considering cameras, the potential advantages of these devices are mainly related to high-resolution outputs and relatively straight-forward identification of humans. However, cameras can compromise privacy as these devices are expected to be installed in private areas such as bedrooms and bathrooms (Demiris et al., 2009). Therefore, this constraint could block the usage of cameras for monitoring the older population. Wearable sensors are an interesting and well-researched alternative to cameras, which have been deployed in many ap-

2

plications. However, similarly to cameras, they come with their own disadvantages. More specifically, the limited battery life of wearables can pose a significant issue especially if they have to be worn for long periods of time (Baig et al., 2019). In addition to this, older adults can feel uncomfortable wearing these devices, which represents another disadvantage. Therefore, this chapter will consider infrared sensors and Doppler radars as ambient sensors, which are seen as non-intrusive, i.e., individuals cannot be identified from the recordings, and these devices do not directly interfere with humans.

Infrared sensors and Doppler radars are an appealing solution for smart monitoring of the older population, which have seen numerous discoveries and applications. Both types of devices produce recordings, where individuals cannot be identified (Karayaneva et al., 2018; Li, Tan and Piechocki, 2018). This is a significant advantage compared to cameras, and as such, it easily allows these devices to be deployed in private areas. In comparison with wearable devices, infrared sensors and Doppler radars can also be easily installed on walls and ceilings without interference with the residents. Infrared sensors are capable of detecting temperature and more specifically the human temperature, which is usually around 36° Celsius degrees. Figure 1 depicts a low-resolution infrared sensors installation for human activity monitoring. Moreover, infrared sensors are ideally very low-resolution devices, which significantly reduces the computational power. This advantage can also be viewed as a disadvantage because the low resolution can be a challenge for detecting humans. In addition to this, infrared sensors usually have a low distance coverage, which implies the need for more sensors to be deployed to cover a room. Radars, more specifically Doppler radars are another appealing solution for smart monitoring. Furthermore, these devices have deep penetration, stable performance, and high-distance range.

Figure 1. Low-resolution infrared sensors used for human activity recognition

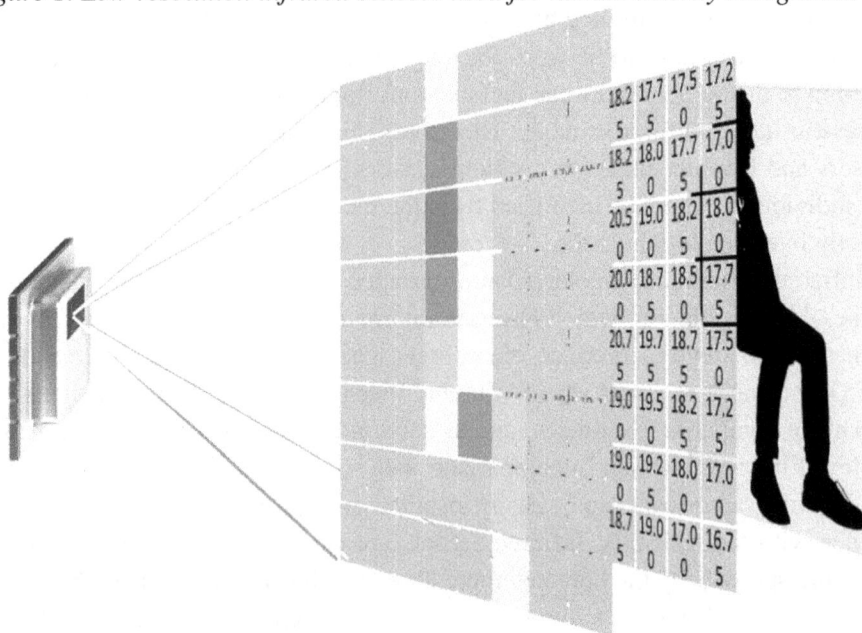

Infrared sensors have been used for human activity recognition, including fall detection, to support the older generation. A number of studies have been undertaken to discover the optimal number of sensors, sensor position and layout (Karayaneva et al., 2023). In terms of methods for predicting human activities, both machine learning and deep learning techniques have been implemented and applied (Yin et al., 2021). Similarly, in terms of radars both machine learning and deep learning techniques have been investigated in the pursuit of the most accurate approach. Unlike infrared sensors, unsupervised human activity recognition using Doppler radars has been deployed in three studies with very interesting findings (Karayaneva et al., 2021; Li et al., 2018; Li et al., 2017).

Amidst the challenges of an ageing population, it has been estimated that development of appropriate robotic technologies that can be used in social care to provide physical, social, and cognitive support could save up to £6 billion in the UK (UK Parliament, 2018). In the context of a 'push' for technology implementation in this sector (Stavropoulos et al., 2020; Abdi et al., 2018), relatively little attention has been paid up to now to which 'pull' factors will influence acceptance by older people, especially the frail super-aged populations living in care homes. Robots and sensors are already being introduced in such settings, but to date social robots like PARO have had limited success, at least partly due to the negative preconceptions of older people (Papadopoulos et al., 2020; Hung et al., 2019). Also, although in-home monitoring technology could increase safety, independence, quality-of-life and mental well-being of elderly people, the adoption rates of such advancements show that these are still undesired by the majority of the population (UK Parliament, 2018). These low adoption rates may be explained by the fact that previous research on technology applications for the elderly has been limited, without serving real user needs.

As a result, there is a gap in the evidence on user acceptance by older people due to a research base consisting of single evaluations of a specific agent following an interaction with no comparators other than 'usual care' (Wu et al., 2014; Beuscher et al., 2017; Heerink et al. 2009). Such an approach excludes any broader comparison of different types of robots (e.g., unobtrusive sensors versus physical robots). Furthermore, the most widely used model for exploring user-acceptance has been developed for other contexts and may not be suitable for this population. The Technology Acceptance Model (TAM) restricts acceptance to two dimensions - perceived usefulness and ease-of-use (Davis, 1989) – while other dimensions may be important for older people. For example, for people living in a care home, additional factors such as perceived impact on physical health and mental well-being as well as cost, physical appearance and functionalities may be important requiring a more comprehensive model to account for observed low technology acceptance. By working with people living in a care home environment, the present study aimed to test the applicability of the TAM model, explore the factors that older people consider important, and produce a more comprehensive framework for assessing the acceptability of prototype sensors and physical robots.

In this chapter, we will describe an exploratory study targeted at older adults which focused on investigating the user acceptance of (1) non-intrusive sensors; and (2) robots with a physical presence. More specifically, 21 adults (3 male and 18 female) were selected and approached in their care home environment to gather data for this study. Residents had the opportunity to complete a questionnaire administered through interview aiming to explore their views and preferences for sensors and robots to be introduced in their care home. As a result, very interesting findings have been identified, including real-world preferences of older people for sensors over robots, as well as clear preferences for a robot's physical appearance type, role, and activities.

2. RELATED WORK

2.1 User Acceptance of Sensors and Robots in Care Homes

A literature review of the acceptability of social robots by older adults including people with dementia or cognitive impairment identified a large number of enablers for successful introduction, including intention to use, ease of-use, usefulness, enjoyment, social presence, sociability, trust and adaptivity, and social influences and facilitating conditions (Whelan et al., 2018). These concepts emerged from the previously defined Almere model for evaluating the acceptance of assistive social devices (Heerink et al., 2010). A subsequent scoping review of the benefits and barriers to using the zoomorphic seal-like social robot PARO in care settings identified social stigma as a major barrier (Hung et al., 2019).

2.1.1 Technology Acceptance Model for User Acceptance of Sensors and Robots

With the advancement and development of new technologies in the modern world, it has become crucial for end users to evaluate these technologies and ultimately show their overall tendency of acceptance. The Technology Acceptance Model (TAM) is an important framework for accepting technologies, which is restricted to two factors – perceived ease-of-use and perceived usefulness (Davis, 1989). The author of the study defined perceived ease-of-use as "the degree to which an individual believes that using a particular system would be free of physical and mental effort." In terms of perceived usefulness, the definition given is "the degree to which an individual believes that using a particular system would enhance his or her job performance". To date, the TAM framework is considered to be fundamental and crucial for the acceptance of any technology regardless of the end users. More specifically, the TAM framework has been researched for assessing the tendency of older adults to accept wearable technologies (Lin et al., 2016; Lazaro et al., 2020). Lin et al. (2016) proposed the use of TAM for evaluating the acceptance of a wearable vest among 50 older adults. Moreover, Lazaro et a., (2020) utilised the framework to evaluate the willingness of older adults to adopt smartwatches (n=76). However, to the best of our knowledge, the investigation of TAM in the domain of accepting ambient sensors by older adults has been largely ignored.

Considering the use of robots, the TAM framework has found more interest compared to ambient sensors. Lee et al. (2020) evaluated the acceptance of older adults towards soft service robots using an extended TAM framework (n=79). In addition to the existing factors i.e., perceived ease-of-use and perceived usefulness, the authors also considered subjective norms, perceived anxiety, and perceived likability in their research. More specifically, the term "subjective norms" is described as the perception of individuals that others consider or think that they should use the technology. As a result, it was found that perceived ease of use, perceived usefulness and subjective norms affected the older adults' acceptance of the soft service robot. Moreover, a humanoid robot named Kabochan was administered among 103 care home residents living with dementia (Ke et al., 2020). The study explored the change of user acceptance over time by considering an extension to the TAM framework. As a result, the study showed the perceived ease-of-use improved over time among the residents. Another study investigated the acceptance of 16 older adults toward a dancing partner robot. Similarly, an extended TAM framework guided the study, where the perceived ease-of-use also increased over time (Chen et al., 2017).

2.1.2 Extended Technology Acceptance Model Including Cost, Physical Appearance and Functionalities for User Acceptance of Sensors and Robots

While the TAM framework is prominent and has found applications in many technology acceptance studies, it is limited to two contributing factors only. As such, it is vital to consider additional factors as these might be highly determinant for the acceptance of new technologies. Therefore, the cost, physical appearance and functionalities will be considered in this section.

2.1.2.1 User Acceptance of Sensors and Robots Based on Cost

Cost is an important factor, which has the potential to influence the adoption of any new technology, especially if it is expected to be fully covered by the end users. A study concerned with the older users' acceptance of wireless sensors networks for health assistance identified the cost to be crucially important (n=13) (Steele et al., 2009). More specifically, the participants indicated that if the system's cost is not affordable, it might not be accepted despite its potential health benefits. In addition to this, the notion of cost was deemed important for the adoption of new technologies if these emerge as cost-saving in small study with 15 older adults (Mihailidis et al., 2008). Ultimately, the acceptance of home monitoring technology investigated in this study came with several conclusions regarding the cost and appearance of the system. More specifically, the ideal monitoring system should be low cost according to the participants. The importance of cost in addition to the widely known factor usefulness was briefly mentioned in a study involving only six older adults (Chung et al., 2017), which investigated the acceptance of home-based sensor system for monitoring.

In terms of robots, the cost is similarly seen as equally important. A study investigating the acceptance of an assistive robot among 11 older adults found the cost to be one of the major themes raised by the participants (Wu et al., 2014). More specifically, the participants were especially concerns whether it would be more reasonable to rent such robots instead of buying them. The cost of robots, and PARO in particular, was seen as a barrier for the acceptance of such technology among 20 care staff workers (Moyle et al., 2016). Furthermore, the acceptance of robotic assistive devices has been further explored among 24 older adults (Shore, De Eyto and O'Sullivan, 2020). More specifically, the cost of such devices was emphasised, which generated some discussions among the participants. Some of them commented that a potential grant from the state could be particularly useful to cover the cost of the robot. The cost was regarded as important in another study concerned with exoskeletons i.e., a subset of assistive robots (Shore et al., 2018). Considering the high significance of the cost, cost-effective, and low-cost robots have been proposed in an attempt to tackle this issue (Sefcik et al., 2018).

2.1.2.2 User Acceptance of Sensors and Robots Based on Physical Appearance

In terms of sensor-based systems' physical appearance, one study indicated that the ideal system should be attractive, small, and discreet in terms of appearance (Mihailidis et al., 2008). In addition to this, a study involving 15 older adults indicated the importance of physical appearance of sensor-based technologies (Bian et al., 2021). More specifically, the participants confirmed they would be more likely to accept a new technology if it is aesthetically pleasing. However, most of the research regarding physical appearance of ambient sensor-based systems is limited, while more attention has been focused on wearable devices. This limitation is understandable as wearable technologies infer directly with the person, while ambient sensors often remain unnoticed by the end users.

Physical appearance may be crucial for acceptance by an older person and, as such, this characteristic has been evaluated in a number of studies concerned with physical robots. A small study (n=11) investigating attitudes to a mechanical human-like robot (Kompai) following one-month of interaction reported mainly negative perceptions (Wu et al., 2014). While the majority of the participants (n=7) admired the humanoid appearance, they found no value in using an assistive robot due to a self-perception of their own independence. In terms of physical appearance, a similar study (n=19) reported a positive response (86%) to the humanoid robot NAO following a short interaction (Beuscher at al., 2017). Another study in France among older adults (n=25) found preferred appearances for socially assistive robots were mechanical human-like, followed by mechanical animal-like, animal-like, and finally machine-like; android and human-like robots were ranked at the bottom of the scale (Pino et al., 2015). An earlier study (n=42) comparing a social robot resembling a cat and a screen monitor robot, found higher preferences for the animal-like robot (Heerink et al., 2009). It appears that android robots and human-like robots may "fall" in Mori's "uncanny valley" (Mori, 1970), and therefore prove to be less desirable for vulnerable older people. The uncanny valley refers to the fact that realism in mechanical humanoid robots may lead users to experience unease and repulsion if robots become too realistic by possessing skin, hair, and nails.

Generally, the literature appears to indicate a preference for humanoid and zoomorphic robots, while mechanoid robots are less admired. However, this preference order was only fully explored in one study (n=25) based in France (Pino et al., 2015). In view of these findings, we included mechanical humanoid robots, mechanical zoomorphic robots, and mechanoid robots for evaluation in our study.

2.1.2.3 User Acceptance of Sensors and Robots Based on Functionalities

2.1.2.3.1 User Acceptance of Sensors Based on Functionalities

Qualitative research into user acceptance of sensor technologies by the older population was found to be relatively limited and mainly focused on results following interaction. A study of implementing monitoring technologies in care homes for people with dementia found that the main enabler identified by older people (n=9) was safety enhancement (Hall et al., 2017). Care home staff (n=24) were concerned about lack of training on how to use the new technology and, although data gathered by sensors could also be used to analyse patterns for improved early diagnosis of illnesses, this was viewed as less useful, largely due to a lack of information about the likely benefits. A study explored social acceptance by senior citizens and caregivers of a fall detection system using sensors in a nursing home (Iio et al., 2016). The highest acceptability was reported for a fall detection system with range sensors compared to a system using out-of-bed sensors for the same purpose.

Other studies mainly focused on community-dwelling participants. A pilot study in 2009 investigated attitudes and preconceptions towards a wireless sensor network for older people (n=13) living in their own homes (Steele et al., 2009). The study involved people with no previous interactions with sensor systems, so views, attitudes and perceptions were not affected by prior experience. The research indicated that in a home-based setting, the main barrier raised by the participants was the cost of the system, and sensor systems that did not require any interaction were preferred. The majority of participants valued the sensor system most highly for emergency situations such as falls. In addition to this, ambient sensors installed in residents' homes (n=8) were found to be non-obtrusive (Reeder et al., 2016). This is due to the fact that residents do not interact directly with the sensors are installed in the rooms. In the same year, another study of older people (n=11) regarding the use of sensor monitoring in their home reported that detecting falls and sense of safety with the sensor system were regarded as important by participants (Pol et al., 2016). Both studies also found that sensors were viewed positively as a tool to enable people to stay in their own home for longer.

In terms of wearable fall detection sensors, a small study (n=5) has reported an overall positive user acceptance of such technology, but it did not provide a comparison between different systems (Wu and Munteanu, 2018). An earlier study of wearable and optical fall prediction and fall detection devices for home use found participants (n=22) to value equally fall prediction and fall prevention systems (Gövercin et al., 2010). A very early 2008 study found that lifestyle monitoring was the least preferred among older adults (n=15), with personal emergency response system and interactive video conferencing highly preferred (Mihailidis et al., 2008). In this same study, fall detection was similarly regarded as an important sensor system feature. A study (n=35) concerned with private residents identified higher preference for health-related activities compared to social activities (Gövercin et al., 2016). A Swiss study (n=34) investigating users' evaluation of a wireless sensor system reported low to moderate interest among the older adults (Cohen, Kamepel and Verloo, 2016). Cost was regarded as crucial for user acceptance based on a study (Puri et al., 2017) concerned with wrist-worn tracker, where the mean age of the participants (n=20) was 64 years. In addition, a more in-depth study (n=146) found that perceived usefulness, compatibility, facilitating conditions, and self-reported health status were linked to older adults' intentions to use new wearable technology (Li et al., 2019).

Overall, the literature identified indicates that sensor systems with less interaction were preferred, with security regarded as more important than privacy. In view of these findings, ambient sensors were included in our study with the main benefit presented to participants being that of non-intrusively detecting falls.

2.1.2.3.2 User acceptance of robots based on roles and functionalities

The role of a robot can largely be described in terms of tasks and capabilities. Socially assistive robots are able to undertake tasks related to communication, entertainment or health-related tasks such as medicines reminders. On the other hand, physical robots are able to perform physical tasks such as cleaning, cooking, washing and environmental navigation, among others. Generally, the literature appears to indicate that older adults prefer robots that undertake everyday living physical tasks and non-intrusive monitoring activities, with a human making decisions for them (Smarr et al., 2012). Additionally, for elderly adults with cognitive impairments a large study (n=83) identified calling for help and moving obstacles as the highest priority (Korchut et al., 2017). A Taiwanese study employed to identify features that enhance acceptance of robots, found that community-dwelling older adults (n=33) expressed a preference for more service-oriented robots rather than companion-oriented robots (Chu et al., 2019). The same study further reported household work as the most preferred robotic function. These findings echo the results of another study (n=21), where household duties were the most preferred robotic activities (Mitzner et al., 2011). A study of retirement home residents (n=32) found detecting falls and calling for help as the most preferred activity (Broadbent et al., 2009). Similarly to previous studies, household duties were found as relevant tasks performed by a robot. A small robot study (n=10) of the Care-O-bot which aids older adults to drink water discovered positive attitudes, despite limited capabilities and slow responses (Bedaf et al., 2018).

In addition, while it has been found that older people prefer activities that require little to no interaction (Ezer, Fisk and Rogers, 2009), social robots still found approval among these populations. A large study (n=115) involved participants with mild to advanced dementia and their interactions with the mechanical humanoid robot Matilda (Khosla, Nguyen and Chu, 2017). In terms of the benefits of interacting with Matilda, participants valued enjoyment more highly (84%) than usefulness (60%). The majority (89%) enjoying the robot dancing, and 60% showed willingness to participate in a group activity with Matilda. Similar findings about sociability were reported in an earlier study (n=46) that employed the social robot Brian 2.1 (Louie, McColl, and Nejat, 2014). The majority of the participants (70%) valued the companionship provided by this robot. An earlier study (n=42) which included comparison between a social robot and a less social robot, found stronger preference for the more social robot (Heerink et al., 2009).

Communicative robots are preferred to non-communicative robots as reported in the findings from two focus groups (n_1=28, n_2=40) (Heerink et al., 2006). A Japanese study of autonomous wheelchair robots to support elderly people (n=28) which considered two versions of the robot: 1) social; and 2) less social, found participants valued the social robot more because it was able to respond to requests made by the older person (Shiomi et al., 2015).

Overall, the evidence indicates that older adults prefer interaction-free robots for monitoring and physical aid. When presented with social robots, participants value social interaction and communication with the robot. In general, usefulness, ease-of-use, trust, and control were also found to be crucial factors for acceptance by older people (Olde Keizer et al., 2019; Piasek and Wieczorowska-Tobis, 2018; Sääskilahti et al., 2012; Whelan et al., 2018; McGlynn et al., 2014). Based on these findings, we not only included factors such as usefulness and ease-of-use contained in the TAM model, but also added further elements such as functionalities, physical appearance, and cost. In addition, because questions of trust and control were identified as crucial in some articles, these were included as part of our evaluation. We included consideration of both social and physical activities.

3. MATERIALS AND METHODS

3.1 Observational Period Setting

'Living Labs' are ethically driven, user-centred design environments. Residential homes based on these principles can provide unique test-beds with the potential for rapid innovation. By living in the care home, observing every-day life and contributing to daily activities, the lead author was able to better understand what types of robot (physical or sensors) might be helpful and to work collaboratively with staff to identify residents' preferences exploring aspects such as preferred appearance, acceptance of robot's physical work or social role, and acceptance of different robot functions; all while reviewing the available research evidence. In preparation for the final stage research examining living lab residents' perceptions of technology, an activity based on delivering an exercise routine performed by the humanoid robot NAO, coherent with the age of the participants, lasting 10 minutes was performed to groups of residents. A further activity involved a presentation about dementia and more specifically its prevention based on guidance provided by the National Health Service (NHS) and the UK Alzheimer's Society. This was delivered in the communal area and coffee shop where residents gather for their morning tea and residents participating actively discussed different factors that are scientifically known to reduce the risk of developing dementia. As a result, residents were familiarized with lifestyle choices that could make a difference to their health and well-being.

3.2 Living Lab Residents' Perceptions of Technology

A cross-section of residents was selected to evaluate their overall perceptions of 1) non-intrusive sensors, and 2) robots with a physical presence, both seen from the perspective of health improvement. A survey questionnaire was designed to explore these factors, piloted before use, and refined following feedback. The questionnaire contained a mix of closed and open-ended questions, presenting practical examples with corresponding images in order to aid understanding. Further clarifications were provided for the questions if needed. The final part of the questionnaire included an open-ended question to identify any activities not included which older people might wish to be performed by a robot. The questionnaire explored two different types of technology: 1) non-intrusive sensing technology; and 2) robots with a physical presence.

Prior to starting the survey, information was provided to familiarise participants with illustrative examples of the two types of technology: 1) ambient sensors which required no interaction e.g., a wall-mounted infrared sensor capable of detecting various movements such as falls, a major adverse event among older adults (Dionyssiotis, 2012). It was also explained that because infrared sensors capture extremely low-resolution temperature images, no one could not be identified, ensuring confidentiality); 2) for robots, a similar approach was adopted with examples given for different types of robots based on their physical appearance, role, and tasks. User acceptance of sensors and robots was evaluated from the perspective of health improvements for both. Regarding health, physical health and mental health were studied as two distinct benefits offered by the two types of technology.

The survey was undertaken during the period of September 2019 - October 2019. All the participants were approached in their own bedrooms or communal living areas of the care home. The survey was administered in the form of a one-to-one interview, where the older adult had the opportunity to ask questions for clarification purposes. This form of survey administration allowed the inclusion of participants who may have various impairments. The participants could answer questions either in writing, or verbally with their answers entered by the interviewer. Each interview lasted approximately 1 hour.

3.3 Setting

The research was undertaken in the new, state-of-the-art 84-bed residential care home owned by WCS Care in Kenilworth, England. Residents live in family groups of 6-8 people, each with their own bedroom and a common kitchen, dining area and entertainment space. In addition, there are communal areas such as a café, shop, cinema and gardens. As well as providing a living lab environment, dissemination of innovation and technology transfer was provided through an embedded innovation hub and national visitor programme (Szczepura et al., 2018). Innovations introduced into the organization included acoustic monitoring (NHS England Transformation Directorate, 2020) circadian lighting (Baandrup and Jennum, 2021), and care planning intervention (Taylor et al., 2023). Thus, in WCS the Living Lab approach supported the management and development of existing facilities and helped to create a blueprint for future innovations.

3.4 User Sample

The final number of residents who took part in the study was 21 (18 female and 3 male). The demographics are presented in Table 1. The gender breakdown reflects the fact that residents in UK care homes are mostly women (McCann, Donnelly and O'Reilly, 2012). All male residents in the care home were approached, but the remaining male residents had chronic conditions which prevented them from participating.

Table 1. Participants' demographic details

GENDER	NUMBER	MEAN AGE±SD	AGE RANGE
Female	18	90±4.65	81-99
Male	3	93±1.41	91-94

3.5 User Acceptance of Sensors

When considering non-intrusive ambient sensors, participants were asked whether the technology could improve 1) their physical well-being; and 2) their mental well-being. With regard to physical well-being, the example given was the rapid detection of a fall by a sensor or sensor array. An example of improved mental well-being was a resident feeling more secure and stable with this sensing technology in place. A breakdown of responses is shown in Figure 2.

Figure 2. Well-being improvement based on sensing technology

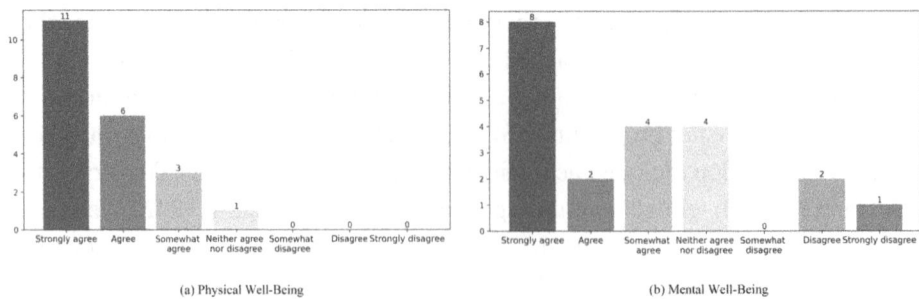

(a) Physical Well-Being   (b) Mental Well-Being

3.6 Factors Affecting the User Acceptance of Robots

The two characteristics in the classical TAM framework (perceived ease-of-use and usefulness) were extended in the survey questionnaire to include three additional characteristics - functionalities, physical appearance, and cost - with respondents having the opportunity to select more than one characteristic. A comparison of the relative importance of these five robot characteristics is shown in Figure 3. Perceived usefulness was considered as the most important robotic feature, with ease-of-use slightly ahead of the other three.

Figure 3. Relative importance of five robot characteristics

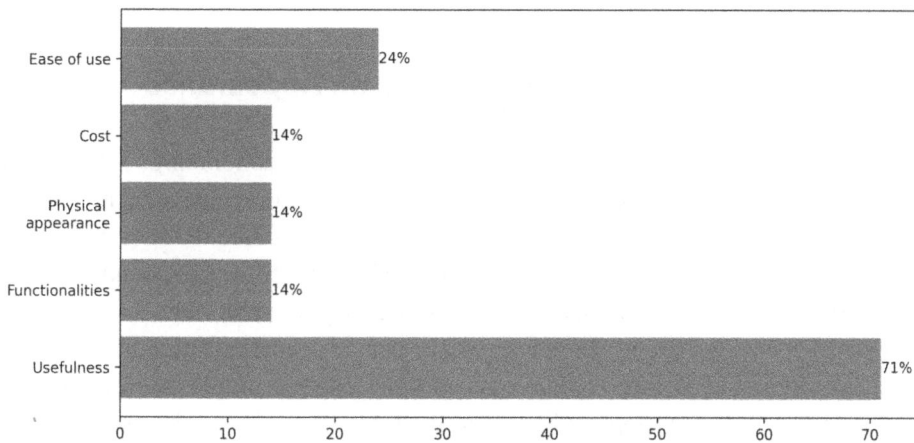

In order to evaluate the willingness of residents to have a robot in their current home (i.e., LTC facility), respondents were asked how far they agreed with the statement "I am likely to use robots in my home". Responses were mixed as shown in Figure 4a: 6 disagreed and 3 strongly disagreed; while only 5 demonstrated strong acceptance and 1 was uncertain (neither agreed nor disagreed). This is perhaps because only a few residents had any previous experience (solely interacting with Amazon Alexa).

To explore the question of whether residents would trust a robot to make decisions for them, the examples given were those which related directly to a resident's health. The results are shown in Figure 4b.

Figure 4. User acceptance of a robot at home and trusting the robot for making decisions

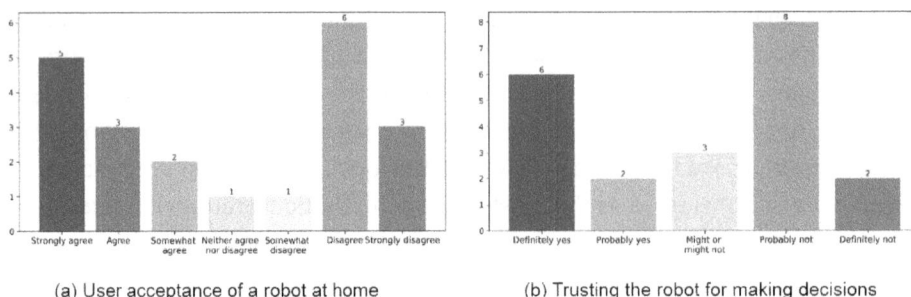

(a) User acceptance of a robot at home

(b) Trusting the robot for making decisions

3.7 User Acceptance of Robots Based on Appearance

Three main types of robots were presented in the questionnaire: mechanical humanoid, zoomorphic (animal-like), and machine-like. For mechanical humanoid robots, only examples made of steel and plastic were presented. Robots with skin, hair, nails, etc. were excluded since these might "fall" into Mori's "uncanny valley" (Mori, 1970). The three humanoid robot examples presented were the Softbank Robotics – NAO (SoftBank Robotics, 2020), Pepper (SoftBank Robotics, 2020), and Romeo (Guizzo, 2010). The three zoomorphic robot examples presented were AIBO (dog-like), MiRo (donkey-like), and PARO (seal-like). For the machine-like robots, although these are widely used in manufacturing, they can also be applied in elderly care homes. The examples given were Baxter and OSARO which can be used for work such as serving meals, or for human navigation through environments. None of the illustrated robots were familiar to the care home residents.

The residents' responses demonstrated that they had a significant preference for humanoid robots (13) over zoomorphic ones (4), as seen in Figure 5. In addition, zoomorphic robots had a small advantage over machine-like robots (2). The latter did not find sympathy with many respondents; one female resident commented on the industrial robot Baxter. "It is awful! It looks like a spider". Two residents (a male and a female) stated that they had no strong interest in a robot's appearance.

Figure 5. User acceptance of robots based on physical appearance

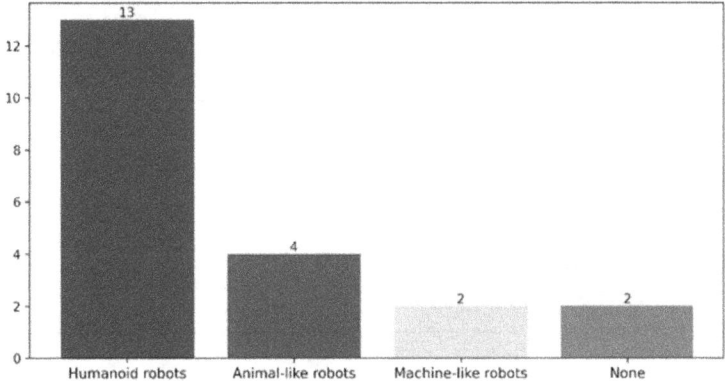

3.8 User Acceptance of Robots Based on Role and Functions of Robot

Activities which might be performed by a robot were differentiated for physical robots and socially-assisting robots. For physical robots, activities such as cooking (A1), cleaning (A2), and environmental navigation (A4) were presented. For socially-assisting robots, the activities were medicines reminders (A3), entertainment such as singing and dancing (A5), communication with the robot (A6), and enabling communication with relatives (A7). The respondents had the opportunity to select more than one answer. The results shown in Figure 6 indicate that the activity most strongly preferred was cleaning (A2), with over half of the residents identifying this as important. The social activity of communication with the robot (A6) was ranked second, followed by activities such as cooking (A1), medicines reminders (A3), and environmental navigation (A4), where the last two were also strongly linked to a resident's health and well-being. The least preferred activities were the provision of entertainment (A5) and communication with relatives (A7). In terms of entertainment, residents felt that a robot could not entertain them, and would instead prefer old-fashioned activities from their youth such as knitting and crafting. A robot's role in communicating with relatives also did not seem important, perhaps due to the fact that most of the residents had their own mobile phone, desktop computer or laptop.

Figure 6. User acceptance of robots based on functions

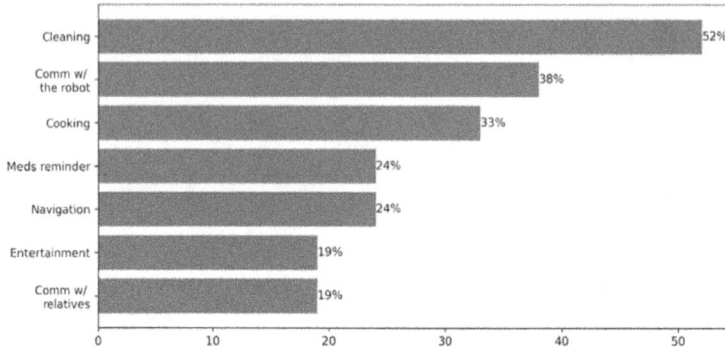

Linked to the previous question, residents were asked whether they considered performance of these activities would improve their physical or mental well-being. The results were mixed as seen in Figure 7, with approximately half the residents agreeing to a differing extent, while the remaining disagreed.

Figure 7. Well-being improvement based on robot's activities

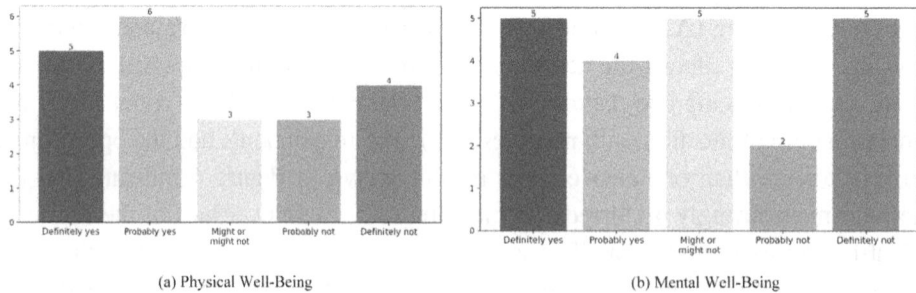

(a) Physical Well-Being   (b) Mental Well-Being

3.9 User Acceptance of Robots Based on Cost of the Robot

Cost was clearly regarded as less important than usefulness, as shown in Figure 3. Some residents commented that, as long as they did not pay for it, they did not consider price important. However, cost was considered to be as important as physical appearance and functionalities.

3.10 Open-Text Comments

Most participants (14) chose to leave the final open-ended question blank. The seven responses mostly focused on comments about cleaning activities, including a smart vacuum cleaner. Other residents commented on a desire for a robot to act as a personal secretary or to possess the ability to wash an individual. Although the environmental navigation activity was included in the questionnaire, one resident left the comment "Help me walk".

3.11 Comparison Between User Acceptance of Sensors and Robots

Figure 2a shows that older respondents exhibited a strong user acceptance of sensors for physical health improvement. At the same time, these residents had some reservations in the area of mental health, as seen in Figure 2b.

In terms of user acceptance of robots, the results for both physical health and mental health were very mixed, as shown in Figure 7a and Figure 7b respectively.

4. DISCUSSION

In addition to the general challenges of an ageing population, the current chapter highlights those associated with a super-ageing group of increasingly frail older people aged 85+ years. The UK currently has the fastest growing population world-wide in this population group, with a predicted doubling in size of those aged 85+ years by 2041 and trebling by 2066 (Office for National Statistics, 2021). The present study provides much needed research evidence on how older people aged 81-99 years living in a long-term residential care facility, or care home, value robots, including those with a physical presence as well as non-intrusive sensing technology. Although sensor systems for human monitoring and recognition have been widely researched for healthcare purposes (Karayaneva et al., 2018; Mashiyama, Hong and Ohtsuki, 2015; Karayaneva et al., 2023), research in care homes is limited. On the other hand, robots with a physical presence with diverse capabilities have been tested in care homes (Trainum et al., 2023), but long-term usage is still to be successfully introduced. Although the current study sample was relatively small, the size is similar to that reported in other studies identified in the literature review. However, the study is unique in that it was carried out in a living lab environment, following an observational period during which the lead author was embedded living full-time in this care home. Evidence from the literature review was combined with first-hand experience to produce the questionnaire administered by interview.

Residents contributed their views to produce the final framework for exploring user-acceptance co-designed with residents. The concept of 24/7 living labs is now being introduced in Japan, the country with the most rapidly ageing society in the world. In 2020, the Japanese Government's Ministry of Health, Labour and Welfare announced a strategy to develop 'care science', following this by needs matched support for development, demonstration, and dissemination of nursing care robots as living labs (or open labs). The aim is to address key issues (needs) faced by care sites across the country with products and technologies held by development companies (Science Council of Japan, 2020). Eight organizations including universities, government's research labs, R&D divisions of care companies, and a local authority have been funded as living labs. These include Care Tech Zenkoukai Lab (R&D division of a network of state-owned care homes) (Zenkoukai, 2024), and Future Care Lab in Japan (R&D division of a network of private care homes owned by insurance company, Sompo) (Future Care Lab in Japan, 2024).

4.1 User Acceptance of Non-Intrusive Sensing Technology

Older people participating in our study consistently showed a very strong preference for non-intrusive sensor technology that could improve their physical health and well-being, with some commenting that as long as the technology was helping them, they were supportive. This echoes the findings of one of the few published studies on the acceptability of assistive technology which found that older people valued 'felt need' and 'product quality' when presented with a new technology (McCreadie and Tinker, 2005). However, residents in the present study provided a mixed response when asked to consider any potential benefits in terms of their mental health and well-being (rather than physical health). A recent scoping review reported that older people's desire to portray themselves as independent and self-reliant will impact upon their adoption patterns for assistive technology (Astell, McGrath and Dove, 2020). Hence, responses in the present study may be indicative of residents' desire to consider that they are fully in control of their own moods and mental health. Alternatively, considering the age of the residents, it may be that mental health was a 'taboo' topic surrounded by stigma (Rössler, 2016).

4.2 Older People's Acceptance of Robots

Our research identified that application of the TAM model confirmed that both perceived ease-of-use and usefulness are considered important characteristics in a robot. For older residents, however, additional characteristics such as physical appearance, roles and functions, and cost also play an important role. Although our study identified humanoid physical appearances as the most popular, examples presented which resembled a human were chosen so as not to "fall" into the "uncanny valley", thus ensuring the robot would engender feelings of sympathy and familiarity among the residents (Mori, 1970). Zoomorphic robots were the next preferred appearance above machine-like robots, a finding in line with previous research in a similar size sample (n=25) which identified the same preference order (Pino et al., 2015).

In terms of the preferred role for social robots, our finding of a preference for cleaning is novel and has not been reported elsewhere. Many older people who move into long-term residential care will have physical problems affecting their ability to perform basic domestic tasks such as cleaning and cooking (Seidel et al., 2010; Ma et al., 2011). Thus, it is not surprising that the residents identified cleaning as important. Interestingly, cooking and communication with the robot were the second most preferred activities. While loneliness among older adults living on their own is recognised to be a major issue, it could become even worse for adults in care homes (Brownie and Horstmanshof, 2011). In line with these findings, the observational period identified that residents spent a large amount of time alone in their own rooms, as has been reported in other household studies (Peak et al., 2019). So, a robot could help by providing companionship.

4.3 Acceptance and Trust of Robot in own Home

Studies have discovered that trust is an important factor for user acceptance of robots (Stuck and Rogers, 2018) and of home monitoring systems (Lie, Lindsay and Brittain, 2016). Residents in our study were largely cautious in their responses to the questions of trusting and accepting a robot in the care home where they were living, with the most common response being to not accept a robot in this setting and probably not trust it to make decisions. This contrasts with previous research with 21 older adults (Age=80.25±7.19) who were identified as generally willing to accept a robot at home (Smarr et al., 2012). However, it is worth noting that our participants were a decade older (Age=90.42±4.46), which might potentially affect their acceptance and trust of robots. Also, views were elicited in structured interviews by a researcher who had been living alongside them. The complexity of understanding the acceptance of robots has been considered by other researchers, with findings identifying the fact that the word "robot" can engender feelings of unease and fear (Johansson-Pajala and Gustafsson, 2022).

4.4 Comparison Between Acceptance of Sensors and Robots

This study discovered stronger preferences for sensor-based monitoring systems compared to robots with a physical presence. Acceptance of interaction-free sensors is in line with previous research, where a similar preference has been reported

(Steele et al., 2009). While robots with a physical presence can potentially allow person-technology interaction, this form of relationship was found to have less support among residents in the present study. The fact that cleaning, identified as the most valued activity, requires no participation by the resident, would appear to substantiate this. However, the concept of "weak" or "vulnerable" robots needs to be considered as part of any person-technology interaction for both social and physical duties (Laitinen, Niemelä and Pirhonen, 2019; Traeger et al., 2020; Parviainen and Pirhonen, 2017). It appears that this is strongly correlated with older adults' dignity and self-esteem. Dignity is a fundamental human right, which could be considered under threat in long-term care settings in regard to robotic care (Laitinen, Niemelä and Pirhonen, 2019). A vulnerable robot serves as a tool for retaining a reasonable level of independence and dignity, whilst providing necessary social or physical robotic care. Thus, robotic cleaners can elicit an older person's interest and engagement by requiring them to help, such as by moving items (Smarr et al., 2014). As such, an individual may feel they have a more meaningful role in the activity, which is reported as beneficial for their self-esteem (Laitinen and Pirhonen, 2019). In addition, physical robots can offer an opportunity for staff, reducing the manual work of human carers and allowing them to focus on the emotional and social aspects of their duties (Parviainen and Pirhonen, 2017). However, other physical tasks undertaken by robots, such as lifting and moving people, could reduce human contact, another important human right (Nwosu et al., 2019).

4.5 Limitations and Strengths of Study

Certain limitations should be borne in mind when considering these research findings. First, the participants may not be representative of the wider population nationally because they were recruited from a single care home. Also, although great care was taken to recruit a wide age range (81-99 years), there were fewer male residents. This generally reflects the UK care home population (McCann, Donnelly, and O'Reilly, 2012), but the sample size meant that gender differences could not be explored. Finally, the fact that individuals living with dementia were not recruited to contribute to this study means the preferences of these individuals could not be explored. The robot examples presented in the questionnaire were also necessarily ones which are commercially available with set physical appearances, roles, and functions, so not allowing for future novel designs and functions. Finally, although the greatest care was taken in the questionnaire design, as with all surveys that record individuals' views, the validity and reliability of the data could not be tested independently.

5. CONCLUSIONS

Although it is assumed that unobtrusive sensors and physical robots will eventually address the challenge of providing care for a super-ageing society with a declining birthrate, research into factors influencing older users' acceptance of such technologies has received far less attention to date than robot development. This is partly due to challenges in accessing these populations in a cost-effective and reliable manner. The present study has successfully explored older people's preferences through in-depth research undertaken in a UK care home 'living lab' environment with a researcher first living alongside residents in order to better understand their lived experience. The findings demonstrates that a range of factors, beyond the two dimensions generally accepted (usefulness and ease-of-use) affect technology acceptance by older adults aged 81-99 years. Elements such as appearance, role, and functions; impact on physical health and mental well-being; and trust towards the robot have been identified, and compared between acceptance of sensors and physical robots, forming the foundation for a more comprehensive, tailored framework for assessing the acceptability of prototype sensors and physical robots. To our knowledge, such an analysis has not been undertaken in previous studies with this population.

By extending the research to older adults in other living lab environments in the UK to newly created living labs in Japan, it should be possible to discover the degree to which culture influences response patterns, and also what impact demographic factors such as education, level of disability, and psychological profile have on acceptance patterns. The use of co-design approaches in controlled environments such as living labs will be necessary if technology development is to successfully meet world-wide market needs through the design of future generations of social care robots.

REFERENCES

Abdi, J., Al-Hindawi, A., Ng, T., & Vizcaychipi, M. P. (2018). Scoping review on the use of socially assistive robot technology in elderly care. *BMJ Open*, 8(2), e018815. DOI: 10.1136/bmjopen-2017-018815 PMID: 29440212

Alzheimer's Society. (2024). Local dementia statistics. URL: https://www.alzheimers.org.uk/about-us/policy-and-influencing/local-dementia-statistics

Astell, A. J., McGrath, C., & Dove, E. (2020). 'That's for old so and so's!': Does identity influence older adults' technology adoption decisions? *Ageing and Society*, 40(7), 1550–1576. DOI: 10.1017/S0144686X19000230

Baandrup, L., & Jennum, P. J. (2021). Effect of a dynamic lighting intervention on circadian rest-activity disturbances in cognitively impaired, older adults living in a nursing home: A proof-of-concept study. *Neurobiology of Sleep and Circadian Rhythms*, 11, 100067. DOI: 10.1016/j.nbscr.2021.100067 PMID: 34095610

Baig, M. M., Afifi, S., GholamHosseini, H., & Mirza, F. (2019). A systematic review of wearable sensors and IoT-based monitoring applications for older adults–a focus on ageing population and independent living. *Journal of Medical Systems*, 43(8), 1–11. DOI: 10.1007/s10916-019-1365-7 PMID: 31203472

Bedaf, S., Marti, P., Amirabdollahian, F., & de Witte, L. (2018). A multi-perspective evaluation of a service robot for seniors: The voice of different stake-holders. *Disability and Rehabilitation. Assistive Technology*, 13(6), 592–599. DOI: 10.1080/17483107.2017.1358300 PMID: 28758532

Beuscher, L. M., Fan, J., Sarkar, N., Dietrich, M. S., Newhouse, P. A., Miller, K. F., & Mion, L. C. (2017). Socially assistive robots: Measuring older adults' perceptions. *Journal of Gerontological Nursing*, 43(12), 35–43. DOI: 10.3928/00989134-20170707-04 PMID: 28700074

Bian, C., Ye, B., Hoonakker, A., & Mihailidis, A. (2021). Attitudes and perspectives of older adults on technologies for assessing frailty in home settings: A focus group study. *BMC Geriatrics*, 21(1), 298. DOI: 10.1186/s12877-021-02252-4 PMID: 33964887

Broadbent, E., Tamagawa, R., Kerse, N., Knock, B., Patience, A., & MacDonald, B. (2009, September). Retirement home staff and residents' preferences for healthcare robots. In RO-MAN 2009-The 18th IEEE International Symposium on Robot and Human Interactive Communication (pp. 645-650). IEEE.

Brownie, S., & Horstmanshof, L. (2011). The management of loneliness in aged care residents: An important therapeutic target for gerontological nursing. *Geriatric Nursing*, 32(5), 318–325. DOI: 10.1016/j.gerinurse.2011.05.003 PMID: 21831481

Chen, T. L., Bhattacharjee, T., Beer, J. M., Ting, L. H., Hackney, M. E., Rogers, W. A., & Kemp, C. C. (2017). Older adults' acceptance of a robot for partner dance-based exercise. *PLoS One*, 12(10), e0182736. DOI: 10.1371/journal.pone.0182736 PMID: 29045408

Chu, L., Chen, H. W., Cheng, P. Y., Ho, P., Weng, I. T., Yang, P. L., Chien, S.-E., Tu, Y.-C., Yang, C.-C., Wang, T.-M., Fung, H. H., & Yeh, S. L. (2019). Identifying features that enhance older adults' acceptance of robots: A mixed methods study. *Gerontology*, 65(4), 441–450. DOI: 10.1159/000494881 PMID: 30844813

Chung, J., Demiris, G., Thompson, H. J., Chen, K. Y., Burr, R., Patel, S., & Fogarty, J. (2017). Feasibility testing of a home-based sensor system to monitor mobility and daily activities in Korean American older adults. *International Journal of Older People Nursing*, 12(1), e12127. DOI: 10.1111/opn.12127 PMID: 27431567

Cohen, C., Kampel, T., & Verloo, H. (2016). Acceptability of an intelligent wireless sensor system for the rapid detection of health issues: Findings among home-dwelling older adults and their informal caregivers. *Patient Preference and Adherence*, •••, 1687–1695. PMID: 27660417

Davis, F. (1989). Perceived Usefulness, Perceived Ease of Use, and User Acceptance of Information Technology. *Management Information Systems Quarterly*, 13(3), 319–340. DOI: 10.2307/249008

Demiris, G., Oliver, D. P., Giger, J., Skubic, M., & Rantz, M. (2009). Older adults' privacy considerations for vision based recognition methods of eldercare applications. *Technology and Health Care*, 17(1), 41–48. DOI: 10.3233/THC-2009-0530 PMID: 19478404

Dionyssiotis, Y. (2012). Analyzing the problem of falls among older people. *International Journal of General Medicine*, •••, 805–813. DOI: 10.2147/IJGM.S32651 PMID: 23055770

England Transformation Directorate, N. H. S. (2020). Acoustic monitoring integrated with electronic care planning. Available at: https://transform.england.nhs.uk/ai-lab/explore-all-resources/understand-ai/acoustic-monitoring-integrated-electronic-care-planning/

Ezer, N., Fisk, A. D., & Rogers, W. A. (2009, October). More than a servant: Self-reported willingness of younger and older adults to having a robot perform interactive and critical tasks in the home. [). Sage CA: Los Angeles, CA: SAGE Publications.]. *Proceedings of the Human Factors and Ergonomics Society Annual Meeting*, 53(2), 136–140. DOI: 10.1177/154193120905300206 PMID: 25349553

Future Care Lab in Japan. (living lab): a project of caregiving improvement produced by the Sompo Holdings Group. https://futurecarelab.com/en/about/

Gövercin, M., Költzsch, Y., Meis, M., Wegel, S., Gietzelt, M., Spehr, J., Winkelbach, S., Marschollek, M., & Steinhagen-Thiessen, E. (2010). Defining the user requirements for wearable and optical fall prediction and fall detection devices for home use. *Informatics for Health & Social Care*, 35(3-4), 177–187. DOI: 10.3109/17538157.2010.528648 PMID: 21133771

Gövercin, M., Meyer, S., Schellenbach, M., Steinhagen-Thiessen, E., Weiss, B., & Haesner, M. (2016). SmartSenior@ home: Acceptance of an integrated ambient assisted living system. Results of a clinical field trial in 35 households. *Informatics for Health & Social Care*, 41(4), 430–447. DOI: 10.3109/17538157.2015.1064425 PMID: 26809357

Guizzo, E. (2010). *France developing advanced humanoid robot Romeo*. IEEE Spectrum Automaton Blog.

Hall, A., Wilson, C. B., Stanmore, E., & Todd, C. (2017). Implementing monitoring technologies in care homes for people with dementia: A qualitative exploration using normalization process theory. *International Journal of Nursing Studies*, 72, 60–70. DOI: 10.1016/j.ijnurstu.2017.04.008 PMID: 28494333

Heerink, M., Kröse, B., Evers, V., & Wielinga, B. (2010). Assessing acceptance of assistive social agent technology by older adults: the almere model.

Heerink, M., Kröse, B., Wielinga, B., & Evers, V. (2009, September). Measuring the influence of social abilities on acceptance of an interface robot and a screen agent by elderly users. In *People and Computers XXIII Celebrating People and Technology*. BCS Learning & Development. DOI: 10.14236/ewic/HCI2009.54

Heerink, M., Kröse, B., Wielinga, B. J., & Evers, V. (2006). Studying the acceptance of a robotic agent by elderly users. *International Journal of Assistive Robotics and Mechatronics*, 7(3), 33–43.

Hung, L., Liu, C., Woldum, E., Au-Yeung, A., Berndt, A., Wallsworth, C., Horne, N., Gregorio, M., Mann, J., & Chaudhury, H. (2019). The benefits of and barriers to using a social robot PARO in care settings: A scoping review. *BMC Geriatrics*, 19(1), 1–10. DOI: 10.1186/s12877-019-1244-6 PMID: 31443636

Iio, T., Shiomi, M., Kamei, K., Sharma, C., & Hagita, N. (2016). Social acceptance by senior citizens and caregivers of a fall detection system using range sensors in a nursing home. *Advanced Robotics*, 30(3), 190–205. DOI: 10.1080/01691864.2015.1120241

Ince Yenilmez, M. (2015). Economic and social consequences of population aging the dilemmas and opportunities in the twenty-first century. *Applied Research in Quality of Life*, 10(4), 735–752. DOI: 10.1007/s11482-014-9334-2

Johansson-Pajala, R. M., & Gustafsson, C. (2022). Significant challenges when introducing care robots in Swedish elder care. *Disability and Rehabilitation. Assistive Technology*, 17(2), 166–176. DOI: 10.1080/17483107.2020.1773549 PMID: 32538206

Karayaneva, Y., Baker, S., Tan, B., & Jing, Y. (2018, July). Use of low-resolution infrared pixel array for passive human motion movement and recognition. In Proceedings of the 32nd international BCS human computer interaction conference. BCS Learning & Development. DOI: 10.14236/ewic/HCI2018.143

Karayaneva, Y., Sharifzadeh, S., Jing, Y., & Tan, B. (2023). Human activity recognition for AI-enabled healthcare using low-resolution infrared sensor data. *Sensors (Basel)*, 23(1), 478. DOI: 10.3390/s23010478 PMID: 36617075

Karayaneva, Y., Sharifzadeh, S., Li, W., Jing, Y., & Tan, B. (2021). Unsupervised Doppler radar based activity recognition for e-healthcare. *IEEE Access : Practical Innovations, Open Solutions*, 9, 62984–63001. DOI: 10.1109/ACCESS.2021.3074088

Ke, C., Lou, V. W. Q., Tan, K. C. K., Wai, M. Y., & Chan, L. L. (2020). Changes in technology acceptance among older people with dementia: The role of social robot engagement. *International Journal of Medical Informatics*, 141, 104241. DOI: 10.1016/j.ijmedinf.2020.104241 PMID: 32739611

Khosla, R., Nguyen, K., & Chu, M. T. (2017). Human robot engagement and acceptability in residential aged care. *International Journal of Human-Computer Interaction*, 33(6), 510–522. DOI: 10.1080/10447318.2016.1275435

Korchut, A., Szklener, S., Abdelnour, C., Tantinya, N., Hernández-Farigola, J., Ribes, J. C., Skrobas, U., Grabowska-Aleksandrowicz, K., Szczęśniak-Stańczyk, D., & Rejdak, K. (2017). Challenges for service robots—Requirements of elderly adults with cognitive impairments. *Frontiers in Neurology*, 8, 228. DOI: 10.3389/fneur.2017.00228 PMID: 28620342

Laitinen, A., Niemelä, M., & Pirhonen, J. (2019). Recognizing Vulnerability, Agency, and Subjectivity in Robot-based, Robot-assisted, and Teleoperated Elderly Care. *Techné: Research in Philosophy and Technology*.

Laitinen, A., & Pirhonen, J. (2019). Ten forms of recognition and misrecognition in long-term care for older people. *Sats*, 20(1), 53–78. DOI: 10.1515/sats-2016-0017

Lazaro, M. J. S., Lim, J., Kim, S. H., & Yun, M. H. (2020). Wearable Technologies: Acceptance Model for Smartwatch Adoption Among Older Adults. In Gao, Q., & Zhou, J. (Eds.), Lecture Notes in Computer Science: Vol. 12207. *Human Aspects of IT for the Aged Population. Technologies, Design and User Experience. HCII 2020*. Springer. DOI: 10.1007/978-3-030-50252-2_23

Lee, L. Y., Lim, W. M., Teh, P. L., Malik, O. A. S., & Nurzaman, S. (2020). Understanding the interaction between older adults and soft service robots: Insights from robotics and the technology acceptance model. *AIS Transactions on Human-Computer Interaction*, 12(3), 125–145. DOI: 10.17705/1thci.00132

Li, J., Ma, Q., Chan, A. H., & Man, S. (2019). Health monitoring through wearable technologies for older adults: Smart wearables acceptance model. *Applied Ergonomics*, 75, 162–169. DOI: 10.1016/j.apergo.2018.10.006 PMID: 30509522

Li, W., Tan, B., & Piechocki, R. (2018). Passive radar for opportunistic monitoring in e-health applications. *IEEE Journal of Translational Engineering in Health and Medicine*, 6, 1–10. DOI: 10.1109/JTEHM.2018.2791609 PMID: 29456898

Li, W., Tan, B., Xu, Y., & Piechocki, R. J. (2018). Log-likelihood clustering-enabled passive RF sensing for residential activity recognition. *IEEE Sensors Journal*, 18(13), 5413–5421. DOI: 10.1109/JSEN.2018.2834739

Li, W., Xu, Y., Tan, B., & Piechocki, R. J. (2017, June). Passive wireless sensing for unsupervised human activity recognition in healthcare. In 2017 13th International Wireless Communications and Mobile Computing Conference (IWCMC) (pp. 1528-1533). IEEE. DOI: 10.1109/IWCMC.2017.7986511

Lie, M. L., Lindsay, S., & Brittain, K. (2016). Technology and trust: Older people's perspectives of a home monitoring system. *Ageing and Society*, 36(7), 1501–1525. DOI: 10.1017/S0144686X15000501

Lin, W.-Y., Chou, W.-C., Tsai, T.-H., Lin, C.-C., & Lee, M.-Y. (2016). Development of a Wearable Instrumented Vest for Posture Monitoring and System Usability Verification Based on the Technology Acceptance Model. *Sensors (Basel)*, 16(12), 2172. DOI: 10.3390/s16122172 PMID: 27999324

Louie, W. Y. G., McColl, D., & Nejat, G. (2014). Acceptance and attitudes toward a human-like socially assistive robot by older adults. *Assistive Technology*, 26(3), 140–150. DOI: 10.1080/10400435.2013.869703 PMID: 26131794

Ma, W. T., Yan, W. X., Fu, Z., & Zhao, Y. Z. (2011). A Chinese cooking robot for elderly and disabled people. *Robotica*, 29(6), 843–852. DOI: 10.1017/S0263574711000051

Mashiyama, S., Hong, J., & Ohtsuki, T. (2015, June). Activity recognition using low resolution infrared array sensor. In *2015 IEEE International Conference on Communications (ICC)* (pp. 495-500). IEEE. DOI: 10.1109/ICC.2015.7248370

McCann, M., Donnelly, M., & O'Reilly, D. (2012). Gender differences in care home admission risk: Partner's age explains the higher risk for women. *Age and Ageing*, 41(3), 416–419. DOI: 10.1093/ageing/afs022 PMID: 22510517

McCreadie, C., & Tinker, A. (2005). The acceptability of assistive technology to older people. *Ageing and Society*, 25(1), 91–110. DOI: 10.1017/S0144686X0400248X

McGlynn, S. A., Kemple, S. C., Mitzner, T. L., King, C. H., & Rogers, W. A. (2014, September). Understanding older adults' perceptions of usefulness for the paro robot. []. Sage CA: Los Angeles, CA: SAGE Publications.]. *Proceedings of the Human Factors and Ergonomics Society Annual Meeting*, 58(1), 1914–1918. DOI: 10.1177/1541931214581400 PMID: 31320791

Mihailidis, A., Cockburn, A., Longley, C., & Boger, J. (2008). The acceptability of home monitoring technology among community-dwelling older adults and baby boomers. *Assistive Technology*, 20(1), 1–12. DOI: 10.1080/10400435.2008.10131927 PMID: 18751575

Mitzner, T. L., Smarr, C. A., Beer, J. M., Chen, T. L., Springman, J. M., Prakash, A., & Rogers, W. A. (2011). *Older adults' acceptance of assistive robots for the home*. Georgia Institute of Technology.

Mori, M. (1970). The uncanny valley. *Energy*, 7(4), 33–35.

Moyle, W., Bramble, M., Jones, C., & Murfield, J. (2016). Care staff perceptions of a social robot called Paro and a look-alike Plush Toy: A descriptive qualitative approach. *Aging & Mental Health*, 22(3), 330–335. DOI: 10.1080/13607863.2016.1262820 PMID: 27967207

Nwosu, A. C., Sturgeon, B., McGlinchey, T., Goodwin, C. D., Behera, A., Mason, S., Stanley, S., & Payne, T. R. (2019). Robotic technology for palliative and supportive care: Strengths, weaknesses, opportunities and threats. *Palliative Medicine*, 33(8), 1106–1113. DOI: 10.1177/0269216319857628 PMID: 31250734

Office for National Statistics. Living longer: how our population is changing and why it matters. Overview of population ageing in the UK and some implications for the economy, public services, society and the individual. Office for National Statistics. https://www.ons.gov.uk/peoplepopulationandcommunity/birthsdeathsandmarriages/ageing/articles/livinglongerhowourpopulationischangingandwhyitmatters/2018-08-13. Census 2021. Accessed 26 October 2022.

Olde Keizer, R. A., van Velsen, L., Moncharmont, M., Riche, B., Ammour, N., Del Signore, S., Zia, G., Hermens, H., & N'Dja, A. (2019). Using socially assistive robots for monitoring and preventing frailty among older adults: A study on usability and user experience challenges. *Health and Technology*, 9(4), 595–605. DOI: 10.1007/s12553-019-00320-9

Papadopoulos, I., Koulouglioti, C., Lazzarino, R., & Ali, S. (2020). Enablers and barriers to the implementation of socially assistive humanoid robots in health and social care: A systematic review. *BMJ Open*, 2020(1), 10. DOI: 10.1136/bmjopen-2019-033096 PMID: 31924639

Parliament, U. K. Parliamentary Office of Science & Technology (POST). Robotics in Social Care. 2018 (12 December). Available from: https://post.parliament.uk/research-briefings/post-pn-0591

Parviainen, J., & Pirhonen, J. (2017). Vulnerable bodies in human–robot interactions: Embodiment as ethical issue in robot care for the elderly.

Peak, J., Barrett, H., Halloran, J., & Szczepura, A. (2019). All for one and one for all? Can communities in care homes support ageing in place? National Seminar, Possibilities of DDRI in Senior People's Care in Japan, (Poster).

Piasek, J., & Wieczorowska-Tobis, K. (2018, July). Acceptance and long-term use of a social robot by elderly users in a domestic environment. In 2018 11th international conference on human system interaction (HSI) (pp. 478-482). IEEE. DOI: 10.1109/HSI.2018.8431348

Pino, M., Boulay, M., Jouen, F., & Rigaud, A. S. (2015). "Are we ready for robots that care for us?" Attitudes and opinions of older adults toward socially assistive robots. *Frontiers in Aging Neuroscience*, 7, 141. DOI: 10.3389/fnagi.2015.00141 PMID: 26257646

Pol, M., Van Nes, F., Van Hartingsveldt, M., Buurman, B., De Rooij, S., & Kröse, B. (2016). Older people's perspectives regarding the use of sensor monitoring in their home. *The Gerontologist*, 56(3), 485–493. DOI: 10.1093/geront/gnu104 PMID: 25384761

Puri, A., Kim, B., Nguyen, O., Stolee, P., Tung, J., & Lee, J. (2017). User acceptance of wrist-worn activity trackers among community-dwelling older adults: Mixed method study. *JMIR mHealth and uHealth*, 5(11), e8211. DOI: 10.2196/mhealth.8211 PMID: 29141837

Reeder, B., Chung, J., Joe, J., Lazar, A., Thompson, H. J., & Demiris, G. (2016). Understanding older adults' perceptions of in-home sensors using an obtrusiveness framework. In Foundations of Augmented Cognition: Neuroergonomics and Operational Neuroscience: 10th International Conference, AC 2016, Held as Part of HCI International 2016, Toronto, ON, Canada, July 17-22, 2016 [Springer International Publishing.]. *Proceedings*, 10(Part II), 351–360.

Rössler, W. (2016). The stigma of mental disorders: A millennia-long history of social exclusion and prejudices. *EMBO Reports*, 17(9), 1250–1253. DOI: 10.15252/embr.201643041 PMID: 27470237

Sääskilahti, K., Kangaskorte, R., Pieskä, S., Jauhiainen, J., & Luimula, M. (2012). Needs and user acceptance of older adults for mobile service robot. 2012 IEEE RO-MAN: The 21st IEEE International Symposium on Robots and Human Interactive Communication (pp. 559-564). Paris, France: IEEE. Paris, France: IEEE.

Science Council of Japan. (2020). *Clinical Medicine Committee/Health/Life Science Committee Joint Care Science Subcommittee in an Aging Society with a Declining Birthrate, Recommendation: Forming the Foundation of Care Science and Creating a Future Society*. Science Council of Japan. (in Japanese)

Sefcik, J. S., Johnson, M. J., Yim, M., Lau, T., Vivio, N., Mucchiani, C., & Cacchione, P. Z. (2018). Stakeholders' perceptions sought to inform the development of a low-cost mobile robot for older adults: A qualitative descriptive study. *Clinical Nursing Research*, 27(1), 61–80. DOI: 10.1177/1054773817730517 PMID: 28918654

Seidel, D., Richardson, K., Crilly, N., Matthews, F. E., Clarkson, P. J., & Brayne, C. (2010). Design for independent living: Activity demands and capabilities of older people. *Ageing and Society*, 30(7), 1239–1255. DOI: 10.1017/S0144686X10000310

Shiomi, M., Iio, T., Kamei, K., Sharma, C., & Hagita, N. (2015). Effectiveness of social behaviors for autonomous wheelchair robot to support elderly people in Japan. *PLoS One*, 10(5), e0128031. DOI: 10.1371/journal.pone.0128031 PMID: 25993038

Shore, L., de Eyto, A., & O'Sullivan, L. (2022). Technology acceptance and perceptions of robotic assistive devices by older adults–implications for exoskeleton design. *Disability and Rehabilitation. Assistive Technology*, 17(7), 782–790. DOI: 10.1080/17483107.2020.1817988 PMID: 32988251

Shore, L., Power, V., De Eyto, A., & O'Sullivan, L. W. (2018). Technology acceptance and user-centred design of assistive exoskeletons for older adults: A commentary. *Robotics (Basel, Switzerland)*, 7(1), 3. DOI: 10.3390/robotics7010003

Smarr, C. A., Mitzner, T. L., Beer, J. M., Prakash, A., Chen, T. L., Kemp, C. C., & Rogers, W. A. (2014). Domestic robots for older adults: Attitudes, preferences, and potential. *International Journal of Social Robotics*, 6(2), 229–247. DOI: 10.1007/s12369-013-0220-0 PMID: 25152779

Smarr, C. A., Prakash, A., Beer, J. M., Mitzner, T. L., Kemp, C. C., & Rogers, W. A. (2012, September). Older adults' preferences for and acceptance of robot assistance for everyday living tasks. []. Sage CA: Los Angeles, CA: Sage Publications.]. *Proceedings of the Human Factors and Ergonomics Society Annual Meeting*, 56(1), 153–157. DOI: 10.1177/1071181312561009 PMID: 25284971

Softbank Robotics. "NAO the humanoid and programmable robot" (2020). Available: https://www.softbankrobotics.com/emea/en/nao

Softbank Robotics. "Pepper the humanoid and programmable robot" (2020). Available: https://www.softbankrobotics.com/emea/en/pepper

Stavropoulos, T. G., Papastergiou, A., Mpaltadoros, L., Nikolopoulos, S., & Kompatsiaris, I. (2020). IoT Wearable Sensors and Devices in Elderly Care: A Literature Review. *Sensors (Basel)*, 20(10), 2826. DOI: 10.3390/s20102826 PMID: 32429331

Steele, R., Lo, A., Secombe, C., & Wong, Y. K. (2009). Elderly persons' perception and acceptance of using wireless sensor networks to assist healthcare. *International Journal of Medical Informatics*, 78(12), 788–801. DOI: 10.1016/j.ijmedinf.2009.08.001 PMID: 19717335

Stuck, R. E., & Rogers, W. A. (2018). Older adults' perceptions of supporting factors of trust in a robot care provider. *Journal of Robotics*, 2018(1), 6519713. DOI: 10.1155/2018/6519713

Szczepura, A., Collinson, M., Moody, L., Jing, Y., Ward, G., Bul, K., Arnab, S., Asbury, C., Russell, E., Gibbons, C., & Dashwood, R. (2018). PP89 Living Lab Concept: An Innovation Hub For Elderly Residential Care. *International Journal of Technology Assessment in Health Care*, 34(S1), 99–100. DOI: 10.1017/S0266462318002362

Taylor, J. P., Smith, N., Prato, L., Damant, J., Jasim, S., Toma, M., Hamashima, Y., McLeod, H., Towers, A.-M., Keemink, J., Nwolise, C., Giebel, C., & Fitzpatrick, R. (2023). Care planning interventions for care home residents: A scoping review. *Journal of Long-Term Care*. Advance online publication. DOI: 10.31389/jltc.223

Traeger, M. L., Strohkorb Sebo, S., Jung, M., Scassellati, B., & Christakis, N. A. (2020). Vulnerable robots positively shape human conversational dynamics in a human–robot team. *Proceedings of the National Academy of Sciences of the United States of America*, 117(12), 6370–6375. DOI: 10.1073/pnas.1910402117 PMID: 32152118

Trainum, K., Tunis, R., Xie, B., & Hauser, E. (2023). Robots in Assisted Living Facilities: Scoping Review. *JMIR Aging*, 6, e42652. DOI: 10.2196/42652 PMID: 36877560

United Nations. (2022). *World Population Prospects 2022*. Department of Economic and Social Affairs, Population Division.

Whelan, S., Murphy, K., Barrett, E., Krusche, C., Santorelli, A., & Casey, D. (2018). Factors affecting the acceptability of social robots by older adults including people with dementia or cognitive impairment: A literature review. *International Journal of Social Robotics*, 10(5), 643–668. DOI: 10.1007/s12369-018-0471-x

Wu, A. Y., & Munteanu, C. (2018, April). Understanding older users' acceptance of wearable interfaces for sensor-based fall risk assessment. In *Proceedings of the 2018 CHI conference on human factors in computing systems* (pp. 1-13). DOI: 10.1145/3173574.3173693

Wu, Y. H., Wrobel, J., Cornuet, M., Kerhervé, H., Domene, S., & Rigaud, A. S. (2014). Acceptance of an assistive robot in older adults: A mixed-method study of human–robot interaction over a 1-month period in the Living Lab setting. *Clinical Interventions in Aging*, ●●●, 801–811. DOI: 10.2147/CIA.S56435 PMID: 24855349

Yin, C., Chen, J., Miao, X., Jiang, H., & Chen, D. (2021). Device-free human activity recognition with low-resolution infrared array sensor using long short-term memory neural network. *Sensors (Basel)*, 21(10), 3551. DOI: 10.3390/s21103551 PMID: 34065183

Zenkoukai: Social Welfare Corporation & Zenkoukai Research Institute. https://zenkou-lab.co.jp/

Chapter 2
The Impact of the Internet of Things in Healthcare Delivery:
A Systematic Literature Review

Omar F. El-Gayar
https://orcid.org/0000-0001-8657-8732
Dakota State University, USA

Giridhar Reddy Bojja
Michigan Tech, USA

Loknath Sai Ambati
Oklahoma City University, USA

James Boit
Grand Valley State University, USA

Nevine Nawar
Alexandria University, Egypt

ABSTRACT

The increasing demand for efficient healthcare has spurred the adoption of IoT technologies, promising reduced costs and improved outcomes. This study addresses the integration of IoT in healthcare, focusing on patient-centered applications across prevention, diagnosis, and treatment. We explore three research questions concerning the main IoT applications, their drivers and challenges, and their impact on healthcare delivery. This systematic literature review synthesizes evidence from the literature to identify trends and mappings in IoT applications. The review includes a

DOI: 10.4018/979-8-3693-5237-3.ch002

comprehensive framework for IoT in healthcare, enhancing patient engagement and care delivery. The study is structured first to define IoT paradigms and technologies, followed by proposing a healthcare framework, describing our methodology, and discussing the implications of our findings on future healthcare innovations.

INTRODUCTION

The demand for a more efficient, faster and better medical services has accelerated the rise of Internet of Things (IoT) enabled technologies in the healthcare domain. While traditionally IoT technologies have often been associated with smart homes of the future, retail, and manufacturing industries, the rapid adoption of IoT in the healthcare industry is gaining prominence. The innovations in IoT technology promises to dramatically reduce costs, improve services and enhance patient outcomes. Furthermore, the evolution in mobile network technologies, such as 5G, acts as a catalyst for increased development of applications of IoT in healthcare (Sodhro & Shah, 2017), specifically, in processes like imaging, treatment and diagnosis (Magsi et al., 2018). In a broader sense, IoT is transforming the healthcare industry at a fast pace including significant advancements in remote health and monitoring, patient tracking and staff inventory, improved drug management, chronic disease management, and reduction in emergency room wait times. The ubiquitous nature of IoT means much more connectivity, increased data sources, and thus the potential for better patient outcomes.

With continuous collection and measurement of individual's data in near real time fashion, the network of IoT devices can significantly contribute towards better prediction of diagnosis, selection of treatment approaches, and through proactive health systems result in low marginal errors. The impact of IoT in healthcare is far reaching, for example, through remote monitoring, patients can cut down hospital visits thus reducing their overall re-admission footprint. From a physician's perspective, the personalized patient engagement and experience metrics offered by IoT can translate to high quality care. This way, the objective of the health continuum is achieved through reduced costs, improved treatment, and enhanced patient outcomes. IoT could, therefore, potentially revolutionize the healthcare industry in service delivery and improvement of patient outcomes by empowering stakeholders such as patients to actively join as valuable partners in the healthcare continuum to track and take ownership of their health journey. Moreover, the exponential growth in wearable devices, ubiquitous and mobile computing, and high global internet connectivity has affected global clinical health services such as prevention, monitoring, and detection thus dramatically increasing the wide adoption of IoT in healthcare.

A recent survey of IoT in healthcare indicates that it is a growing phenomenon with a tendency to focus on patient monitoring (Din, Almogren, et al., 2019). This has also been explored in another survey on IoT applications evaluating the potential for health-care monitoring (Asghari et al., 2019b). The survey by Din et al. (Din, Guizani, et al., 2019), provides a summary of enabling technologies for IoT such as fog computing and argues that sensor devices are key technology drivers for a proposed smart health care system. The survey by Sadoughi et al. (Sadoughi et al., 2020) reviewed IoT developments in medicine. Other surveys of IoT in healthcare focused on cyber-physical systems (Gatouillat et al., 2018; Plaza et al., 2018); Network and IoT architectures (Ahmadi et al., 2018; Ray, 2018; Riazul Islam et al., 2015); IoT-related applications in medicine (Din, Almogren, et al., 2019); applications of IoT in healthcare (Ahmadi et al., 2018; Atzori et al., 2010; Hu et al., 2013); enabling technologies (Ahmadi et al., 2018; Atzori et al., 2010; Din, Guizani, et al., 2019; Riazul Islam et al., 2015); nursing care (Mieronkoski et al., 2017); security and privacy (Ahmadi et al., 2018; Aleisa & Renaud, 2017; Riazul Islam et al., 2015); wireless body area networks (Cavallari et al., 2014; Ghamari et al., 2016); Big Data (Dimitrov, 2016); and wireless sensor networks(Ko et al., 2010). Overall, these studies almost exclusively focused on specific or holistic aspects of enabling technologies, network or cloud architectures, and general to specific applications of IoT in healthcare.

This study complements prior research by emphasizing individual and patient-centered applications along the clinical processes of prevention, diagnosis, and treatment. For the purpose of this research, we adopt the US National Institute of Health (NIH) (NIH, 2001) notion of patient-centered care reflecting *"healthcare that establishes a partnership among practitioners, patients and their families (when appropriate) to ensure that decisions respect patients' wants, needs and preferences and solicit patients' input on the education and support they need to make decisions and participate in their own care"*. Specifically, and in the context of patient-centered care where the individual is central to the application and use of IoT in a manner that transcends traditional healthcare provider setting, the study addresses the following research questions:

RQ1: What are the main IoT applications in healthcare?

RQ2: What are the major IoT technologies used in supporting healthcare activities?

RQ3: What are the main drivers, challenges and issues surrounding the applications of IoT for healthcare and wellbeing?

The remainder of this paper is organized as follows. Section 2 presents the background of IoT as a paradigm and its corresponding definitions, features, related technologies, and communication models while section 3 describes the proposed framework. Section 4 describes the research methodology applied in this study. Section 5 presents the results obtained from the systematic review process. Section

6 discusses the implications of the results, while sections 7 and 8 present the drivers and challenges of IoT applications in healthcare, respectively. Finally, Section 9 concludes the paper by explaining the future trends and contemporary research directions.

BACKGROUND AND RELATED WORK

IoT as a Paradigm, Definition, and Components

IoT is a paradigm where objects situated in our everyday lives have the capability to sense, gather, process and communicate data with other devices over the Internet to achieve a specific goal. Over the last decade, the advancement in smart object technology and availability of ubiquitous Internet-enabled devices have produced significant successes in IoT applications in industries such as retail, manufacturing, and healthcare. IoT as a paradigm is guided by the convergence of three visions: 1). Network oriented, 2). Things oriented, and 3). Semantic oriented perspectives, creating a modern disruptive innovation that brings enhancement to the value network (Atzori et al., 2010). The multi-vision nature of IoT implies an architecture for both virtual and physical objects to communicate with each other seamlessly while operating in an intelligent environment. IoT models around the use of radio-frequency identification (RFID) and tracking technologies allowing manufacturers, retailers and distributors with the benefit of improved efficiency, real-time information feedback, and reduction in labor costs (S. Li et al., 2015). The idea behind IoT is to enable cooperative interconnection and integration of physical objects in the real-world environment over the Internet.

Despite the current popularity and trends on the Internet of Things adoption, there seems to be no universally acceptable definition of the IoT concept. In fact, many definitions have been used or proposed to explain the different perspectives of IoT in terms of usage, protocols, standards or even characteristics. Table 1 presents a number of definitions of IoT with varying emphasis or focus.

Table 1. Different definitions of the IoT paradigm

Author	Definition	Focus	References
Merriam-Webster Dictionary	"the networking capability that allows information to be sent to and received from objects and devices (such as fixtures and kitchen appliances) using the Internet"	IoT as a vehicle or feature for connectivity	*(Internet Of Things | Definition of Internet Of Things by Merriam-Webster*, n.d.)
Atzori et. al	IoT is a network of "things" where objects are connected to a server that offers appropriate services and can be uniquely identified	Network of "things"	(Atzori et al., 2010)
The Internet Architecture Board (IAB) begins RFC 7452	"The term "Internet of Things" (IoT) denotes a trend where a large number of embedded devices employ communication services offered by the Internet protocols. Many of these devices, often called "smart objects," are not directly operated by humans, but exist as components in buildings or vehicles, or are spread out in the environment"	Connectivity of Smart objects	(Tschofenig et al., 2015)
International Telecommunication Union (ITU) ITU–T	A global infrastructure for the information society, enabling advanced services by interconnecting (physical and virtual) things based on existing and evolving interoperable information and communication technologies.	Interconnectivity	(ITU, 2012)
IEEE Communications Magazine	"The Internet of Things (IoT) is a framework in which all things have a representation and a presence in the Internet. More specifically, the Internet of Things aims at offering new applications and services bridging the physical and virtual worlds, in which Machine-to-Machine (M2M) communications represent the baseline communication that enables the interactions between Things and applications in the cloud."	Cloud Services	(Rose et al., 2015)

With the lack of a universal definition of IoT, the everyday activities are dotted with smart objects that can identify, sense, network, process and communicate with other objects and services over the internet to accomplish a specific goal (Whitmore et al., 2015). Many attempts have been made to define IoT as its application and adoption gains momentum. Recent literature, seeks to bring clarity to the key defining features of IoT from several sources including whitepapers, books, National activities, Industrial activities, research projects, and a comprehensive review of currently used standards (Minerva et al., 2015). An all-inclusive IoT definition is given from both small and large system perspectives. Table 2 depicts the salient features of IoT (Minerva et al., 2015).

Table 2. Key features of the IoT paradigm

Feature	Description
Interconnection of Things	Refers to any physical object ("Thing") from a user or application viewpoint.
Connection of Things to the Internet	The system of Things is connected to the Internet and does not refer to Intranet or Extranet of Things.
Uniquely identifiable Things	Refers to unique identity of physical objects in IoT system.
Ubiquity	The network is available where it is needed ("anywhere") and when it is needed ("anytime")
Sensing/Actuation capability	The connection of sensors/actuators to physical objects brings smartness of the physical objects.
Interoperable communication capability	The IoT system communication is guided by standards and interoperable protocols.
Programmability	The ability of a physical object to take a variety of user's commands without requiring physical changes.
Small environment scenario	For small systems, it refers to the lowest complexity of an IoT system that have programmable, sensing/actuation and unique identification capabilities, for example, Static data stored in RFID tags, so that data can be available anywhere, at any time, by anything.
Large environment scenario	Refers to a large quantity of interconnected physical objects that can support, deliver services and execute complex processes thus increasing the level of complexity for managing the IoT system at this level. Additionally, the physical objects have unique identification, programmable and sensing/actuation capabilities with a management focus on security concerns due the interaction of large complexity of physical objects.

We endeavor to provide a holistic and futuristic perspective to the definition of IoT in the context of healthcare application. For the purposes of this paper and in view of the definition of IoT and its key features summarized in Table 2, the terms "Internet of Things" and "IoT" in healthcare is broadly used to refer to a collection of physical objects communicating over the Internet towards provision of healthcare services that achieve patient-centric goals by fostering interaction between health practitioners, patients, and healthcare providers.

IoT Architecture and Supporting Communication Models

Recent advances in information technology in terms of improved speed, reduced cost, increased storage, among others coupled with the wide adoption of internet-enabled devices provide opportunities to transform healthcare processes and activities. From a broader perspective, these technologies enable easier and affordable interconnection of smart devices further contributing towards the overarching IoT vision. In essence, IoT is comprised of multiple layers of distributed systems, ranging from sensors, smart devices, microcontrollers, wired and wireless network, Internet for connectivity, cloud for storage, and analytics. With a unique set of features and characteristics, each layer has its own functionality. Although various architectures were proposed for IoT (Al-Fuqaha et al., 2015; Miao Wu et al., 2010; Said & Masud, 2013; Touati & Tabish, 2013), we use a three-layer architecture comprised of a perception layer, a gateway layer and a cloud layer (Al-Fuqaha et al., 2015; Touati & Tabish, 2013).

The perception layer, otherwise called the edge layer is closest to the 'Things' of IoT or it is regularly depicted in the terms of sensor capabilities. The perception layer is responsible for collecting health and ecological data from a variety of monitoring entities including patients, clinicians, and medical devices with the help of heterogeneous sensors. The gateway layer, otherwise called as network layer allows the communication of data provided by the perception layer to the cloud using cellular, wireless, wired, and internet technologies. The IoT nodes in this layer are known as gateways. Gateways allows continuous and seamless communication from the perception layer or sensors to the cloud. As the data is transferred through this layer, gateways have the capability to filter and aggregate the data. The cloud layer, otherwise referred as the application layer, is the third and most sophisticated layer in IoT system. Data collected by the sensors in the perception layer is transferred to the cloud systems via gateways. The cloud layer for a specific IoT system may vary from one or more public or private clouds. Private clouds can be local servers connected to the hospital information systems whereas public clouds can be obtained by third-party vendors and can be accessed using the Internet. The cloud layer provides additional capabilities by leveraging data fusion, analysis and advanced analytics to further process and make sense of the data. The outcome of the analysis can be used in patient care. Real-time analytics has a capability to leverage value-based care initiatives by providing doctors with the data they need to diagnose or treat a patient at the point of care.

In essence, IoT allows things and people to be connected at anyplace, anytime using any network/path and any service. There are numerous ways to deploy these devices. In this regard, the Internet Architecture Board (IAB), developed an architectural document (RFC 7452) to guide the interconnection of smart objects, herein, referred to as the four common IoT communication models (Tschofenig et al., 2015) . The following discussion briefly demonstrates the main characteristics of each model as defined in the architectural framework. Appendix I provides a list of definitions for key technologies and terms related to IoT.

Device-to-Device Communications

In a device-to-device communication model (Figure 1), two or more heterogenous devices/sensors/things that collect environmental and comprehensive health data connect directly and communicate between one another rather than through an intermediary layer. In this model, the devices typically communicate using protocols such as Bluetooth or Zigbee. This model is frequently used in scenarios where the amount of data that need to be transferred between the devices is low and data rate is not an issue. Security is less of an issue compared to other models as devices directly interact with each other. Some examples of applications that utilize this communication model are home automation and emergency communications (Rose et al., 2015).

Figure 1. Example of a device-device communication model

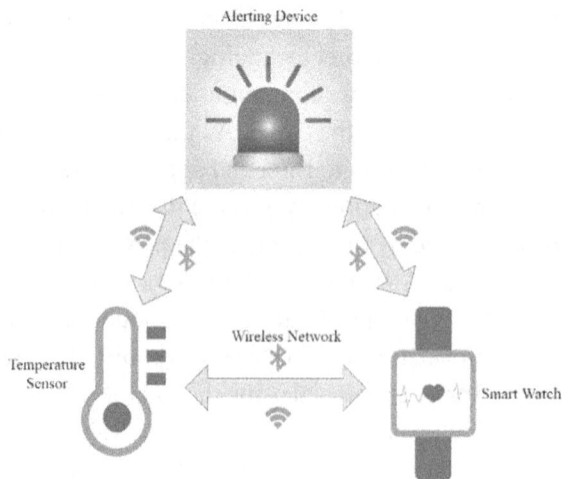

(Rose et al., 2015)

Device-to-Cloud Communications

In a Device-to-Cloud communication model (Figure 2), the heterogenous devices connect directly to the cloud layer rather than through an intermediary layer. Communication technologies such as Ethernet and cellular radio facilitate communication between the devices and cloud layer. The main advantage of this model is to enable the user to access the devices remotely. Interoperability and security are key factors that need to be considered for this model. Compared to D2D model, the security considerations are complex, as there is an additional layer. When implementing this model, the heterogenous devices need to be compatible with the cloud layer, thus, it is often suggested to utilize the devices and cloud services provided by the same vendor.

Figure 2. Example of a device-cloud communication model

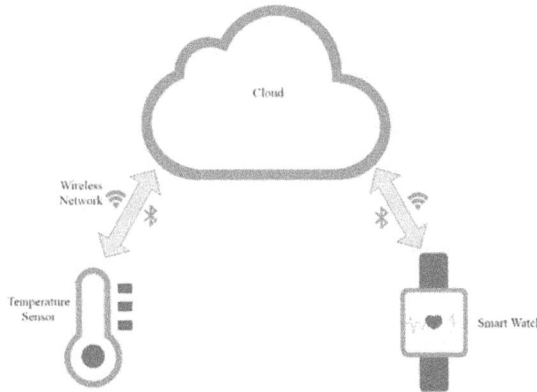

(Rose et al., 2015)

Device-to-Gateway Communications

In this communication model (Figure 3), the heterogenous devices access the cloud layer with the help of an intermediary layer. This intermediary layer is often called a gateway, which in many scenarios is a smartphone. The main advantage of this model is its capability to tackle the interoperability issue raised from the D2C model, by mitigating compatibility issues between the devices and cloud services. Usually, this model employs the usage of a mobile application for the user to access the data (Rose et al., 2015). Fitness tracking is a common application that employs this communication model.

Figure 3. Example of a device-to-gateway model

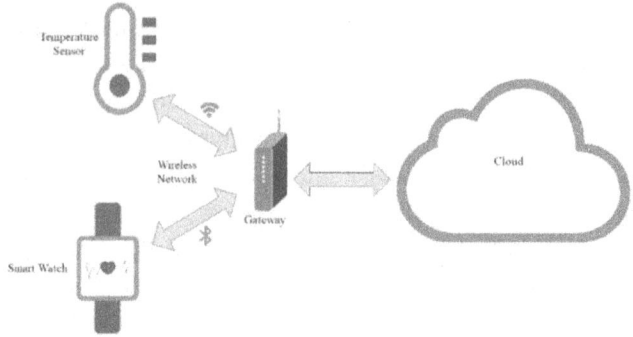

2.2.4 Back-end Data Sharing Model

The back-end data sharing model is an extension to the D2C communication model. In this model, the user can authorize access for heterogenous device data to a third party. As shown in Figure 4, this model allows the aggregation of data from multiple sources along with the heterogenous device data to analyze in the cloud layer. This model is efficient when the use case requires analyzing the device data in combination with other data source (Rose et al., 2015).

Figure 4. Example of a Back-End Data Sharing Model

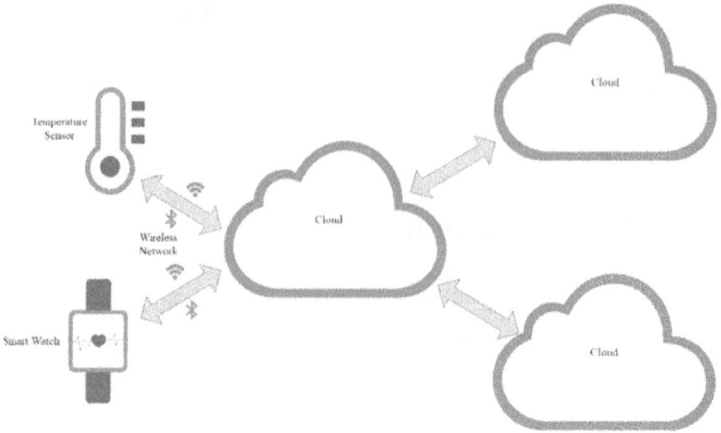

In a smart object environment, it is feasible that one or more of the communication patterns can be utilized at the same time. The IoT communication model provides interoperability to IoT vendors regardless of device manufacturer's' specifications thus enabling a level of flexibility for interaction of IoT devices for healthcare applications.

Healthcare Activities and Supporting IoT Applications

Clinical activities of prevention, diagnosis, and treatment are largely driven and shaped by knowledge, both clinical as well as contextual. To understand these healthcare activities and supporting IoT applications, we relied on the Unified Medical Language Systems (UMLS) (Bodenreider, 2004). We classified healthcare processes and activities into two types, primary healthcare processes and secondary healthcare processes. Table 3 lists the primary healthcare processes: Prevention (primary, secondary, and tertiary), Diagnosis and Treatment, while Table 4 lists the secondary healthcare activities: Disease Management, Assisted Living, Emergency Health Services, Fall Prevention, Medication Management, Child Health, Rehabilitation Therapy, and Preventive Monitoring.

Table 3. Definitions of primary healthcare processes and activities

Primary Healthcare Activities	Definition
Primary Prevention	Prevention of disease or mental disorders in susceptible individuals or populations through promotion of health, including mental health, and specific protection, as in immunization, as distinguished from the prevention of complications or after-effects of existing disease.
Secondary Prevention	A procedure performed to avoid a subsequent occurrence of a disease condition or processes to prevent complications.
Tertiary Prevention	Measures aimed at providing appropriate supportive and rehabilitative services to minimize morbidity and maximize quality of life after a long-term disease or injury is present.
Diagnosis	The investigation, analysis and recognition of the presence and nature of disease, condition, or injury from expressed signs and symptoms; also, the scientific determination of any kind; the concise results or summary of such an investigation.
Treatment	Any action or process to improve or remedy a syndrome, disease, or condition.

(Bodenreider, 2004)

Table 4. Definitions of secondary healthcare processes and activities

Secondary Healthcare Activities	Definition
Assisted Living	Assisted living is for adults who need help with everyday tasks. They may need help with dressing, bathing, eating, or using the bathroom, but they don't need full-time nursing care.
Child Health	The concept covering the physical and mental conditions of children.
Disease Management	A broad approach to appropriate coordination of the entire disease treatment process that often involves shifting away from more expensive inpatient and acute care to areas such as preventive medicine, patient counseling and education, and outpatient care.
Emergency Health Services	Services specifically designed, staffed and equipped for the emergency care of patients; includes services such as ambulances, helicopters, facilities, etc., that specifically provide emergency care.
Fall Prevention	Instituting special precautions with patient at risk for injury from falling.
Medication Management	Managing and/or monitoring a patient's use of medication and/or prescription drug(s) to avoid complications.
Preventive Monitoring	Act of overseeing, tracking, observing, or supervising something over a period of time in order to see how it develops, so that any necessary changes can be identified and made, whether performed by a person, device or system.
Rehabilitation Therapy	Restoration of the ability to function in a normal or near normal manner following disease, illness, or injury.

(Bodenreider, 2004)

Primary and secondary healthcare activities may appear to overlap. For example, fall prevention is under both primary prevention as well as secondary prevention. Yet, fall prevention under primary prevention focuses on precautions and measures to prevent a fall whereas fall prevention under secondary prevention emphasize measures and precautions taken when a fall is detected to prevent complications. With respect to preventive monitoring, most of these applications focus on monitoring and analyzing any health vulnerabilities in order to prevent any health conditions (primary), prevent complications (secondary), or maximize quality of life after a long-term disease or injury is present (tertiary).

Framework

Figure 5 depicts a conceptual framework for IoT in healthcare. The communication layer refers to the various communication models for IoT solutions i.e., the pipeline by which information is collected and securely transmitted/received. The next layer refers to the IoT architecture. Together, the communication model and IoT architecture layers provide the underlying information technology foundation for supporting various healthcare activities. These activities are captured in the third (and top-most) layer. We grouped health processes into two types – Primary healthcare processes and secondary healthcare processes. We have a number of s secondary IoT healthcare activities associated with the three different primary healthcare processes namely, Prevention, Diagnosis and Treatment.

Figure 5. Proposed framework classifying IoT architecture layers along with IoT communication models across the healthcare processes and healthcare activities

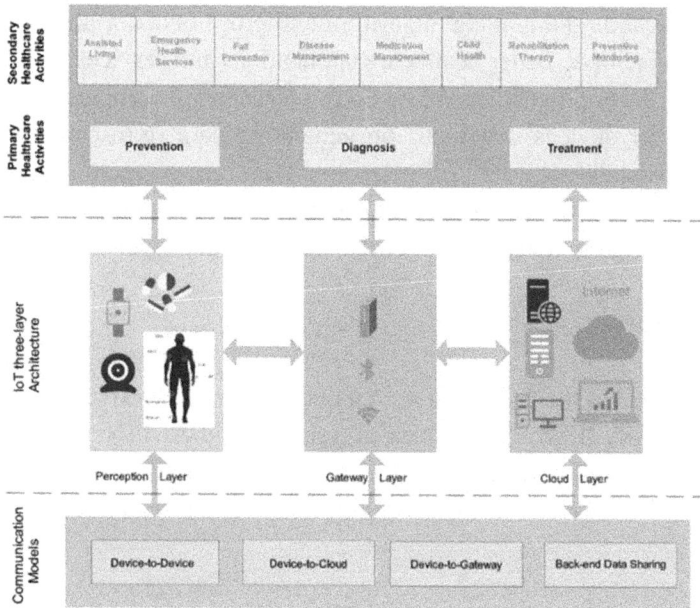

Methodology

We used the Preferred Reporting Items for Systematic Reviews and Meta-Analysis (PRISMA) principles to guide our review (Moher et al., 2009). We conducted a systematic search of articles from selected scientific and journal online databases that included IEEE, ACM digital library, PubMed, and web of science ranging from January 1, 2010 to June 30, 2020. For our search strategy, we used both inclusion and exclusion criteria as follows:

Inclusion criteria (IC):
- Articles addressing individual or patient-centric IoT applications or architectures for health and wellbeing.

Exclusion Criteria (EC):

- Articles not specific to healthcare regardless of focus on engineering/ technical aspects such as security protocols, or behavioral aspects such as user adoption.
- Articles focusing on engineering or technical aspects that are related to IoT but not necessarily specific to IoT e.g., minimizing power consumption or signal reconstruction.
- Articles discussing the analytics or other aspects of IoT regardless of application domain e.g. algorithmic improvements of analyzing IoT data to facilitate better healthcare applications and services.
- Articles describing WSN, body area network articles, e.g., ECG and other devices that focus on generating data from equipment's inside hospitals.
- Articles presenting survey or reviews of IoT applications.
- Articles in languages other than English language.

Search Query

We then created the following search queries across the five online databases, namely: PubMed, IEEE, ACM, Web of Science, and ABI/INFORM which were selected for their relevance to the research questions and domain topic. Moreover, the articles were extracted from the databases using the search terms summarized in Table 5.

Table 5. Summary of search query across the online databases

Type of Database	Search Query
PUBMED	(((internet of things[Title/Abstract]) OR IoT[Title/Abstract]) AND ((healthcare[Title/Abstract]) OR medic*[Title/Abstract]))
IEEE	(("Document Title":"Internet of Things" OR "Document Title":"IoT" OR "IEEE Terms":"Internet of Things" OR "IEEE Terms":"IoT") AND ("Document Title":"healthcare" OR "IEEE Terms":"healthcare" OR "IEEE Terms":"medic*"))
ACM	acmdlTitle:(+"Internet of Things" "IoT" +"Healthcare" "medic*") OR recordAbstract:(+"Internet of Things" "IoT" +"Healthcare" "medic*") - syntax change acmdlTitle:(+"Internet of Things" +"Healthcare" "IoT" "medic*") OR recordAbstract:(+"Internet of Things" +"Healthcare" "IoT" "medic*")
Web of Science	(((TS = "internet of things" OR TS = "IoT") AND (TS = "healthcare" OR TS = "medic*")))
ABI/INFORM	noft(((((ab("internet of things") OR ab("IoT") OR ti("internet of things") OR ti("IoT")) AND (ab("healthcare") OR ti("healthcare") OR ab("medic*") OR ti("medic*")))))))

Data Collection and Analysis

In the data collection phase, the search query created in Table 5 was used to extract relevant articles across the selected online databases following the IC and EC criteria and the results were updated using the PRISMA diagram shown in Fig.6. Furthermore, we reviewed the results from the search process using the inter-rater reliability test to ensure consistency and validity of the results. During the analysis of gathered articles, two raters used Cohen's kappa statistical measure to measure the inter-rater reliability of relevant articles by utilizing a contingency table as shown and explained in the results section. Cohen's kappa (K) is a statistic measure that is used to measure inter-rater reliability. It is a measure of agreement between the two reviewers who each classify N items into C mutually exclusive categories. The main idea of using Inter-rater reliability is to ensure consistency, reproducibility and validity of the results.

Results

As shown in Fig.6, a total of 82 articles were identified based on the Systematic Literature Review (SLR) conducted. The SLR was conducted in a comprehensive manner following certain steps. Initially, five databases were targeted to search for relevant articles namely ABI Inform, ACM Digital Library, IEEE Xplore, PubMed, and Web of Science. A sum of 3,125 peer-reviewed articles were obtained from the five databases based on the search criteria. Initially, 459 duplicate articles were removed. After removing the duplicates, 2,666 articles remained and were further reviewed for relevance by reading the article title and abstract. Based on the EC, 2,176 articles were removed from the 2,666 articles. The remaining 490 articles were further reviewed for relevance by reading the full text of the articles. Based on the EC, 408 additional articles were removed, yielding a final selection of 82 articles. These 82 peer-reviewed articles were thoroughly read to answer the "research questions". Relevant information to answer the research questions were carefully extracted from the resultant articles based on the proposed framework. Figure 6 depicts the resultant numbers and method followed for the SLR process.

Figure 6. Systematic literature review process

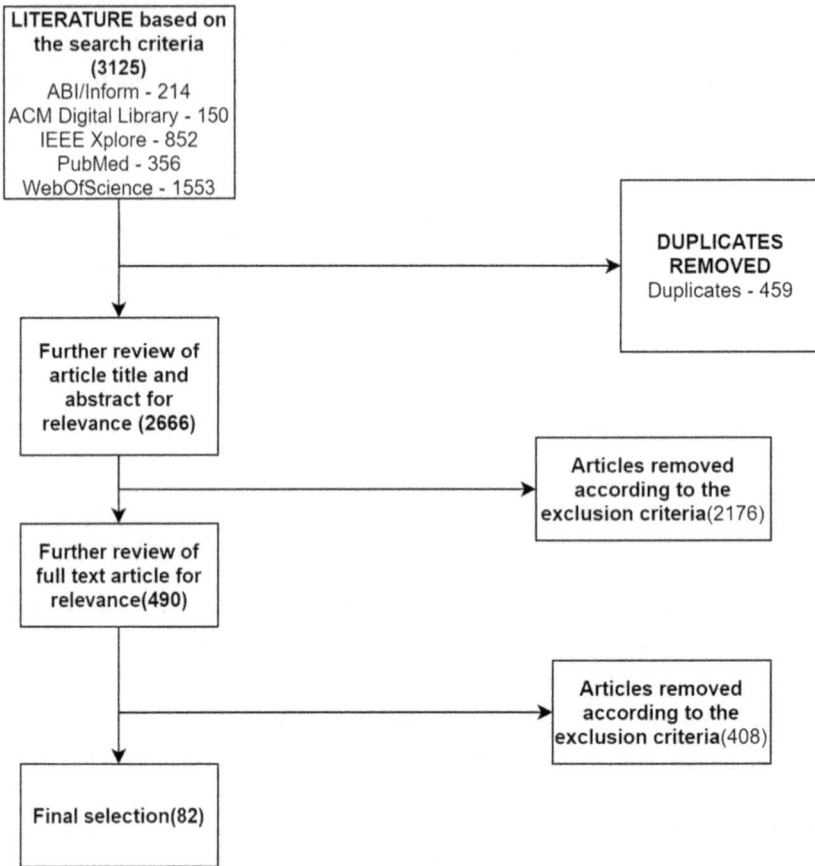

Two reviewers performed two iterations of inter-rater reliability testing using Cohen's Kappa (K) (Cohen, 1960). Cohen's Kappa (K) can be interpreted by the guideline table, proposed by(Landis & Koch, 1977). After computing the contingency matrix for iteration 1, we achieved an inter-rater reliability K of 0.419 which is moderate acceptance with an 86% of agreement. For iteration 2, we achieved a K value of 0.834 with a 95% agreement which makes our agreement almost perfect. The results of the inter-rater reliability measure were acceptable with over 80% agreement of analysis of articles under review. All authors were involved in discussing and resolving any disagreements.

Figure 7 represents the publication frequency of the resultant articles by year. As shown, IoT in healthcare was addressed more prevalently during the last three years as compared to the first six years (2010 – 2016).

Figure 7. Publication frequency of the resultant articles by year

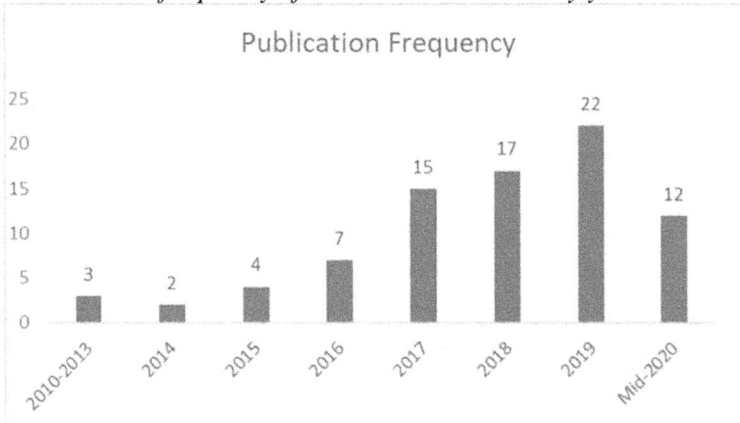

Table 6 shows the distribution of articles by publication source. Research papers were found in 36 different journals and conferences. IEEE conferences represented 17.1% of the sources. Other conferences such as, but not limited to, ACM Proceedings represented 15.9%. IEEE Internet of Things Journal published 7.3% of total articles related to IoT in healthcare. IEEE Access Journal published 6.1% of the sources. SENSORS journal published 4.9% of total articles related to IoT in healthcare. Whereas, IEEE Communications Magazine, and Future Generation Computer Systems contributed 3.7% each. EURASIP Journal on Wireless Communications and Networking, Computers in Industry, Journal of Medical Systems, Wireless Networks, Multimedia Tools and Applications contributed 2.4% each. The rest of the other sources contributed 1.2% each.

Figure 8 represents the number of articles based on healthcare processes. From the chart, Primary Prevention is the most popular area. Diagnosis is the second most prevalent area that papers have addressed. Secondary Prevention, Tertiary Prevention and Treatment have the least number of papers when compared to others.

Table 6. Distribution of articles by publication source

Journal or conference	Type of article	Frequency	Percentage
IEEE Conferences	Conference	14	17.1%
Other Conferences	Conference	13	15.9%
IEEE Internet of Things Journal	Journal	6	7.3%
IEEE Access	Journal	5	6.1%
SENSORS	Journal	4	4.9%

continued on following page

Table 6. Continued

Journal or conference	Type of article	Frequency	Percentage
Future Generation Computer Systems	Journal	3	3.7%
IEEE Communications Magazine	Magazine	3	3.7%
EURASIP Journal on Wireless Communications and Networking	Journal	2	2.4%
Computers in Industry	Journal	2	2.4%
Journal of Medical Systems	Journal	2	2.4%
Wireless Networks	Journal	2	2.4%
Multimedia Tools and Applications	Journal	2	2.4%
Other IEEE journals	Journal	4	4.9%
Other computing/engineering related journals	Journal	14	17.1%
Other health/medical related journals	Journal	5	6.1%
Emergence of Pharmaceutical Industry Growth with Industrial IoT Approach	Book chapter	1	1.2%
Total		82	100%

Figure 8. Types of primary healthcare applications

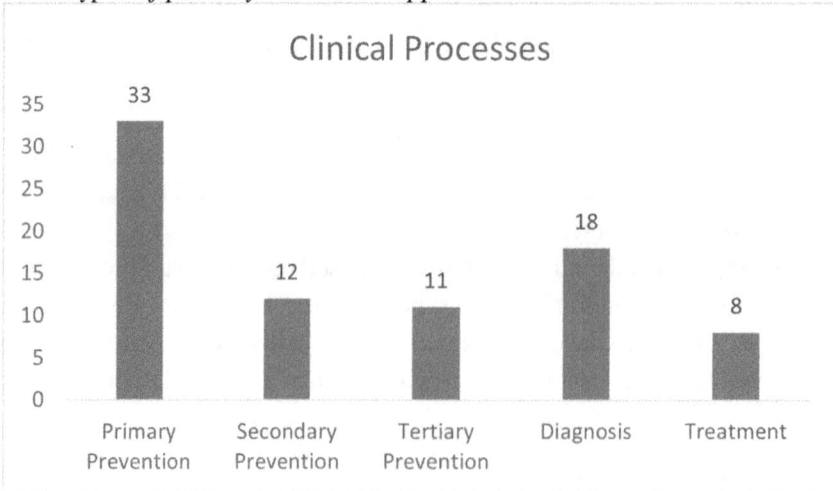

Figure 9 shows that Wi-FI, RFID, and mobile networks usage is declining in the healthcare applications, whereas Bluetooth and especially other IoT technologies usage is increasing. New technologies such as, but not limited to, LoRaWAN, Sigfox, and Wireless Local Area Network (WLAN) are being adopted in the healthcare applications.

Figure 9. Usage of IoT technologies by year

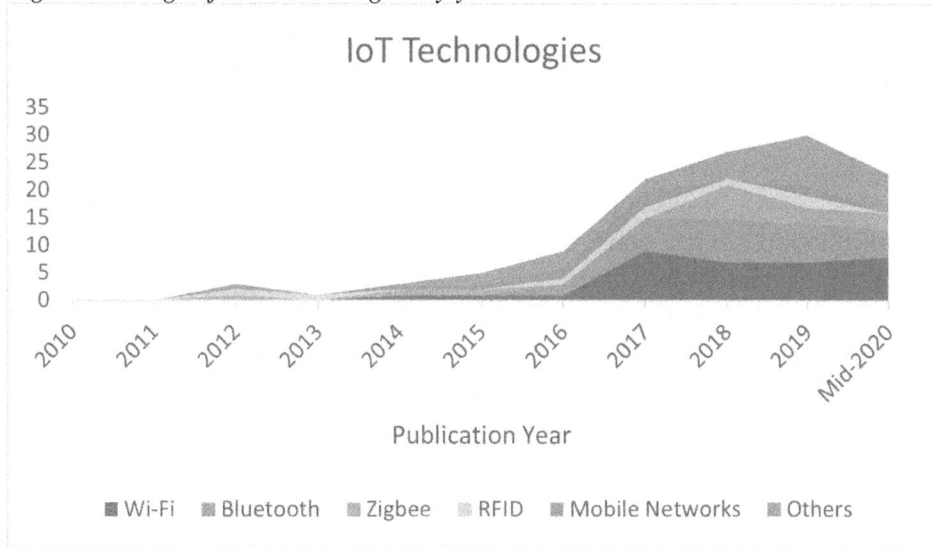

Appendix II lists all relevant articles grouped by the supported primary and secondary healthcare activities. Most of the IoT solutions targeted elderly and adult individuals and covered 29 countries. Primary prevention by far represented the largest healthcare activity supported (33 articles). These articles covered a variety of secondary healthcare activities including assisted living, child health, disease management, fall prevention, and preventive monitoring. Most assisted living applications targeted the elderly and people with disabilities to aid in performing their daily activities efficiently. For example, a virtual caregiver as cyber physical smart home was proposed to support the daily life activities of elderly people through their gestures (Md. A. Rahman & Hossain, 2019). Similarly, some assisted living applications employ wearable technologies (Wan et al., 2018), which can aid elderly individuals with customized services depending on their physical and cognitive disabilities (Al-Khafajiy et al., 2019; Mincolelli et al., 2019). Overall, assisted living healthcare interventions aim to help elderly people with performing their daily routines independently at home by providing customized services along with vitals anomaly detection such that the need for joining a nursing home can be delayed as long as possible (Basanta et al., 2016; Hussain et al., 2015; Pham et al., 2018; H.-T. Wu & Tsai, 2018). Other secondary healthcare activities under primary prevention included child health activities aimed at monitoring children's vitals to detect any abnormalities in their early stages to reduce child mortality rates (Kadarina & Priambodo, 2017; Nyasulu, 2016) Also included were disease management activities, fall prevention (Aljahdali et al., 2018), and preventive monitoring of disease conditions such as cancer (Onasanya et al., 2019), diabetes (Rghioui et al., 2019), dementia (Enshaeifar et al., 2018), and emotions (Chen et al., 2017). Secondary prevention was addressed in 12 articles that supported a variety of secondary healthcare activities including assisted living, disease management, emergency services, and fall prevention. Assisted living activities focused on detecting high risk situations and improving the quality of life (Addante et al., 2019; Pace et al., 2019). Disease management activities aimed to reduce and prevent the complications of disease conditions such as cardiovascular diseases (Kario et al., 2017), non-communicable diseases (Y. Liu et al., 2014), epilepsy (Hayek et al., 2020), congestive heart failure (Abawajy & Hassan, 2017) and other diseases (La et al., 2015). Emergency healthcare activities mainly focused on emergency medical services using vital signs collected from sensors (Gusev et al., 2017; Rathore et al., 2016). Fall prevention activities aimed to detect falls and inform the respective authorities or family members regarding the incidents (Gutierrez-Madronal, La Blunda, et al., 2019; Luo et al., 2012; Manatarinat et al., 2019).

Tertiary prevention had a total of 11 articles and covered three types of secondary healthcare activities namely, assisted living, child health, and rehabilitation therapy. For assisted living activities, the main goal was to support the daily activities of healthcare assistants who work in assisted living facilities for people with physical or cognitive disabilities (Corno et al., 2016). Under Child health activities, the aim was to support children in managing disease conditions such as diabetes. Rehabilitation therapy focuses on helping patients recover from particular health conditions.

Diagnosis was the focus of 18 articles that supported two secondary healthcare activities namely, assisted living and disease management. For assisted living activities, the main aim was to continuously monitor the vital signs in an assistive environment for diagnosis and detection of anomalies (Jara et al., 2012). For disease management, the goal was to continuously monitor and diagnose the onset of a disease condition.

Treatment was the focus of eight articles that supported three secondary healthcare activities including disease management, medication management, and rehabilitation therapy. For disease management activities, the main goal was to detect and treat healthcare conditions such as sleep apnea (Yacchirema et al., 2018a, 2018b) and muscle fatigue (Ma et al., 2019).For medication management, the aim was to provide medication adherence to improve the medication self-management for people suffering from any health condition (Chang et al., 2020; Latif et al., 2020; Toh et al., 2016; Yang et al., 2014). Rehabilitation therapy focused on people suffering from health conditions such as Obsessive-compulsive disorder (OCD) (Suraki & Suraki, 2013).

DISCUSSION

Healthcare activities

Many IoT applications in healthcare focused on the design and implementation of continuous monitoring of patients to collect data on vitals such as blood glucose, temperature, pulse, ECG, and potentially sharing the data with clinicians in real-time thus facilitating a timely evaluation of individuals' health (Haghi et al., 2020; I. Khan et al., 2019; S. F. Khan, 2017; Nasri & Mtibaa, 2017; Nduka et al., 2019; Neto et al., 2018; Rahmani et al., 2018; Saha et al., 2018; Subhedar et al., 2018; T. Wu et al., 2020). Key features of preventive monitoring such as remote monitoring and trend analysis of physiological parameters, enable early detection of sickness which contributes towards a reduction in hospital visits and hospitalization (Vavilis et al., 2012). Further, preventive monitoring aims to motivate individuals to undertake self-care and track their well-being (Maksimović et al., 2016). Despite the advancement in IoT technologies, preventive monitoring systems are yet to gain wide adoption. It turns out that some of the main obstacles to mainstream adoption include the costs associated with implementation and the lack of potential payment mechanism included in the pay for service systems (Berenson & Rich, 2010). Further, in the absence of an individual's preparedness and readiness to actively participate in monitoring their well-being, the objectives of preventive monitoring are unattainable.

Another emergent perspective on primary prevention is related to assisted living (Basanta et al., 2016; Hussain et al., 2015; Mincolelli et al., 2019; Pham et al., 2018; Md. A. Rahman & Hossain, 2019; Tun et al., 2020; Wan et al., 2018; H.-T. Wu & Tsai, 2018). Assisted Living Systems (ALS) enhance the living experience of elderly people and individuals with disabilities by leveraging technologies that simplify daily activities and to an extent support self-dependence. Techniques and methods used in assisted living support a user-centric approach to health monitoring and are integrated into the living environment of the individuals with the objectives of providing emergency support and enhancing active participation in physical activities (Hussain et al., 2015). It is evident that ALS allow older and physically challenged people to improve their quality of care through increased mobility in their environments while minimizing their dependence on several caregivers. Although the beneficial aspects of assisted living have been elucidated, the availability of trained personnel to support assisted living systems remains a challenge thus impeding the wide of adoption of such systems due to expensive costs of implementation and maintenance.

Secondary prevention applications mainly focused on providing IoT-based solutions with the aim of reducing the occurrence and complications of disease or injury with several papers tackling the issue of disease management. Disease management was very prominent in many papers with efforts utilizing IoT-based solutions to address and improve programs that involved the management of chronic diseases (Abawajy & Hassan, 2017; Hayek et al., 2020; Kario et al., 2017; La et al., 2015; Y. Liu et al., 2014). Overall, IoT has shown promise in assisting with improving the wellbeing of patients with chronic conditions.

Another dimension of secondary prevention, fall prevention, used low-cost IoT systems, such as *SensFall* to automatically detect elderly falls and trigger an alert mechanism to promptly notify family members and caregivers (Gutierrez-Madronal, Luigi La Blunda, et al., 2019; Luo et al., 2012; Manatarinat et al., 2019). . Unlike in the traditional fall detection systems which rely on pushbuttons to sound an alarm, IoT-based fall detection systems are autonomous and can immediately trigger alerts even when an individual becomes unconscious. With regard to the use of fall detection systems, older people reported an increased confidence in their day-to-day activities, enhanced safety, and independence that reflected in their perception of an increased quality of life (Brownsell & Hawley, 2004). Overall, the success of fall prevention systems will depend on the availability of reliable, low-cost, and accurate deployment of IoT based solutions. Despite the potential benefits of automatic fall detection systems, their performance still exhibits high incidences of false positives and false negatives. Further, their field performance is ambiguous as most of these systems are programmed and tested under controlled conditions (Gutierrez-Madronal, La Blunda, et al., 2019; Manatarinat et al., 2019). Several papers in tertiary prevention aimed to address rehabilitation therapy where the objective was to develop solutions that help patients improve their quality of life in the event of an illness or injury using rehabilitation systems (Alexandre & Postolache, 2018; de la Iglesia et al., 2020; Jiang et al., 2017; Md. A. Rahman & Hossain, 2018; Vukicevic et al., 2016). For example, IoT-based therapy and rehabilitation could improve the life quality of stroke patients (Yang et al., 2018).

Rehabilitation can be demanding, and patients' adherence to rehabilitation regiment can be problematic due to lack of motivation. In that regard, recent advances in IoT technologies aimed to engage patients to participate in therapy by integrating augmented reality and virtual reality games making it more interactive and user friendly (Cano Porras et al., 2018). IoT applications for rehabilitation therapy faces a greater challenge for its widespread adoption. Most notably is the difficulty to demonstrate medical efficacy and to obtain the necessary regulatory and clinical acceptance of these systems (Mills et al., 2017).

Diagnostic applications represent IoT-based solutions aimed at determining the presence of any disease, illness, or injuries based on signs and symptoms. Many of these applications use analytic techniques to analyze and recognize disease conditions, for example dengue and chikungunya (Bhatia et al., 2020; M. K. Hassan et al., 2019; N. H. Hassan et al., 2018; Sood & Mahajan, 2017, 2019). Other studies propose wearable sensors that can help diagnose disease (N. H. Hassan et al., 2018;

B. Li et al., 2019) and demonstrate the potential for wearables coupled with analytical capabilities to improve the diagnosis process.

IoT promotes the transition of routine health checks from being hospital-centric to being home-centric and can potentially reduce the need for hospitalization (Matthews & Industry Voice, 2020). With the increasing number of IoT applications, it is possible to better understand health behavior by maintaining a repository of personal health conditions. IoT with artificial intelligence capabilities can help diagnose diseases and complicated health conditions by analyzing the extensive data collected, streamlining the diagnostic process, and reducing medical errors by integrating patient-specific data (Dimitrov, 2016). IoT solutions such as chatbot shows evidence in reducing the diagnostic errors and would be a probable mainline solution in the future for diagnostic healthcare (Faggella, 2020). Most IoT applications supporting the treatment processes aim to address disease management. One example is the provision of IoT-based solutions to treat sleep apnea and muscle fatigue using big data analytics (Ma et al., 2019; Yacchirema et al., 2018a, 2018b). Besides, our findings revealed that applications focused on medication management (Toh et al., 2016; Yang et al., 2014) and used IoT-based solutions to promote medication adherence. According to the CDC, 50% of patients with chronic diseases such as cardiovascular, hypertension, and cancer do not adhere to treatment plans (Neiman et al., 2018). Lower adherence makes disease management difficult and thereby increases the cost for healthcare and results in serious adverse effects (HCPO, 2013). IoT could potentially mitigate the medical adherence challenge by sending reminders, monitoring conditions, and providing health updates.

IoT technologies

Healthcare IoT architecture can be broadly classified into three layers: perception layer, gateway layer and cloud layer. The perception layer is considered the physical layer where sensors are used to collect information on the environment. These sensors detect physical parameters such as temperature, heartbeat, motion, location, and acceleration etc. They can be broadly classified into devices worn on the wrist, head, body clothes, and other devices.

Wrist-worn devices have been developed for physiological monitoring with improved battery life as well as hardware miniaturization for transmission of data. Wrist-based devices such as fitness trackers and smart watches range from simple smart pedometers focused on accelerometers to biometric sensing. These devices perform two functions: 1) monitoring individual physiological and activity signals and 2) communicating with other electronic devices (Seneviratne et al., 2017). Blood pressure, heart rate, and body temperature are the physiological measurements most frequently monitored by wrist-based devices (Al-Khafajiy et al., 2019; Basanta et al., 2016; Bhatia & Sood, 2017; Chen et al., 2017; B. Li et al., 2019; Manatarinat et al., 2019; Wan et al., 2018). Head- worn devices include smart glasses and augmented reality. Smart glasses have several features that allow users to both view and analyze the information related to their environment. In an article by Chang et al., wearable smart glasses were designed for drug image acquisition and transmission to the AI-based intelligent drug pill recognition box (Chang et al., 2020). Virtual or augmented reality provides contextual details and allow users to control their environment visually. (Alexandre & Postolache, 2018; de la Iglesia et al., 2020) used augmented reality for rehabilitation purposes. Body clothes or smart clothing are enhanced with technology, adding functionality to the conventional use. These devices are equipped with sensors at various parts of garments or sewn into fabric. (Alexandre & Postolache, 2018) reported the use of smart gloves to perform training sessions for hand motor rehabilitation. (Ikram et al., 2015) used smart cloths to monitor the health of footballers and reduce the occurrence of adverse health conditions. Other portable sensors and devices include smart chest straps, smart toilets, and smart pills (Bhatia et al., 2020; T. Wu et al., 2020; Yang et al., 2014).

With the most recent advances in sensor innovation, microelectronics, communication technologies, and data analytics, attachable devices are the future of IoT. Specifically, the miniaturization of the electronic devices has been a significant piece of the advancement of attachable devices. More powerful and efficient devices with smaller footprints coupled with improved edge processing will prompt improved self-quantification and also enhance the ability of providers and facilities to keep track of patients.

The gateway layer, also known as the network layer, is used for transmitting sensor data as well as connecting devices and services with each other while acting as a network bridge for packets transfer between various sources and destinations. For the three healthcare processes, i.e., prevention (primary, secondary, tertiary), diagnosis, and treatment, most of the studies leveraged device-to-gateway as its communication model (see Appendix II). Mobile devices and applications as a gateway emerged as a dominant method to connect to the cloud. The choice of these methods is deemed suitable for overcoming the interoperability issues usually experienced during technology transition (Rose et al., 2015). Vital to the field is the system used to connect IoT devices, a role that a multitude of wired and wireless technologies are used to play. For example, Bluetooth is considered a mature IoT technology used for short-range connectivity requiring low-power consumption and at a low-cost. It is ideal and widely adopted for IoT applications in preventive monitoring and appears to be the current technology used in wearables and fitness devices which monitor physiological metrices such as blood glucose, ECG, and heart rate (I. Khan et al., 2019; Krishnan et al., 2016; Neto et al., 2018; T. Wu et al., 2020).

Another IoT technology is Wi-Fi, a popular wireless technology in home healthcare providing medium range connectivity thus allowing higher data throughput for low-powered sensor devices. Wi-Fi technology is widely adopted among healthcare activities such as assisted living and disease management (Abawajy & Hassan, 2017; Hayek et al., 2020; Hussain et al., 2015; Mumtaj & Umamakeswari, 2017; Md. A. Rahman & Hossain, 2019). IoT devices based on Wi-Fi connectivity need to seamlessly connect with and disconnect from various Wi-Fi networks with every movement the user makes (Sethi & Sarangi, 2017). Technologies such as LoRaWAN, Sigfox, and WLAN provide long-range connectivity with moderate power consumption (Krishnan et al., 2016; Manatarinat et al., 2019; Onasanya et al., 2019). These IoT technologies are capable of connecting millions of devices through cloud technologies and can support developments of smart hospitals, smart homes, and smart cities (Cheruvu et al., 2020). Ultimately, the choice of a healthcare activity is dependent on requirements such as IoT sensor device connectivity, power consumption, IoT technology, and the financial resources available to implement an IoT based healthcare system.

Finally, the cloud layer also known as the application layer offers flexibility and scalability for IoT healthcare by providing software, storage, data fusion, machine learning, and intelligent decision-making capabilities. Cloud computing overcome the constraints related to traditional storage and real-time data capture and processing (Abawajy & Hassan, 2017; Buzachis et al., 2018; Jiang et al., 2017). Fog computing as an extension of cloud computing, permits the decentralization of devices and allows higher levels of security and privacy. Further fog computing provides edge analytics capabilities that enable real-time data processing with increased privacy, reduced latency, cost, and resource usage (Rahmani et al., 2018; Sood & Mahajan, 2017; Vijayakumar et al., 2019). Our literature review identified few techniques for data extraction such as Hadoop batch processing and Apache Spark but no metrics related to data quality (Rathore et al., 2016; Yacchirema et al., 2018a). Data quality is of vital importance given the sensitivity of patients' health-related data. Future research could focus on data extraction methods to enhance the quality of data extracted from the IoT devices.

Drivers for IoT in healthcare

In this section, we provide a discussion on several drivers for IoT in healthcare based on the analysis and results of the review process. The main drivers (healthcare, and technology) are further sub-divided into two sections. In the first sub-section, the healthcare drivers associated with changes in the healthcare industry are discussed. Secondly, we discuss the technology drivers of IoT in healthcare.

Healthcare drivers

Cost of healthcare: The healthcare expenditure in the USA and other developed countries is significantly higher than the rest of the world (Baltagi et al., 2017; CMS, 2019). Healthcare activities, such as remote health monitoring, assisted living, medication management, in conjunction with wearable fitness trackers have tremendous potential to minimize healthcare costs resulting in a lower number of outpatient visits to various healthcare providers. These healthcare activities help mitigate and diagnose possible health complications (Nedungadi et al., 2017). The cost-savings are highlighted in a recent survey conducted by Accenture Consulting, where 33% of healthcare providers and 42% of payers reported extensive operational and medical savings resulting from the use of IoT based remote patient monitoring programs (HITInfrastructure, 2017).

Insurance: The application of IoT systems has empowered the healthcare insurance industry to go past conventional solutions of offering customization and flexibility of services (Silvello, 2017). For example, a Canadian-based health insurance provider had stopped offering traditional health insurance and instead started selling only interactive policies to track health and fitness data through wearables devices (Jeong, 2019). These IoT-based solutions have increased benefits to health insurance providers by better assessing risks and enabling caregivers to develop a comprehensive and a much more personalized approach to care that revolves around individuals. Moreover, the insurers can leverage the vast amounts of health data generated from connected devices to create customized products and policy packages targeted to specific customers based on their individual behavior and lifestyle.

Workforce optimization: Optimization of healthcare workers' productivity is one of the critical elements driving IoT applications in healthcare (Dash et al., 2019). With the current digital revolution, IoT devices can assist in the automatic collection and transmission of continuous streams of healthcare data. The data collected by the IoT medical devices can be directly transmitted and stored in electronic medical records. Using technologies such as remote health monitoring, clinicians can track a patient's health progress and provide diagnosis and treatment plans, thus reducing hospital visits (Jacobson & Karjalainen, 2019).

Self-management: The use of wearable devices could potentially assist in reducing the need for regular health checkups (Piwek et al., 2016). The data obtained from these wearable devices enable patients to monitor and analyze the progress of their health and better manage their medical conditions (El-Gayar et al., 2020). Self-management interventions are predicted to significantly reduce hospital expenses incurred by patients during hospital visits (Panagioti et al., 2014).

Accessibility: In remote health monitoring applications, IoT integration helps improve accessibility to health services by enabling doctors to access data from medical devices (Zhang & Zhang, 2011). According to a study conducted by Market Research Future (Market Research Future, 2018), remote health monitoring programs are increasing rapidly due to the increased demand for healthcare services in rural areas, and the market is expected to see a 16.5% annual growth of remote health services from the year 2017 until 2023.

Health awareness: The increasing trend of adopting fitness/activity trackers such as Fitbit shows self-care intent among individuals, which fuels the growth of the wearable market (Correa, 2019) This increase in demand for wearable fitness/activity trackers has enticed several big organizations to enter the IoT and healthcare market to develop products for specific medical applications. For example, Microsoft has developed an azure cloud platform for delivering multiple cloud-based healthcare services. Apple started to develop its portable health hubs based on its consumer products (Meola, 2020).

Medication non-adherence: Lower adherence makes disease management difficult, which significantly increases the cost for healthcare. Some research reports that lack of adherence will cause an average of 125,000 deaths every year and contributes to 70% of hospitalizations in the united states (HCPO, 2013). Although some studies tried to improve medication management using IoT technologies, there still remains some adherence aspects that need to be addressed and are driving further interest in IoT interventions (Toh et al., 2016; Yang et al., 2014).

Emerging diseases and epidemics: With the application of IoT, AI, and ubiquitous connectivity of smart devices, surveillance systems can curb the spread of infectious diseases (Kaushalya et al., 2019). At Virginia tech laboratories, an IoT-based monitoring system 'Epicaster" used population data, social media streams, GIS data, land use information, and other sources to identify and track emerging public health threats such as Zika and H1N1 (Deodhar et al., 2015). Similarly, the South Korean government utilized transaction data, phone location logs, and surveillance camera footage to detect, trace, and stop the spread of COVID-19 with a view to flatten the soaring curve of coronavirus cases (Fendos, 2020). Although researchers are rapidly developing new IoT-based tools and applications to monitor the spread of coronavirus (Fatima, 2020), other researchers are employing IoT-based drone technology to detect and diagnose cases (Mohammed et al., 2020). Additional research needs to focus on developing efficient and automated alert systems for early and timely detection of outbreaks resulting in lower morbidity and mortality rates through early diagnosis and treatment interventions (Md. S. Rahman et al., 2020).

Technology drivers

Cost of technology: The cost of hardware and devices used in IoT systems are increasingly affordable, paving the way for wider access and adoption. According to (McKinsey Global Institute, 2015), in the last decade, the price of sensors has declined by 50%, and bandwidth now costs 40 times less. The steady decline in the cost of technology, it has opened the door to widespread adoption of IoT-based healthcare outside the hospital setting (Balandina et al., 2015).

Seamless connectivity: Increased connectivity and improved communication mechanisms are key factors that drive IoT innovations (Cheruvu et al., 2020). The emergence of newer technologies such as 5G networks, LoRa, Sigfox, and device-to-gateway mechanisms promises to offer faster speeds, lower cost of operations, and lower latency ensuring that a large number of connected devices can leverage a more reliable and efficient channel of communication, therefore, accelerating a wider adoption of IoT in healthcare.

Edge analytics: Analyzing data in the cloud presents various issues, including latency, reliability, and bandwidth congestion, which can adversely affect health outcomes (Yu et al., 2017). Adopting edge technology offers a significant advantage by analyzing and providing insights immediately at the point of collection. Advances in edge analytics will allow for locally processing, filtering, and securing the collected data before transmission to the cloud, thus reducing transfer and storage costs (M. K. Hassan et al., 2019).

Storage: The IoT is expanding at a phenomenal growth, with over 50 billion connected devices expected by the end of 2020. These connected devices are predicted to generate petabytes and zettabytes of data, mostly in unstructured forms, presenting challenges in collecting, storing, and managing the data. However, the advent of big data in healthcare provides compelling opportunities for innovative solutions through predictive and personalized medicine powered by AI (M. A. Khan et al., 2014). With voluminous data, cloud-based solutions provide a flexible and, ubiquitous platform to manage the data. In the last decade, the cost of cloud computing has dramatically decreased by 58% while providing increased processing power leading to improved customer value (Supernor, 2018).

Form factor: Users prefer IoT devices that are relatively small, easy to use, and portable. Miniaturization enables IoT devices to be cost-effective, robust, and efficient (Blowers et al., 2016). while maximizing the trade-off between form factor (size and weight) and power consumption at an affordable cost.

Challenges to IoT applications in healthcare

This section offers a discussion of the challenges facing the implementation and adoption of IoT applications in the healthcare domain. The challenges are broadly categorized into two sections: healthcare and technology related challenges affecting IoT in healthcare.

Healthcare challenges

User adoption and retention: A recent study mined user tweets (El-Gayar et al., 2019) and demonstrated that people tend to terminate the usage of devices that lack features such as dialog, credibility, social support, integration with other systems, and issues related to wearing these devices on a daily basis. Other studies argued that the factors associated with wearable technology adoption and retention are different. For example, the capability to collect and analyze activity data play a pivotal role in adoption whereas resilience and device portability are the key factors related to user retention (Canhoto & Arp, 2017).

Clinician adoption: Clinicians' motivation can be one of the most significant barriers facing IoT technologies today. As with any new technological advancement in medical sciences, it is vital for clinicians to learn, trust, and not be threatened by IoT-based systems (De Grood et al., 2016). Another barrier is the potential reduction in the interaction between clinicians and patients, which may be viewed as detrimental to providing an optimum patient care (Biran Achituv & Haiman, 2016).

Efficacy: Despite the potential for IoT in healthcare and the proliferation of IoT-based interventions, the availability of randomized control trials demonstrating the efficacy of these interventions is rather limited (Inan et al., 2020; Klímová & Kuča, 2019). Without RCT trials, the credibility of potential IoT-based healthcare interventions for improving health and wellbeing remain questionable, limiting their adoption by care providers and users alike.

Payment structure: The traditional fee-for-service model does not create the incentive structure for providers to support IoT-based interventions particularly those aimed at providing the user with increased autonomy and shifting the care structure upstream (Tai et al., 2014). While the shift to an outcome-based model is likely to result in a better aligned incentive structure, there are several challenges with respect to the potential for inducing a challenging work environment for healthcare professionals and complicating the payment system between the provider, patient, and the insurer (Vlaanderen et al., 2019).

Legal and regulatory issues: IoT devices in healthcare may require clearance or approval from regulatory bodies such as the Food and Drug Administration (FDA) (Ahmed, 2019). An individual-centric device that is utilized for prevention, diagnosis, treatment, monitoring or alleviating a disease, is considered a medical device and should pass regulatory and compliance regimes. (Caddy, 2019). IoT devices' most common regulatory issues are Corrective and Preventive Action (CAPA) issues, inadequate purchasing controls, errors in compliant procedures, and faulty document control (Fenton, 2019).

Technology challenges:

Data interoperability and heterogeneity: IoT platforms and IoT vendors with different communication standards and protocols (e.g., Bluetooth, RFID, LoRaWAN) raise data interoperability concerns (Pace et al., 2019; Pal et al., 2018; Rahmani et al., 2018). Efforts such as the development of the D2G communication model have focused on addressing these interoperability issues between heterogenous IoT devices (Yacchirema et al., 2018b). However, the potential to improve data interoperability while maintaining data quality from heterogenous IoT devices remains an open research area.

Energy consumption: Typically, an IoT healthcare connected device provides a wireless connection to connect patients and doctors over a device to gateway model. Although the analysis is performed in the cloud layer, due to continuous and seamless data transfer, these IoT devices run into power efficiency problems (Nugraha et al., 2017). The challenge is to develop innovative solutions of IoT systems that maximize the trade-offs between improving energy efficiency and functionality of the connected devices (Luo et al., 2012; Rahmani et al., 2018).

Privacy and security: The rapid evolution in the healthcare industry to integrate IoT systems and other connected devices to share healthcare data across many endpoint devices has increased the magnitude of cybersecurity threats. A recent survey revealed that data breaches cost the healthcare industry approximately $6.5 billion every year (Landi, 2019). Another study found that security vulnerabilities such as clear-text login information and clear text HTTP data processing are prevalent in IoT solutions where device sensors are socially connected to the internet (Borgohain et al., 2015), subjecting the privacy and information of users to increased risks. To mitigate these emerging cybersecurity threats, health organizations must be proactive in deploying advanced security technologies and robust cybersecurity measures to detect, protect, and respond to cyber-attacks.

CONCLUSION

This research provides a systematic review of the use of IoT in healthcare. On a self-care continuum (Self Care Forum, 2020), the review focuses on exploring and understanding healthcare activities outside a hospital or a healthcare facility setting that is supported by the recent developments of IoT solutions. A primary objective is to depict current state-of-the-art IoT solutions that could allow individuals an increased responsibility for healthcare activities as well as shed insight regarding major drivers and impediments for large-scale diffusion and adoption of the technological paradigm. A framework is proposed to characterize the IoT paradigm and supported healthcare activities. In this framework, we identified three primary healthcare activities namely, prevention (primary, secondary, and tertiary), diagnosis and treatment, and eight secondary healthcare activities namely, Disease Management, Assisted Living, Emergency Health Services, Fall Prevention, Medication Management, Child Health, Rehabilitation Therapy, and Preventive Monitoring. The review revealed that primary prevention and preventive monitoring are the main primary and secondary healthcare activities, respectively, that are supported by IoT technologies outside of a hospital or a healthcare facility. Innovations related to diagnosis and treatment are still emerging. The Device to Gateway communication model was adopted in most of the reviewed studies. A key factor is its scalability and flexibility. Further, there was a significant increase in the use of newer technologies such as LoRaWAN, Sigfox and WLAN. Most notable technology drivers for IoT support for healthcare activities include, cost of technology, seamless connectivity, edge analytics, storage and form factor. Most notable healthcare drivers include cost, insurance, workforce optimization, self-management, accessibility, health awareness, and emerging diseases and epidemics. Technology challenges include interoperability, data heterogeneity, energy consumption, and security and privacy. Healthcare challenges includes technology adoption and retention, payment structure, clinician adoption, efficacy, regulations, and medical non-adherence.

In summary, this research provides a snapshot of current IoT developments in healthcare, emphasizing the potential for shifting the responsibility of care further upstream, i.e., the individual. While the review affirms such potential from a technology perspective, there appears to be a gap with respect to the healthcare efficacy for such solutions, particularly for large-scale adoption. From a theoretical perspective, further research is needed to address this gap. For example, to what extent are healthy individuals or patients ready or willing to adopt such IoT-based solutions? What are the factors driving or impeding such adoption and continued use (retention)? What are the supportive structural changes, including business models, that are needed to ensure seamless integration with the healthcare systems (providers, insurers, government, and individuals)? And last but not least, what is the healthcare outcome from such use? From a practical perspective, the review depicts examples of implementations that support various healthcare activities. These examples can serve as a blueprint or a starting point for healthcare providers and practitioners envisioning the development of similar interventions. Such implementations can also provide insights for policymakers into understanding the salient issues surrounding IoT adoption in healthcare outside a traditional healthcare setting. Examples include issues related to data privacy and security, liability, and supporting business (payment) models.

The following limitations of the study should be acknowledged. Our review followed a traditional disease-orientated (pathogenic) model of health, thus omitting the salutogenic factors such as but not limited to empathy, resilience, quality of life, and social capital. Future research that can include salutogenic factors will improve the scope of the research and reach broader audiences. It should be also noted that the scope of this systematic review is limited to peer-reviewed articles indexed in scholarly databases and published in the English language. Future research could expand the scope to capture implementations and development published in other languages. This could provide further insight into factors that may be affected by context and cultural elements, e.g., user behavior and expectations, alternative business models, and supporting information technology infrastructure. Given the rapidly developing technological landscape, future reviews could also attempt to incorporate 'gray' literature from non-peer-reviewed sources.

Internet of Things plays a viable role in the healthcare Industry. It created avenues for smarter devices to deliver more valuable information, decreased the need for patient-physicians direct interaction, and provided efficiency in healthcare processes. With the technological developments in the last decade, IoT has become a topic of interest for researchers and healthcare providers and it is expected to play a major role in the quest for improved health and wellbeing along the line of the self-care continuum.

REFERENCES

Abawajy, J. H., & Hassan, M. M. (2017). Federated Internet of Things and Cloud Computing Pervasive Patient Health Monitoring System. *IEEE Communications Magazine*, 55(1), 48–53. DOI: 10.1109/MCOM.2017.1600374CM

Abdel-Basset, M., Abduallah Gamal, Gunasekaran Manogaran, Le Hoang Son, & Long, H. V. (. (2019). A novel group decision making model based on neutrosophic sets for heart disease diagnosis. *Multimedia Tools and Applications*, ●●●, 1–26. DOI: 10.1007/s11042-019-07742-7

Abdur Rahman, M., Rashid, M. M., Le Kernec, J., Philippe, B., Barnes, S. J., Fioranelli, F., Yang, S., Romain, O., Abbasi, Q. H., Loukas, G., & Imran, M. (2019). A Secure Occupational Therapy Framework for Monitoring Cancer Patients' Quality of Life. *Sensors (Basel)*, 19(23), 5258. Advance online publication. DOI: 10.3390/s19235258 PMID: 31795384

Addante, F., Gaetani, F., Patrono, L., Sancarlo, D., Sergi, I., & Vergari, G. (2019). An Innovative AAL System Based on IoT Technologies for Patients with Sarcopenia. *Sensors (Basel)*, 19(22), 4951. Advance online publication. DOI: 10.3390/s19224951 PMID: 31739396

Ahmadi, H., Arji, G., Shahmoradi, L., Safdari, R., Nilashi, M., & Alizadeh, M. (2018). The application of internet of things in healthcare: A systematic literature review and classification. *Universal Access in the Information Society*. Advance online publication. DOI: 10.1007/s10209-018-0618-4

Ahmed, S. (2019). BYOD, Personal Area Networks (PANs) and IOT: Threats to Patients Privacy. In Visvizi, A., & Lytras, M. D. (Eds.), *Research & Innovation Forum 2019* (pp. 403–410). Springer International Publishing., DOI: 10.1007/978-3-030-30809-4_36

Al-Fuqaha, A., Guizani, M., Mohammadi, M., Aledhari, M., & Ayyash, M. (2015). Internet of Things: A Survey on Enabling Technologies, Protocols, and Applications. *IEEE Communications Surveys Tutorials, 17*(4), 2347–2376. *IEEE Communications Surveys and Tutorials*. Advance online publication. DOI: 10.1109/COMST.2015.2444095

Al-Khafajiy, M., Baker, T., Chalmers, C., Asim, M., Kolivand, H., Fahim, M., & Waraich, A. (2019). Remote health monitoring of elderly through wearable sensors. In *Multimedia Tools and Applications* (Vol. 78, Issue 17, pp. 24681–24706). SPRINGER. DOI: 10.1007/s11042-018-7134-7

Al-Taee, M. A., Al-Nuaimy, W., Muhsin, Z. J., & Al-Ataby, A. (2017). Robot Assistant in Management of Diabetes in Children Based on the Internet of Things. *IEEE Internet of Things Journal*, 4(2), 437–445. DOI: 10.1109/JIOT.2016.2623767

Aleisa, N., & Renaud, K. (2017). Privacy of the Internet of Things: A Systematic Literature Review. *Proceedings of the 50th Hawaii International Conference on System Sciences*, 10. DOI: 10.24251/HICSS.2017.717

Alexandre, R., & Postolache, O. (2018). Wearable and IoT Technologies Application for Physical Rehabilitation. *2018 International Symposium in Sensing and Instrumentation in IoT Era (ISSI)*, 1–6. DOI: 10.1109/ISSI.2018.8538058

Aljahdali, M., Abokhamees, R., Bensenouci, A., Brahimi, T., & Bensenouci, M. (2018). IoT based assistive walker device for frail &visually impaired people. *2018 15th Learning and Technology Conference (L&T)*, 171–177. DOI: 10.1109/LT.2018.8368503

Asghari, P., Rahmani, A. M., & Javadi, H. H. S. (2019a). A medical monitoring scheme and health-medical service composition model in cloud-based IoT platform. *Transactions on Emerging Telecommunications Technologies*, 30(6), e3637. Advance online publication. DOI: 10.1002/ett.3637

Asghari, P., Rahmani, A. M., & Javadi, H. H. S. (2019b). Internet of Things applications: A systematic review. *Computer Networks*, 148, 241–261. DOI: 10.1016/j.comnet.2018.12.008

Atzori, L., Iera, A., & Morabito, G. (2010). The Internet of Things: A survey. *Computer Networks*, 54(15), 2787–2805. DOI: 10.1016/j.comnet.2010.05.010

Azimi, I., Anzanpour, A., Rahmani, A. M., Pahikkala, T., Levorato, M., Liljeberg, P., & Dutt, N. (2017). HiCH: Hierarchical Fog-Assisted Computing Architecture for Healthcare IoT. *ACM Transactions on Embedded Computing Systems, 16*(5, SI). DOI: 10.1145/3126501

Bae, J.-H., & Lee, H.-K. (2018). User Health Information Analysis With a Urine and Feces Separable Smart Toilet System. *IEEE Access : Practical Innovations, Open Solutions*, 6, 78751–78765. DOI: 10.1109/ACCESS.2018.2885234

Balandina, E., Balandin, S., Koucheryavy, Y., & Mouromtsev, D. (2015). IoT Use Cases in Healthcare and Tourism. *2015 IEEE 17th Conference on Business Informatics, 2*, 37–44. DOI: 10.1109/CBI.2015.16

Baltagi, B. H., Lagravinese, R., Moscone, F., & Tosetti, E. (2017). Health Care Expenditure and Income: A Global Perspective. *Health Economics*, 26(7), 863–874. DOI: 10.1002/hec.3424 PMID: 27679983

Basanta, H., Huang, Y., & Lee, T. (2016). Intuitive IoT-based H2U healthcare system for elderly people. *2016 IEEE 13th International Conference on Networking, Sensing, and Control (ICNSC)*, 1–6. DOI: 10.1109/ICNSC.2016.7479018

Berenson, R. A., & Rich, E. C. (2010). US Approaches to Physician Payment: The Deconstruction of Primary Care. *Journal of General Internal Medicine*, 25(6), 613–618. DOI: 10.1007/s11606-010-1295-z PMID: 20467910

Bhatia, M., Kaur, S., & Sood, S. K. (2020). IoT-Inspired Smart Toilet System for Home-Based Urine Infection Prediction. *ACM Transactions on Computing for Healthcare*, 1(3), 1–25. DOI: 10.1145/3379506

Bhatia, M., & Sood, S. K. (2017). A comprehensive health assessment framework to facilitate IoT-assisted smart workouts: A predictive healthcare perspective. *Computers in Industry*, 92–93, 50–66. DOI: 10.1016/j.compind.2017.06.009

Biran Achituv, D., & Haiman, L. (2016). Physicians' attitudes toward the use of IoT medical devices as part of their practice. [OJAKM]. *Online Journal of Applied Knowledge Management*, 4(2), 128–145. DOI: 10.36965/OJAKM.2016.4(2)128-145

Bisio, I., Garibotto, C., Lavagetto, F., & Sciarrone, A. (2019). Towards IoT-Based eHealth Services: A Smart Prototype System for Home Rehabilitation. *2019 IEEE Global Communications Conference (GLOBECOM)*, 1–6. DOI: 10.1109/GLOBE-COM38437.2019.9013194

Blowers, M., Iribarne, J., Colbert, E., & Kott, A. (2016). The Future Internet of Things and Security of its Control Systems. *arXiv:1610.01953[Cs]*. http://arxiv.org/abs/1610.01953 DOI: 10.1007/978-3-319-32125-7_16

Bodenreider, O. (2004). The Unified Medical Language System (UMLS): Integrating biomedical terminology. *Nucleic Acids Research*, 32(Database issue), D267–D270. DOI: 10.1093/nar/gkh061 PMID: 14681409

Borgohain, T., Kumar, U., & Sanyal, S. (2015). Survey of Security and Privacy Issues of Internet of Things. *arXiv:1501.02211[Cs]*. http://arxiv.org/abs/1501.02211

Brownsell, S., & Hawley, M. S. (2004). Automatic fall detectors and the fear of falling. *Journal of Telemedicine and Telecare*, 10(5), 262–266. DOI: 10.1258/1357633042026251 PMID: 15494083

Buzachis, A., Bernava, G. M., Busa, M., Pioggia, G., & Villari, M. (2018). Towards the Basic Principles of Osmotic Computing: A Closed-Loop Gamified Cognitive Rehabilitation Flow Model. *2018 IEEE 4th International Conference on Collaboration and Internet Computing (CIC)*, 446–452. DOI: 10.1109/CIC.2018.00067

Caddy, B. (2019, September 19). *Wearable tech and regulation: What laws do wearables need to follow?* Wareable. https://www.wareable.com/health-and-wellbeing/wearable-tech-and-regulation-5678

Canhoto, A. I., & Arp, S. (2017). Exploring the factors that support adoption and sustained use of health and fitness wearables. *Journal of Marketing Management*, 33(1–2), 32–60. DOI: 10.1080/0267257X.2016.1234505

Cano Porras, D., Siemonsma, P., Inzelberg, R., Zeilig, G., & Plotnik, M. (2018). Advantages of virtual reality in the rehabilitation of balance and gait: Systematic review. *Neurology*, 90(22), 1017–1025. DOI: 10.1212/WNL.0000000000005603 PMID: 29720544

Cavallari, R., Martelli, F., Rosini, R., Buratti, C., & Verdone, R. (2014). A Survey on Wireless Body Area Networks: Technologies and Design Challenges. *IEEE Communications Surveys and Tutorials*, 16(3), 1635–1657. DOI: 10.1109/SURV.2014.012214.00007

Chang, W.-J., Chen, L.-B., Hsu, C.-H., Chen, J.-H., Yang, T.-C., & Lin, C.-P. (2020). MedGlasses: A Wearable Smart-Glasses-Based Drug Pill Recognition System Using Deep Learning for Visually Impaired Chronic Patients. *IEEE Access : Practical Innovations, Open Solutions*, 8, 17013–17024. DOI: 10.1109/ACCESS.2020.2967400

Chen, M., Ma, Y., Li, Y., Wu, D., Zhang, Y., & Youn, C.-H. (2017). Wearable 2.0: Enabling Human-Cloud Integration in Next Generation Healthcare Systems. *IEEE Communications Magazine*, 55(1), 54–61. DOI: 10.1109/MCOM.2017.1600410CM

Cheruvu, S., Kumar, A., Smith, N., & Wheeler, D. M. (2020). Connectivity Technologies for IoT. In Cheruvu, S., Kumar, A., Smith, N., & Wheeler, D. M. (Eds.), *Demystifying Internet of Things Security: Successful IoT Device/Edge and Platform Security Deployment* (pp. 347–411). Apress., DOI: 10.1007/978-1-4842-2896-8_5

Choi, A., Noh, S., & Shin, H. (2020). Internet-Based Unobtrusive Tele-Monitoring System for Sleep and Respiration. *IEEE Access : Practical Innovations, Open Solutions*, 8, 76700–76707. DOI: 10.1109/ACCESS.2020.2989336

CMS. (2019). *Historical National Health Expenditure Accounts*. Centers for Medicare & Medicaid Services. https://www.cms.gov/Research-Statistics-Data-and-Systems/Statistics-Trends-and-Reports/NationalHealthExpendData/NationalHealthAccountsHistorical

Cohen, J. (1960). A Coefficient of Agreement for Nominal Scales. *Educational and Psychological Measurement*, 20(1), 37–46. Advance online publication. DOI: 10.1177/001316446002000104

Corno, F., Russis, L. D., & Roffarello, A. M. (2016). A Healthcare Support System for Assisted Living Facilities: An IoT Solution. *2016 IEEE 40th Annual Computer Software and Applications Conference (COMPSAC), 1*, 344–352. DOI: 10.1109/ COMPSAC.2016.29

Correa, D. (2019). *Fitness Trackers Market Projected To Display A Robust Growth With a CAGR of 19.6% by 2023.* MarketWatch. https://www.marketwatch.com/press -release/fitness-trackers-market-projected-to-display-a-robust-growth-with-a-cagr -of-196-by-2023-2019-09-18

Dash, S., Shakyawar, S. K., Sharma, M., & Kaushik, S. (2019). Big data in healthcare: Management, analysis and future prospects. *Journal of Big Data, 6*(1), 1–25. DOI: 10.1186/s40537-019-0217-0

De Grood, C., Raissi, A., Kwon, Y., & Santana, M. J. (2016). Adoption of e-health technology by physicians: A scoping review. *Journal of Multidisciplinary Healthcare, 9*, 335–344. DOI: 10.2147/JMDH.S103881 PMID: 27536128

de la Iglesia, D. H., Sales Mendes, A., Villarrubia Gonzalez, G., Jimenez-Bravo, D. M., & de Paz Santana, J. F. (2020). Connected Elbow Exoskeleton System for Rehabilitation Training Based on Virtual Reality and Context-Aware. In *Sensors* (Vol. 20, Issue 3). MDPI. DOI: 10.3390/s20030858

Deodhar, S., Chen, J., Wilson, M., Bisset, K., Barrett, C., & Marathe, M. (2015). EpiCaster: An integrated web application for situation assessment and forecasting of global epidemics. *Proceedings of the 6th ACM Conference on Bioinformatics, Computational Biology and Health Informatics*, 156–165. DOI: 10.1145/2808719.2808735

Dimitrov, D. V. (2016). Medical Internet of Things and Big Data in Healthcare. *Healthcare Informatics Research, 22*(3), 156. DOI: 10.4258/hir.2016.22.3.156 PMID: 27525156

Din, I., Almogren, A., Guizani, M., & Zuair, M. (2019). A Decade of Internet of Things: Analysis in the Light of Healthcare Applications. *IEEE Access : Practical Innovations, Open Solutions, 7*, 89967–89979. DOI: 10.1109/ACCESS.2019.2927082

Din, I., Guizani, M., Hassan, S., Kim, B., Khan, M. K., Atiquzzaman, M., & Ahmed, S. H. (2019). The Internet of Things: A Review of Enabled Technologies and Future Challenges. *IEEE Access : Practical Innovations, Open Solutions, 7*, 7606–7640. DOI: 10.1109/ACCESS.2018.2886601

El-Gayar, O., Ambati, L. S., & Nawar, N. (2020). Wearables, Artificial intelligence, and the Future of Healthcare. In *AI and Big Data's Potential for Disruptive Innovation* (pp. 104–129). IGI GLOBAL., DOI: 10.4018/978-1-5225-9687-5.ch005

El-Gayar, O., Nasralah, T., & Elnoshokaty, A. (2019, January 8). Wearable Devices for Health and Wellbeing: Design Insights from Twitter. *HICSS 52. Hawaii International Conference on System Sciences.* DOI: 10.24251/HICSS.2019.467

Enshaeifar, S., Barnaghi, P., Skillman, S., Markides, A., Elsaleh, T., Acton, S. T., Nilforooshan, R., & Rostill, H. (2018). The Internet of Things for Dementia Care. *IEEE Internet Computing*, 22(1), 8–17. DOI: 10.1109/MIC.2018.112102418

Faggella, D. (2020, March). *Machine Learning for Medical Diagnostics—4 Current Applications.* Emerj. https://emerj.com/ai-sector-overviews/machine-learning-medical-diagnostics-4-current-applications/

Fatima, S. A. (2020). IoT enabled Smart Monitoring of Coronavirus empowered with Fuzzy Inference System. *International Journal of Advance Research. Ideas and Innovations in Technology*, 6(1), 8.

Fendos, J. (2020, April 29). How surveillance technology powered South Korea's COVID-19 response. *Brookings.* https://www.brookings.edu/techstream/how-surveillance-technology-powered-south-koreas-covid-19-response/

Fenton, R. (2019, November). 5 Common Medical Device Regulatory Compliance Problems Faced in 2019 [Qualio]. *Medical-Device-Regulatory-Compliance.* https://www.qualio.com/blog/medical-device-regulatory-compliance

Gatouillat, A., Badr, Y., Massot, B., & Sejdic, E. (2018). Internet of Medical Things: A Review of Recent Contributions Dealing With Cyber-Physical Systems in Medicine. *IEEE Internet of Things Journal*, 5(5), 3810–3822. DOI: 10.1109/JIOT.2018.2849014

Ghamari, M., Janko, B., Sherratt, R., Harwin, W., Piechockic, R., & Soltanpur, C. (2016). A Survey on Wireless Body Area Networks for eHealthcare Systems in Residential Environments. *Sensors (Basel)*, 16(6), 831. DOI: 10.3390/s16060831 PMID: 27338377

Gusev, M., Ristov, S., Prodan, R., Dzanko, M., & Bilic, I. (2017). Resilient IoT eHealth solutions in case of disasters. *2017 9th International Workshop on Resilient Networks Design and Modeling (RNDM)*, 1–7. DOI: 10.1109/RNDM.2017.8093024

Gutierrez-Madronal, L., La Blunda, L., Wagner, M. F., & Medina-Bulo, I. (2019). Test Event Generation for a Fall-Detection IoT System. *IEEE Internet of Things Journal*, 6(4), 6642–6651. DOI: 10.1109/JIOT.2019.2909434

Gutierrez-Madronal, L., La Blunda, L., Wagner, M. F., & Medina-Bulo, I. (2019). Test Event Generation for a Fall-Detection IoT System. *IEEE Internet of Things Journal*, 6(4), 6642–6651. DOI: 10.1109/JIOT.2019.2909434

Hadi, M. S., Lawey, A. Q., El-Gorashi, T. E. H., & Elmirghani, J. M. H. (2019). Patient-Centric Cellular Networks Optimization Using Big Data Analytics. *IEEE Access : Practical Innovations, Open Solutions*, 7, 49279–49296. DOI: 10.1109/ACCESS.2019.2910224

Haghi, M., Neubert, S., Geissler, A., Fleischer, H., Stoll, N., Stoll, R., & Thurow, K. (2020). A Flexible and Pervasive IoT Based Healthcare Platform for Physiological and Environmental Parameters Monitoring. *IEEE Internet of Things Journal*, 7(6), 1–1. DOI: 10.1109/JIOT.2020.2980432

Hassan, M. K., El Desouky, A. I., Elghamrawy, S. M., & Sarhan, A. M. (2019). A Hybrid Real-time remote monitoring framework with NB-WOA algorithm for patients with chronic diseases. *Future Generation Computer Systems*, 93, 77–95. DOI: 10.1016/j.future.2018.10.021

Hassan, N. H., Salwana, E., Drus, S., Maarop, N., Samy, G. N., & Ahmad, N. A. (2018). Proposed Conceptual Iot-Based Patient Monitoring Sensor for Predicting and Controlling Dengue. *International Journal of Grid and Distributed Computing*, 11(4), 127–134. DOI: 10.14257/ijgdc.2018.11.4.11

Hayek, A., Telawi, S., Boercsoek, J., Daou, R. A. Z., & Halabi, N. (2020). Smart wearable system for safety-related medical IoT application: Case of epileptic patient working in industrial environment. *Health and Technology, 10*(1, SI), 363–372. DOI: 10.1007/s12553-019-00335-2

HCPO. (2013). *Pharmaceutical Compliance and Adherence Packaging Trade Organizations*. https://www.hcponline.org/

HITInfrastructure. (2017, May 15). *Remote Monitoring, Operations Drive Healthcare IoT Adoption*. HITInfrastructure. https://hitinfrastructure.com/news/remote-monitoring-operations-drive-healthcare-iot-adoption

Hu, F., Xie, D., & Shen, S. (2013). On the Application of the Internet of Things in the Field of Medical and Health Care. *2013 IEEE International Conference on Green Computing and Communications and IEEE Internet of Things and IEEE Cyber, Physical and Social Computing*, 2053–2058. DOI: 10.1109/GreenCom-iThings-CPSCom.2013.384

Hussain, A., Wenbi, R., da Silva, A. L., Nadher, M., & Mudhish, M. (2015). Health and emergency-care platform for the elderly and disabled people in the Smart City. *Journal of Systems and Software*, 110, 253–263. DOI: 10.1016/j.jss.2015.08.041

Ikram, M. A., Alshehri, M. D., & Hussain, F. K. (2015). Architecture of an IoT-based system for football supervision (IoT Football). *2015 IEEE 2nd World Forum on Internet of Things (WF-IoT)*, 69–74. DOI: 10.1109/WF-IoT.2015.7389029

Inan, O. T., Tenaerts, P., Prindiville, S. A., Reynolds, H. R., Dizon, D. S., Cooper-Arnold, K., Turakhia, M., Pletcher, M. J., Preston, K. L., Krumholz, H. M., Marlin, B. M., Mandl, K. D., Klasnja, P., Spring, B., Iturriaga, E., Campo, R., Desvigne-Nickens, P., Rosenberg, Y., Steinhubl, S. R., & Califf, R. M. (2020). Digitizing clinical trials. *Digital Medicine*, 3(1), 1. Advance online publication. DOI: 10.1038/s41746-020-0302-y PMID: 32821856

Internet Of Things | Definition of Internet Of Things by Merriam-Webster. (n.d.). Retrieved January 29, 2020, from https://www.merriam-webster.com/dictionary/Internet%20of%20Things

ITU. (2012, June 15). *Overview of the Internet of Things.* https://Www.Itu.Int/ITU-T/Recommendations/Rec.Aspx?rec=Y.2060

Jacobson, C., & Karjalainen, P. (2019). *Embracing Internet of Medical Things: A multiple case study of contextual factors' influence on the implementation of IoT healthcare solutions* [Gothenburg University]. https://gupea.ub.gu.se/handle/2077/61406

Jara, A. J., Zamora, M. A., & Skarmeta, A. F. (2012). Knowledge Acquisition and Management Architecture for Mobile and Personal Health Environments Based on the Internet of Things. *2012 IEEE 11th International Conference on Trust, Security and Privacy in Computing and Communications*, 1811–1818. DOI: 10.1109/TrustCom.2012.194

Jeong, S. (2019). Insurers Want to Know How Many Steps You Took Today. *The New York Times*, 3.

Jiang, Y. (2020). Combination of wearable sensors and internet of things and its application in sports rehabilitation. In *Computer Communications* (Vol. 150, pp. 167–176). ELSEVIER., DOI: 10.1016/j.comcom.2019.11.021

Jiang, Y., Qin, Y., Kim, I., & Wang, Y. (2017). Towards an IoT-based upper limb rehabilitation assessment system. *2017 39th Annual International Conference of the IEEE Engineering in Medicine and Biology Society (EMBC)*, 2414–2417. DOI: 10.1109/EMBC.2017.8037343

Kadarina, T. M., & Priambodo, R. (2017). Preliminary design of Internet of Things (IoT) application for supporting mother and child health program in Indonesia. *2017 International Conference on Broadband Communication, Wireless Sensors and Powering (BCWSP)*, 1–6. DOI: 10.1109/BCWSP.2017.8272576

Kang, J. J., Adibi, S., Larkin, H., & Luan, T. (2015). Predictive data mining for Converged Internet of Things: A Mobile Health perspective. *2015 International Telecommunication Networks and Applications Conference (ITNAC)*, 5–10. DOI: 10.1109/ATNAC.2015.7366781

Kario, K., Tomitani, N., Kanegae, H., Yasui, N., Nishizawa, M., Fujiwara, T., Shigezumi, T., Nagai, R., & Harada, H. (2017). Development of a New ICT-Based Multisensor Blood Pressure Monitoring System for Use in Hemodynamic Biomarker-Initiated Anticipation Medicine for Cardiovascular Disease: The National IMPACT Program Project. *Progress in Cardiovascular Diseases*, 60(3), 435–449. DOI: 10.1016/j.pcad.2017.10.002 PMID: 29108929

Kaushalya, S. A. D. S., Kulawansa, K. A. D. T., & Firdhous, M. F. M. (2019). Internet of Things for Epidemic Detection: A Critical Review. In Bhatia, S. K., Tiwari, S., Mishra, K. K., & Trivedi, M. C. (Eds.), *Advances in Computer Communication and Computational Sciences* (pp. 485–495). Springer., DOI: 10.1007/978-981-13-6861-5_42

Khan, I., Zeb, K., Mahmood, A., Uddin, W., & Khan, M. A. Saif-ul-Islam, & Kim, H. J. (2019). Healthcare Monitoring System and transforming Monitored data into Real time Clinical Feedback based on IoT using Raspberry Pi. *2019 2nd International Conference on Computing, Mathematics and Engineering Technologies (iCoMET)*, 1–6. DOI: 10.1109/ICOMET.2019.8673393

Khan, M. A., Uddin, M. F., & Gupta, N. (2014). Seven V's of Big Data understanding Big Data to extract value. *Proceedings of the 2014 Zone 1 Conference of the American Society for Engineering Education*, 1–5. DOI: 10.1109/ASEEZone1.2014.6820689

Khan, S. F. (2017). Health care monitoring system in Internet of Things (IoT) by using RFID. *2017 6th International Conference on Industrial Technology and Management (ICITM)*, 198–204. DOI: 10.1109/ICITM.2017.7917920

Klímová, B., & Kuča, K. (2019). Internet of things in the assessment, diagnostics and treatment of Parkinson's disease. *Health and Technology*, 9(2), 87–91. DOI: 10.1007/s12553-018-0257-z

Ko, J., Lu, C., Srivastava, M. B., Stankovic, J. A., Terzis, A., & Welsh, M. (2010). Wireless Sensor Networks for Healthcare. *Proceedings of the IEEE*, 98(11), 1947–1960. DOI: 10.1109/JPROC.2010.2065210

Krishnan, B., Babu, S., Shaji, S. P., Tamanampudi, A. S. R., & Sanagapati, S. S. S. (2016). Software based gateway with distributed flow environment for medical IoT in rural areas. *2016 IEEE International Conference on Advanced Networks and Telecommunications Systems (ANTS)*, 1–5. DOI: 10.1109/ANTS.2016.7947858

La, H. J., Jung, H. T., & Kim, S. D. (2015). Extensible Disease Diagnosis Cloud Platform with Medical Sensors and IoT Devices. *2015 3rd International Conference on Future Internet of Things and Cloud*, 371–378. DOI: 10.1109/FiCloud.2015.65

Landi, H. (2019). *Healthcare data breaches cost an average $6.5M: Report*. Fierce Healthcare. https://www.fiercehealthcare.com/tech/healthcare-data-breach-costs -average-6-45m-60-higher-than-other-industries-report

Landis, J. R., & Koch, G. G. (1977). The Measurement of Observer Agreement for Categorical Data. *Biometrics*, 33(1), 159–174. DOI: 10.2307/2529310 PMID: 843571

Latif, G., Shankar, A., Alghazo, J. M., Kalyanasundaram, V., Boopathi, C. S., & Jaffar, M. A. (2020). I-CARES: advancing health diagnosis and medication through IoT. In *Wireless Networks* (Vol. 26, Issues 4, SI, pp. 2375–2389). Springer. DOI: 10.1007/s11276-019-02165-6

Li, B., Dong, Q., Downen, R. S., Tran, N., Jackson, J. H., Pillai, D., Zaghloul, M., & Li, Z. (2019). A wearable IoT aldehyde sensor for pediatric asthma research and management. *Sensors and Actuators. B, Chemical*, 287, 584–594. DOI: 10.1016/j. snb.2019.02.077 PMID: 31938011

Li, S., Xu, L. D., & Zhao, S. (2015). The internet of things: A survey. *Information Systems Frontiers*, 17(2), 243–259. DOI: 10.1007/s10796-014-9492-7

Liu, Y., Niu, J., Yang, L., & Shu, L. (2014). eBPlatform: An IoT-based system for NCD patients homecare in China. *2014 IEEE Global Communications Conference*, 2448–2453. DOI: 10.1109/GLOCOM.2014.7037175

Luo, X., Liu, T., Liu, J., Guo, X., & Wang, G. (2012). Design and implementation of a distributed fall detection system based on wireless sensor networks. *EURASIP Journal on Wireless Communications and Networking*, 2012(1), 1–13. DOI: 10.1186/1687-1499-2012-118

Ma, B., Li, C., Wu, Z., Huang, Y., van der Zijp-Tan, A. C., Tan, S., Li, D., Fong, A., Basetty, C., Borchert, G. M., Benton, R., Wu, B., & Huang, J. (2019). Muscle fatigue detection and treatment system driven by internet of things. In *BMC Medical Informatics and Decision Making* (Vol. 19, Issues 7, SI). BMC. DOI: 10.1186/ s12911-019-0982-x

Magsi, H., Sodhro, A. H., Chachar, F. A., Abro, S. A. K., Sodhro, G. H., & Pirbhu-lal, S. (2018). Evolution of 5G in Internet of medical things. *2018 International Conference on Computing, Mathematics and Engineering Technologies (iCoMET)*, 1–7. DOI: 10.1109/ICOMET.2018.8346428

Maksimović, D., Vujovic, V., & Perisic, B. (2016). Do It Yourself solution of Internet of Things Healthcare System: Measuring body parameters and environmental parameters affecting health. *Journal of Information Systems Engineering & Management*, 1(1), •••. DOI: 10.20897/lectito.201607

Manatarinat, W., Poomrittigul, S., & Tantatsanawong, P. (2019). Narrowband-Internet of Things (NB-IoT) System for Elderly Healthcare Services. *2019 5th International Conference on Engineering, Applied Sciences and Technology (ICEAST)*, 1–4. DOI: 10.1109/ICEAST.2019.8802604

Market Research Future. (2018, April). *Telemedicine Market Size, Trends, Growth, Share, Industry Forecast Till 2023*. https://www.marketresearchfuture.com/reports/telemedicine-market-2216

Matthews, K., & Industry Voice. (2020, April 3). *How AI and IoT Are Changing Daily Operations in Hospitals*. Healthcare Innovation. https://www.hcinnovationgroup.com/analytics-ai/article/21132663/how-ai-and-iot-are-changing-daily-operations-in-hospitals

McKinsey Global Institute. (2015, June). *The Internet of Things: Mapping the Value Beyond the Hype*. McKinsey & Company. https://www.mckinsey.com/~/media/McKinsey/Industries/Technology%20Media%20and%20Telecommunications/High%20Tech/Our%20Insights/The%20Internet%20of%20Things%20The%20value%20of%20digitizing%20the%20physical%20world/The-Internet-of-things-Mapping-the-value-beyond-the-hype.ashx

Meola, A. (2020). *IoT Healthcare in 2020: Companies, devices, use cases and market stats*. Business Insider. https://www.businessinsider.com/iot-healthcare

Mieronkoski, R., Azimi, I., Rahmani, A. M., Aantaa, R., Terävä, V., Liljeberg, P., & Salanterä, S. (2017). The Internet of Things for basic nursing care-A scoping review. *International Journal of Nursing Studies*, 69, 78–90. DOI: 10.1016/j.ijnurstu.2017.01.009 PMID: 28189116

Mills, J.-A., Marks, E., Reynolds, T., & Cieza, A. (2017). Rehabilitation: Essential along the Continuum of Care. In Jamison, D. T., Gelband, H., Horton, S., Jha, P., Laxminarayan, R., Mock, C. N., & Nugent, R. (Eds.), *Disease Control Priorities: Improving Health and Reducing Poverty* (3rd ed.). The International Bank for Reconstruction and Development / The World Bank., https://www.ncbi.nlm.nih.gov/books/NBK525298/ DOI: 10.1596/978-1-4648-0527-1_ch15

Mincolelli, G., Imbesi, S., Marchi, M., & Giacobone, G. A. (2019). New Domestic Healthcare. Co-designing Assistive Technologies for Autonomous Ageing at Home. *The Design Journal*, 22(1), 503–516. DOI: 10.1080/14606925.2019.1595435

Minerva, R., Biru, A., & Rotondi, D. (2015). Towards a definition of the Internet of Things (IoT). *IEEE Internet Initiative*, 1, 1–86.

Mohammed, M. N., Hazairin, N. A., Al-Zubaidi, S., Mustapha, S., & Yusuf, E. (2020). Toward a Novel Design for Coronavirus Detection and Diagnosis System Using IoT Based Drone Technology. *International Journal of Psychosocial Rehabilitation*, 24(7), 10.

Moher, D., Liberati, A., Tetzlaff, J., Altman, D. G., & Group, T. P. (2009). Preferred Reporting Items for Systematic Reviews and Meta-Analyses: The PRISMA Statement. *PLoS Medicine*, 6(7), e1000097. DOI: 10.1371/journal.pmed.1000097 PMID: 19621072

Mora, H., Gil, D., Terol, R. M., Azorin, J., & Szymanski, J. (2017). An IoT-Based Computational Framework for Healthcare Monitoring in Mobile Environments. *Sensors (Basel)*, 17(10), 2302. Advance online publication. DOI: 10.3390/s17102302 PMID: 28994743

Muhammad, G., Rahman, S. M. M., Alelaiwi, A., & Alamri, A. (2017). Smart Health Solution Integrating IoT and Cloud: A Case Study of Voice Pathology Monitoring. *IEEE Communications Magazine*, 55(1), 69–73. DOI: 10.1109/MCOM.2017.1600425CM

Mumtaj, S. Y., & Umamakeswari, A. (2017). Neuro fuzzy based healthcare system using IoT. *2017 International Conference on Energy, Communication, Data Analytics and Soft Computing (ICECDS)*, 2299–2303. DOI: 10.1109/ICECDS.2017.8389863

Nasri, F., & Mtibaa, A. (2017). Smart Mobile Healthcare System based on WBSN and 5G. *International Journal of Advanced Computer Science and Applications*, 8(10), 147–156. DOI: 10.14569/IJACSA.2017.081020

Nduka, A., Samual, J., Elango, S., Divakaran, S., & Umar, U., & SenthilPrabha, R. (2019). Internet of Things Based Remote Health Monitoring System Using Arduino. *2019 Third International Conference on I-SMAC (IoT in Social, Mobile, Analytics and Cloud) (I-SMAC)*, 572–576. DOI: 10.1109/I-SMAC47947.2019.9032438

Nedungadi, P., Jayakumar, A., & Raman, R. (2017). Personalized Health Monitoring System for Managing Well-Being in Rural Areas. *Journal of Medical Systems*, 42(1), 22. DOI: 10.1007/s10916-017-0854-9 PMID: 29242996

Neiman, A. B., Ruppar, T., Ho, M., Garber, L., Weidle, P. J., Hong, Y., George, M. G., & Thorpe, P. G. (2018). CDC Grand Rounds: Improving medication adherence for chronic disease management — Innovations and opportunities. *American Journal of Transplantation*, 18(2), 514–517. DOI: 10.1111/ajt.14649 PMID: 29381269

Neto, M. M., Coutinho, E. F., Moreira, L. O., de Souza, J. N., & Agoulmine, N. (2018). A Proposal for Monitoring People of Health Risk Group Using IoT Technologies. *2018 IEEE 20th International Conference on E-Health Networking, Applications and Services (Healthcom)*, 1–6. DOI: 10.1109/HealthCom.2018.8531196

NIH. (2001, July 31). *PA-01-124: Patient-Centered Care: Customizing Care to Meet Patients' Needs*. https://grants.nih.gov/grants/guide/pa-files/PA-01-124.html

Nugraha, B., Ekasurya, I., Osman, G., & Alaydrus, M. (2017). Analysis of Power Consumption Efficiency on Various IoT and Cloud-Based Wireless Health Monitoring Systems: A Survey. *International Journal of Information Technology and Computer Science*, 9(5), 31–39. DOI: 10.5815/ijitcs.2017.05.05

Nyasulu, T. (2016). Smart under-five health care system. *2016 IST-Africa Week Conference*, 1–8. DOI: 10.1109/ISTAFRICA.2016.7530674

Onasanya, A., Lakkis, S., & Elshakankiri, M. (2019). Implementing IoT/WSN based smart Saskatchewan Healthcare System. *Wireless Networks*, 1(7), 3999–4020. Advance online publication. DOI: 10.1007/s11276-018-01931-2

Oriwoh, E., & Conrad, M. (2015). *'Things' in the Internet of Things: Towards a Definition*. 5.

Pace, P., Aloi, G., Caliciuri, G., Gravina, R., Savaglio, C., Fortino, G., Ibanez-Sanchez, G., Fides-Valero, A., Bayo-Monton, J., Uberti, M., Corona, M., Bernini, L., Gulino, M., Costa, A., De Luca, I., & Mortara, M. (2019). INTER-Health: An Interoperable IoT Solution for Active and Assisted Living Healthcare Services. *2019 IEEE 5th World Forum on Internet of Things (WF-IoT)*, 81–86. DOI: 10.1109/WF-IoT.2019.8767332

Pal, A., Rath, H. K., Shailendra, S., & Bhattacharyya, A. (2018). *IoT Standardization: The Road Ahead. Internet of Things - Technology*. Applications and Standardization., DOI: 10.5772/intechopen.75137

Panagioti, M., Richardson, G., Murray, E., Rogers, A., Kennedy, A., Newman, S., Small, N., & Bower, P. (2014). *Reducing Care Utilisation through Self-management Interventions (RECURSIVE): A systematic review and meta-analysis*. NIHR Journals Library. https://www.ncbi.nlm.nih.gov/books/NBK263888/

Pham, M., Mengistu, Y., Do, H., & Sheng, W. (2018). Delivering home healthcare through a Cloud-based Smart Home Environment (CoSHE). *Future Generation Computer Systems*, 81, 129–140. DOI: 10.1016/j.future.2017.10.040

Pierleoni, P., Belli, A., Bazgir, O., Maurizi, L., Paniccia, M., & Palma, L. (2019). A Smart Inertial System for 24h Monitoring and Classification of Tremor and Freezing of Gait in Parkinson's Disease. *IEEE Sensors Journal*, 19(23), 11612–11623. DOI: 10.1109/JSEN.2019.2932584

Piwek, L., Ellis, D. A., Andrews, S., & Joinson, A. (2016). The Rise of Consumer Health Wearables: Promises and Barriers. *PLoS Medicine*, 13(2), e1001953. Advance online publication. DOI: 10.1371/journal.pmed.1001953 PMID: 26836780

Plaza, A. M., Díaz, J., & Pérez, J. (2018). Software architectures for health care cyber-physical systems: A systematic literature review. *Journal of Software (Malden, MA)*, 30(7), e1930. DOI: 10.1002/smr.1930

Puri, V., Kumar, R., Le, D. N., Jagdev, S. S., & Sachdeva, N. (2020). BioSenHealth 2.0-a low-cost, energy-efficient Internet of Things-based blood glucose monitoring system. In Balas, V. E., Solanki, V. K., & Kumar, R. (Eds.), *Emergence of Pharmaceutical Industry Growth with Industrial Iot Approach* (pp. 305–324). Academic Press LTD-Elsevier Science LTD., DOI: 10.1016/B978-0-12-819593-2.00011-X

Rahman, Md. A., & Hossain, M. S. (2018). M-Therapy: A Multisensor Framework for in-Home Therapy Management: A Social Therapy of Things Perspective. *IEEE Internet of Things Journal, 5*(4, SI), 2548–2556. DOI: 10.1109/JIOT.2017.2776150

Rahman, M., & Hossain, M. S. (2019). A cloud-based virtual caregiver for elderly people in a cyber physical IoT system. *Cluster Computing*, 22(1), 2317–2330. DOI: 10.1007/s10586-018-1806-y

Rahman, M., Peeri, N. C., Shrestha, N., Zaki, R., Haque, U., & Hamid, S. H. A. (2020, June). S., Peeri, N. C., Shrestha, N., Zaki, R., Haque, U., & Hamid, S. H. A. (2020). Defending against the Novel Coronavirus (COVID-19) Outbreak: How Can the Internet of Things (IoT) help to save the World? *Health Policy and Technology*, 9(2), 136–138. Advance online publication. DOI: 10.1016/j.hlpt.2020.04.005 PMID: 32322475

Rahmani, A. M., Gia, T. N., Negash, B., Anzanpour, A., Azimi, I., Jiang, M., & Liljeberg, P. (2018). Exploiting smart e-Health gateways at the edge of healthcare Internet-of-Things: A fog computing approach. *Future Generation Computer Systems*, 78, 641–658. DOI: 10.1016/j.future.2017.02.014

Raj, S. (2020). An Efficient IoT-Based Platform for Remote Real-Time Cardiac Activity Monitoring. *IEEE Transactions on Consumer Electronics*, 66(2), 106–114. DOI: 10.1109/TCE.2020.2981511

Rathore, M. M., Ahmad, A., Paul, A., Wan, J., & Zhang, D. (2016). Real-time Medical Emergency Response System: Exploiting IoT and Big Data for Public Health. *Journal of Medical Systems*, 40(12), 283. DOI: 10.1007/s10916-016-0647-6 PMID: 27796839

Ray, P. P. (2018). A survey on Internet of Things architectures. *Journal of King Saud University. Computer and Information Sciences*, 30(3), 291–319. DOI: 10.1016/j.jksuci.2016.10.003

Rghioui, A., Lloret, J., Parra, L., Sendra, S., & Oumnad, A. (2019). Glucose Data Classification for Diabetic Patient Monitoring. In *Applied Sciences-Basel* (Vol. 9, Issue 20). MDPI. DOI: 10.3390/app9204459

Riazul Islam, S. M., Daehan Kwak, , Humaun Kabir, M., Hossain, M., & Kyung-Sup Kwak, . (2015). The Internet of Things for Health Care: A Comprehensive Survey. *IEEE Access : Practical Innovations, Open Solutions*, 3, 678–708. DOI: 10.1109/ACCESS.2015.2437951

Rose, K., Eldridge, S., & Chapin, L. (2015). *The Internet of Things: An Overview—Understanding the Issues and Challenges of a More Connected World*. Internet Society.

Sadoughi, F., Behmanesh, A., & Sayfouri, N. (2020). Internet of things in medicine: A systematic mapping study. *Journal of Biomedical Informatics*, 103, 103383. DOI: 10.1016/j.jbi.2020.103383 PMID: 32044417

Saha, J., Saha, A. K., Chatterjee, A., Agrawal, S., Saha, A., Kar, A., & Saha, H. N. (2018). Advanced IOT based combined remote health monitoring, home automation and alarm system. *2018 IEEE 8th Annual Computing and Communication Workshop and Conference (CCWC)*, 602–606. DOI: 10.1109/CCWC.2018.8301659

Said, O., & Masud, M. (2013). *Towards Internet of Things: Survey and Future Vision*. 17.

Self Care Forum. (2020). *What do we mean by self care and why is it good for people?*https://www.selfcareforum.org/about-us/what-do-we-mean-by-self-care -and-why-is-good-for-people/

Seneviratne, S., Hu, Y., Nguyen, T., Lan, G., Khalifa, S., Thilakarathna, K., Hassan, M., & Seneviratne, A. (2017). A Survey of Wearable Devices and Challenges. *IEEE Communications Surveys Tutorials, 19*(4), 2573–2620. *IEEE Communications Surveys and Tutorials*. Advance online publication. DOI: 10.1109/COMST.2017.2731979

Sethi, P., & Sarangi, S. R. (2017). Internet of Things: Architectures, Protocols, and Applications. *Journal of Electrical and Computer Engineering*, 2017, 1–25. DOI: 10.1155/2017/9324035

Silvello, A. (2017). IoT and Connected Insurance Reshaping The Health Insurance Industry. A Customer-centric "From Cure To Care" Approach. *ICST Transactions on Ambient Systems*, 4(15), 153462. DOI: 10.4108/eai.8-12-2017.153462

Sodhro, A. H., & Shah, M. A. (2017). Role of 5G in medical health. *2017 International Conference on Innovations in Electrical Engineering and Computational Technologies (ICIEECT)*, 1–5. DOI: 10.1109/ICIEECT.2017.7916586

Sood, S. K., & Mahajan, I. (2017). Wearable IoT sensor based healthcare system for identifying and controlling chikungunya virus. *Computers in Industry*, 91, 33–44. DOI: 10.1016/j.compind.2017.05.006 PMID: 32287550

Sood, S. K., & Mahajan, I. (2019). IoT-Fog-Based Healthcare Framework to Identify and Control Hypertension Attack. *IEEE Internet of Things Journal*, 6(2), 1920–1927. DOI: 10.1109/JIOT.2018.2871630

Subhedar, M., Jadhav, V., Tekade, S., & Prajapati, M. (2018). A Real Time Healthcare Monitoring System Based on Open Source IoT and ANFIS. *2018 Second International Conference on Intelligent Computing and Control Systems (ICICCS)*, 281–286. DOI: 10.1109/ICCONS.2018.8663037

Supernor, B. (2018). *Why the cost of cloud computing is dropping dramatically*. App Developer Magazine. https://appdevelopermagazine.com/why-the-cost-of-cloud -computing-is-dropping-dramatically/

Suraki, M. Y., & Suraki, M. Y. (2013). Technology therapy for obsessive-compulsive disorder based on Internet of Things. *2013 7th International Conference on Application of Information and Communication Technologies*, 1–4. DOI: 10.1109/ICAICT.2013.6722800

Tai, W., Kalanithi, L., & Milstein, A. (2014). What can be achieved by redesigning stroke care for a value-based world? *Expert Review of Pharmacoeconomics & Outcomes Research*, 14(5), 585–587. DOI: 10.1586/14737167.2014.946013 PMID: 25095813

Tan, E. T., & Halim, Z. A. (2019). Health care Monitoring System and Analytics Based on Internet of Things Framework. In *IETE Journal of Research* (Vol. 65, Issue 5, pp. 653–660). Taylor & Francis LTD. DOI: 10.1080/03772063.2018.1447402

Toh, X., Tan, H., Liang, H., & Tan, H. (2016). Elderly medication adherence monitoring with the Internet of Things. *2016 IEEE International Conference on Pervasive Computing and Communication Workshops (PerCom Workshops)*, 1–6. DOI: 10.1109/PERCOMW.2016.7457133

Touati, F., & Tabish, R. (2013). u-Healthcare system: State-of-the-art review and challenges. *Journal of Medical Systems*, 37(3), 9949. DOI: 10.1007/s10916-013-9949-0 PMID: 23640734

Tschofenig, H., Arkko, J., Thaler, D., & McPherson, D. (2015). *Architectural considerations in smart object networking. RFC 7452.* http://hjp.at/doc/rfc/rfc7452.html

Tun, S. Y. Y., Madanian, S., & Mirza, F. (2020). Internet of things (IoT) applications for elderly care: A reflective review. *Aging Clinical and Experimental Research.* Advance online publication. DOI: 10.1007/s40520-020-01545-9 PMID: 32277435

Vavilis, S., Petković, M., & Zannone, N. (2012). Impact of ICT on Home Healthcare. In M. D. Hercheui, D. Whitehouse, W. McIver, & J. Phahlamohlaka (Eds.), *ICT Critical Infrastructures and Society* (pp. 111–122). Springer. DOI: 10.1007/978-3-642-33332-3_11

Vijayakumar, V., Malathi, D., Subramaniyaswamy, V., Saravanan, P., & Logesh, R. (2019). Fog computing-based intelligent healthcare system for the detection and prevention of mosquito-borne diseases. In *Computers in Human Behavior* (Vol. 100, pp. 275–285). Pergamon-Elsevier Science LTD., DOI: 10.1016/j.chb.2018.12.009

Vlaanderen, F. P., Tanke, M. A., Bloem, B. R., Faber, M. J., Eijkenaar, F., Schut, F. T., & Jeurissen, P. P. T. (2019). Design and effects of outcome-based payment models in healthcare: A systematic review. *The European Journal of Health Economics*, 20(2), 217–232. DOI: 10.1007/s10198-018-0989-8 PMID: 29974285

Vukicevic, S., Stamenkovic, Z., Murugesan, S., Bogdanovic, Z., & Radenkovic, B. (2016). A New Telerehabilitation System Based on Internet of Things. *FACTA Universitatis-Series Electronics and Energetics*, 29(3), 395–405. DOI: 10.2298/FUEE1603395V

Wan, J., Al-awlaqi, M. A. A. H., Li, M., O'Grady, M., Gu, X., Wang, J., & Cao, N. (2018). Wearable IoT enabled real-time health monitoring system. *EURASIP Journal on Wireless Communications and Networking*. Advance online publication. DOI: 10.1186/s13638-018-1308-x

Whitmore, A., Agarwal, A., & Da Xu, L. (2015). The Internet of Things—A survey of topics and trends. *Information Systems Frontiers*, 17(2), 261–274. DOI: 10.1007/s10796-014-9489-2

Wu, H.-T., & Tsai, C.-W. (2018). A home security system for seniors based on the beacon technology. *Concurrency and Computation-Practice & Experience, 30*(15, SI). DOI: 10.1002/cpe.4496

Wu, M., Lu, T.-J., Ling, F.-Y., Sun, J., & Du, H.-Y. (2010). Research on the architecture of Internet of Things. *2010 3rd International Conference on Advanced Computer Theory and Engineering(ICACTE), 5*, V5-484-V5-487. DOI: 10.1109/ICACTE.2010.5579493

Wu, T., Wu, F., Qiu, C., Redoute, J., & Yuce, M. R. (2020). A Rigid-Flex Wearable Health Monitoring Sensor Patch for IoT-Connected Healthcare Applications. *IEEE Internet of Things Journal*, 7(8), 1–1. DOI: 10.1109/JIOT.2020.2977164

Yacchirema, D., Sarabia-Jacome, D., Palau, C. E., & Esteve, M. (2018a). A Smart System for Sleep Monitoring by Integrating IoT With Big Data Analytics. *IEEE Access : Practical Innovations, Open Solutions*, 6, 35988–36001. DOI: 10.1109/ACCESS.2018.2849822

Yacchirema, D., Sarabia-Jacome, D., Palau, C. E., & Esteve, M. (2018b). System for monitoring and supporting the treatment of sleep apnea using IoT and big data. *Pervasive and Mobile Computing*, 50, 25–40. DOI: 10.1016/j.pmcj.2018.07.007

Yang, G., Deng, J., Pang, G., Zhang, H., Li, J., Deng, B., Pang, Z., Xu, J., Jiang, M., Liljeberg, P., Xie, H., & Yang, H. (2018). An IoT-Enabled Stroke Rehabilitation System Based on Smart Wearable Armband and Machine Learning. *IEEE Journal of Translational Engineering in Health and Medicine, 6*, 1–10. *IEEE Journal of Translational Engineering in Health and Medicine*. Advance online publication. DOI: 10.1109/JTEHM.2018.2822681 PMID: 29805919

Yang, G., Xie, L., Mantysalo, M., Zhou, X., Pang, Z., Xu, L. D., Kao-Walter, S., Chen, Q., & Zheng, L.-R. (2014). A Health-IoT Platform Based on the Integration of Intelligent Packaging, Unobtrusive Bio-Sensor, and Intelligent Medicine Box. *IEEE Transactions on Industrial Informatics*, 10(4), 2180–2191. DOI: 10.1109/TII.2014.2307795

Yu, W., Liang, F., He, X., Hatcher, W., Lu, C., Lin, J., & Yang, X. (2017). A Survey on the Edge Computing for the Internet of Things. *IEEE Access, PP*, 1–1. DOI: 10.1109/ACCESS.2017.2778504

Zhang, X. M., & Zhang, N. (2011). An Open, Secure and Flexible Platform Based on Internet of Things and Cloud Computing for Ambient Aiding Living and Telemedicine. *2011 International Conference on Computer and Management (CAMAN)*, 1–4. DOI: 10.1109/CAMAN.2011.5778905

APPENDIX I

Table 7. Key technologies and terms related to IoT

Technology	Description
Device	this is a piece of equipment with the mandatory capabilities of communication and the optional capabilities of sensing, actuation, data capture, data storage and data processing (ITU, 2012)
Things	Things can be anything, for example a physical object, in the healthcare context, a smart device connected to the Internet to enable intelligent communication between or among healthcare stakeholders. (Oriwoh & Conrad, 2015)
Smart objects	These are devices that typically have significant constraints, such as limited power, memory, and processing resources, or bandwidth. (Tschofenig et al., 2015)
WSN	Wireless sensor networks are highly distributed, lightweight nodes, deployed in large numbers to monitor the environment or system.
RFID and NFC	Radio frequency identification is a technology that allows almost any object to be wirelessly identified using data transmitted via radio waves.
Cloud computing	Cloud computing is a pay-per-use model enabling on-demand networks to a shared pool of configurable computing resources such as network, server, storage, and applications, etc. which is available over the internet.
Bluetooth	This is a low-powered wireless communication network developed for short distances with connectivity ranging up to 100m with bandwidth speeds of 3 Mbps or more.
ZigBee	This is another class of wireless communication technology developed and optimized for IoT applications and renowned for its low-cost power consumption with value added feature such as interoperability, network resilience and security.
Wireless Fidelity (Wi-Fi)	This communication technology is the backbone of IoT connectivity and is common in most network topologies and application domains including healthcare, for example, connecting hospital systems in provision of healthcare services.
Mobile Networks	This wireless communication technology is driven by current 4G and 5G generation networks which provide high speed bandwidth and efficient energy consumption for most portable devices, for example, smart phones which are gaining wide application in IoT for healthcare scenarios.
HTTP	Hypertext Transfer Protocol (HTTP) is an application protocol for distributed, collaborative, hypermedia information systems

APPENDIX II

Table 8. Summary of IoT applications organized by healthcare activities

Primary healthcare activity	Secondary healthcare activity	Article	Paper type	Contribution	Sensor/Measurement	Target Group	Country	Comm. model	Limitations
Primary Prevention	Assisted Living	(Hussain et al., 2015)	J	A platform aimed to monitor health of the elderly and disabled person and provide them with a service-oriented emergency response in case of abnormal health condition.	Activity (smartphone), ECG and GPS	E	China	D2G	-
Primary Prevention	Assisted Living	(Basanta et al., 2016)	P	The IoT system increases accessibility, efficiency, and also lower the health expenses to improve the comfort and safety as well as management of daily routines of an elderly life.	BP, blood sugar, heart rate, body temperature and body weight	E	Taiwan	D2G	The symptom checker needs to be optimized.
Primary Prevention	Assisted Living	(H.-T. Wu & Tsai, 2018)	J	This study uses the beacon device to position the location of elderly people in their residence and alerts if any unusual behavior is detected.	Heart rate and location sensors	E	Taiwan	D2C	System need to be installed in home environments of elderly people and update it according to their feedback.
Primary Prevention	Assisted Living	(Pham et al., 2018)	J	A Cloud-Based Smart Home Environment for home healthcare for providing contextual information to health data that can help better understand caretaker's health status.	ECG (smart garment), blood oxygen concentration (Pulse oximeter), respiration rate, audio (acoustic sensor), and motion (smart watch), human activity (IMU).	A/E	USA	D2G	No alert system and low battery life.
Primary Prevention	Assisted Living	(Wan et al., 2018)	J	The WISE (Wearable IoT-cloud-Based health monitoring system), using body area sensor network for real-time personal health monitoring.	Heartbeat, body temperature and BP sensors	A/E	China	D2G	Sensor data filtering mechanism and sophisticated data transmission need be addressed.
Primary Prevention	Assisted Living	(Md. A. Rahman & Hossain, 2019)	J	A virtual caregiver (VCareGiver) as a cyber-physical smart home (CPSH) companion to support the daily life activities of elderly people through their gestures.	Gesture recognition (MYO arm band, Kinect 2.0 and LEAP)	E	Saudi Arabia	D2C	As a product, it needs to go through a lot of cycles of validity such as privacy, performance testing, reliability, ease of use, etc.
Primary Prevention	Assisted Living	(Mincolelli et al., 2019)	J	An assistive IoT ecosystem, which provides a customizable healthcare service to the elderly and a home care management system to their caregivers.	No specific device mentioned	E	Italy	D2G	Real-time implementation of the system would give more insights for understanding the design features.

continued on following page

Table 8. Continued

Primary healthcare activity	Secondary. healthcare activity	Article	Paper type	Contribution	Sensor/ Measurement	Target Group	Country	Comm. model	Limitations
Primary Prevention	Assisted Living	(Al-Khafajiy et al., 2019)	J	This study proposes a smart healthcare monitoring system, which can observe elderly people remotely by tracking a person's physiological data to detect specific disorders which can aid in Early Intervention Practices.	Blood oxygen saturation, skin temperature and heart-rate sensors	E	UK	D2G	There is scope for extending the study to include machine learning techniques and other sensors to train the data collected and predict the patient behavior.
Primary Prevention	Child Health	(Nyasulu, 2016)	P	An IoT architecture for monitoring of growth and vital parameters of under-five children, alerts sent for under-weight cases or abnormal readings of vital parameters.	height (ultrasonic sensor), body temperature, respiration rate, and pulse rate.	C	UK	D2G	Only one sensor node is utilized for ambient monitoring and can include growth monitoring as well, using the vital parameters.
Primary Prevention	Child Health	(Kadarina & Priambodo, 2017)	P	This IoT system is designed to enable remote monitoring and early detection by medical specialist and physicians at the clinic for mother and child preventive care.	Weight, height, heartbeat, breathing and temperature.	C	Indonesia	D2G	There is still scope for development for each module of the personal mobile system for mother and child.
Primary Prevention	Disease Management	(Chen et al., 2017)	M	Proposed system consists of washable smart clothing, which consists of sensors to collect users' physiological data and receive the analysis results of users' health and emotional status.	ECG, ambient data (not mentioned), physiological data (not mentioned).	C/A/E	China	D2G	-
Primary Prevention	Disease Management	(Enshaeifar et al., 2018)	J	Technology integrated health management uses a set of machine-learning techniques and healthcare professionals to generate notifications regarding the well-being of the patients.	humidity, temperature conditions, appliance usage, BP and pulse.	E	UK	D2G	-
Primary Prevention	Disease Management	(Onasanya et al., 2019)	J	A Smart Saskatchewan Healthcare System based on IoT in the context of four services, namely: business analytics and cloud services, cancer care services, emergency services, and operational services.	No specific device mentioned	A/E	Canada	D2G	A lot of scope to increase the health services (limited services).
Primary Prevention	Disease Management	(Rghioui et al., 2019)	J	This study proposes a patient monitoring system based on Internet of Things (IoT) and a diagnostic prediction tool for diabetic patients.	Blood glucose sensor	A	Morocco	D2G	The solution is solely based on the blood glucose sensor values, integration of additional sensors could improve the scope of the objective.

continued on following page

Table 8. Continued

Primary healthcare activity	Secondary healthcare activity	Article	Paper type	Contribution	Sensor/ Measurement	Target Group	Country	Comm. model	Limitations
Primary Prevention	Fall Prevention	(Aljahdali et al., 2018)	P	A smart assistive walker device for frail & visually impaired people to reduce the risk of falling and the costly emergency interventions and hospitalizations.	Speaker, location sensor and proximity sensor (IR sensor)	A/E	Saudi Arabia	D2G	Lack of alert or notification feature in the system.
Primary Prevention	Preventive Monitoring	(Ikram et al., 2015)	P	Monitor the health of footballers and reduce the occurrence of adverse health conditions using embedded sensing devices.	Human activity, ECG, BP and amount of oxygen in blood.	A	Australia	D2G	Framework will need to be adjusted when used in real situations or simulated on TinyOS.
Primary Prevention	Preventive Monitoring	(Kang et al., 2015)	P	Inference system is proposed, so that life-threatening situations can be prevented in advance based on a short- and long-term health status prediction.	BP, Pulse, Temperature and Breathing	A	Australia	D2G	security and privacy of the generated data need to be addressed.
Primary Prevention	Preventive Monitoring	(Krishnan et al., 2016)	P	IoT based patient health monitoring system to follow up with patients in rural parts of India. Real-time vital monitoring and alerts sent to doctor when anomalies are detected.	Body temperature, heart rate, BP and pulse oximetry	A	India	D2G	Miniaturization of sensors and their wearability need to be addressed along with the security and privacy issues of the data.
Primary Prevention	Preventive Monitoring	(Bhatia & Sood, 2017)	J	Intelligent healthcare framework to analyze real time health conditions during workouts and predict probabilistic health state vulnerability.	Redmi Mi wrist band (heart rate, number of steps, calorie burnt and distance covered), 3D accelerometer, BodyMedia sensor (skin and ambient temperature and Galvanic Skin Response), Zephyr (Breath rate and skin temperature), cosmed calorimeter (Respiration rate), other ambient sensors (Noise, Humidity, room temperature and other ambient sensors).	A	India	D2C	-

continued on following page

Table 8. Continued

Primary healthcare activity	Secondary healthcare activity	Article	Paper type	Contribution	Sensor/ Measurement	Target Group	Country	Comm. model	Limitations
Primary Prevention	Preventive Monitoring	(Mora et al., 2017)	J	A distributed framework based on the internet of things paradigm is proposed for monitoring human biomedical signals in activities involving physical exertion.	ECG, Physical exertion time, ambient temperature, ambient humidity, altitude, and distance covered.	A	Switzerland	D2G	Technology and formalization of the domain knowledge are the limitations and framework will need to be adjusted when used in real situations.
Primary Prevention	Preventive Monitoring	(S. F. Khan, 2017)	P	Proposes a complete monitoring existence cycle and effective healthcare monitoring system designed by using the IoT and RFID tags for weighting the health status of patients in medical emergencies.	ECG, Body temperature, BP, Blood Glucose, Motion and Relay (alert).	A/E	Oman	D2G	-
Primary Prevention	Preventive Monitoring	(Nedungadi et al., 2017)	J	This patient-centric integrated healthcare system is designed to manage the overall health of villagers with real-time health monitoring of patients and to offer guidance on preventive care at an affordable price.	ECG, Pulse, BP, Blood glucose, Oxygen in blood, Weight scale and Body temperature.	A	India	D2C	Need to evaluate the system with real-time implementation in rural villages (collaborate with health centers)
Primary Prevention	Preventive Monitoring	(Nasri & Mtibaa, 2017)	J	Smart mobile IoT healthcare system for monitoring patients' risk, using a smart phone and 5G.	Body temperature, BP, pulse and oxygen in blood	A	Tunisia	D2G	-
Primary Prevention	Preventive Monitoring	(Neto et al., 2018)	P	Monitoring people who are part of risk groups, for example, sedentary people, using IoT technologies using physiological data by healthcare professionals to establish new activities for the user.	Accelerometer, Gyro meter, Magnetometer and ECG. (step count and calorie count)	A/E	Brazil	D2G	Improve the interface, design, and perform a case study to implement the strategy in wearable devices.
Primary Prevention	Preventive Monitoring	(Subhedar et al., 2018)	P	This system provides a reliable, accurate and real time data of patients continuously, and transmits the prioritized data (depending on patient situation) during emergency.	Temperature sensor, accelerometer, and pulse sensor.	A/E	India	D2C	System can be designed and trained for specific disease by monitoring variety of body parameters and integrating medical and engineering knowledge.
Primary Prevention	Preventive Monitoring	(Saha et al., 2018)	P	The proposed system generates an alarm to provide the prescribed medicine to the patient in time.	Heart rate, blood pressure, respiration, temperature, blood sugar level, movement of the patient (IR sensor) and saline level.	A/E	India	D2G	Implementation of the system using mobile application would be more efficient.

continued on following page

Table 8. Continued

Primary healthcare activity	Secondary healthcare activity	Article	Paper type	Contribution	Sensor/ Measurement	Target Group	Country	Comm. model	Limitations
Primary Prevention	Preventive Monitoring	(Rahmani et al., 2018)	J	IoT-based remote health monitoring system with enhanced overall system intelligence, energy efficiency, mobility, performance, interoperability, security, and reliability.	ECG, BP, Oxygen saturation, Body temperature, Respiration rate, Ambient (humidity, light and temperature), step count and human activity.	A/E	Finland	D2G	-
Primary Prevention	Preventive Monitoring	(I. Khan et al., 2019)	P	IoT-based, intelligent health monitoring system which continuously monitors patient's health parameters to get feedback from doctors accordingly.	BP, heartbeat, body temperature, Pi camera and ECG sensor	A/E	South Korea	D2G	Lack of alert system and can include patient - doctor communication using camera.
Primary Prevention	Preventive Monitoring	(Hadi et al., 2019)	J	a system for that employs big data from the outpatient's medical records and body connected medical IoT sensors to predict the likelihood of a life-threatening medical condition such as an imminent stroke.	BP, sugar level, cholesterol, and smoking rate	A	UK	D2C	Real-time implementation of the system can address more limitations such as decision-making entity and routing issues.
Primary Prevention	Preventive Monitoring	(Nduka et al., 2019)	P	This study proposes a Remote Health Monitoring (RHM) system that can sense certain human vital signs which is connected in real time environment that is further designed in a way that physicians can view patient's vital sign reading in real-time irrespective of their geographical location.	Temperature sensor, Heartbeat sensor and respiration sensor.	A/E	Malaysia	D2G	There is scope for extending the study to include machine learning techniques and other sensors to train the data collected and predict the patient behavior.
Primary Prevention	Preventive Monitoring	(Haghi et al., 2020)	J	This study developed an innovative wrist-worn prototype for ambient monitoring and a flexible IoT gateway.	Gas sensor, UV sensor, noise sensor, pressure sensor, temperature sensor, accelerometer, gyroscope, and magnetometer.	C/A/E	USA	D2G	-
Primary Prevention	Preventive Monitoring	(T. Wu et al., 2020)	J	Designed a compact wearable sensor patch is presented for measurements of different physiological signals for remote health monitoring	BP sensor, ECG, PPG, heart rate, and body temperature sensors.	A	Australia	D2G	More edge computing functions can be utilized on the gateway for the proposed healthcare platform.

continued on following page

Table 8. Continued

Primary healthcare activity	Secondary. healthcare activity	Article	Paper type	Contribution	Sensor/ Measurement	Target Group	Country	Comm. model	Limitations
Primary Prevention	Preventive Monitoring	(Choi et al., 2020)	J	This study proposes an ubiquitous central monitoring system that links an existing, personal use, unobtrusive measurement system to cloud-based systems via WIFI transmission and simultaneously collects, stores, and displays the data from multiple devices.	On bed strip sensor	A	South Korea	D2G	There is scope for extending the study to include machine learning techniques and other physiological sensors to train the data collected.
Secondary prevention	Assisted Living	(Pace et al., 2019)	P	INTER-Health (Horizon 2020) European project is focused on providing value added assisted living mobile health services in terms of faster detection and correction of wrong lifestyles or high-risk critical situations.	Body weight, BP, physical activity and eating habits.	A/E	Italy	D2G	-
Secondary prevention	Assisted Living	(Addante et al., 2019)	J	This work is focused on the use of combined hardware and software technologies, enabling the IoT, in order to monitor people suffering from sarcopenia by offering a high value-added service in the field of AAL.	EMG sensor, strength sensor, accelerometer, and gyroscope.	E	Italy	D2G	This study can introduce human activity recognition features for improving the proposed IoT solution.
Secondary prevention	Disease Management	(Y. Liu et al., 2014)	P	eBPlatform, an information system based on IoT for homecare of the non-communicable disease patients.	BP, blood sugar and ECG measurement	A/E	China	D2G	-
Secondary prevention	Disease Management	(La et al., 2015)	P	a cloud platform which helps to enable personal medical diagnosis and prognosis over the network.	body temperature, blood pulse, blood oxygen, and blood pressure	A	South Korea	D2G	-
Secondary prevention	Disease Management	(Kario et al., 2017)	J	A multisensory home and ambulatory blood pressure (BP) monitoring system for monitoring 24-h central and brachial BP variability concurrent with physical activity (PA), temperature, and atmospheric pressure.	BP, Temperature, Illumination, Humidity and Physical Activity.	A/E	Japan	D2G	Could try predicting the BP surges using historic data and risk conditions.
Secondary prevention	Disease Management	(Abawajy & Hassan, 2017)	M	A persuasive patient health monitoring system is tested with a case study for real-time monitoring of a patient suffering from congestive heart failure using ECG.	ECG	A/E	Australia	D2C	The proposed system needs to be tested by implementing in real-life.

continued on following page

Table 8. Continued

Primary healthcare activity	Secondary. healthcare activity	Article	Paper type	Contribution	Sensor/ Measurement	Target Group	Country	Comm. model	Limitations
Secondary prevention	Disease Management	(Hayek et al., 2020)	J	This study proposes an IoT based application that targets epileptic patients working in an industrial environment to capture continuously the vital signs of the patient for problem detection.	EEG, ECG, BP sensor, accelerometer, and gyroscope.	A	Germany	D2D	The whole system needs to be tested with epileptic patients for sustainability.
Secondary prevention	Emergency Health Services	(Rathore et al., 2016)	J	A real-time medical emergency response system for analysis and decision making based on vital signs data.	Heart rate, respiration rate, arterial pressure, oxygen saturation, activity recognition.	A	South Korea	D2G	-
Secondary prevention	Emergency Health Services	(Gusev et al., 2017)	P	eHealth IoT solution to manage the consequences after a natural or any other disaster as a kind of a technology-enabled crisis management.	Body temperature, heart rate, ECG scan and respiratory rate	A	Macedonia	D2C	The real-time implementation and challenges associated to the designed solution need to be addressed.
Secondary prevention	Fall Prevention	(Luo et al., 2012)	J	Design and implementation of fall detection system called SensFall	Movement (IR sensor)	A/E	China	D2G	-
Secondary prevention	Fall Prevention	(Manatarinat et al., 2019)	P	Narrow band –IoT device to assist medical patients, the elderly, and disabled people that are susceptible to falling. Detect Falls and alerts required people with location information.	GPS, heart rate and activity (accelerometer and gyroscope)	E	Thailand	D2G	-
Secondary prevention	Fall Prevention	(Gutierrez-Madronal, La Blunda, et al., 2019)	J	Analysis of the fall-involved events based on an IoT prototype, the event patterns to detect the falls and their test using the IoT-test event generator (IoT-TEG) tool.	3D accelerometer.	E	Spain	D2G	Various post-fall postures need to be analyzed, security and privacy issues need to be addressed.
Tertiary prevention	Assisted Living	(Corno et al., 2016)	P	A system capable of supporting the daily activities of healthcare assistants that operate in assisted living facilities for people with physical or cognitive disabilities.	Smart Watch	E	Italy	D2G	People with severe physical disabilities hardly interact with wearable and mobile devices.
Tertiary prevention	Child Health	(Al-Taee et al., 2017)	J	eHealth platform incorporating humanoid robots to support an emerging multidimensional care approach for the treatment of diabetes in children.	Blood glucose monitor, BP, pulse rate and weight scale.	C	UK	D2G	Can enhance the cognitive capabilities of the virtual objects to improve the system.

continued on following page

Table 8. Continued

Primary healthcare activity	Secondary healthcare activity	Article	Paper type	Contribution	Sensor/Measurement	Target Group	Country	Comm. model	Limitations
Tertiary prevention	Rehabilitation Therapy	(Vukicevic et al., 2016)	J	A telerehabilitation system that uses wearable muscle sensor and Microsoft Kinect to create interactive personalized physical therapy that can be carried out at home.	Muscle sensor, Kinect (sound sensor)	A	Serbia	D2G	-
Tertiary prevention	Rehabilitation Therapy	(Jiang et al., 2017)	P	An IoT-based upper limb rehabilitation assessment system for stroke survivors based on wireless sensing sub-system, data cloud, computing cloud and software based on Android platform.	Accelerometer, ECG, and body temperature.	A	China	D2G	The sensing sub system and computing ability can be improved.
Tertiary prevention	Rehabilitation Therapy		J	Multisensory therapy (m-Therapy) framework, in which multiple gesture-tracking sensors and environmental sensors are used to collect therapy and ambient data to guide them in therapy exercises.	Audio, video, text, motion (Kinect) and hand gestures (Leap).	A	Saudi Arabia	D2C	User interface is not tested, other technologies such as augmented reality and virtual reality can be explored.
Tertiary prevention	Rehabilitation Therapy	(Buzachis et al., 2018; Md. A. Rahman & Hossain, 2018)	P	A closed-loop osmotic computing flow model applied to a gamified cognitive rehabilitation which allows the patient to carry out physical and cognitive rehabilitation therapies using a natural user interface based on Microsoft Kinect. eas.	Motion (Kinect sensor)	A	Italy	D2G	The system performance needs to be evaluated.
Tertiary prevention	Rehabilitation Therapy	(Alexandre & Postolache, 2018)	P	smart gloves to be used for natural interactions with therapeutic serious games for upper limb rehabilitation, and to perform training sessions for hands and fingers motor rehabilitation.	Accelerometer, gyro meter, Magnetometer (IMU), gesture/force (piezo-resistive force sensors) and head rotation.	A/E	Portugal	D2C	Specific games can be built with respect to the therapy or rehabilitation.
Tertiary prevention	Rehabilitation Therapy	(Abdur Rahman et al., 2019)	J	This study proposes a blockchain and off-chain-based framework, which will allow multiple medical and ambient intelligent Internet of Things sensors to capture the QoL information from one's home environment and securely share it with their community of interest.	EEG and EMG tracker, body joint tracker, hand joint tracker, and eye tracker.	A	Saudi Arabia	D2G	There is a need to implement the framework in clinical trials for real life data collection to assess the sustainability of the framework for widespread usage.

continued on following page

95

Table 8. Continued

Primary healthcare activity	Secondary. healthcare activity	Article	Paper type	Contribution	Sensor/ Measurement	Target Group	Country	Comm. model	Limitations
Tertiary prevention	Rehabilitation Therapy	(Bisio et al., 2019)	P	This study proposes a SmartPANTS framework, an IoT-based wireless system specifically designed for the rehabilitation of lower limbs to be employed during the physical therapy for patients recovering from a brain stroke condition.	IMU sensors and pressure sensors	A	Italy	D2G	Additional investigation needs to be done on possible tensor decomposition and regression techniques to the purpose of estimating the distribution of the patient's load only from accelerometer and gyroscope data.
Tertiary prevention	Rehabilitation Therapy	(Jiang, 2020)	J	This study proposes a sports rehabilitation monitoring system based on wearable sensors and IoT technology.	Motion position sensors, myoelectric sensor, temperature, and ECG.	A	China	D2G	-
Tertiary prevention	Rehabilitation Therapy	(de la Iglesia et al., 2020)	J	This study presents a low-cost exoskeleton for the elbow that is connected to a Context-Aware architecture a VR system with which, the patient can perform rehabilitation exercises in an interactive way.	Exoskeleton sensors (load cell, engine position, battery level) and e-health sensors (pulse sensor).	A	Spain	D2G	The solution has a complex backend configuration and would be more sustainable if a greater number of patients are included in the study.
Diagnosis	Assisted Living	(Jara et al., 2012)	P	Proposes a knowledge acquisition and management architecture for continuous monitored vital signs, the capabilities for diagnosis and detection of anomalies.	ECG and oxygen saturation (pulse oximeter)	A/E	Spain	D2G	overload for a light version of IPv6 for Wireless Sensor Networks need to be considered for improving the system.
Diagnosis	Disease Management	(Azimi et al., 2017)	J	Proposes a hierarchical computing architecture for continuous remote health monitoring and tested on a case study focusing on arrhythmia detection for patients suffering from Cardiovascular diseases.	ECG	A	Finland	D2G	-
Diagnosis	Disease Management	(Mumtaj & Umamakeswari, 2017)	P	The proposed system monitors the patients' physiological parameters as well as supports the medical professionals to diagnose the diseases as early as possible.	Temperature and ECG.	A/E	India	D2C	security and privacy of the generated data need to be addressed.
Diagnosis	Disease Management	(Muhammad et al., 2017)	M	a voice pathology detection system is proposed inside the monitoring framework (Easy to use) and an extreme learning machine classifier to detect the pathology with high accuracy.	voice, body temperature, electrocardiogram, and ambient humidity.	A	Saudi Arabia	D2G	Can integrate different input modalities of the voice for dynamic scalability.

continued on following page

Table 8. Continued

Primary healthcare activity	Secondary healthcare activity	Article	Paper type	Contribution	Sensor/Measurement	Target Group	Country	Comm. model	Limitations
Diagnosis	Disease Management	(Sood & Mahajan, 2017)	J	IoT and fog-based healthcare system is proposed to identify and control the outbreak of Chikungunya virus	Ambient temperature, humidity, precipitation, atmospheric pressure, wind speed and direction (climate meter), body temperature (touch free thermometer), GPS and mosquito sensor (BG counter).	A	India	D2C	-
Diagnosis	Disease Management	(N. H. Hassan et al., 2018)	J	A conceptual IoT-based patient monitoring sensor were proposed comprising three different sensors to further work with analytical tools for dengue prediction pattern.	Temperature, humidity, rainfall, air quality, body temperature, heart rate and BP.	A	Malaysia	D2G	Need to cover in depth architectural elements of the IoT design and implement in healthcare industry.
Diagnosis	Disease Management	(Bae & Lee, 2018)	J	sensor-based urine and feces separating toilet, which applies various scenarios and analyses of the urine components for diagnosing health conditions to transmit data from the smart toilet to the user.	IR sensors, color sensing (RGB sensor).	A	South Korea	D2G	-
Diagnosis	Disease Management	(M. K. Hassan et al., 2019)	J	A hybrid real-time remote monitoring framework is proposed to predict the health status of patients suffering from BP disorders accurately.	Heart rate, BP, Respiratory rate, Oxygen saturation, Room Temperature, and activity recognition	A/E	Egypt	S2S	The need of usage of HRMM in monitoring different illnesses, the observation of context domains that may affect patients' vital signs, and the adoption of different bio-inspired algorithms instead of WOA.
Diagnosis	Disease Management	(Asghari et al., 2019a)	J	A medical monitoring scheme for effective disease diagnosis from IoT devices and medical records to offer composite medical prescription.	Respiratory rate, Heart rate, BP, Oral temperature, oxygen saturation and blood sugar	A	Iran	D2G	The statistical extents can be developed from the suggested architecture in deployment and implementing in the real physical environment.
Diagnosis	Disease Management	(B. Li et al., 2019)	J	A cloud based wearable IoT sensor system which can measure an asthma patient's exposure to aldehydes, a known class of airway irritants, in real-life settings.	Temperature, relative humidity, and aldehyde level.	A	USA	D2G	Real-time implementation of sensor for personalized asthma management.

continued on following page

Table 8. Continued

Primary healthcare activity	Secondary healthcare activity	Article	Paper type	Contribution	Sensor/ Measurement	Target Group	Country	Comm. model	Limitations
Diagnosis	Disease Management	(Sood & Mahajan, 2019)	J	IoT-fog-based healthcare system is proposed for continuous monitoring and analysis of BP statistics to predict hypertensive users.	Activity (accelerometer), GPS, room temperature, air quality, noise level, humidity, BP, heart rate, anxiety level, restlessness, diet type, diet quantity, cholesterol, and lipoprotein	A/E	India	D2C	Security and privacy of the generated data need to be addressed.
Diagnosis	Disease Management	(Abdel-Basset et al., 2019)	J	This study proposes a Remote Health Monitoring (RHM) system that can sense certain human vital signs such as, temperature, respiration, and heartbeat (pulse) which is connected in real time environment.	Temperature sensor, Heartbeat sensor and respiration sensor	A	Egypt	D2G	-
Diagnosis	Disease Management	(Pierleoni et al., 2019)	J	This study developed a system that is appropriate for use in the real-time monitoring of neurodegenerative diseases such as Parkinson's for both outpatient diagnosis and home monitoring.	Accelerometer, gyroscope, and magnetometer.	A/E	Italy	D2G	There is scope for extending the study to include machine learning techniques to train the data collected and predict the patient behavior.
Diagnosis	Disease Management	(Vijayakumar et al., 2019)	J	This study proposes an intelligent system to detect and control the mosquito-borne diseases at the early stage using wearable and IoT sensors to gather the required information and fog computing to analyze, categorize and share medical information among the user and healthcare service providers.	Wireless mosquito sensors, Contextual sensors (location, humidity, temperature, and CO2 sensors), and physiological sensors (heartbeat, blood pressure, body temperature, humidity, and oxygen supply sensors).	A	India	D2G	An unsecured channel is employed for data transfer, a more secured channel needs to be utilized to ensure data integrity and privacy.
Diagnosis	Disease Management	(Tan & Halim, 2019)	J	This study presents the prototyping of an embedded health care monitoring system based on the IoT paradigm, and health care analytical framework for anomalies related to diabetes and kidney disease.	Body temperature, pulse rate and blood pressure sensors.	A	Malaysia	D2G	The solution needs to be verified with real time data or a clinical test for sustainability.

continued on following page

Table 8. Continued

Primary healthcare activity	Secondary. healthcare activity	Article	Paper type	Contribution	Sensor/ Measurement	Target Group	Country	Comm. model	Limitations
Diagnosis	Disease Management	(Raj, 2020)	J	This study presents an Internet-of-Things (IoT) based embedded platform to monitor and analyze the ECG of cardiac outpatients for improving healthcare services.	ECG	A	India	D2G	-
Diagnosis	Disease Management	(Puri et al., 2020)	B	This study presents a low-cost energy efficient prototype of an IoT-based glucose testing meter that can connect with cloud services.	Glucose strip and electrodes	A	Vietnam	D2G	-
Diagnosis	Disease Management	(Bhatia et al., 2020)	J	This study proposes a framework for an IoT-based smart toilet system, which enables home-based determination of Urinary Infection (UI) efficaciously for an individual to monitor his or her health on daily basis and predict UI so that precautionary measures can be taken at early stages.	Electronic hydrometer, e-urine strips, and multi-analyte sensors.	A/E	India	D2G	In the case of urine containing poop, appropriate mechanical components such as strainers and pipes must embedded to ensure enhanced performance.
Treatment	Disease Management	(Yacchirema et al., 2018a)	J	Detect and support of treatment of OSA of elderly people by monitoring multiple factors such as sleep environment, sleep status, physical activities, and physiological parameters as well as the use of open data available in smart cities.	Body weight scale, heart rate sensor, MEMS sensor (sleep environment), LM 393 (snoring intensity) and Fitbit flex bangle (physical activity and sleep status).	A/E	Ecuador	D2G	Integrate the system with other solutions applied to the healthcare domain derived from Inter-IoT project to facilitate the delivery of elderly smart healthcare services.
Treatment	Disease Management	(Yacchirema et al., 2018b)	J	Detect events that might endanger elderly health and act on it, improve the health professionals' decision making to monitor and guide sleep apnea treatment, as well as improving elderly people's quality of life.	Pulse, humidity, temperature, and snoring (sound sensor), step count, weight, sleep stages (activity sensors such as gyroscope, accelerometer, GPS and actinometrical).	A/E	Spain	D2G	ML techniques can be utilized to predict to predict sleep apnea.
Treatment	Disease Management	(Ma et al., 2019)	J	An IoT based fatigue detection and recovery system is introduced in this paper to help alleviate muscle fatigue.	EMG sensor and PWM sensor	A/E	Spain	D2G	There is a need to integrate additional sensors in determining muscle fatigue

continued on following page

Table 8. Continued

Primary healthcare activity	Secondary healthcare activity	Article	Paper type	Contribution	Sensor/ Measurement	Target Group	Country	Comm. model	Limitations
Treatment	Medication Management	(Yang et al., 2014)	J	This paper proposes an open-platform-based intelligent medicine box (iMedBox) with enhanced connectivity and interchangeability for the integration of devices and services.	RFID, BioPatch (ECG and Body Temperature)	E	China	D2G	Non-bendable silicon chip, limited form of communication (short messages phone calls and notifications) and better user-friendly GUI.
Treatment	Medication Management	(Toh et al., 2016)	P	monitor medication adherence and detect changes in medication consumption patterns among the elderly, thus enabling timely interventions by caregivers to take place.	Normally closed Reed switch.	E	Singapore	D2G	The duration and scale of the study can be increased to more elderly participants to derive both longitudinal and transversal insights in medication adherence.
Treatment	Medicine Management	(Latif et al., 2020)	J	This study proposes a novel approach is developed with IoT prototype of Wireless Sensor Network and Cloud based system to provide continuous monitoring of a patient's health status, ensuring timely scheduled and unscheduled medicinal dosage based on real-time patient vitals measurement, life-saving emergency prediction and communication.	ECG, pulse rate, blood pressure, body temperature, stress level, SpO2 and GPS location sensors.	A/E	Malaysia	D2G	The proposed system needs to implement in large scale for truly understanding its potential.
Treatment	Medicine Management	(Chang et al., 2020)	J	This study proposes a wearable smart-glasses-based drug pill recognition system using deep learning, named MedGlasses, for visually impaired people to improve their medication-use safety.	Wearable smart glasses, image sensor, and an AI-based intelligent drug pill recognition box	E	Taiwan	D2G	The circuit complexity of this system is complex and there is a scope for addition of other physiological sensors.
Treatment	Rehabilitation Therapy	(Suraki & Suraki, 2013)	P	assist the treatment of OCD patients, improve the behavior of the patients and to help the therapists.	No specific device mentioned	A	Iran	D2C	security and privacy of the generated data need to be addressed.

Note: The paper type is represented as follows: 'B' – Book section; 'J' – Journal; 'M' – Magazine; 'P' – Proceedings.
The target group is represented as follows: 'A' – Adults; 'C' – Children; 'E' – Elderly

Chapter 3
Artificial Intelligence, Decision–Making, 6G, and Wearable IoT:
The Next Generation´s Backbone for Digital Smart Healthcare Services

William Alberto Cruz Castañeda
https://orcid.org/0000-0002-9803-1387
Universidade Tecnológica Federal do Paraná, Brazil

ABSTRACT

Healthcare is facing challenges, such as the rising cost of care, an increase in the elderly population, and the prevalence of chronic diseases. To address these challenges, there is a need to transform healthcare from a hospital-centered to a patient-centered model focused on disease management to improve well-being. To achieve this, decentralized healthcare services are integrated with the Internet of Things and cloud technologies. As a result, cost-effective digital healthcare services have emerged. These digital services use body sensor networks and wearable devices for health monitoring, ensuring access to health data. Nevertheless, data from several digital services is difficult to handle using conventional analysis procedures. Thus, this chapter proposes small-scale and large-scale digital smart healthcare service architectures to allow autonomy and decision-making founded on artificial intelligence, multiple criteria decisions, sixth-generation communication, cloud technologies, and wearable Internet of Things for point-of-care and chronic disease management.

DOI: 10.4018/979-8-3693-5237-3.ch003

INTRODUCTION

Prevalence of chronic diseases on a global scale demands the transformation of healthcare from a hospital-centered system to a patient-centered environment focused on disease management and well-being (Bennett, et al., 2018) (World Health Organization, 2022). Healthcare systems worldwide, to face these challenges, have created decentralized health services that can provide patient care at home through support from digital health technology (DHT). Digital health is a global trend adopted to transform healthcare delivery through DHT, such as personal mobile devices, smartphones, tablets, or wearables, to monitor and manage healthcare quality. (Vansimaeys, Benamar, & Balagué, 2021) (Tsoi & Wong, 2021). The association between decentralized health service and DHT improves traditional health care delivery to redefine the patient chronic disease self-management, creating digital health services (DHS) that establish a model that promotes continuously patient-centered care as a medium of sensing, interaction, and communication everywhere. Thus, conventional healthcare services integrate ubiquitous and pervasive computing paradigms, and consequently, cost-effective and smart healthcare services emerge.

According to (Solanas, et al., 2014), smart health (s-health) defines the provision of health services using a context-aware network and sensing infrastructure of smart cities. Thus, a DHS provided by s-health, or a Smart Digital Health Service (SDHS), includes medical wearable devices, monitoring devices (such as digital thermometers, smart glucometers, and blood pressure monitors), the Internet of Things (IoT), wireless networks, body area networks, extensive area networks, and ambient-assisted living for health monitoring. Therefore, the SDHS aim is to provide healthcare solutions and services focused on disease prevention, diagnosis, and treatment. It ensures that healthcare resources create awareness among individuals about daily health and self-checkups to enable them to self-manage during medical emergencies (Vyas & Bhargava, 2021). A Smart Healthcare System (SHS) obtains benefits from SDHS to ensure pervasive access to health monitoring, information, and services. Integration of several SDHS into a large-scale solution brings benefits in scalability and storage together with enabling heterogeneous devices to transmit and process large amounts of data without requiring rigorous explicit human-to-human and human-to-machine interactions.

Technologies such as wearable IoT (wIoT), cloud technologies (cloud computing, fog computing, and edge computing), artificial intelligence (AI), multi-criteria decision methods, and sixth-generation (6G) communication constitute the cornerstone of large-scale SDHS at homes to implement remote services and monitor patient health. In health facilities, those technologies integrate management and collect information for assisted decision-making. With these technologies, SHS could improve the utilization of medical resources, promote self-service medical care, and make personalized medical services ubiquitous. Using wIoT and its applications could improve the quality of patient care while reducing the cost of care outside of healthcare facilities performing health maintenance and patient disease management (Iqbal, Mahgoub, Du, Leavitt, & Asghar, 2021) (Lou, Wang, Jiang, Wei, & Shen, 2020). 6G enables wireless healthcare with intelligent wIoT to transform s-health into intelligent health (i-health). Thus, SDHS will be a data-driven environment that allows machine learning (ML) or deep learning (DL) solutions in a heterogeneous and scalable network (Deng, et al., 2020).

However, collecting the data generated by wIoT devices from several SDHS is challenging with conventional computational approaches. Data will be analyzed and shared in real-time. Cloud computing offers real-time storage and processing. Fog computing optimizes performance by placing analytic services closer to where they're needed, reducing distance, and improving speed and overall network performance. Edge computing offers solutions associated with data acquisition generated in SDHS, transferring the processing power, intelligence, and communication capabilities directly into devices (Atieh, 2021). As a result, AI systems (machine and deep learning solutions) analyze, learn, and interpret data by recognizing underlying patterns and trends. The goal is to identify patterns in data and perform inferences using those patterns learned (Wang, et al., 2021).

Nevertheless, if considering the high growth of healthcare data generated and flowing into a large-scale SHS is appropriated to devise methodologies for better decision-making implemented based on existing values, multiple criteria decision analysis, and AI methods, which are capable enough to deal with the data from its origination to processing and from processing to analysis and decision-making.

This chapter aims to guide researchers or professionals to the fundamentals of an SDHS as a next-generation healthcare delivery service. The chapter describes an integrated architecture based on AI, multi-criteria decision methods, 6G communication, wIoT, and cloud technologies to establish large-scale and small-scale architectures to allow autonomy and decision-making for point-of-care and chronic disease management in long-term services. Its look first related works section describes current scientific literature to understand the evolution of all these technologies into healthcare. Afterward, the next-generation healthcare service architecture section describes a unified architecture for small-scale and large-scale SDHS. Finally, the conclusion and further research directions highlight the key challenges and opportunities.

SCIENTIFIC RELATED WORKS

In healthcare, currently, diagnostic tools offer information that is essentially a snapshot in time. The next great challenge for managing chronic diseases is prevention through patient monitoring of physiological parameters continuously, under natural physiological conditions, and in any environment (Vansimaeys, Benamar, & Balagué, 2021) (Nittas, et al., 2023). However, chronic disease is just a component of complex comorbidities characterized by cardiovascular diseases, pulmonary hypertension, ischemic heart disease, heart failure, atrial fibrillation, lung cancer, osteoporosis, depression, anxiety, metabolic syndrome, diabetes, and systemic effects. Integrating conventional care services with ubiquitous and pervasive computing paradigms can provide a model of s-health services and systems that include data collection from on-body sensors to facilitate continuous patient-centered care of long-term events as a medium of sensing, interaction, and communication everywhere. The essential elements in SHS include digital and mobile health services, electronic records, smart homes, and connected intelligent medical devices. Thus, cloud computing technologies, IoT, AI, and 6G networks enable SHS to be manageable and functional (Vyas & Bhargava, 2021).

(Akhtar, Haleem, & Javaid, 2024) analyses medical 4.0 development using bibliometric analysis of scientific publications. Medical 4.0 involves the integration of digital technologies, data analytics, automation, and AI into healthcare practices. Key elements include digital health records, telemedicine, IoT, big data analytics, AI, robotics, pharmaceutical innovation, patient engagement, and cybersecurity. The study identifies that the enabling technologies are AI Applications, big data analytics, IoT, and nanotechnology. (Iqbal, Mahgoub, Du, Leavitt, & Asghar, 2021) review different types of wearable devices used in healthcare. It also highlights their efficacy in monitoring different diseases and applications for diagnostic and treatment purposes. Include different noninvasive wearables (skin-based, biofluidic-based) and applications for drug delivery systems.

(Raoof & Durai, 2022) summarize the technologies for an SHS. AI technologies such as ML and DL algorithms work with structured and unstructured data that provide different healthcare problem solutions. ML and DL achieved enhanced performance for disease identification, disease prediction, medical image diagnosis, personalized medication, robotic surgeries, cancer detection, oral disease detection, and classification tasks. IoT models work well for health monitoring and reporting the patient's condition, where a general IoT architecture comprises the layers of data management, application, middleware, network, and perception. Cloud computing analyzes, stores, and processes data to provide services to manage real-time software and applications. Cloud-based IoT system characteristics include cloud data storage, processing and analysis, data cleaning, and emergency alerts. Fog computing, considered a platform to support IoT, is another technology that extends cloud services in a decentralized computing environment.

(Tuli, et al., 2019) describe and explain a conceptual model that brings together all technologies that mark the Industry 4.0 revolution to provide a single end-to-end integrated solution for healthcare. The main components of this model leverage state-of-the-art technologies in IoT devices, cloud technologies, and AI. The IoT comprises devices with associated healthcare sensors and actuators. These devices collect data and package them to the IoT-Fog broker. IoT-Edge Broker is the core component of the model, which is responsible for perceiving the context of IoT devices and application scenarios, monitoring the performance of Edge nodes, resource discovery, and planning for advanced resource configuration. At this level, DL models, databases, and services maintain the integrity of the sensor data and the model parameters.

(Pal, Saha, Sen, Saif, & Biswas, 2022) describe cloud and edge-based s-health architectures that consist of a sensor layer, edge layer, cloud layer, network layer, and medical layer. One of them is a system that comprises an implementation layer (sensors that separate the data from its storage and analysis), an evaluation layer (guarantees the improvement of the medical administrations), a feedback layer, and a security layer of the data client as well as medical services staff. Another one is a hybrid model with a wireless body area network. This model consists of a perception layer that collects patient-related data, a network layer that sends the data, and a cloud layer that stores and deals with the information for different medical services applications.

(Tian, et al., 2019) list the key technologies that support s-health from the point of view of multiple participants (doctors, patients, hospitals, research institutions) involving multiple dimensions (disease prevention and monitoring, diagnosis and treatment, hospital management, health decision-making, and medical research). Define that information technologies, such as IoT, mobile Internet, cloud computing, big data, 5G, microelectronics, AI, and biotechnology constitute the cornerstone of s-health. From the patient's perspective, wearable devices monitor their health, seek medical assistance through virtual assistants, and use remote homes to implement remote services. From the doctor's perspective, intelligent clinical decision support systems assist and improve diagnosis. From the hospital's perspective, the technology manages materials and supports decision-making. From the research institutions' perspective, it is possible to implement ML techniques to find suitable subjects using big data.

(Quy, Hau, Anh, & Ngoc, 2022) present a common architectural framework based on fog computing for Internet of Health Things applications. The architecture consists of three layers: the thing layer, the fog layer, and the cloud layer. The Thing layer includes end-user devices such as sensors, wearable IoT devices,

Arduino motherboards, and actuators to collect body data. The Fog layer involves the internet gateway, local router, and fog servers. This layer communicates and transfers data between the thing and cloud layers. The Cloud layer includes servers with storage, processing, and analysis capabilities that help medical staff make treatment decisions for patients.

(Seng, Ang, & Ngharamike, 2022) inspect recent developments in AI and IoT architectures, techniques, and hardware platforms; sensors, devices, and energy approaches; communication and networking; and applications. The study also discusses the association of smart sensors, edge computing, and software-defined networks as enabling technologies. (Singh, Mallesha, Vijayaragavan, Sureshbabu, & Alsekait, 2022) explain the integration of AI with IoT in a medical services framework and its effect on a few clinical fields using 6G technology and DL techniques. (Onakpojeruo, Al-Turjman, Mustapha, Altrjman, & Ozsahin, 2022) summarize the architecture, roles, and trends of AI and cloud computing in current medical and healthcare applications. Cloud technologies involve federation, edge, fog, and mobile computing interaction and trends into delivery models, smart-working models, compliance/security, and innovation/application development. Cloud-smart working models involve IoT, data analysis, AI, ML, and DL.

(Upadhyay, et al., 2023) discuss and analyze the performance of IoT systems for deployment in s-health systems using cloud features. It also addressed the design of an IoT system for efficient monitoring of various healthcare issues in elderly patients and the limitations of resources, power absorption, and security when implemented in different devices. The survey of (Popov, et al., 2022) explores and highlights state-of-the-art digitalization of medicine and healthcare and alludes to the sharp transition while moving towards Industry 5.0. The survey also discusses the trends in digital medicine and healthcare. Detect that the ingredients of an Industry 4.0 healthcare system are IoT, 5G technology, AI, big data analytics, digital manufacturing and advanced materials processing, augmented reality and virtual reality, and wearable medical devices.

(Wang, et al., 2023) review state-of-the-art edge computing methods (for collection, transmission, and processing of health data) and wireless sensor technologies for s-health development, where big data in the cloud involves storage, retrieval, and processing. Combining cloud and s-health improves health services to solve big data and performance problems. But cloud alone is not enough. s-health services require edge networking devices to include three main aspects: acquisition, calculation, and wireless transmission technology. (Prasad, Bhavsar, & Tanwar, 2019) discusses techniques for monitoring edge and fog computing and its advantages in the healthcare system. Propose an architecture that consists of four components. Sensor data which sense and communicate signals from patients' bodies to the control room. Smart e-health network gateway that forms the fog and receives the data from different networks. Backend system that implements storage and data analytics. Smart e-health at the fog level that performs local pre-processing of the sensor data.

Multiple healthcare domains face problems for which there are no mono-causal solutions because there are no known possible paths due to the numerous multidimensional variables involved. AI as a solution requires a large amount of data to mimic human decisions. (Liao, He, Wu, Wu, & Bausys, 2023) present the application of AI techniques in multi-criteria decision-making (MCDM). (Ali, Hussain, Nazir, Khan, & Khan, 2023) explore the integration of ML and MCDM in the medical field. The objective is to analyze state-of-the-art research methods used in intelligent decision support systems to identify their application areas, the significance of decision support systems, and the methods, approaches, frameworks, or algorithms exploited to solve complex problems. Results of the study show that the AI algorithms and MCDM methods used in the medical field are long-short-term-memory (LSTM) based anomaly detection algorithms, logistic classifiers, TOPSIS, naïve Bayes algorithm, support vector machine (SVM), artificial neural network (ANN), Model of Original Multi-objective Decision-making (MODM), Analytical Hierarchy Process (AHP), genetic support vector machines (GSVM), and ELECTRE II method.

The research works of (Gupta, Saini, & Verma, 2022) (Shankar, Perumal, & Gupta, 2021) include healthcare solutions with ML and Informatics. The authors present AI and IoT-based solutions for medical image analysis, medical big-data processing, and disease predictions. The effective integration of AI and IoT in the healthcare sector avoids unplanned downtime, improves operating efficiency, en-ables new products and services, and increases risk management. (Vyas, Upadhyaya, Bhargava, & Shukla, 2023) explain the concepts and issues in edge AI and the future developments with ML, DL, IoT, and blockchain in healthcare. (Nijhawan & Bhatia, 2023) establish a generic edge-IoT s-health architecture with three levels. First, IoT body sensors at the edge node level perform low-level processing. Second, fog nodes collect data from IoT field sensors and edge devices. Third, servers and stores local processing, where information is captured and stored on the cloud.

The work of (Baker & Xiang, 2023) explores the field of the AI of Things (AIoT) for healthcare to establish a unified architecture, including sensors and devices, communication technologies, and cross-layer AI. The AIoT architecture consists of a three-layer computational hierarchy (embedded computing layer, edge computing layer, cloud computing layer) and application layer, which includes a variety of healthcare domains that will utilize AIoT. This scientific literature indicates a general acceptance of IoT, cloud technologies, AI, and 6G as tools across the community that reflects a general awareness of the state-of-the-art to assist and support s-health services and systems.

In this fashion, is proposed a technological architecture establishing small-scale and large-scale digital s-health services that allow autonomy and decision-making for point-of-care and chronic disease management in long-term services founded on AI, MCDM, 6G communication, wIoT, and cloud technologies.

NEXT GENERATION HEALTHCARE DELIVERY SERVICE ARCHITECTURE

The proposed unified architecture for SDHS establishes fundamental technologies such as AI, MCDM, 6G communication, cloud, and wIoT. As a result, these technologies deliver health care everywhere with a small-scale and large-scale substructure where the technologies are intertwined to construct an advanced infrastructure. WIoT and AI proliferation require real-time learning and inference in a small-scale technological environment. The 6G communication and cloud technologies allow data transmission. AI and MCDM services could leverage this infrastructure to fully unleash the potential of cloud technology related to data and computing capability in a large-scale technological environment. Easy deployment is essential to attach new environments. Then, 6G and edge computing allow deployment of large-scale environments with service migration and resource converges.

Small-scale Architecture

Oriented 6G technologies such as long-range low-power communications, ultra-reliable low-latency communications, and in-network intelligent computing services accelerated the development of smart wearables and personal ecosystems. These fundamental technologies can be used for health care delivery at a small scale through two elements to encompass autonomy and mobility: wearable data acquisition and edge-AI. Figure 1 depicts the small-scale architecture and the element's interaction.

Figure 1. Small-scale smart digital health-care service architecture to allow autonomy and mobility

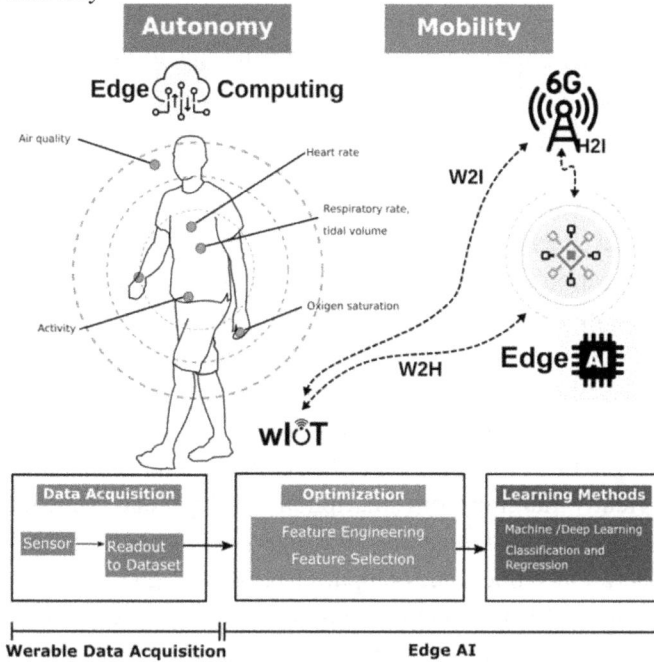

A set of sensors for disease management (heart rate, respiratory rate, tidal volume, oxygen saturation, blood pressure, air quality, bio-impedance, and movement or vibration for activity measurements) involves the implementation of wearable sensors for data transmission with body sensor networks that make use of 6G communication to send to an edge-AI device these data. Since the 6G infrastructure has a convenient medium for wIoT devices to access the network, small-scale environments exploit these facilities to establish their interconnections through three topologies: wearable-to-wearable (W2W), wearable-to-Hub (W2H), and wearable-to-Infrastructure (W2I).

A W2W topology implies a connection association, where wearables directly communicate to exchange information with short-range communication technologies (Bluetooth low energy, infrared wireless, ZigBee, and wifi direct). A wIoT device performs 1:1 or 1:n transmission modes following selective unicast, multicast, and broadcast protocols via one-hop or multi-hop delivery paths. In addition, W2W establishes a resource allocation procedure to self-negotiate between two participating wIoT devices or with an edge-AI device.

A W2H topology aims to gather wIoT data at an edge-AI device to send data for training and inference and to relay Internet connections. The edge-AI device provides at least two interfaces: one for the wIoT device interaction and the other for the Internet. In this context, wIoT devices acquire information and send this data to the edge-AI device. Meanwhile, the edge-AI device possesses an outstanding computing capacity for further data processing activities such as information fusion, information presentation, data storage, data distribution, training, and inference. On the other hand, H2I topology supports wireless technologies such as WiFi and 6G.

In this respect, data acquisition with wearable devices is the sampling of real data sensing applications that generate patient data managed by a large-scale SDHS. The result is a dataset of features extracted from wearable devices and processed in edge-AI for health analysis. In this dataset, the edge-AI device applies two learning methods: classification and regression. The first method categorizes labeled classes, while the second method models continue-valued functions for approximating the target variable.

The edge-AI element focused on developing and implementing lightweight edge and embedded cross-layer AI algorithms. Nonetheless, edge-AI resources operate one step away from the wearable device. The computational capabilities of edge-AI devices vary greatly, ranging from smartphones to high-end embedded microcontrollers. Their advantages are that different layers of learning offer low latency and high data preservation, while cloud computing provides higher computational power.

Pre-processing and feature engineering tasks run in edge-AI devices to obtain an optimized dataset. Feature selection methods consist of reducing the number of features without incurring a degradation in the performance of the automatic AI algorithm. It serves two purposes: it makes training more efficient and increases the model performance by avoiding over-fitting. Feature selection techniques are filters, wrappers, and embedded methods. Both wrappers and embedded methods have the risk of over-fitting when having more features than samples. Consequently, filters allow the reduction of data dimensionality without compromising the time and memory requirements of machine learning algorithms.

Large-scale Architecture

Healthcare delivery at a large scale involves the ubiquitousness and pervasiveness of the fundamental technologies to collect data and select actions to arrive at specific desired outcomes. The aim is that decisions result in a fusion of AI algorithms and Human Intelligence (HI) to find a state midway contribution between them. A large-scale architecture has six components integrated into three elements: Interfaces and Interconnectivity, Infrastructure and Interoperability, and Intelligence and Decision to improve healthcare delivery. Figure 2 shows this large-scale architecture for a smart digital healthcare delivery implementation.

Figure 2. Large-scale architecture to allow smart digital healthcare service delivery

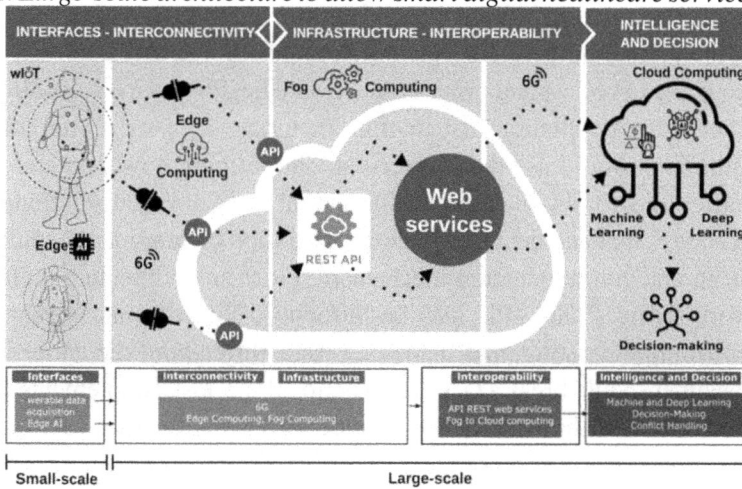

The interfaces and interconnectivity element entail sensor interface management and integration of low-power wearable devices for recovering information related to health in daily life. Additionally, it aims to establish a standard way of interconnecting Body Sensor Networks devices using 6LowPan protocols. As for communication technology, 6G provides the infrastructure for wireless health by integrating with the Internet and treating the human body as part of the Internet. 6G technology centers on how to link and manage billions of units, from macro to micro to nano, offering a significant performance improvement using terahertz (THz) bands from 100 Giga hertz to 10 THz. Here, the essential role of wIoT and 6G involves building an infrastructure with access to cloud computing resources that are very close to end users. This infrastructure meets the industry standards for computing capabilities and connectivity resources (from clouds, edge devices, and fog base stations) required to run AI and MCDM services. AI and MVDM services that run on this infrastructure will bring many advantages, as follows. From global AI to local AI (or combined), reduce power consumption, and from offline AI and MCDM to real-time and distributed training and inference.

Data collected from wearable devices needs to be processed and stored somewhere. The Infrastructure and Interoperability element consists of hardware and software resources that enable technological solutions for DSHS. Multi-layered cloud, fog, and edge technologies provide a scalable task-oriented solution to implement interoperable and intelligent embedded services. The information collected from edge-level devices is pre-processed and stored at the fog level. At the cloud level, high-performance processing provides reliable remote storage and reliability. REST web services API promotes interaction between edge and fog levels to obtain sensing datasets and convert them into new datasets through a feature selection optimization process. Here, task-oriented solutions involves a different design where connections are established based on what the network provides for the users. For example, an AI task would be to collect and process data over a health service according to user mobility, real-time population distribution, or usage intensity. Public or private health institutions would use the service without defining how data are collected from specific users to obtain certain information. Task-oriented solutions include four aspects: task management, resource orchestration or runtime scheduling, data management, and communication mechanism. From an architectural perspective, new network services and APIs may be introduced for task management, which involves defining, operating, and managing tasks throughout the entire lifecycle. Task management could break a task into functional sub-tasks implemented through various methods due to the heterogeneous type of access and formats. From a resource perspective, a task involves a computation and a communication task established across clouds, cloud edges, fog base stations, and devices. The resource schedule, provided by the system, establishes a session for two parties to communicate and perform a specific task. Regarding performing tasks, data management explores the areas of data availability and quality, information storage, network capability, and knowledge management. For example, among wIoT and edge/fog computing devices, a task involving flexible and efficient multi-user, multi-access, and multi-computing collaboration.

Intelligent healthcare is required instead of one-to-one interaction with patients. The Intelligence and Decision element helps manage proper services, reduce costs, and improve scalability. AI-driven healthcare improves clinical diagnosis and decision-making by performing tasks in real time. Supervised learning maps between input features and output labels to predict the new data. For instance, DL does not require data preprocessing and can process original health data directly. Another AI algorithm explored in health data is deep reinforcement learning, which computes an optimal decision based on observations. In addition, multi-criteria decision analysis methods formulate a set of alternatives (classifier) and criteria (performance measures), evaluate performance measures, and provide ranking lists. Thus, a decision matrix represents those performance measures of the alternatives in each criterion. In the decision-making process, weights are given arbitrarily to each criterion to reflect its relative importance, and weighted preference scores are derived based on the criteria weights and scores. In case of existing disagreements between these methods, conflict handling provides a single ranking. Conflict handling furnishes different methods to choose an approximate solution to these conflicts. One of these methods is Spearman's rank correlation nonparametric technique for evaluating the degree of linear association or correlation between two independent variables.

Edge devices become essential for future developments. It extends computing capabilities from a small-scale environment to the edge of the large-scale system, thereby delivering flexibility in data processing and network performance. 6G communication system is used for both broad and local-scope networks based on independent but controllable edge devices. The efficient synchronization of data and services, runtime scheduling, selection of suitable resources, and identification of local applications are essential aspects of this architecture. In a large-scale network via edge devices, it is possible to perform healthcare service delivery by combining local and global AI and decision-making. AI and decision-making operations and management are aspects considered for the architecture design. The architecture facilitates the seamless integration and deployment of AI and decision-making services. The AI and decision-making management services include data workflow, computing, and communication resource organization.

CONCLUSION AND FURTHER RESEARCH DIRECTIONS

This chapter proposes a small-scale and large-scale SDHS architecture. The lowering costs of wearable sensor devices, the data that these devices can provide, and cloud technologies represent an opportunity to open new perspectives in chronic disease monitoring and management. Deploying small or large SDHS based on solutions like wIoT, 6G, edge, fog, and cloud computing allows data retrieval to support the prediction of possible disease breakouts. The inception of BANs and wearable devices for health analysis in healthcare has resulted in increased data volumes and the number of features. A potential area to emphasize is the creation and optimization of health datasets. The reliability of healthcare data not only ensures the accuracy of the monitoring procedures but can also lead to efficiency with effective dimension-reduction techniques applied to the data.

This book chapter also showcased some solutions for using AI-based systems using health data to improve healthcare delivery. The subject of HI–MI decision-making is an emerging area, and an innovative technological methodology proposes a conceptual framework to support HI-MI decisions based on a multi-criteria decision-making approach. Several healthcare areas and applications have risen in HI-MI systems, and there is an emerging need for developing new quantitative models to support HI-MI decisions. Adopting large-scale or small-scale SDHS approaches is also proposed as a tool to model HI-MI decisions by developing cause-and-effect models. wIoT, AI, 6G, MCDM, and cloud computing technologies expect to benefit each other. If AI and Edge are well integrated, they can offer great potential for innovative applications. Several AI applications in healthcare require edge computing platforms to ensure millisecond-level interaction delay. In addition, edge perception is more conducive to analyzing the health environment around the patient, thus enhancing care safety.

On the other hand, 6G creates an AI-driven communication technology to enable intelligent and mobile connectivity development for smart devices capable of forecasting, choosing, and sharing their expertise with other devices. As a result, the use of 6G communication technologies is causing a paradigm change from the smart to the intelligent era. SHS is an evolution from conventional systems to a disseminated approach to better patient assistance. Hence, two types of technological expansion can exist for s-health: a) transferring maintenance functions outside the SHS using IoT and wIoT. These techniques allow the composition of an SHS, irrespective of the patient location, and b) ML or DL analytical capabilities predominant in s-health environments.

REFERENCES

Akhtar, M., Haleem, A., & Javaid, M. (2024). Exploring the advent of Medical 4.0: A bibliometric analysis systematic review and technology adoption insights. Informatics and Health, 16-28. DOI: 10.1016/j.infoh.2023.10.001

Ali, R., Hussain, A., Nazir, S., Khan, S., & Khan, H. (2023). Intelligent Decision Support Systems—An Analysis of Machine Learning and Multicriteria Decision-Making Methods. *Applied Sciences (Basel, Switzerland)*, 13(22), 12426. Advance online publication. DOI: 10.3390/app132212426

Atieh, A. (2021). The Next Generation Cloud technologies: A Review On Distributed Cloud, Fog And Edge Computing and Their Opportunities and Challenges. ResearchBerg Review of Science and Technology, 1-15. Retrieved from https://www.researchberg.com/index.php/rrst/article/view/18

Baker, S., & Xiang, W. (2023). Artificial Intelligence of Things for Smarter Healthcare: A Survey of Advancements, Challenges, and Opportunities. *IEEE Communications Surveys and Tutorials*, 25(2), 1261–1293. DOI: 10.1109/COMST.2023.3256323

Bennett, J., Stevens, G., Mathers, C., Bonita, R., Rehm, J., Kruk, M., . . . Ezzati, M. (2018). NCD Countdown 2030: worldwide trends in non-communicable disease mortality and progress towards Sustainable Development Goal target 3.4. The Lancet, 0140-6736. DOI: 10.1016/S0140-6736(18)31992-5

Deng, S., Zhao, H., Fang, W., Yin, J., Dustdar, S., & Zomaya, A. (2020). Edge Intelligence: The Confluence of Edge Computing and Artificial Intelligence. *IEEE Internet of Things Journal*, 7(8), 2327–4662. DOI: 10.1109/JIOT.2020.2984887

Gupta, P., Saini, D., & Verma, R. (2022). *Healthcare Solutions Using Machine Learning and Informatics*. Auerbach Publications., DOI: 10.1201/9781003322597

Iqbal, S., Mahgoub, I., Du, E., Leavitt, M., & Asghar, W. (2021). Advances in healthcare wearable devices. npj Flexible Electronics, 2397-4621. DOI: 10.1038/s41528-021-00107-x

Liao, H., He, Y., Wu, X., Wu, Z., & Bausys, R. (2023). Reimagining multi-criterion decision making by data-driven methods based on machine learning: A literature review. *Information Fusion*, 12, 101970. Advance online publication. DOI: 10.1016/j.inffus.2023.101970

Lou, Z., Wang, L., Jiang, K., Wei, Z., & Shen, G. (2020). Reviews of wearable healthcare systems: Materials, devices and system integration. *Materials Science and Engineering R Reports*, 24, 100523. Advance online publication. DOI: 10.1016/j.mser.2019.100523

Nijhawan, R., & Bhatia, S. (2023). Edge-AI tools and techniques for healthcare. In Vyas, S., Upadhyaya, A., Bhargava, D., & Shukla, V. (Eds.), *Edge-AI in Healthcare Trends and Future Perspectives* (p. 14). CRC Press. DOI: 10.1201/9781003244592-2

Nittas, V., Zecca, C., Kamm, C., Kuhle, J., Chan, A., & Wyl, V. (2023). Digital health for chronic disease management: An exploratory method to investigating technology adoption potential. *PLoS One*, 18(4), e0284477. Advance online publication. DOI: 10.1371/journal.pone.0284477 PMID: 37053272

Onakpojeruo, E., Al-Turjman, F., Mustapha, M., Altrjman, C., & Ozsahin, D. (2022). Emerging AI and cloud computing paradigms applied to healthcare. International Conference on Forthcoming Networks and Sustainability (p. 2022.2557). Cyprus: IET. DOI: 10.1049/icp.2022.2557

Pal, T., Saha, R., Sen, S., Saif, S., & Biswas, S. (2022). Architecture for Smart Healthcare: Cloud Versus Edge. In S. Biswas, C. Chowdhury, B. Acharya, & C. Liu, Internet of Things Based Smart Healthcare-Intelligent and Secure Solutions Applying Machine Learning Techniques (pp. 23-48). Singapore: Springer Singapore. DOI: 10.1007/978-981-19-1408-9_2

Popov, V., Kudryavtseva, E., Katiyar, N., Shishkin, A., Stepanov, S., & Goel, S. (2022). Industry 4.0 and Digitalisation in Healthcare. *Materials (Basel)*, 15(6), 2140. Advance online publication. DOI: 10.3390/ma15062140 PMID: 35329592

Prasad, V., Bhavsar, M., & Tanwar, S. (2019). Influence of Montoring: Fog and Edge Computing. Scalable Computing: Practice and Experience. DOI: 10.12694/scpe.v20i2.1533

Quy, V., Hau, N., Anh, D., & Ngoc, L. (2022). Smart healthcare IoT applications based on fog computing: Architecture, applications and challenges. *Complex & Intelligent Systems*, 8(5), 3805–3815. DOI: 10.1007/s40747-021-00582-9 PMID: 34804767

Raoof, S., & Durai, M. (2022). A Comprehensive Review on Smart Health Care: Applications, Paradigms, and Challenges with Case Studies. *Contrast Media & Molecular Imaging*, 18(1), 4822235. Advance online publication. DOI: 10.1155/2022/4822235

Seng, K., Ang, L., & Ngharamike, E. (2022). Artificial intelligence Internet of Things: A new paradigm of distributed sensor networks. *International Journal of Distributed Sensor Networks*, 18(3). Advance online publication. DOI: 10.1177/15501477211062835

Shankar, K., Perumal, E., & Gupta, D. (2021). *Artificial Intelligence for the Internet of Health Things*. CRC Press., DOI: 10.1201/9781003159094

Singh, C., Mallesha, M., Vijayaragavan, M., Sureshbabu, J., & Alsekait, D. (2022). IoT BASED SECURED HEALTHCARE USING 6G TECHNOLOGY AND DEEP LEARNING TECHNIQUES. *Journal of Pharmaceutical Negative Results*, ●●●, 462–472. DOI: 10.47750/pnr.2022.13.S09.053

Solanas, A., Patsakis, C., Conti, M., Vlachos, I., Ramos, V., Falcone, F., Postolache, O., Perez-martinez, P., Pietro, R., Perrea, D., & Martinez-Balleste, A. (2014). Smart health: A context-aware health paradigm within smart cities. *IEEE Communications Magazine*, 52(8), 1558–1896. DOI: 10.1109/MCOM.2014.6871673

Tian, S., Yang, W., Grange, J., Wang, P., Huang, W., & Ye, Z. (2019). Smart healthcare: Making medical care more intelligent. *Global Health Journal (Amsterdam, Netherlands)*, 62-65(3), 62–65. Advance online publication. DOI: 10.1016/j.glohj.2019.07.001

Tsoi, K., & Wong, M. (2021). Digital health for chronic disease management. In Fong, B., & Wong, M. (Eds.), *The Routledge Handbook of Public Health and the Community* (p. 12). Routledge., DOI: 10.4324/9781003119111-24-28

Tuli, S., Tuli, S., Wander, G., Wander, P., Gill, S., Dustdar, S., & Rana, O. (2019). Next generation technologies for smart healthcare: Challenges, vision, model, trends and future directions. *Internet Technology Letters*, 15. Advance online publication. DOI: 10.1002/itl2.145

Upadhyay, S., Kumar, M., Upadhyay, A., Verma, S., Kavita, M., Khurma, R., & Castillo, P. (2023). Challenges and Limitation Analysis of an IoT-Dependent System for Deployment in Smart Healthcare Using Communication Standards Features. Sensors, 11. doi:https://www.mdpi.com/1424-8220/23/11/5155

Vansimaeys, C., Benamar, L., & Balagué, C. (2021). Digital health and management of chronic disease: A multimodal technologies typology. *The International Journal of Health Planning and Management*, 36(4), 1107–1125. DOI: 10.1002/hpm.3161 PMID: 33786849

Vyas, S., & Bhargava, D. (2021). *Smart Health Systems - Emerging Trends*. Springer Singapore., DOI: 10.1007/978-981-16-4201-2

Vyas, S., Upadhyaya, A., Bhargava, D., & Shukla, V. (2023). *Edge-AI in Healthcare-Trends and Future Perspectives*. CRC Press., DOI: 10.1201/9781003244592

Wang, H., Dauwed, M., Khan, I., Sani, N., Omar, H., Amano, H., & Mostafa, S. (2023). MEC-IoT-Healthcare: Analysis and Prospects. *Computers, Materials & Continua*, 32. Advance online publication. DOI: 10.32604/cmc.2022.030958

Wang, X., Han, Y., Leung, V., Niyato, D., Yan, X., & Chen, X. (2021). *Edge AI - Convergence of Edge Computing and Artificial Intelligence*. Springer Singapore., DOI: 10.1007/978-981-15-6186-3

World Health Organization. (2022). Noncommunicable diseases: progress monitor 2022. Genevra: WHO. Retrieved from https://iris.who.int/handle/10665/353048

KEY TERMS AND DEFINITIONS

Digital Health Service: a model that promotes patient-centered care as a medium of sensing, interaction, and communication everywhere. Conventional healthcare services integrate digital health technologies and computing paradigms for cost-effective healthcare service delivery.

Digital Health Technology: an approach that includes personal mobile devices, such as smartphones, tablets, or wearables to transform how health is monitored and managed to offer and deliver decentralized health care quality services.

Edge Artificial Intelligence: a combination of artificial intelligence and edge computing technologies that implements machine learning or deep learning to deploy intelligent solutions on hardware devices to locally curate, analyze, and produce advanced analytical methods with power efficiency, scalable reduced costs, and increased real-time processing and decisions.

Large-Scale Digital Health Service: a standard way of interconnecting body sensor network devices using 6G communication technology infrastructure with multi-layered cloud technologies to provide scalable, distributed, and interoperable services where intelligence and decision help manage proper services, reduce costs, and improve scalability.

Small-Scale Digital Health Service: oriented 6G communication personal ecosystem that includes intelligent computing services for healthcare delivery to encompass patient autonomy and mobility

Smart Health (s-health): provision of health services using context-aware networks and sensing infrastructure of a smart environment or smart city. Include medical wearable devices, monitoring devices, the Internet of Things, wireless networks, body area networks, extensive area networks, and Ambient-Assisted Living to enable health monitoring and self-manage during medical emergencies.

Smart Healthcare System: scalable and distributed s-health that provides healthcare solutions and quality services for daily personal and clinical care, focused on management, prevention, diagnosis, and treatment of disease through the deployment of digital health services.

Chapter 4
Accelerating Healthcare Outcomes Uplifting Patient Experiences Pairing Artificial intelligence (AI):
Transforming the Healthcare Industry in the Digital Arena

Bhupinder Singh
https://orcid.org/0009-0006-4779-2553
Sharda University, India

Christian Kaunert
https://orcid.org/0000-0002-4493-2235
Dublin City University, Ireland

ABSTRACT

Artificial Intelligence encompasses a range of technologies which includes machine learning, natural language processing and predictive analytics and all of which are being integrated into healthcare systems. These applications are optimizing clinical workflows, aiding in more accurate diagnoses and providing data-driven insights that enhance decision-making for healthcare professionals. The diagnostic tools powered by AI are proving instrumental in early detection of diseases ultimately leading to improved treatment plans and outcomes. With accelerating outcomes, improving patient experiences and transforming traditional approaches, AI is reshaping the healthcare industry in profound ways. This chapter provides in-depth exploration

DOI: 10.4018/979-8-3693-5237-3.ch004

into the transformative impact of Artificial Intelligence on healthcare outcomes, specifically focusing on enhancing the patient experience in the digital era. It also explores the multifaceted ways in which AI is accelerating healthcare outcomes and reshaping patient experiences which contributing to the overall transformation of the healthcare industry.

1. INTRODUCTION

The capacity of AI to improve patient experience is the most important contributions to healthcare because AI-powered solutions provide tailored treatment regimens that consider the unique qualities, medical background and preferences of each patient (Basulo-Ribeiro & Teixeira, 2024) (El Zein et al., 2024). Artificial intelligence (AI)-powered chatbots and virtual health assistants facilitate better patient-provider interactions by providing real-time information and assistance (Holt, 2022) (Liu et al., 2023). This guarantees a more interesting and knowledgeable healthcare experience while also empowering patients (Singh & Kaunert, 2024). From the automating routine tasks to analyzing vast datasets for precision medicine, AI is enhancing the speed and accuracy of healthcare delivery (Singh et al., 2024). There is a global scarcity of healthcare professionals, especially physicians, as a result of the growing demand for healthcare services (Singh & Kaunert, 2024). Healthcare organizations face difficulties in keeping up with technology developments and satisfying patients higher expectations for treatment and results (Taghian et al., 2021). Through health tracking applications and search portals, on-demand healthcare services are now possible thanks to the advancement of wireless technology and smartphones (Ray et al., 2023) (Arpaia et al., 2021). This has led to the development of a new method of delivering healthcare that enables interactions to take place remotely at any time and from any location (Jadhakhan et al., 2022) (Reger, 2020). These services are particularly important for underprivileged areas without access to experts, as they save costs and reduce the risk of contracting infectious diseases at clinics (Singh, 2024) (Singh et al., 2024) (Singh & Kaunert, 2024).

Since infrastructure can be adjusted to meet current demands, telehealth technology is important for emerging countries looking to grow their healthcare systems (Marvaso et al., 2022). Though conceptually straightforward, many treatments require significant independent validation to prove their effectiveness and safety for patients (Drigas et al., 2022). The importance of AI-powered tools in the next generation of healthcare technology is becoming increasingly apparent throughout the healthcare ecosystem (Elor & Kurniawan, 2020). It is thought that artificial intelligence (AI) can improve a number of healthcare delivery and operational systems (Ebert et al., 2019). Notably, one of the main drivers behind the adoption of AI technologies in the healthcare sector is the potential cost savings (Patangia et al., 2021). The shift in the healthcare model from a reactive to a proactive one, prioritizing health maintenance above illness treatment, is largely responsible for these cost savings (Midha & Singh, 2023). It is anticipated that this change would result in fewer hospital stays, fewer medical visits and fewer treatments (Singh, 2024). Artificial Intelligence (AI) has the potential to significantly contribute to health maintenance by means of ongoing coaching and monitoring, early diagnosis, individualized treatment plans and more effective follow-ups (Singh & Kaunert, 2024).

1.1 Background of the Study

Artificial intelligence (AI) is the umbrella term for a variety of technologies intended to do tasks like voice recognition, visual perception, and decision-making that has historically required human intellect. AI has a lot of potential uses in the healthcare industry that might improve patient care (Singh, 2024). It might have a positive effect on treatment protocols, reduce the amount of labor that healthcare professionals have to do and generally improve how well healthcare practitioners and institutions use resources (Singh, 2023). This might thus result in possible financial savings or better health results. But given the wide range of ways AI is being used to improve health and healthcare decision-making, moral, legal and societal issues are bound to come up (Thompson, 2021).

Despite rising prices and rising demand, improving the quality and efficiency of care delivery presents several obstacles for healthcare services. Internal inefficiencies affect patient safety, staff and patient happiness, overall quality of treatment and results. The example of an internal inefficiency is inadequate patient flow. There are inherent complications in the field of mental health and the combination of growing healthcare needs and scarce resources has made it possible for technology and digital solutions most notably artificial intelligence (AI) to solve some of these issues. Artificial Intelligence (AI) has the ability to improve population health, guarantee patient safety, cut expenses and advance research (Cotler et al., 2017).

1.2 Objectives of the Chapter

This chapter aims to:
- examine the current landscape of AI applications in healthcare.
- analyze the impact of AI on accelerating healthcare outcomes.
- evaluate the role of AI in enhancing patient experiences.
- consider challenges and ethical considerations in AI-driven healthcare.
- propose recommendations for optimizing AI integration in the healthcare sector.

Figure 1. Objectives of the chapter (Original)

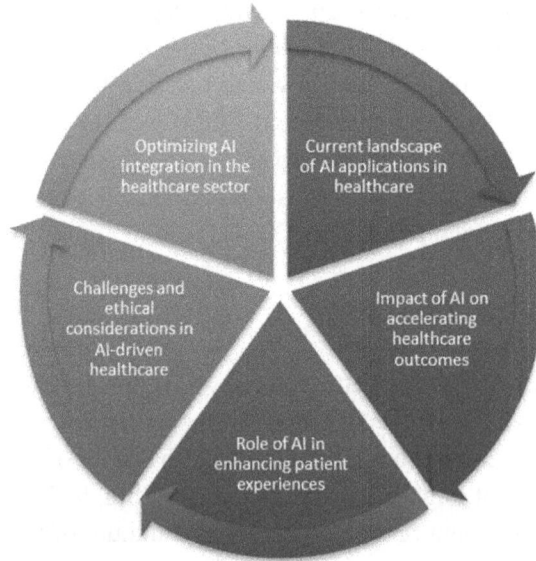

1.3 Structure/ Flow of the Chapter

This chapter comprehensively explores the diverse arena for Accelerating Healthcare Outcomes Uplifting Patients Experience Coupling Artificial intelligence (AI) which Transforming Healthcare Industry in Digital Landscapes. Section 2 elaborates the Current Landscape of AI Applications in Healthcare. Section 3 expresses the Accelerating Healthcare Outcomes. Section 4 highlights the Enhancing Patient Experiences. Section 5 specifies the Challenges and Ethical Considerations. Section 6 travels the Advancements in AI Technology. Finally, Section 7 Conclude the Chapter with Future Scope.

Figure 2. Organization of the chapter (Original)

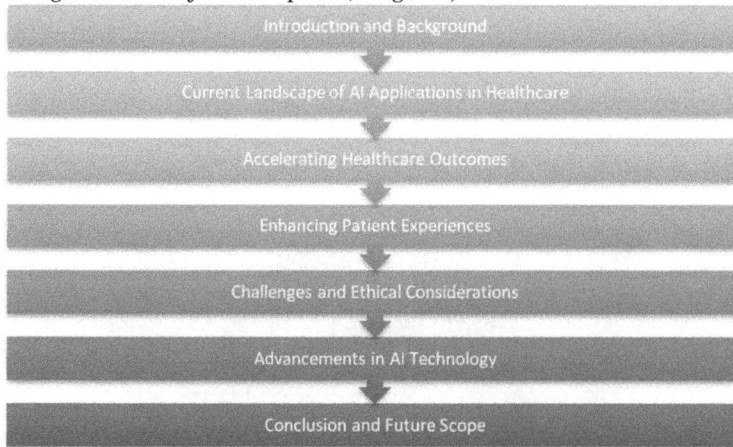

2. ARTIFICIAL INTELLIGENCE APPLICATIONS IN HEALTHCARE: CURRENT LANDSCAPE

Artificial intelligence (AI) in medicine refers to systems and algorithms that assess symbolic disease models and how they relate to patient symptoms. AI integration is now essential for improving and changing medical diagnostics and healthcare. AI technology is revolutionizing illness diagnosis, prognosis and treatment in the healthcare sector, benefiting patients as well as healthcare professionals (Cheng et al., 2019). Cloud computing, IoT, machine learning, and digital data capture have all advanced recently, making it easier to apply AI-based algorithms in the healthcare industry. AI technology may greatly improve a number of elements of healthcare systems such as- health forecasts, patient involvement and adherence, diagnostic and treatment suggestions and more. Maintaining quality and patient satisfaction throughout the treatment process depends on patient flow, which is described as the capacity of healthcare systems to manage patients effectively and with minimal delays as they progress through phases of care (Banos et al., 2021). As a result, the idea of using patient flow to improve treatment has drawn more attention, especially in relation to cutting down on patient wait times for elective and emergency care. Even though applying AI to patient-facing environments has received a lot of attention "back-end" operations and service delivery still have room for improvement (Miner, 2022).

Figure 3. Applications of artificial intelligence in healthcare (Original)

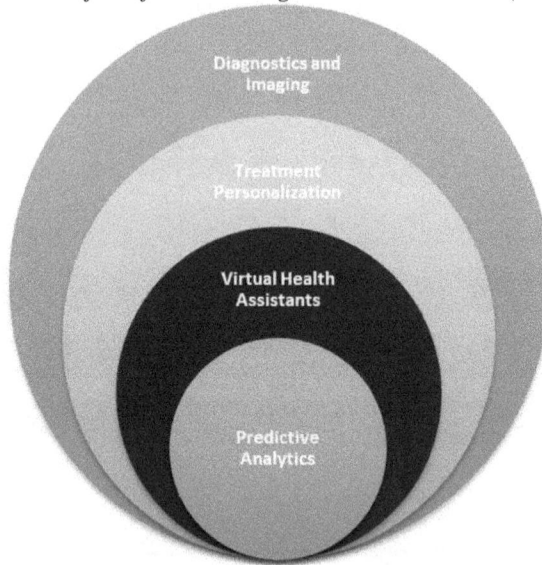

2.1 Diagnostics and Imaging

Artificial intelligence (AI) can automatically recognize and classify structures in medical photographs, such as tumors and organs, saving time and effort for human healthcare workers. AI is also capable of doing quality control evaluations on medical pictures to make sure they meet the requirements needed for precise diagnosis and therapy. AI simplifies accessibility for healthcare practitioners by handling and organizing massive amounts of medical imaging data. This provides a thorough overview of the patient's medical history and imaging data to healthcare practitioners, facilitating improved accuracy and efficiency in diagnosis and treatment.

AI-powered routine job automation in medical imaging reduces workload for healthcare practitioners while improving patient outcomes. However, it is crucial to prioritize patient privacy and safety while developing and using AI algorithms in a responsible and ethical manner. Technological developments have resulted in the growing incorporation of AI for risk assessment and prediction via medical imaging. Artificial Intelligence is utilized in the analysis of medical pictures, such CT or MRI scans to discover early stages of illnesses like Alzheimer's disease or to detect indicators of cancer. AI is also used in risk assessment in medical imaging (Singh & Kaunert, 2024). To identify risk factors that lead to certain medical disorders, AI models are trained on large datasets of medical pictures and related patient data (Singh, 2024). Healthcare professionals can use this knowledge to reduce the risk of certain illnesses by implementing preventative measures or by making well-informed judgments about treatment alternatives. It is important to recognize that artificial intelligence (AI) does not take the role of healthcare professionals, even if one benefit of AI in medical imaging is its capacity to quickly and effectively evaluate vast datasets. While AI helps with picture analysis, healthcare professionals ultimately make the decisions about diagnosis and treatment, taking into account all relevant data (Durnell, 2018).

2.2 Treatment Personalization

Customizing medical care to a patient's specific genetic and molecular traits is known as personalized medicine and the use of AI has great promise to advance this sector. The main difficulty is in efficiently evaluating large datasets in order to develop individualized treatment plans. The infrastructure of healthcare must be modified in order to integrate AI into tailored therapy. When patients come, the AI system is updated with their approved personal data as well as clinical information, such as photos, electrophysiological results, genetic information, blood pressure readings and physician notes (Singh, 2022). The AI system then makes use of this patient-specific data to offer suggestions for medical treatment, supporting medical practitioners in their clinical decision-making. Beyond the technology that makes it possible, the idea of customized medicine requires adjustments to the pharmaceutical and diagnostic industries business structures, government and private payers' payment systems, and the regulatory supervision framework. With changing the roles of doctors and patients, this method replaces reactive illness treatment in medicine with proactive healthcare management, which includes screening, early treatment, and prevention. In an industry that has generally been averse to information technology, it will also result in a greater dependence on electronic medical records and decision support systems (Choukou et al., 2022).

2.3 Virtual Health Assistants

AI-powered healthcare virtual assistants can effectively handle routine duties, freeing up highly skilled medical practitioners to devote their time to more complex activities within their areas of expertise. Medical virtual assistants' main duties include asking simple questions, such what symptoms, like fever, cold, or bodily soreness, a patient is experiencing, and how long the symptoms have persisted. The virtual assistant then uses inputs from the user to analyze and propose voice or text answers. These suggestions might be for things like getting enough sleep, scheduling doctor's visits or guiding to emergency treatment. This job division streamlines the process and frees up qualified medical experts to concentrate on more intricate facets of their responsibilities (Singh, 2023).

2.4 Predictive Analytics

Predictive analytics is a subset of data analytics that primarily utilizes machine learning, artificial intelligence, data mining, and modeling approaches. In order to forecast future occurrences, this discipline looks at data that is both historical and current. Predictive analytics as used in the healthcare industry is the study of historical and present healthcare data to help clinicians and administrators make better clinical and operational choices, anticipate trends, and stop the spread of illness in advance. Information on a person's or a group's health is included in healthcare data, which can be obtained via patient and disease registries, administrative and medical records, health surveys, claims-based datasets and electronic health records (EHRs) (Singh, 2024).

3. ACCELERATING HEALTHCARE OUTCOMES COUPLING ARTIFICIAL INTELLIGENCE (AI): TRANSFORMING HEALTHCARE INDUSTRY

Artificial intelligence (AI) has the potential to revolutionize the provision of healthcare to improve patient experience, care results and accessibility to healthcare services. Artificial Intelligence (AI) enables healthcare systems to provide better and more efficient care to a larger population by increasing productivity and optimizing care delivery. AI also helps to improve the experience of medical professionals by allowing them to devote more time to overseeing patient care and lowering the likelihood of burnout. Modern healthcare is a remarkable success story, as rising medical research breakthroughs have extended life expectancy worldwide. However, despite its success, healthcare systems face difficulties as a result of growing patient demands, soaring prices and a staff that finds it difficult to adapt to changing patient needs. The aging of the population, changing patient expectations, changes in lifestyle preferences and an ongoing cycle of innovation are just a few of the unstoppable elements contributing to the spike in demand. This requires healthcare systems to change in order to accommodate more patients with complex demands. In addition to being expensive, managing these patients calls for a shift from an episodic care-based strategy to a more proactive one that emphasizes long-term care management.

Healthcare might undergo a revolution thanks to artificial intelligence (AI) which can also help with the issues in healthcare delivery. AI which is a computer program has capacity to carry out operations and thought processes that are normally associated with the human intellect. AI in healthcare has the potential to improve patient outcomes, increase the effectiveness and productivity of care delivery and enhance the quality of life for medical professionals on a daily basis. Consequently, this raises staff morale and retention by enabling practitioners to devote more time to patient care. Artificial Intelligence has the capacity to accelerate the release of therapies that save lives. However, there are continuous ethical discussions about the proper application of AI and the data that supports it, raising worries about the influence of AI on patients, practitioners and health systems (Singh, 2024).

Figure 4. Healthcare outcomes coupling artificial intelligence (Original)

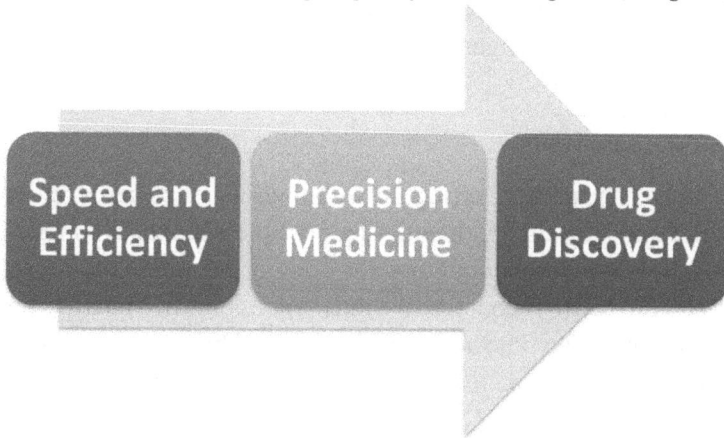

3.1 Speed and Efficiency

The growth of artificial intelligence in the healthcare industry has been driven by significant expenditures from both public and commercial sectors. There are advancements in the in areas like- diagnosis, planning and implementation of treatment, population health management, reduction of administrative load, delivery of individualized care, increased precision and better prognostication for illness treatment and prevention among other areas. Healthcare uses AI to meet the industry's constant need for efficiency, precision and speed. With the use of machine learning, computer vision, context-aware computing and natural language processing, artificial intelligence (AI) has a lot to offer the healthcare industry (Singh, 2024).

3.2 Precision Medicine

The advancement of medicines and precision medicine is being accelerated by AI techniques. An examination of genetic, behavioral, and environmental data combined with machine learning enables more precise illness risk prediction and tailored treatment outcomes. This eliminates the need for the prior one-size-fits-all strategy and opens the door for more precisely targeted therapy. Precision medicine and artificial intelligence (AI) together have the potential to drastically change healthcare. The goal of precision medicine techniques is to identify patient phenotypes that require specific care or have unusual therapy responses. AI enables the system to reason and learn by using sophisticated computing and inference to obtain insights. This in turn uses augmented intelligence to improve clinical decision-making.

3.3 Drug Discovery

AI is essential for quickly sorting through millions of chemical compounds in the drug development field and identifying possible candidates for additional research. AI is also capable of simulating the consequences of structural alterations on potency and efficacy by modeling the interactions between pharmaceuticals and bio-molecular target. The time and costs involved in bringing new medications to market are significantly being reduced by these developments.

4. ENHANCING PATIENT EXPERIENCES WITH ARTIFICIAL INTELLIGENCE IN HEALTHCARE SECTOR

The strategic benefits of AI apps that customize the patient experience are becoming more widely recognized by healthcare businesses. These applications result in higher engagement, more unique encounters and better health outcomes. When leaders are able to properly manage the associated risks, these applications show to be especially advantageous for firms that are just beginning their road towards adopting AI. AI-enabled patient engagement covers a broad spectrum of interactions and has several advantages for companies and the patients they serve (Mer & Virdi, 2023).

Facilitating more frequent and customized conversations: With improving the frequency and caliber of communications, AI solutions helps to create longer-lasting and better patient connections. By tailoring interaction to patients' language choices, reading abilities, and health literacy, organizations may improve adherence to treatment programs and prescription regimens.

Summarizing significant points from patient talks: AI systems may condense the content of conversations, giving patients the opportunity to learn important lessons from their care team and the team the opportunity to recognize important points that the patient brought up. This makes it easier to have more organic, insightful talks that record important details.

Simplifying the patient intake process: Patients and the care team often become frustrated with the many questions that are asked during traditional patient intake procedures (Singh et al., 2024). AI technologies can verify a patient's medical history and present state of health, negating the necessity for pointless inquiries. This guarantees a deeper conversation on any changes since the last visit between the patient and the care team (Drigas et al., 2022).

Achieving a balance between practical guidance and compassion: AI helps physicians communicate more empathetically and even helps them break bad medical news (Singh, 2022). The technology may convert difficult medical ideas into communications that patients can readily grasp, increasing patient participation overall (D'Errico et al., 2023).

Helping patients comprehend cost estimates and advantages: Artificial intelligence (AI) technologies make it simpler for patients to appreciate the benefits of their own health plans. Also, these systems provide simple messages to convey service cost estimations, enabling patients to take advantage of advantageous and economical healthcare solutions. Artificial intelligence (AI) apps for patient interaction have several benefits, which makes them an important tool for healthcare companies looking to improve results and customization (Hagege et al., 2023).

Artificial intelligence (AI) is playing a big part in how the healthcare sector is adjusting to new developments as the world continues to change. AI is becoming a common topic of conversation in technology and has a big influence on a lot of different businesses. Its innovative models stand out in particular because they can make art and visuals that closely resemble real human works, participate in genuine conversations, and produce easily understandable textual content. AI integration in healthcare enables quick and accurate data collection by medical professionals, resulting in prompt diagnosis and improved patient outcomes. AI enables healthcare organizations to refocus their attention from unproven, long-term solutions to immediate advantages. Improving the patient experience is one of the most significant changes artificial intelligence has brought about in the healthcare industry. Patients can receive individualized care that is catered to their specific requirements because of AI. Customizing treatment approaches, anticipating patient requirements, and spotting potential health hazards are all made possible by this technology. As a result, patients gain from a more tailored approach to care, which promotes improved results and a satisfying experience with healthcare in general (Singh & Kaunert, 2024).

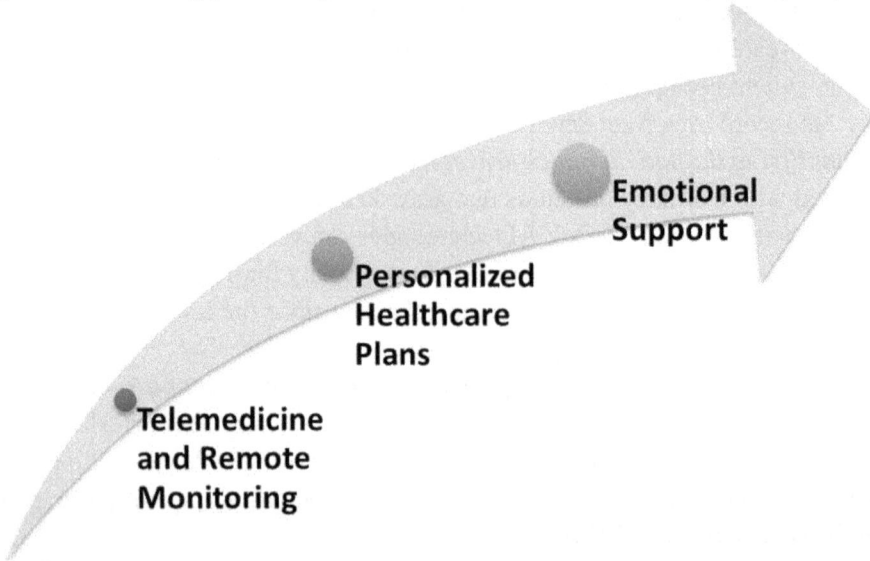

Figure 5. Enhancing patient experiences via AI in health industry (Original)

4.1 Telemedicine and Remote Monitoring

The common healthcare application is remote patient monitoring (RPM) which helps doctors monitor patients with acute or chronic diseases from a distance. It also helps with elderly patients who are hospitalized or getting in-home care. The effectiveness of conventional patient monitoring systems depends on how well staff members manage their time, which is impacted by their workload (Singh, 2024). In contrast to traditional patient monitoring techniques which entail intrusive procedures needing skin contact for monitoring health status, AI is used in RPM for a variety of tasks, including vital sign monitoring in emergency situations, chronic illness monitoring, and physical activity classification. AI-enabled RPM designs have transformed applications for healthcare monitoring. The particularly impressive are their abilities to recognize patterns in human behavior using techniques like reinforcement learning, tailor individual patient health parameter monitoring through federated learning, and identify early deterioration in patients' health (Jopowicz, 2022).

4.2 Personalized Healthcare Plans

AI algorithms are essential in helping medical professionals create individualized treatment programs that consider the unique qualities of every patient. These treatment plans, which are based on particular and unique facts, may include suggestions for therapy, alterations to lifestyle and customized pharmaceutical doses (Marossi et al., 2023). The notion of customized healthcare has surfaced as a potentially effective approach to augment patient outcomes by tailoring medical interventions to the distinct requirements and attributes of every individual. Healthcare providers may now use patient data to create more individualized treatment regimens that take into consideration lifestyle, genetics, and medical history thanks to artificial intelligence (AI) (Singh, 2023).

4.3 Emotional Support

Robots and AI-powered lifestyle management software provide round-the-clock patient monitoring, doing away with the necessity for nurses and doctors to be there all the time (Singh, 2023). The front camera on a smartphone is used by a number of real-time applications to track patient behavior in real time (Sharma & Singh, 2022). The efficacy of drug adherence is increased when lifestyle and monitoring applications are integrated with AI which has already improved face and medical recognition skills. As a result, it guarantees that patients are adhering to their recommended schedules (Than, 2023). The ability to customize care to meet each patient's unique requirements is a major benefit of personalized healthcare (Cotler, 2016). Large-scale patient data sets, including genetic information, environmental variables, and electronic health records, may be analyzed by AI algorithms. Healthcare providers can personalize treatments and improve patient outcomes and quality of life by recognizing distinctive patterns and trends linked to each patient (Chen & Ibrahim, 2023).

5. CHALLENGES AND ETHICAL CONSIDERATIONS

The application of AI in healthcare raises questions about data breaches and possible inaccuracy. The use of electronic health records can contribute to scientific research and improve the quality of healthcare, but it also increases the risk of data breaches and abuse for improper reasons (Naylor et al., 2020). The ownership of a person's medical records, who may access them, when data exchange occurs, and whether or not express agreement is necessary are all matters of ethics (Liao et al., 2019). The expected use of artificial intelligence to expedite and streamline the drug development process poses ethical concerns. With using data processing, robotics, and models of genetic targets, organs, medications, and illness development, artificial intelligence (AI) has the potential to completely transform the drug discovery process (Singh, 2022). Notwithstanding the enormous potential for enhancing patient recuperation, there is continuous discussion about whether or not new regulation is necessary to handle the ethical issues raised by AI in healthcare, or if the current legal framework is adequate (Singh, 2024).

The ethical concerns associated with the application of artificial intelligence in healthcare include important factors including gaining informed permission for the use of data, guaranteeing safety and transparency, resolving algorithmic biases and fairness, and protecting data privacy (Singh et al., 2024). To make sure that the advantages of AI outweigh the hazards involved, policymakers are required to proactively address these ethical issues. In AI-driven healthcare, the collection and use of patient data raises a number of ethical concerns (Singh & Kaunert, 2024). Ensuring the privacy and security of patient data is a top priority in order to protect people from the negative consequences that might result from data breaches and unauthorized access. It is crucial to let patients know how their data will be used in AI applications (Macorano, 2020). Regarding the patients' understanding of the consequences of sharing their data with AI systems, assumptions should not be made. Rather, people ought to be given concise justifications and the choice to decline these kinds of data-sharing agreements (Singh et al., 2024).

Figure 6. Challenges and concerns (Original)

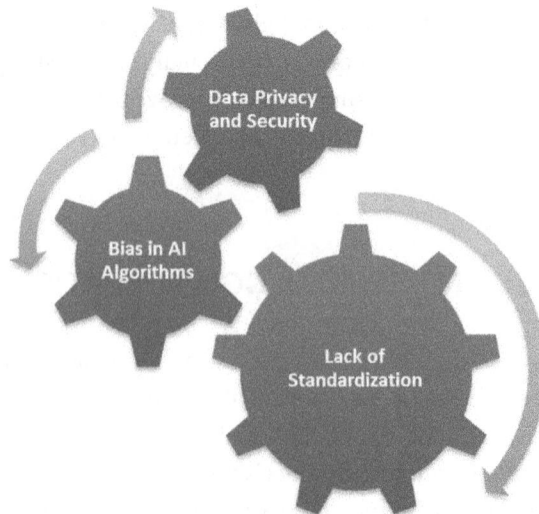

5.1 Data Privacy and Security

When AI-based solutions are adopted, worries about data security and privacy increase. When there is a data breach, hackers find health records to be appealing targets due to their significance and susceptibility. Maintaining the privacy of medical records becomes crucial as users may incorrectly believe artificial systems to be human, thereby consenting to covert data gathering (Singh et al., 2024). This creates privacy concerns as AI advances (Singh, 2022). Given that medical professionals may permit the wide use of patient data for AI research without the express agreement of the patients, patient consent becomes a crucial factor in data privacy issues. In order to provide accurate and representative results, artificial intelligence frequently requires large amounts of data, which raises serious privacy problems. Using preventative and investigative measures is a reasonable strategy for protecting Protected Health Information (Singh, 2019). In order to maintain the security, confidentiality and integrity of information systems and datasets, these controls must be carefully designed. Extensive datasets are necessary for Machine Learning (ML) and Deep Learning (DL) models to accurately classify or forecast across a variety of domains (Quintero, 2019). Notably, industries where large datasets are easily accessible have made notable progress in improving machine learning algorithms. Because patient records are sensitive, the healthcare sector has particular challenges with data accessibility. Because patient privacy is a concern, institutions are reluctant to share health data (Singh, 2024).

5.2 Bias in AI Algorithms

Unfortunately, biases can have a significant impact on AI algorithms used in healthcare. The healthcare system already has racial and socioeconomic inequities that might be made worse by the application of AI algorithms (Singh, 2024). These algorithms may generate suggestions for different treatment choices based on a patient's membership in a certain group if they are trained on biased data (Singh, 2022). A situation like this might lead to the continuation of uneven access to healthcare, with some groups benefiting from preferential treatment and others suffering from worse health results (Singh, 2020).

5.3 Lack of Standardization

It takes more than simply data diversity based on equal or relative representation to provide equitable outcomes. There could be underlying biases in the way the data on these people is portrayed, even in databases that proportionately represent individuals (Singh, 2023). For example, a dataset may contain people from an ethnic group that matches the national census data as numerical representation; however, these people may be more likely to receive a false positive than the sampled population which would skew the insights drawn from the data. Although we focus on variety of data, it also emphasizes a more comprehensive view of representativeness in health data (Singh, 2019). This entails recognizing the constraints on data gathering, guaranteeing data correctness, and resolving moral issues with data use among marginalized and underprivileged populations (Richer et al., 2022).

6. ADVANCEMENTS IN AI TECHNOLOGY

Artificial Intelligence has the ability to completely transform healthcare in the upcoming decades. Globally, patients stand to benefit much from more accurate diagnosis, individualized care, sophisticated robotics, and data-driven insights (Schneider, 2020). However, in order to minimize any potential negative effects, it is imperative that this technology be properly shaped and regulated. AI has the ability to bring in a new age of better health outcomes for everyone if it is used carefully (Folland et al., 2024). Early in the twenty-first century, significant advances in data analysis and technology attracted attention to AI's introduction into the medical field (Igwaran & Okoh, 2019). Increased computer power, the accessibility of large datasets as Big Data and significant advancements in machine learning techniques all came together in this age (Ji et al., 2023). A turning point was reached when it became clear how AI might help with important healthcare issues including operational efficiency, individualized therapy, and accurate diagnosis (Leen & Juurlink, 2019).

The benefits of AI in healthcare were immediately obvious as beyond human capability, technology was able to handle and analyze large amounts of medical data, which was vital for illness diagnosis, outcome prediction, and therapy recommendations (Sanyoalu et al., 2019). Compared to human radiologists, AI systems significantly outperformed them in terms of speed and accuracy when interpreting medical imaging like MRIs and X-rays, frequently identifying illnesses like cancer at an earlier stage. The uses of AI in healthcare go beyond diagnosis. Artificial Intelligence has the potential to transform customized medicine and diagnostics (Shaw et al., 2024). Patient care management is changing as a result of AI-driven chatbots and virtual health assistants that improve patient involvement and adherence to treatment plans. Artificial intelligence (AI) in drug research shortens the duration of clinical trials by anticipating drug responses, which speeds up the development process (Eger et al., 2024).

7. CONCLUSION AND FUTURE SCOPE

The rise of AI in healthcare has the potential to improve patient outcomes and change the way healthcare is delivered. AI is now being used in the healthcare industry to do activities including managing electronic health data, interpreting medical imaging, developing customized treatment plans, progressing drug research and offering virtual help. Artificial Intelligence (AI) trend in healthcare looks promising with possible improvements in diagnosis promptness and accuracy as well as in personalized treatment regimens all leading to better patient outcomes. Healthcare organizations, hospitals, doctors, physicians, psychologists, pharmacists, pharmaceutical companies and other healthcare stakeholders can all benefit from the use of healthcare analytics, which helps to improve the quality of care provided.

With continued breakthroughs in AI, there is an increasing chance that it may improve its capacity to more accurately forecast health outcomes and provide more customized treatment regimens for individuals. But as AI spreads throughout the healthcare industry, worries about data security, privacy and ethics must be systematically addressed in tandem with these breakthroughs. Healthcare AI is gaining traction and drawing significant investment, while being in its early phases. As the healthcare industry experiences a digital revolution, both long-standing participants and recent arrivals are aggressively seeking their positions. Future developments in AI, large multimodal data resources, and more processing capacity will open up possibilities that are presently only in the realm of human imagination. The increasing use of AI in healthcare presents promising opportunities to improve patient accessibility and quality of care.

REFERENCES

Arpaia, P., D'Errico, G., De Paolis, L. T., Moccaldi, N., & Nuccetelli, F. (2021). A narrative review of mindfulness-based interventions using virtual reality. *Mindfulness*, 1–16.

Baños, R. M., Etchemendy, E., Carrillo-Vega, A., & Botella, C. (2021). Positive psychological interventions and information and communication technologies. In *Research Anthology on Rehabilitation Practices and Therapy* (pp. 1648–1668). IGI Global.

Basulo-Ribeiro, J., & Teixeira, L. (2024). The Future of Healthcare with Industry 5.0: Preliminary Interview-Based Qualitative Analysis. *Future Internet*, 16(3), 68. DOI: 10.3390/fi16030068

Chen, X., & Ibrahim, Z. (2023). A Comprehensive Study of Emotional Responses in AI-Enhanced Interactive Installation Art. *Sustainability (Basel)*, 15(22), 15830. DOI: 10.3390/su152215830

Cheng, V. W. S., Davenport, T., Johnson, D., Vella, K., & Hickie, I. B. (2019). Gamification in apps and technologies for improving mental health and well-being: Systematic review. *JMIR Mental Health*, 6(6), e13717. DOI: 10.2196/13717 PMID: 31244479

Choukou, M. A., Zhu, X., Malwade, S., Dhar, E., & Abdul, S. S. (2022). Digital Health Solutions Transforming Long-Term Care and Rehabilitation. In *Healthcare Information Management Systems: Cases, Strategies, and Solutions* (pp. 301–316). Springer International Publishing. DOI: 10.1007/978-3-031-07912-2_19

Cotler, J. L. (2016). *The impact of online teaching and learning about emotional intelligence, Myers Briggs personality dimensions and mindfulness on personal and social awareness*. State University of New York at Albany.

Cotler, J. L., DiTursi, D., Goldstein, I., Yates, J., & Del Belso, D. (2017). A mindful approach to teaching. *Information Systems Education Journal*, 15(1), 12.

D'Errico, G., Barba, M. C., Gatto, C., Nuzzo, B. L., Nuccetelli, F., Luca, V. D., & Paolis, L. T. D. (2023, September). Measuring the Effectiveness of Virtual Reality for Stress Reduction: Psychometric Evaluation of the ERMES Project. In *International Conference on Extended Reality* (pp. 484-499). Cham: Springer Nature Switzerland. DOI: 10.1007/978-3-031-43401-3_32

Drigas, A., Mitsea, E., & Skianis, C. (2022). Virtual reality and metacognition training techniques for learning disabilities. *Sustainability (Basel)*, 14(16), 10170. DOI: 10.3390/su141610170

Drigas, A., Mitsea, E., & Skianis, C. (2022). Subliminal Training Techniques for Cognitive, Emotional and Behavioral Balance. The Role of Emerging Technologies. *Technium Soc. Sci. J.*, 33, 164.

Durnell, L. A. (2018). *Emotional Reaction of Experiencing Crisis in Virtual Reality (VR)/360* (Doctoral dissertation, Fielding Graduate University).

Ebert, D. D., Harrer, M., Apolinário-Hagen, J., & Baumeister, H. (2019). Digital interventions for mental disorders: key features, efficacy, and potential for artificial intelligence applications. *Frontiers in Psychiatry: Artificial Intelligence, Precision Medicine, and Other Paradigm Shifts*, 583-627.

Eger, H., Chacko, S., El-Gamal, S., Gerlinger, T., Kaasch, A., Meudec, M., Munshi, S., Naghipour, A., Rhule, E., Sandhya, Y. K., & Uribe, O. L. (2024). Towards a Feminist Global Health Policy: Power, intersectionality, and transformation. *PLOS Global Public Health*, 4(3), e0002959. DOI: 10.1371/journal.pgph.0002959 PMID: 38451969

El Zein, B., Elrashidi, A., Dahlan, M., Al Jarwan, A., & Jabbour, G. (2024). Nano and Society 5.0: Advancing the Human-Centric Revolution.

Elor, A., & Kurniawan, S. (2020). The ultimate display for physical rehabilitation: A bridging review on immersive virtual reality. *Frontiers in Virtual Reality*, 1, 585993. DOI: 10.3389/frvir.2020.585993

Folland, S., Goodman, A. C., & Stano, M. (2024). *The economics of health and health care: Pearson new international edition*. Routledge.

Hagège, H., Ourmi, M. E., Shankland, R., Arboix-Calas, F., Leys, C., & Lubart, T. (2023). Ethics and Meditation: A New Educational Combination to Boost Verbal Creativity and Sense of Responsibility. *Journal of Intelligence*, 11(8), 155. DOI: 10.3390/jintelligence11080155 PMID: 37623538

Holt, S. (2022). Virtual reality, augmented reality and mixed reality: For astronaut mental health; and space tourism, education and outreach. *Acta Astronautica*.

Igwaran, A., & Okoh, A. I. (2019). Human campylobacteriosis: A public health concern of global importance. *Heliyon*, 5(11), e02814. DOI: 10.1016/j.heliyon.2019.e02814 PMID: 31763476

Jadhakhan, F., Blake, H., Hett, D., & Marwaha, S. (2022). Efficacy of digital technologies aimed at enhancing emotion regulation skills: Literature review. *Frontiers in Psychiatry*, 13, 809332. DOI: 10.3389/fpsyt.2022.809332 PMID: 36159937

Ji, X., Chun, S. A., Wei, Z., & Geller, J. (2023). Twitter sentiment classification for measuring public health concerns. *Social Network Analysis and Mining*, 5, 1–25. PMID: 32226558

Jopowicz, A., Wiśniowska, J., & Tarnacka, B. (2022). Cognitive and physical intervention in metals' dysfunction and neurodegeneration. *Brain Sciences*, 12(3), 345. DOI: 10.3390/brainsci12030345 PMID: 35326301

Leen, J. L., & Juurlink, D. N. (2019). Carfentanil: A narrative review of its pharmacology and public health concerns. *Canadian Journal of Anaesthesia*, 66(4), 414–421. DOI: 10.1007/s12630-019-01294-y PMID: 30666589

Liao, D., Shu, L., Liang, G., Li, Y., Zhang, Y., Zhang, W., & Xu, X. (2019). Design and evaluation of affective virtual reality system based on multimodal physiological signals and self-assessment manikin. *IEEE Journal of Electromagnetics, RF and Microwaves in Medicine and Biology*, 4(3), 216–224. DOI: 10.1109/JERM.2019.2948767

Liu, K., Madrigal, E., Chung, J. S., Parekh, M., Kalahar, C. S., Nguyen, D., & Harris, O. A. (2023). Preliminary Study of Virtual-reality-guided Meditation for Veterans with Stress and Chronic Pain. *Alternative Therapies in Health and Medicine*, 29(6). PMID: 34559692

Maçorano, R. D. N. A. (2020). *Exploratory Psychometric Validation and Efficacy Assessment Study of Social Phobia Treatment based on Augmented and Virtual Reality Serious Games and Biofeedback* (Doctoral dissertation, Universidade de Lisboa (Portugal)).

Marossi, C., Mariani, V., Arenas, A., Brondino, M., de Carvalho, C. V., Costa, P., . . . Pasini, M. (2023, July). Mindfulness Lessons in a Virtual Natural Environment to Cope with Work-Related Stress. In *International Conference in Methodologies and intelligent Systems for Techhnology Enhanced Learning* (pp. 227-238). Cham: Springer Nature Switzerland. DOI: 10.1007/978-3-031-41226-4_24

Marvaso, G., Pepa, M., Volpe, S., Mastroleo, F., Zaffaroni, M., Vincini, M. G., & Jereczek-Fossa, B. A. (2022). Virtual and Augmented Reality as a Novel Opportunity to Unleash the Power of Radiotherapy in the Digital Era: A Scoping Review. *Applied Sciences (Basel, Switzerland)*, 12(22), 11308. DOI: 10.3390/app122211308

Mer, A., & Virdi, A. S. (2023). Navigating the paradigm shift in HRM practices through the lens of artificial intelligence: A post-pandemic perspective. *The Adoption and Effect of Artificial Intelligence on Human Resources Management, Part A*, 123-154.

Midha, S., & Singh, K. (2023). Happiness-Enhancing Strategies Among Indians. In *Religious and Spiritual Practices in India: A Positive Psychological Perspective* (pp. 341–368). Springer Nature Singapore. DOI: 10.1007/978-981-99-2397-7_15

Miner, N. (2022). *Stairway to Heaven: Breathing Mindfulness into Virtual Reality* (Doctoral dissertation, Northeastern University).

Naylor, M., Ridout, B., & Campbell, A. (2020). A scoping review identifying the need for quality research on the use of virtual reality in workplace settings for stress management. *Cyberpsychology, Behavior, and Social Networking*, 23(8), 506–518. DOI: 10.1089/cyber.2019.0287 PMID: 32486836

Patangia, B., Sankruthyayana, R. G., Sathiyaseelan, A., & Balasundaram, S. (2021). How could Mindfulness Help? A Perspective on the Applications of Mindfulness in Enhancing Tomorrow's Workplace. *i-Manager's. Journal of Management*, 16(3), 52.

Quintero, L. (2019). *Facilitating Technology-based Mental Health Interventions with Mobile Virtual Reality and Wearable Smartwatches* (Doctoral dissertation, Department of Computer and Systems Sciences, Stockholm University).

Radovic, , ABadawy, , S. M. (2020). Technology use for adolescent health and wellness. *Pediatrics*, 145(Supplement_2), S186–S194.

Ray, J., Kumar, S., Pandey, S., & Akram, S. V. (2023, June). The Role of Augmented Reality and Virtual Reality in Shaping the Future of Health Psychology. In *2023 3rd International Conference on Pervasive Computing and Social Networking (ICPCSN)* (pp. 1604-1608). IEEE. DOI: 10.1109/ICPCSN58827.2023.00268

Reger, G. M. (Ed.). (2020). *Technology and mental health: a clinician's guide to improving outcomes*. Routledge. DOI: 10.4324/9780429020537

Richir, S., Kadri, A., & Ribeyre, N. (2022). Virtual Reality and Augmented Reality to Fight Effectively against Pandemics. In *The Nature of Pandemics* (pp. 311–348). CRC Press. DOI: 10.4324/9781315170220-20

Sanyaolu, A., Okorie, C., Qi, X., Locke, J., & Rehman, S. (2019). Childhood and adolescent obesity in the United States: a public health concern. *Global pediatric health, 6*, 2333794X19891305.

Schneider, M. J. (2020). *Introduction to public health*. Jones & Bartlett Learning.

Sharma, A., & Singh, B. (2022). Measuring Impact of E-commerce on Small Scale Business: A Systematic Review. *Journal of Corporate Governance and International Business Law*, 5(1).

Shaw, F. E., Asomugha, C. N., Conway, P. H., & Rein, A. S. (2024). The Patient Protection and Affordable Care Act: Opportunities for prevention and public health. *Lancet*, 384(9937), 75–82. DOI: 10.1016/S0140-6736(14)60259-2 PMID: 24993913

Singh, B. (2022). Understanding Legal Frameworks Concerning Transgender Healthcare in the Age of Dynamism. *Electronic Journal Of Social And Strategic Studies*, 3(1), 56–65. DOI: 10.47362/EJSSS.2022.3104

Singh, B. (2022). Relevance of Agriculture-Nutrition Linkage for Human Healthcare: A Conceptual Legal Framework of Implication and Pathways. *Justice and Law Bulletin*, 1(1), 44–49.

Singh, B. (2023). Unleashing Alternative Dispute Resolution (ADR) in Resolving Complex Legal-Technical Issues Arising in Cyberspace Lensing E-Commerce and Intellectual Property: Proliferation of E-Commerce Digital Economy. *Revista Brasileira de Alternative Dispute Resolution-Brazilian Journal of Alternative Dispute Resolution-RBADR*, 5(10), 81–105. DOI: 10.52028/rbadr.v5i10.ART04.Ind

Singh, B. (2023). Blockchain Technology in Renovating Healthcare: Legal and Future Perspectives. In *Revolutionizing Healthcare Through Artificial Intelligence and Internet of Things Applications* (pp. 177-186). IGI Global.

Singh, B. (2023). Federated Learning for Envision Future Trajectory Smart Transport System for Climate Preservation and Smart Green Planet: Insights into Global Governance and SDG-9 (Industry, Innovation and Infrastructure). *National Journal of Environmental Law*, 6(2), 6–17.

Singh, B. (2024). Evolutionary Global Neuroscience for Cognition and Brain Health: Strengthening Innovation in Brain Science. In Prabhakar, P. (Ed.), *Biomedical Research Developments for Improved Healthcare* (pp. 246–272). IGI Global., DOI: 10.4018/979-8-3693-1922-2.ch012

Singh, B. (2024). Featuring Consumer Choices of Consumable Products for Health Benefits: Evolving Issues from Tort and Product Liabilities. *Journal of Law of Torts and Consumer Protection Law*, 7(1), 53–56.

Singh, B. (2024). Green Infrastructure in Real Estate Landscapes: Pillars of Sustainable Development and Vision for Tomorrow. *National Journal of Real Estate Law*, 7(1), 4–8.

Singh, B. (2024). Legal Dynamics Lensing Metaverse Crafted for Videogame Industry and E-Sports: Phenomenological Exploration Catalyst Complexity and Future. *Journal of Intellectual Property Rights Law*, 7(1), 8–14.

Singh, B. (2024). Transformative Wave of IoMT, EHRs, RPM Technologies to Revolutionize Public Health. *Indian Journal of Health and Medical Law*, 7(2), 22–26.

Singh, B. (2024). Lensing Legal Dynamics for Examining Responsibility and Deliberation of Generative AI-Tethered Technological Privacy Concerns: Infringements and Use of Personal Data by Nefarious Actors. In Ara, A., & Ara, A. (Eds.), *Exploring the Ethical Implications of Generative AI* (pp. 146–167). IGI Global., DOI: 10.4018/979-8-3693-1565-1.ch009

Singh, B. (2024). Biosensors in Intelligent Healthcare and Integration of Internet of Medical Things (IoMT) for Treatment and Diagnosis. *Indian Journal of Health and Medical Law*, 7(1), 1–7.

Singh, B. (2024). Evolutionary Global Neuroscience for Cognition and Brain Health: Strengthening Innovation in Brain Science. In Prabhakar, P. (Ed.), *Biomedical Research Developments for Improved Healthcare* (pp. 246–272). IGI Global., DOI: 10.4018/979-8-3693-1922-2.ch012

Singh, B., Dutta, P. K., & Kaunert, C. (2024). Replenish Artificial Intelligence in Renewable Energy for Sustainable Development: Lensing SDG 7 Affordable and Clean Energy and SDG 13 Climate Actions With Legal-Financial Advisory. In Derbali, A. (Ed.), *Social and Ethical Implications of AI in Finance for Sustainability* (pp. 198–227). IGI Global., DOI: 10.4018/979-8-3693-2881-1.ch009

Singh, B., Jain, V., Kaunert, C., Dutta, P. K., & Singh, G. (2024). Privacy Matters: Espousing Blockchain and Artificial Intelligence (AI) for Consumer Data Protection on E-Commerce Platforms in Ethical Marketing. In Saluja, S., Nayyar, V., Rojhe, K., & Sharma, S. (Eds.), *Ethical Marketing Through Data Governance Standards and Effective Technology* (pp. 167–184). IGI Global., DOI: 10.4018/979-8-3693-2215-4.ch015

Singh, B., Jain, V., Kaunert, C., & Vig, K. (2024). Shaping Highly Intelligent Internet of Things (IoT) and Wireless Sensors for Smart Cities. In *Secure and Intelligent IoT-Enabled Smart Cities* (pp. 117-140). IGI Global.

Singh, B., & Kaunert, C. (2024). Future of Digital Marketing: Hyper-Personalized Customer Dynamic Experience with AI-Based Predictive Models. *Revolutionizing the AI-Digital Landscape: A Guide to Sustainable Emerging Technologies for Marketing Professionals*, 189.

Singh, B., & Kaunert, C. (2024). Salvaging Responsible Consumption and Production of Food in the Hospitality Industry: Harnessing Machine Learning and Deep Learning for Zero Food Waste. In *Sustainable Disposal Methods of Food Wastes in Hospitality Operations* (pp. 176-192). IGI Global.

Singh, B., & Kaunert, C. (2024). Revealing Green Finance Mobilization: Harnessing FinTech and Blockchain Innovations to Surmount Barriers and Foster New Investment Avenues. In Jafar, S., Rodriguez, R., Kannan, H., Akhtar, S., & Plugmann, P. (Eds.), *Harnessing Blockchain-Digital Twin Fusion for Sustainable Investments* (pp. 265–286). IGI Global., DOI: 10.4018/979-8-3693-1878-2.ch011

Singh, B., & Kaunert, C. (2024). Harnessing Sustainable Agriculture Through Climate-Smart Technologies: Artificial Intelligence for Climate Preservation and Futuristic Trends. In Kannan, H., Rodriguez, R., Paprika, Z., & Ade-Ibijola, A. (Eds.), *Exploring Ethical Dimensions of Environmental Sustainability and Use of AI* (pp. 214–239). IGI Global., DOI: 10.4018/979-8-3693-0892-9.ch011

Singh, B., & Kaunert, C. (2024). Computational Thinking for Innovative Solutions and Problem-Solving Techniques: Transforming Conventional Education to Futuristic Interdisciplinary Higher Education. In Fonkam, M., & Vajjhala, N. (Eds.), *Revolutionizing Curricula Through Computational Thinking, Logic, and Problem Solving* (pp. 60–82). IGI Global., DOI: 10.4018/979-8-3693-1974-1.ch004

Singh, B., & Kaunert, C. (2024). Integration of Cutting-Edge Technologies such as Internet of Things (IoT) and 5G in Health Monitoring Systems: A Comprehensive Legal Analysis and Futuristic Outcomes. *GLS Law Journal*, 6(1), 13–20. DOI: 10.69974/glslawjournal.v6i1.123

Singh, B., & Kaunert, C. (2024). Aroma of Highly Smart Internet of Medical Things (IoMT) and Lightweight Edge Trust Expansion Medical Care Facilities for Electronic Healthcare Systems: Fortified-Chain Architecture for Remote Patient Monitoring and Privacy Protection Beyond Imagination. In Hassan, A., Bhattacharya, P., Tikadar, S., Dutta, P., & Sagayam, M. (Eds.), *Lightweight Digital Trust Architectures in the Internet of Medical Things (IoMT)* (pp. 196–212). IGI Global., DOI: 10.4018/979-8-3693-2109-6.ch011

Singh, B., & Kaunert, C. (2024). Augmented Reality and Virtual Reality Modules for Mindfulness: Boosting Emotional Intelligence and Mental Wellness. In Hiran, K., Doshi, R., & Patel, M. (Eds.), *Applications of Virtual and Augmented Reality for Health and Wellbeing* (pp. 111–128). IGI Global., DOI: 10.4018/979-8-3693-1123-3.ch007

Singh, B., & Kaunert, C. (2024). Future of Digital Marketing: Hyper-Personalized Customer Dynamic Experience with AI-Based Predictive Models. In *Revolutionizing the AI-Digital Landscape* (pp. 189–203). Productivity Press. DOI: 10.4324/9781032688305-14

Singh, B., & Kaunert, C. (2024). Salvaging Responsible Consumption and Production of Food in the Hospitality Industry: Harnessing Machine Learning and Deep Learning for Zero Food Waste. In Singh, A., Tyagi, P., & Garg, A. (Eds.), *Sustainable Disposal Methods of Food Wastes in Hospitality Operations* (pp. 176–192). IGI Global., DOI: 10.4018/979-8-3693-2181-2.ch012

Singh, B., Kaunert, C., & Vig, K. (2024). Reinventing Influence of Artificial Intelligence (AI) on Digital Consumer Lensing Transforming Consumer Recommendation Model: Exploring Stimulus Artificial Intelligence on Consumer Shopping Decisions. In Musiolik, T., Rodriguez, R., & Kannan, H. (Eds.), *AI Impacts in Digital Consumer Behavior* (pp. 141–169). IGI Global., DOI: 10.4018/979-8-3693-1918-5.ch006

Singh, B., Vig, K., & Kaunert, C. (2024). Modernizing Healthcare: Application of Augmented Reality and Virtual Reality in Clinical Practice and Medical Education. In Modern Technology in Healthcare and Medical Education: Blockchain, IoT, AR, and VR (pp. 1-21). IGI Global.

Taghian, A., Abo-Zahhad, M., Sayed, M. S., & Abdel-Malek, A. (2021, December). Virtual, Augmented Reality, and Wearable Devices for Biomedical Applications: A Review. In *2021 9th International Japan-Africa Conference on Electronics, Communications, and Computations (JAC-ECC)* (pp. 93-98). IEEE.

Than, N. N. (2023). *Journey to Wellbeing: Seeing Beyond the Mind's Eye Through Story in a Virtual Therapeutic Space* (Doctoral dissertation, New York University Tandon School of Engineering).

Thompson, A. H. (2021). A Holistic Approach to Employee Functioning: Assessing the Impact of a Virtual-Reality Mindfulness Intervention at Work.

Chapter 5
Modelling and Optimizing the Decontamination Process of Surgical Instruments

Tracey England

https://orcid.org/0000-0001-7565-4189

Southampton University, UK

Doris A. Behrens

Universität für Weiterbildung Krems, Austria

Thomas Davies

Cardiff University, UK

Daniel Gartner

https://orcid.org/0000-0003-4361-8559

Cardiff University, UK

ABSTRACT

In the age of multi-resistant bacteria and viruses, sterilizing surgical instruments effectively and efficiently impacts hospital-acquired infections. In a hospital sterilization and decontamination unit (HSDU), contaminated equipment arrives after their use in the operating theatre, intensive care unit, diagnostics facilities, and wards. Items are unpacked, checked, inventoried, washed, dried and packed. Each activity requires resources and inefficient management can lead to increasing lead times for items to be processed and, thus, poses an increased risk of hospital-acquired infections. A simulation model was developed for the National Health Service in

DOI: 10.4018/979-8-3693-5237-3.ch005

the U.K. Data relating to staffing levels and machine availability has been collected and the arrival patterns of items are considered. A heuristic simulation-optimization approach was employed to produce an improved staffing pattern that meets the required service level. Furthermore, the output ensures that instruments are processed within a 5-hour target time and is developed and applied to real-world scenarios.

1. INTRODUCTION

The management and decontamination of surgical instruments are key components in the delivery of safe interventional care that minimizes risk to patients. Guidelines such as Health Technical Memoranda (HTM) advocate a full assessment of the volume and types of surgical services provided, (Rutala & Weber, 2008). To ensure that surgery is delivered in a timely, efficient, and effective way, it is essential that the demand placed on the decontamination unit is well understood so that effective planning decisions can be made in relation to the available resources. In hospitals, the decontamination of medical devices is undertaken by a Hospital Sterilization and Decontamination Unit (HSDU). In ensuring that they are safe for further use, instruments are required to undergo a process of decontamination. This includes cleaning and disinfection, and sterilization which is used to render instruments free from all microorganisms, (Fraise, 2013). However, before sterilization happens, contaminated items are washed to remove loose debris and surface contamination. Figure 1 shows the decontamination life cycle which includes all the activities undertaken in an orderly manner to ensure that items are fit for re-use before returning them to their respective areas.

Figure 1. Decontamination life cycle

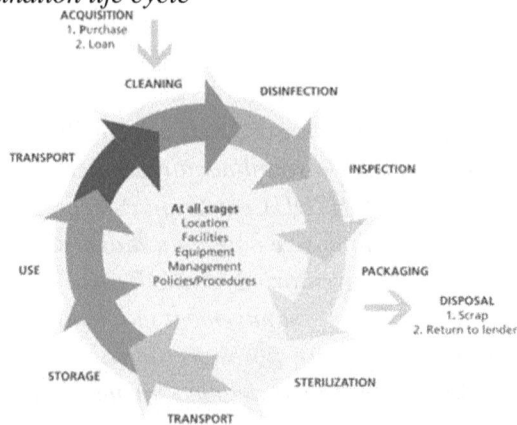

A HSDU requires staff to clean devices to an appropriate level using a combination of manual and automated methods. Validated washer disinfectors are used that must be configured with appropriate chemistry to achieve the required standards prior to sterilization. A process map is shown in Figure 2. Both priority and non-priority items move through the system, each with a different requirement on their 5-hour target turnaround time within the system. Instruments that are contaminated with high-risk pathogens as well as medical items, such as loans sets and trauma sets, are considered high priority items. They need to be decontaminated as quickly as possible to prevent drying of proteins and to ensure the efficient running of Operating Theatres.

Figure 2. Process mapping of an HSDU

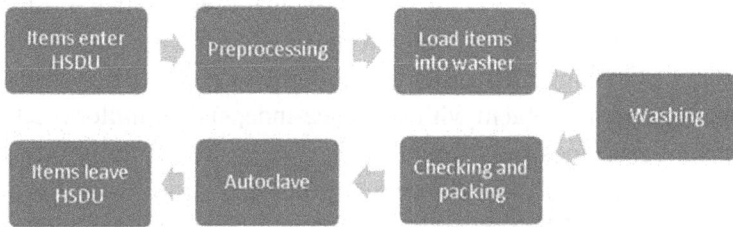

In this chapter, a heuristic simulation-optimization approach are developed to produce an efficient staffing model to ensure target turnaround time requirements. Our modelling follows a two-stage process. Firstly, a Discrete-Event Simulation (DES) model is used to mimic the aforementioned process mapping. Furthermore, a simulation-optimization heuristic ensures that improved staffing patterns are generated without compromising the turnaround targets.

Our results reveal that, using current staffing levels and a high demand scenario, as few as 67.4% of high priority items leave the system within the 5-hour target after entering the HSDU.

In contrast, using our proposed methodology and schedule, more than 80% of high priority items would leave the system within the 5-hour target.

The remainder of this paper is structured as follows. In the next section, we highlight related work in this field followed by an algebraic model description as well as an overview of our simulation model. In section 4, our simulation model is validated using real-world data. We also evaluate the influence of different demand scenarios on the turnaround times. Finally, we close our book chapter with a discussion, a summary and generalizability statements.

2. RELATED WORK

Volland *et al.* (2017) provide a literature review on material logistics in hospitals and our planning problem can be categorized into the following echelon: Distribution and scheduling decisions of sterile medical devices. In the remainder of this section, we will highlight similarities and differences of our work with respect to publications in the field of sterile medical devices.

Di Mascolo and Gouin (2013) develop a generic simulation model for hospital sterilization. The difference to our model is, however, that our items have different priority levels which means that medical items which were used to treat patients with infectious diseases are prioritized over other items. Furthermore, our approach determines staffing levels which can also be seen as an extension of Di Mascolo and Gouin (2013). Finally, our model allows HSDU managers to trade-off turnaround times broken down by priority classes and staffing levels.

Di Mascolo and Gouin (2013) model the problem of sterilizing medical items as a flexible flow shop problem with sequence-independent uniform setup times, parallel batching machines and parallel batches. They use a deterministic model in which jobs are processed in parallel batches by multiple identical parallel machines. Our problem differs to their approach because our objective is to find a minimum number of staff that covers all the workstations. Furthermore, we develop a discrete event simulation model that can handle uncertainty in arrivals and activity durations such as pre-processing the arriving items.

Similar to Rossi, Puppato, and Lanzetta (2013), Ozturk, Begen, and Zaric (2014) formulate the sterilization process as a job shop scheduling problem. They present a branch-and-bound based heuristic method and compare it to a linear model and two other heuristics from the literature. Again, the difference to our approach is that we use simulation-optimization to find the minimum number of staff required such that turnaround targets are satisfied.

Lau *et al.* (2015) develop a simulation model for the thermal energy consumption of a sterilization device. Their model is used to predict the actual transient temperature and pressure profiles and the details of the mass transfers in the autoclave during a sterilization cycle, among others. The purpose of their simulation model is different than ours because we are looking more at the entire sterilization process from the arrival of items to their packing and, again, our objectives are rather operational and not the total steam consumption as they have.

In terms of simulation-optimisation methodology, one related paper is Omar, Augusto, and Xie (2015) who focus on the organisation of human resources in an Emergency Department. The authors seek to optimally balance service quality and working conditions. They address this issue by optimising the shift distribution among employees and minimise total expected patient waiting time. Similar to our work,

Omar, Augusto, and Xie (2015) propose a stochastic mixed-integer programming model that is solved by a sample average approximation approach.

Possik *et al.* (2022) discuss the use of distributed simulation (DS) in healthcare, specifically in the context of a hospital's intensive care unit (ICU) ward for COVID-19 patients. The simulation employs the AnyLogic platform for agent-based and discrete event modeling to depict physical contacts between healthcare providers and patients. The high-level architecture of the DS system enhances training and assesses managerial decisions for minimizing contacts and disease transmission. In contrast, our chapter focuses on the sterilization and decontamination process of surgical instruments in a hospital sterilization and decontamination unit (HSDU). It addresses the challenge of efficiently managing resources to minimize lead times for processing items and reduce the risk of hospital-acquired infections. Utilizing a simulation model based on real-world practices, our study employs a mathematical model and heuristic simulation-optimization approach to optimize staffing patterns, ensuring that instruments are processed within a 5-hour target time, in accordance with WHO guidelines, and applied to a practical scenario within the National Health Service in the U.K.

Brittin, Ramirez-Nafarrate, and Huang (2021) study the impact of built-environment changes on human behaviour and health, emphasizing the growing recognition of systems approaches for scenario testing in public health interventions. Similar to our chapter, the authors use a computer simulation approach, but their focus is on the potential positive impact of dynamic furniture, promoting micromovement, on energy expenditure among elementary school children and its potential role in reducing childhood obesity.

Rosales, Magazine, and Rao 2019) discusses hospitals investing in technology to enhance inventory visibility and control to address rising supply chain costs, presenting a dual-source hybrid inventory system as an example. The focus is on optimizing inventory policies to reduce costs and improve availability through a simulation-based approach. In contrast, our chapter emphasizes the impact of

efficient sterilization on hospital-acquired infections, detailing activities in a sterilization and decontamination unit and highlighting the need for optimal staffing and turnaround times based on WHO guidelines and a simulation-optimization approach. While Rosales, Magazine, and Rao (2019) addresses technology driven inventory optimization in response to supply chain costs, our chapter focuses on the efficient sterilization of surgical instruments to mitigate the risk of infections.

In conclusion, the models proposed in this chapter can be categorized into and differentiated from the literature on scheduling sterilization processes as follows. First, we model the problem as a stochastic program which is similar to Omar, Augusto, and Xie (2015). Second, in terms of scheduling methods, we use a heuristic algorithm which is similar to Ozturk, Begen, and Zaric (2014). However, their heuristic is based on a job shop scheduling model formulation rather than a staffing problem. Finally, we compare the staffing patterns currently in use with the staffing pattern produced by our simulation-optimization approach.

3. METHODS

Simulation Models

A Discrete Event Simulation (DES) Model was employed to solve the problem of planning the most efficient staffing levels. The model was developed in the Discrete Event Simulation software called Simul8. Details of this are available in the Technical Appendix. The model enables the investigation of various inputs, such as differing arrival patterns, processing times and staff shifts. It was then used to investigate the effects that a new shift pattern would have on different demand patterns. This was then verified respectively with HSDU staff and validated by comparing the turnaround times of items from the simulation with actual data obtained from the HSDU.

Di Mascolo and Gouin (2013) provide a generic structure for a hospital sterilization simulation. Their model breaks down the system into five steps:

1) Pre-disinfection and transfer
2) Rinsing
3) Automatic washing
4) Packing
5) Autoclaving

Due to limitations on the data collected, the model used here will be structured as four steps:

1) Pre-processing
2) Automatic washing
3) Packing
4) Autoclaving

Di Mascolo and Gouin (2013) also make an assumption that there is no item priority due to only a small proportion of autoclave cycles containing priority items. This assumption is not used in this model due to the interest in this study being that priority items must be processed within a different time to non-priority items.

Packing in their model is also broken into bags and containers, in which items are packed into. Since items within the data are recorded as trays with no distinction between the numbers of items on the tray, packing is simply taken as the time taken to pack a tray. Storage capacity while waiting for the next step is assumed to be un-limited as visits to the sterilization system seemed to demonstrate enough capacity to prevent any blockages. Items are processed in a FirstIn-First-Out (FIFO) manner, though priority items will always go before non-priority items.

A Discrete Event Simulation model of the sterilization system was created. It could take various inputs for investigation, such as different arrival patterns, activity times and staff shift. This model was used to investigate what effects the new shift pattern would have on different demand patterns and was validated by comparing the turnaround times of items from the simulation to a real week's turnaround times.

The model which is shown in Figure 3 simulates a total period of two weeks, with results being collected for one week across the second week. This is done to provide a warmup time for the simulation. In the real-life system, it's possible that items can be left over from the previous week which then need to be processed in the following week. The one-week warm up time allows the simulation to account for this, leading to more accurate results. It simulates one week since the shift schedule being built will be a weekly schedule.

Figure 3. Simulation model overview

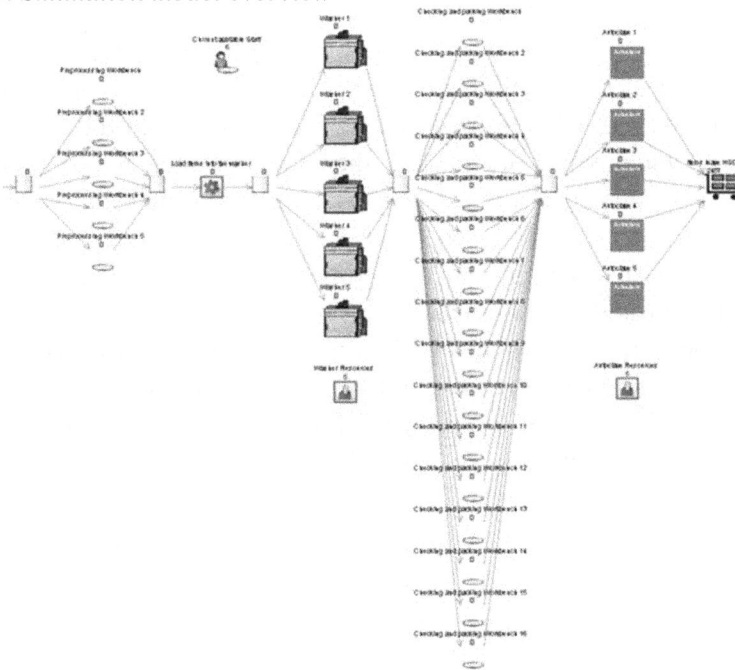

Modelling Assumptions

The model is based on the following assumptions:

- Priority items are always processed before non-priority items in the queue. Within each priority class, items are processed based on a First-In-First-Out policy.
- Maintenance and breakdowns of machines are not considered in the simulation model.
- No items going into the unit require repair.
- The sterilization or decontamination process cannot be interrupted.
- Staff are available for their entire shift.

4. A SIMULATION-OPTIMIZATION HEURISTIC

A new shift schedule was created using a heuristic algorithm that is described in more detail in the Technical Appendix. Essentially, a heuristic approach is a practical method that aims to find a close-to-optimal solution for a complex optimization problem. Given that shifts can start at one out of multiple start times during a day and that multiple workers can be assigned to shifts, determining optimal staffing patterns is complex.

For the model that was built in Simul8, we first divide the staff schedule into 6 different shift types: 3 shifts for the weekdays and 3 for the weekends. The heuristic then starts with an initial staff scenario which ensures that 100% of the items are processed within target times. Then, the total number of employees assigned to shift types is gradually decreased using a randomized Greedy approach. In each iteration when a new staff shift schedule solution representation is generated, we run the simulation to determine whether items are processed within target times. If the new shift schedule maintains the 100% target times, then it is accepted as a new solution. If the target time goes below 100% then the schedule was rejected, and the previous solution was kept. A different shift schedule would then be selected from the old solution to be reduced by one to test to see if it could be improved. This then continued until a schedule was discovered that could not be reduced further, which was accepted as the final solution.

5. RESULTS

In this section, we describe the parameters that we used to carry out our study, followed by a presentation of our results. The results are measured using the percentage of all items during the week which met the target turnaround times. This is done because the focus of this work is on maximizing the percentage of items which meet the time target.

A. Model Validation

To ensure that the discrete-event simulation model is a valid representation of the real-world sterilization and decontamination process, we carried out a validation step, see Law and Kelton (2000). A week representing an average demand scenario was selected in which 2,401 items entered the HSDU. As validation metric, we chose the turnaround times in seconds that items require to be processed in the system.

The results are shown in Figure 4. On the left-hand side, the turnaround times produced by the simulation is shown whereas on the right-hand side the real-world turnaround times are given. The comparison shows that in both outputs there are 3 turnaround time peaks happening at, approximately, 400s, 1,500s and 2,700s. Another observation is that the median turnaround times are 1,531s and 1,348s for the simulation model and the real-world observations, respectively.

Figure 4. Model validation results

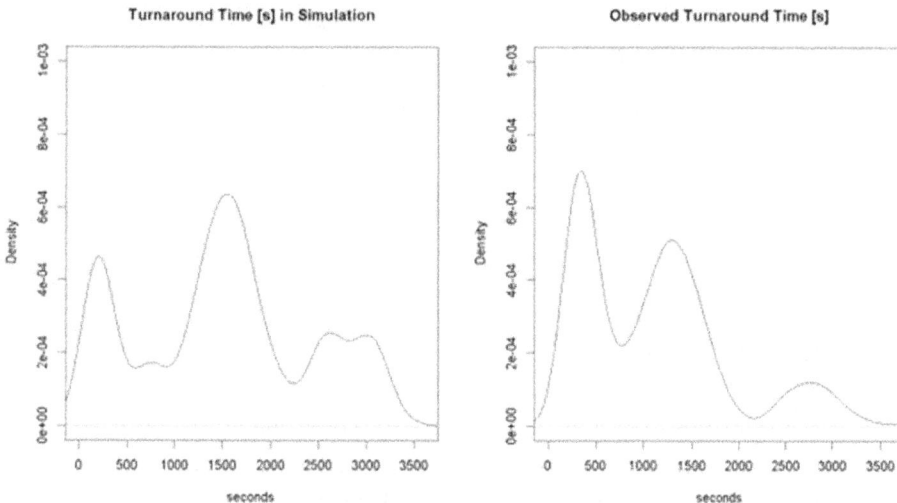

B. Proposed Shift Schedule

We ran our heuristic algorithm which suggested the following pattern: On weekdays, we schedule 5, 11 and 11 staff members for the 6am, 8am and 4pm shift, respectively. On weekends, we schedule 2, 8 and 6 staff members for the 6am, 8am and 4pm shifts, respectively. Figure 5 shows a comparison of the number of staff allocated to the time intervals currently employed and using the proposed shift schedule from the heuristic optimization approach. The results of the simulation which are shown in Figure 5 reveal that the new shift schedule would be capable of 99.5% of items meeting the target turnaround times on an average week. To compare this to the current shift schedule, a representative week was selected. The results also showed that 64.2% of items could meet the turnaround targets in the real-life situation using the current schedule, much lower than the proposed schedule.

Figure 5. Current vs. proposed shift schedule

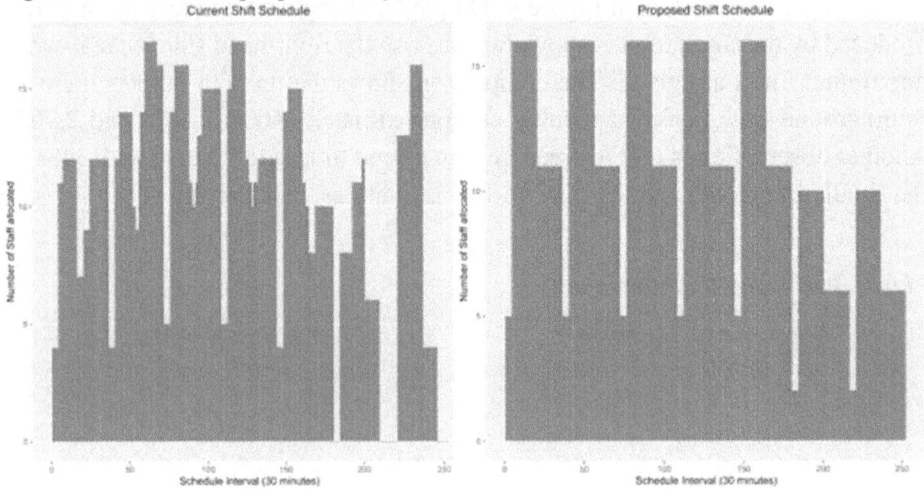

C. Scenario Analysis

The current shift schedule and the new proposed shift schedule were tested in two different scenarios: The Low Demand Scenario and The High Demand Scenario. The scenarios look at the upper and lower bounds of item arrivals for a week, with results being collected for the item turnaround time distribution. This was used in order to determine the percentage of items unable to meet the target turnaround times.

Low Demand Scenario: A low demand week in which 2,124 items arrived was chosen. The simulation was run and the turnaround times for the current and new shift schedule were reported. The data showed that the percentage of items that met the target turnaround times was 78.8% using the current shift schedule. In contrast, the simulation results from using the new shift schedule revealed that 99.2% of items met the target turnaround times.

High Demand Scenario: This scenario looks at how the staff schedule performs in a high demand week. The corresponding item arrival function was selected from the week before Easter 2016 in which 3,093 items arrived. The result of simulating the high demand scenario is shown in Figure 6. Again, we compare the relative frequency of items processed within the turnaround times using the current and the proposed shift schedule. The results reveal that the number of items that met the turnaround target times was 67.4% from the current shift schedule. In contrast, the proposed shift schedule was able to meet the target turnaround times 80.4% of the time.

6. DISCUSSION

A. Limitations

Our simulation model doesn't consider planned and unplanned downtimes of machines which could be added in a next stage of the simulation. Planned downtimes are typically scheduled on a cyclic pattern, e.g., every morning before the ramp up of the demand curve. Unscheduled downtimes, e.g., when a machine randomly breaks down, could be incorporated into the simulation model by using a probability distribution with a machine-dependent mean time to failure.

The model also doesn't consider that items going through the HSDU may fail to be processed at different stages of the sterilization process (e.g., ripped packaging). This could also be considered in the next development of the simulation model.

Figure 6. High demand scenario results

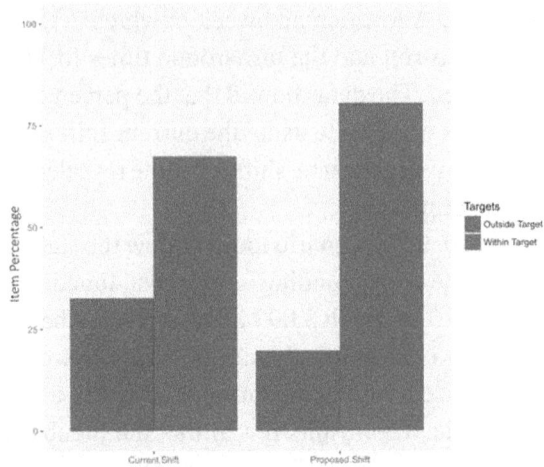

B. Discussion of Modelling HSDU-Acquired Hospital Infections

The modelling of nosocomial infections and infection epidemics is out of scope of this study. However, our results can be used to extend prior studies of mathematical modelling of hospital acquired infections and infection epidemics, see van Kleef *et al.* (2013) and Behrens, Rauner, and Caulkins (2008), respectively.

C. Discussion of Choosing a Discrete-Event Simulation Model

Because of the stochastic nature in demand, we have chosen to use a discrete-event simulation model as compared to using a deterministic approach such as Linear Programming to determine shift schedules, see Lemmer *et al.* (2004). The combination between these approaches and to provide analytical results using time-dependent queueing models (see, e.g., Sehulster (2004)) is part of our ongoing research.

7. SUMMARY AND GENERALIZABILITY

The aim of this study was to develop a simulation model which can be used to evaluate shift schedules for a sterilization service. A scenario analysis was carried out to observe how robust the solution was under different circumstances and compare it to the current shift schedule. This has practical implications for the delivery of

HSDU services in the collaborating NHS Trust and could provide useful evidence for other organizations.

Using a heuristic method, we created shift schedules requiring 33.4 whole time equivalents. The simulation showed that this model would be sufficient to meet the turnaround target times for items in an average week. It also showed that this shift schedule would be unable to meet the item target times for high demand weeks, which would require additional staff to be assigned to meet the targets. Practicality, a solution could be to deploy temporary staff or utilize overtime to cope with unexpected high demand work. Future work will focus on developing a linear programming model for the optimal planning of shift schedules.

REFERENCES

Behrens, D. A., Rauner, M. S., & Caulkins, J. P. (2008). Modelling the spread of hepatitis c via commercial tattoo parlours: Implications for public health interventions. *OR-Spektrum*, 30(2), 269–288. DOI: 10.1007/s00291-007-0090-7

Di Mascolo, M., & Gouin, A. (2013). A generic simulation model to assess the performance of sterilization services in health establishments. *Health Care Management Science*, 16(1), 45–61. DOI: 10.1007/s10729-012-9210-2 PMID: 22886097

Lau, W. L., Reizes, J., Timchenko, V., Kara, S., & Kornfeld, B. (2015). Heat and mass transfer model to predict the operational performance of a steam sterilisation autoclave including products. *International Journal of Heat and Mass Transfer*, 90, 800–811. DOI: 10.1016/j.ijheatmasstransfer.2015.06.089

Law, A. M., & Kelton, W. D. (2000). *Simulation modeling and analysis* (Vol. 3). McGraw-Hill New York.

Lemmer, K., Mielke, M., Pauli, G., & Beekes, M. (2004). Decontamination of surgical instruments from prion proteins: In vitro studies on the detachment, destabilization and degradation of prpsc bound to steel surfaces. *The Journal of General Virology*, 85(12), 3805–3816. DOI: 10.1099/vir.0.80346-0 PMID: 15557254

Omar, E., Garaix, T., Augusto, V., & Xie, X. (2015). A stochastic optimization model for shift scheduling in emergency departments. *Health Care Management Science*, 18(3), 289–302. DOI: 10.1007/s10729-014-9300-4 PMID: 25270574

Ozturk, O., Begen, M. A., & Zaric, G. S. (2014). A branch and bound based heuristic for makespan minimization of washing operations in hospital sterilization services. *European Journal of Operational Research*, 239(1), 214–226. DOI: 10.1016/j.ejor.2014.05.014

Possik, J., Asgary, A., Solis, A. O., Zacharewicz, G., Shafiee, M. A., Najafabadi, M. M., Nadri, N., Guimaraes, A., Iranfar, H., & Ma, P.. (2021). An agent-based modeling and virtual reality application using distributed simulation: Case of a covid-19 intensive care unit. *IEEE Transactions on Engineering Management*, 2022. Brittin J, Araz O.M., Ramirez-Nafarrate A, and Huang T.T. An agent-based simulation model for testing novel obesity interventions in school environment design. *IEEE Transactions on Engineering Management*.

Rosales, C. R., Magazine, M. J., & Rao, U. S. (2019). Dual sourcing and joint replenishment of hospital supplies. *IEEE Transactions on Engineering Management*, 67(3), 918–931. DOI: 10.1109/TEM.2019.2895242

Rossi, A., Puppato, A., & Lanzetta, M. (2013). Heuristics for scheduling a two-stage hybrid flow shop with parallel batching machines: Application at a hospital sterilisation plant. *International Journal of Production Research*, 51(8), 2363–2376. DOI: 10.1080/00207543.2012.737942

Russell, Hugo & Ayliffe's: Principles and Practice of Disinfection. (2013). (pp. 445–458). Preservation and Sterilization.

Rutala, W. A., & Weber, D. J. (2019). Guideline for disinfection and sterilization in healthcare facilities, 2008. update: May 2019.

Sehulster, L. M. (2004). Prion inactivation and medical instrument reprocessing: Challenges facing healthcare facilities. *Infection Control and Hospital Epidemiology*, 25(4), 276–279. DOI: 10.1086/502391 PMID: 15108722

van Kleef, E., Robotham, J. V., Jit, M., Deeny, S. R., & Edmunds, W. J. (2013). Modelling the transmission of healthcare associated infections: A systematic review. *BMC Infectious Diseases*, 13(1), 1–13. DOI: 10.1186/1471-2334-13-294 PMID: 23809195

Volland, J., Fügener, A., Schoenfelder, J., & Brunner, J. O. (2017). Material logistics in hospitals: A literature review. *Omega*, 69, 82–101. DOI: 10.1016/j.omega.2016.08.004

APPENDIX

We approach the problem of evaluating staffing levels at the HSDU using a discrete-event simulation model. The model was built using the software 'Simul8'. The following assumptions are taken in the simulation model:

- Weekly machine maintenance is not simulated.
- It assumes that no items require repairs or to redo the sterilization process one begun.
- Machines do not suffer breakdowns.
- Priority items will always be processed ahead of non-priority items.

A. Discrete Event Simulation

Simulation Models can be divided into different types such as Agent Based Simulation, Monte Carlo Simulation each of which are useful for solving different problems. The approach employed in our research is Discrete Event Simulation. These types of models are popular within healthcare systems such as hospitals due to their ability to model queueing systems, which is a common problem in these systems. The model breaks down the system structure into two different types, queues and activities. Activities are the steps in the model that an item must undergo. Examples of this in the sterilization system are processes such as item packing or item washing, which are activities that items must undergo to complete the process. Queues are the areas that objects are able to wait within the system until the next activity is ready to receive them. The simulation interprets activities as instantaneous events which have a time before they can be performed, known as the processing time. This processing time can be a fixed time, a known distribution or a distribution created by the user. Items which enter the system are all individually simulated, as opposed to other simulation techniques such as System Dynamics, which looks at the rates of events instead of each individual event. Activities which accept an item and begin processing will become full, meaning that if other items are ready to enter that activity, they will have to wait and the queue will begin to build up. It is through this process that these queueing systems are simulated.

These types of simulation are known as Discrete Event Simulation since time only advances in the simulation when an event occurs, such as an activity being complete, or an item entering the system, unlike continuous models such as System Dynamics, which will advance at each time increment regardless of if anything has occurred. This system of varying time steps is known as the next-event time advance [12]. To keep track of the total time which has passed, a simulation clock is present which counts time based on these variable time steps. There are a number of advantage for these types of model. Since the process is broken into arriving items, queues and activities, it is relatively easy to gather the required data for the simulation. The types of data required, such as the item arrival time, the time for activities to complete and resource allocation, are commonly recorded and easily quantified. The models are often easy to understand, with the model structure generally reflecting the simulated system structure. It also allows individual items to be monitored which makes it simple to find out where errors occur in the simulation and collect data on specific items or item types. Disadvantages of this method are that it can fail to model some processes such as feedback loops, which makes it less ideal for systems where there are effects that are hard to quantify.

B. Simulation model using Simul8

A Discrete Event Simulation model of the sterilization system was created. It could take various inputs for investigation, such as different arrival patterns, activity times and staff shifts. This model was used to investigate what effects the new shift pattern would have on different demand patterns and was validated by comparing the turnaround times of items from the simulation to a real week's turnaround times.

The model which is shown in Figure 3 simulates a total period of two weeks, with results being collected for one week across the second week. This is done to provide a warmup time for the simulation. In the real-life system, it's possible that items can be left over from the previous week which then need to be processed in the following week. The one-week warm up time allows the simulation to account for this, leading to more accurate results. It simulates one week since the shift schedule being built will be a weekly schedule.

C. Heuristic Approach for Solving Shift Schedules

Table 1 shows the initial staff scenario that is improved using our heuristic approach.

Table 1. Initial staff scenario

Weekday 6am	Weekday 8am	Weekday 4pm	Weekend 6am	Weekend 8am	Weekend 4pm
5	15	15	5	15	15

D. Heuristic Algorithm Output

Table 2 provides an overview of the current shift schedule.

Table 2. The current shift schedule

Shift number	Shift time	Shift Day	Number of staff
1	6am - 2pm	Mon - Fri	4
2	6am - 2pm	Wed - Thurs	1
3	8am - 4pm	Mon - Fri	7
4	8am - 4pm	Tues - Thurs	1
5	8am - 4pm	Wed - Sun	1
6	8am - 4pm	Sat-Sun	5
7	8am - 4pm	Sun	3
8	8am - 4pm	Fri - Sun	1
9	8am - 4pm	Mon	1
10	8am - 4pm	Mon, Thurs, Fri	1
11	9:30am - 4pm	Tues - Thurs	1
12	9:30am - 3pm	Tues - Fri	1
13	4pm - 12am	Mon - Fri	1
14	4pm - 12am	Tues - Fri	2
15	4pm - 12am	Mon, Tues, Thurs, Fri	2
16	4pm - 12am	Mon - Thurs	2
17	4pm - 12am	Mon - Wed	3
18	4pm - 12am	Tues - Wed	1
19	4pm - 12am	Mon, Wed, Thurs	1
20	4pm - 12am	Thurs - Fri	1
21	4pm - 12am	Tues, Wed, Fri	2
22	4:30pm - 12am	Tues - Thurs	1
23	4:30pm - 12am	Tues - Wed	1
24	8pm - 12am	Tues - Wed	1
25	8pm - 12am	Mon - Fri	1
26	8pm - 12am	Mon, Fri	1
27	8pm - 10pm	Tues	1
28	8am - 12pm	Sat - Sun	1
29	3pm - 8pm	Sat	1
30	12pm - 8pm	Sat-Sun	4
31	9:30am-2pm/ 6pm - 12am	Mon	1

Using the simulation model, a heuristic approach was used to determine a shift schedule which would meet the target turnaround times for all items while using the lowest possible working staff. This is shown in Table 3.

Table 3. Heuristic procedure for the proposed solution

	6am	8am	4pm	6am	8am	4pm	within target
1	5	15	15	5	15	15	100
2	5	14	15	5	15	15	100
3	5	14	14	5	15	15	100
4	5	14	14	5	14	15	100
5	5	14	14	5	14	14	100
6	5	13	14	5	14	14	100
7	5	13	13	5	14	14	100
8	5	13	13	5	13	14	100
9	5	13	13	5	13	13	100
10	5	12	13	5	13	13	100
11	5	12	12	5	13	13	100
12	5	12	12	5	12	13	100
13	5	12	12	5	12	12	100
14	5	11	12	5	12	12	100
15	5	11	11	5	12	12	100
16	5	11	11	5	11	12	100
17	5	11	11	5	11	11	100
18	5	11	11	5	10	11	100
19	5	11	11	5	10	10	100
20	5	11	11	5	9	10	100
21	5	11	11	5	9	9	100
22	5	11	11	5	8	9	100
23	5	11	11	5	8	8	100
24	5	11	11	4	8	8	100
25	5	11	11	4	8	7	100
26	5	11	11	3	8	7	100
27	5	11	11	2	8	7	100
28	5	11	11	2	8	6	100
29	4	11	11	2	8	6	99
30	5	10	11	2	8	6	99
31	5	11	10	2	8	6	99
32	5	11	11	1	8	6	99
33	5	11	11	2	7	6	99
34	5	11	11	2	8	5	99

Chapter 6
Revolutionizing Skin Cancer Diagnosis With Artificial Intelligence:
Insights Into Machine Learning Techniques

Wasswa Shafik
https://orcid.org/0000-0002-9320-3186

Dig Connectivity Research Laboratory, Kampala, Uganda & School of Digital Science, Universiti Brunei Darussalam, Brunei

ABSTRACT

A frequent cancer worldwide is skin cancer. Non-melanoma exists. Melanoma kills more than non-melanoma skin malignancies. Successful treatment and early diagnosis improve skin cancer survival. Cancer burden and prognosis vary depending on the diagnosis type and stage. The biopsy method used to diagnose skin cancer is imprecise. To diagnose and treat skin cancer early, onco-dermatologists must enhance diagnostic accuracy. Doctors use several tools to diagnose skin lesions. Through image processing, AI has enhanced early skin cancer diagnosis. Radiology adopted artificial intelligence (AI) sooner than dermatology. AI is now more accessible because of technology, AI-powered expert systems can detect skin cancer early. This chapter examines early skin cancer diagnosis using machine learning (ML) models and the problem of automating skin cancer diagnosis with AI algorithms. This study sheds light on past and future efforts to diagnose early skin cancer and other concerns.

DOI: 10.4018/979-8-3693-5237-3.ch006

INTRODUCTION

The uncontrollable growth of skin cells indeed characterizes skin tumours. It occurs when the deoxyribonucleic acid[1] (DNA) in skin cells becomes damaged, and this damage is often attributed to exposure to ultraviolet (UV) radiation from the sun or tanning beds (Shafik et al., 2024a). The damaging effects of UV radiation on DNA can lead to mutations in the genes that regulate cell growth, causing cells to divide and grow uncontrollably, forming tumours. Anyone can get skin cancer; out of that, some are at higher risk than others. Skin cancer varies from person to person due to skin tone, size, type of skin cancer, and location on the body (Saju et al., 2022). Skin cancer is classified into two major categories: melanoma and non-melanoma. Non-melanoma is categorized into squamous cell carcinoma[2] (SCC) and basal cell carcinoma (BCC), which affects more men and is more common in older adults. It is a much more common, less dangerous, and non-deadly type of skin cancer (Vasconcelos et al., 2022). Non-melanoma skin cancer mostly affects the areas, including the face, ears, hands, neck, upper chest, and back, that are regularly exposed to the sun. It is easily treated compared with melanoma cancer, as illustrated in Figure 1.

Figure 1. Types of skin cancers: (a) Basal cell carcinoma (BCC), (b) Squamous cell carcinoma (SCC) and (c) Melanoma

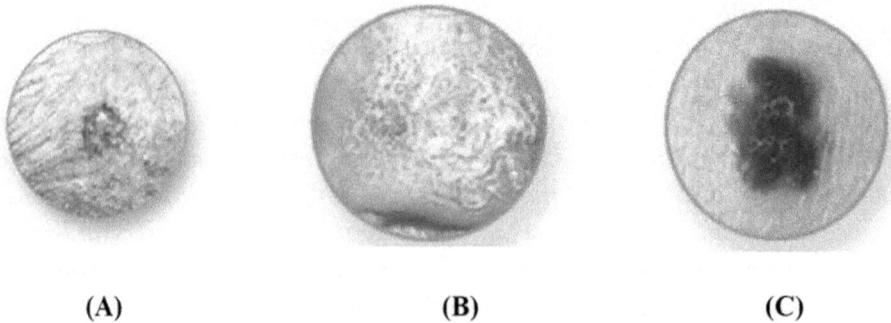

(A)   (B)   (C)

Melanoma or black tumor is much less common than the other types of cancer. It is a hazardous, rare, and deadly cancer. Melanoma develops from cells called melanocytes and can easily attack nearby tissue and spread to other body parts. Most of the deaths because of skin cancer are caused by melanoma (Simango, Mushiri, Yahya, & Nyanduwa, 2023). Any part of the human body may also be affected by melanoma. Melanoma skin cancer mostly affects the areas including the face, ears, hands, and shoulders, among others. It can also come in varying types, such as nodular melanoma, superficial spreading melanoma, acral lentiginous, and lentigo maligna. Melanoma cancer can be treated successfully if diagnosed early unless it spreads to other parts of the body and leads to horrible death. The risk factor that increases the chances of getting skin cancer includes a previous history of skin cancer, family history of skin cancer, pale/fair color skin that affects easily, rare congenital diseases, obesity, a large number of moles, a history of tanning bed issue, living in the location where excess sun exposure, medicines that suppress the immune system, a weak immune system and co-existing medical conditions which suppress the immune system (Singh, Kaushik, Talyan, & Dwivedi, 2022).

According to statistics published by the American Cancer Society[3], 97,160 Americans were diagnosed with skin cancer[4] in 2023. This accounts for approximately 5.0% of all the cancer patients in the United States, and 7990 (5420 men and 2570 women) died because of skin cancer (Rajesh, Murugan, Muruganantham, & Ganesh Kumar, 2020). This accounts for approximately 1.3% of the deaths because of skin cancer in the United States. In 2023, the number of deaths due to melanoma skin cancer increased by 4.4%. Melanoma skin cancer patients are only about 1.7% of all other skin cancer cases, but they account for more skin cancer deaths (Kumar, 2021). Melanoma[5] is the 17th most common type of cancer worldwide. It is the 13th among cancers in men and the 15th in women, as presented in Figure 2.

Figure 2. Global melanoma skin cancer rates during 2020[6]

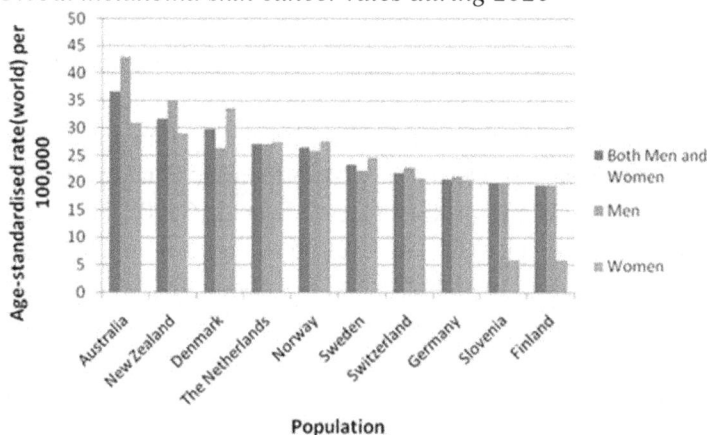

During the year 2020, the new cases of melanoma skin cancer were reported more than 150,000. The average five-year survival rate for melanoma is 93.5%, which is quite high. If melanoma[7] is diagnosed at an early stage, the five-year survival rate of melanoma is 99% (Suhasini et al., 2022). The chances of survival are higher when melanoma has not spread to other parts of the body, but only 77.6% of melanomas are diagnosed at the local level. The number of deaths from melanoma can be reduced if it is diagnosed early. Non-melanoma skin cancer is not included in the cancer statistics report (Bollino et al., 2022). This disease is not reported in all cancer patients globally because it is so common; it often goes undiagnosed, and it is often treated in primary care and is likely to be unreported in national cancer registry data (Rajeshkumar, Ananth, & Mohananthini, 2023). Figure 3 shows the incidence of melanoma globally, among men and women, during the year 2020. Australia, followed by New Zealand, had the highest overall rate of melanoma skin in 2020.

Figure 3. Global non-melanoma skin cancer rates in 2020[8]

Non-melanoma skin cancer rates

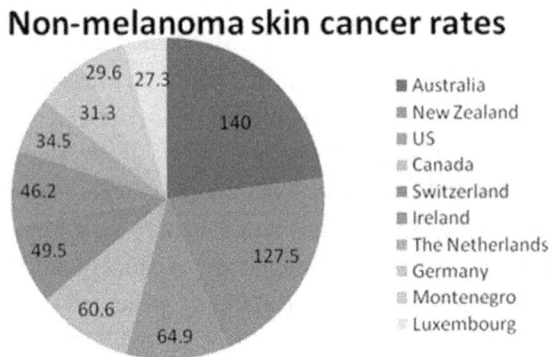

Figure 3 shows the global incidence of non-melanoma skin cancer in 2020. The country with the highest number of non-melanoma cancer cases in 2020 was Australia, followed by New Zealand. Therefore, early diagnosis is important in the treatment of skin cancer. Dermatologists often use visual examination, such as the biopsy method, to diagnose skin cancer (Ma et al., 2020). This system will use samples taken from a suspicious skin lesion for diagnostic purposes to determine whether they are cancerous, with an accuracy of about 60%. The process is painful, slow, and time-consuming.

Dermoscopy is another method commonly used in the diagnosis of skin cancer[9]. The accuracy of cancer diagnosis using dermoscopy reaches 89%. We are also expected to diagnose skin cancer with high sensitivity; dermoscopy was given 82.6% sensitivity in the diagnosis of melanoma, 98.6% sensitivity in the diagnosis of basal cell carcinoma, and 86.5% sensitivity in the diagnosis of squamous cell carcinoma. Dermoscopy has increased the accuracy of melanoma diagnosis, but accurate diagnosis of early melanomas without dermoscopy features remains difficult. Although dermoscopy is very accurate in diagnosing melanoma, it is less suitable for the diagnosis of featureless melanoma, and the accuracy still needs to be further improved to improve patient survival rates. The problems with dermoscopy and the need to improve the accuracy of skin cancer diagnosis further laid the groundwork for the development of computer-aided detection tests for the diagnosis of skin cancer (D. & A.R., 2021).

Computer-aided detection technology provides an easy, inexpensive, and fast way to detect skin cancer symptoms. In general, the steps in computer-aided diagnosis of skin cancer are as follows: image acquisition, preprocessing, segmentation, feature extraction, and classification. The most important steps in computer-aided skin cancer diagnosis are segmentation and classification. Segmentation plays a crucial role because subsequent steps are dependent on the output of this phase. Segmentation can be managed in a controlled manner by taking parameters such as shapes, sizes, and colors depending on skin texture and type. However, it is not easy to diagnose skin cancer using computer-aided methods, and for an accurate diagnosis, we have to consider many factors (S., 2022). For example, artifacts such as hair, loss of vignetting, blisters, scars, ink marks, and ruler marks can lead to misclassification and inaccurate segmentation of skin lesions.

Overall, early diagnosis is important for cancer treatment and skin improvement. Professionals can diagnose cancer accurately, but their numbers are limitations; technologies that can diagnose diseases need to be developed with the aid of automated systems that can improve health hygiene and reduce the financial burden on patients (Maiti, Chatterjee, Ashour, & Dey, 2019). AI could be one of the automated methods for the early detection of skin cancer. Through a comprehensive survey and analysis of existing AI algorithms, this chapter aims to provide valuable insights into the different AI algorithms for skin cancer detection. By combining the findings, dermatologists are guided in selecting the appropriate AI algorithm based on their specific needs (Segall & Sankarasubbu, 2022). The outcomes of this research will not only contribute to the understanding of various machine learning algorithms but also provide a foundation for future advancements and innovations in this rapidly evolving field (Maede Banki, Farhad Farsinia, & Shohreh Ghasemi, 2023). How can Machine Learning (ML) techniques be optimized to overcome current challenges in skin cancer diagnosis, and what future research directions should be pursued to enhance the efficacy of AI-based diagnostic systems? is the major research question as justified below:

- CNNs are highly effective at processing medical images due to their ability to recognize patterns and features, while transfer learning allows the use of pre-trained models, reducing the need for extensive labeled datasets and accelerating the development process.
- Addressing data biases is crucial because it ensures that the ML models are fair and accurate across different demographics, reducing the risk of misdiagnosis and improving the trustworthiness of AI diagnostic tools.

- Integrating diverse data sources can provide a more comprehensive view of a patient's condition, leading to more precise and personalized diagnoses, thereby enhancing the overall effectiveness of AI-based skin cancer diagnostic systems.

MACHINE LEARNING (ML) TECHNIQUES

This section presents ML[10] technologies as they are used in cancer diagnosis.

Decision trees

Decision trees are a popular supervised learning algorithm used for both classification and regression tasks. They are particularly effective for tasks where the goal is to extract information or make decisions based on a set of input features. Decision trees are known for their interpretability and ease of understanding (Panthakkan, Anzar, Jamal, & Mansoor, 2022). The rules inferred from the tree structure are often human-readable, making decision trees a valuable tool for extracting insights from complex datasets. They are widely used in various domains, including finance, healthcare, and natural language processing, where extracting information from patterns in data is a common task (Kiran Kumar & Divya Udayan, 2019). The decision tree starts with the root node, which is split into two or more child nodes that represent all the analyzed data. Create child nodes to increase homogeneity.

The decision tree splits the node into all possible paths and then selects the path that gives the most homogeneous child. The choice of decision algorithm for making a decision depends on changes in the objective, which influences the final correctness of the algorithm. A common algorithm is the Classification and Regression Tree algorithm (Attallah & Sharkas, 2021). The decision tree represents the results of determining whether a treatment is successful for a group of tumors or can be used globally. Decision trees may act as an intermediate process rather than a separate process.

Decision tree models were used to evaluate the worthwhileness of sentinel lymph node biopsy, a novel procedure used in the treatment of melanoma and breast cancer. Validity was calculated using head and neck with respect to cutaneous squamous cell carcinoma, a type of skin cancer (Khanam & Kumar, 2022). The decision trees have also been used to clarify the classification of breast cancer cells. The specificity of the decision tree model is 42%, its sensitivity is 91%, and its accuracy is more than 90%.

Naive Bayes Classifier

Naive Bayes classifiers are based on a family of probability classifiers that are based on the principle of Bayes theorem and are based on supervised learning. It is also called a probability classifier. Naive Bayes classifiers are used to classify clinical images and dermatological diseases in the skin with high accuracy (Fatima, Khan, Shaheen, Almujally, & Wang, 2023). The model uses the key information available to help dermatologists accurately identify and diagnose diseases with an accuracy of ~ 70.15% and specificity of ~73.33%. The Naive Bayes classifiers extend their application by providing a means to diagnose other types of skin diseases (Shastry & Sanjay, 2022).

The posterior probability distribution is obtained for each output of the classification. Repeating this process can eliminate the need for multiple training, thereby reducing computational resources. The closing classification performed in this case includes accessible information on data points used for Bayesian analysis (Suiçmez, Tolga Kahraman, Suiçmez, Yılmaz, & Balcı, 2023). The Bayesian sequential framework has also been used to help the models detect melanoma invading human skin. The model estimates all three model parameters, namely the growth rate of melanoma cells, the diffusion rate of melanoma cells, and finally, a constant that determines the rate of degradation of melanoma cells (Kushimo, Salau, Adeleke, & Olaoye, 2023).

The algorithm learns the data from the sequential method: spatially uniform cell testing, 2D circular barrier testing, and finally, 3D invasion testing. These Bayesian methods can be extracted and applied in other biological contexts. This is often possible mainly in the presence of detailed information on quantitative biological measurements, such as extraction of skin lesions from scientific images (Takiddin, Schneider, Yang, Abd-Alrazaq, & Househ, 2021).

Random Forests

The random forest[11] algorithm is an extension of the decision tree and a supervised learning method. It is based on the ensemble learning method, which uses multiple decision trees; this means that the accuracy of the ensemble model is greater than using a single decision tree and avoids overfitting issues (Du-Harpur, Watt, Luscombe, & Lynch, 2020). It is mostly used for classification problems and Regression problems. Each tree in the random forest outputs a prediction for the specific selected class, and the highest-voted class becomes the model result prediction. Random forests continue their applications to diagnose skin cancer and classify skin diseases (Obayya et al., 2023).

The work of the random forest follows two phases. First, the multiple decision trees are combined to create the random forest, and second, the prediction is made from each tree created in the first phase. Random forest for skin cancer works by first selecting the random subset of samples from the skin sample dataset (Ghaffar Nia, Kaplanoglu, & Nasab, 2023). Then, for each feature in the subset, a decision tree is constructed to obtain an estimate. A voting process is then created for each previous release, and the prediction with the higher votes is selected as the final output. The Random Forest classifier shows up to 70% accuracy, sensitivity, and specificity regardless of features. Based on the dataset used, it can also provide greater accuracy in skin cancer detection (Bhatt, Shah, Shah, Shah, & Shah, 2023).

Artificial Neural Networks

The biological structure of the human brain indeed inspires Artificial Neural Networks[12] (ANNs). ANN is a nonlinear and statistical estimator method. ANNs typically consist of three layers. Neural networks have an input layer; neurons in the input layer transmit data to the neurons in the middle layer (Melarkode, Srinivasan, Qaisar, & Plawiak, 2023). The middle layer is called the hidden layer. A relational Neural Network may have a varying number of hidden layers. Neurons in the hidden layer send data to the neurons in the output layer, referred to as output neurons. Calculations are done on every layer by means of backpropagation, which is used to learn complex links/associations between the input and output layers (Shafik et al., 2024b). It is similar to a neural network. Currently, in computer science, the terms neural network and artificial neural network are used interchangeably. The basic ANN structure is shown in Figure 4.

Figure 4. Basic ANN structure

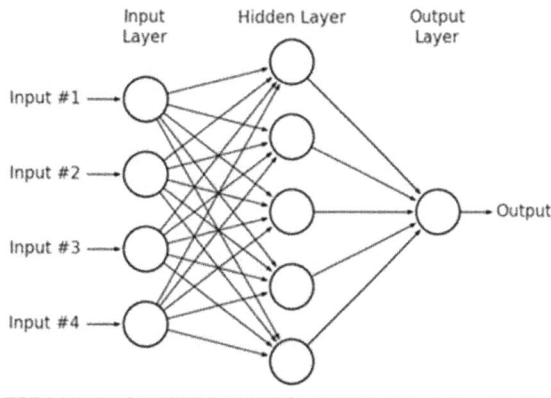

ANN is used for categorization purposes in skin cancer recognition systems. After successful training, the input images from the training set are classified as melanoma or non-melanoma. In ANN, the number of hidden layers sometimes depends directly on the input images—the input layer of the ANN process is connected to the intermediate layer by the first layer data set (Saju et al., 2022). The dataset used in this system can be supervised learning with labeled or unsupervised learning with unlabeled accordingly using an appropriate mechanism. An NN uses backpropagation or feed-forward architecture to train weights present on every network connection line. Both architectures use a pattern that is unlike the one used for the underlying data set (Vasconcelos et al., 2022).

Neural networks based on feed-forward architecture transfer data only in one direction. Data flows only from the first to the last layer. ANNs have been used to predict skin cancer by inputting a set of proven parameters suitable for training, such as gender, movement habits, hypertension, asthma, age, heart disease, etc (Simango et al., 2023). ANN takes the whole data set as input. To improve the accuracy of the model, the inputs are normalized to values between 0 and 1. The outputs are treated as typical classification outputs, which return fractional values between 0 and 1. ANNs can also be used to detect skin cancer by taking an image as input and forwarding it to hidden layers. This process is performed in the following consecutive steps; the first step is the initialization of the random weights to each of its input sets.

Each of the activation values is calculated. Therefore, the magnitude of the error is also known as the change in loss. The scales are updated proportional to the loss. Until the loss reaches a certain lower limit or minimum value, the three steps are repeated. In this area, which is related to skin cancer detection, visual inspection is the initial stage (Singh et al., 2022). This is due to shared similarities between different tumor subcategories, such as color, area, and distribution. For this reason, the use of ANNs is recommended to improve the detection of skin lesions in several classes. ANN is also used to predict various symptoms commonly experienced by cancer patients simultaneously (Rajesh et al., 2020).

The risk of predicted symptoms was an ache, dullness, and weak well-being. The input to the ANN was a list of 39 different covariates. The input characteristics can be divided into five subcategories such as demographic characteristics, such as age and gender; clinical characteristics, such as type and stage of cancer; treatment characteristics, such as radiation treatment and surgical treatment of cancer, reported the underlying patient measurements, such as performance status and symptom burden status and finally health care utilization measures, such as whether or not the patient was hospitalized, live-in caregiver (Kumar, 2021).

ANNs play an important role in predicting skin cancer and the presence of tumors due to their flexible structure and data-driven nature, which makes them a potential modeling approach. ANN systems account for a sensitivity of about ~ 88.5% and a specificity of about ~62.2% for the training set, whereas the validation set demonstrates a comparable sensitivity of ~ 86.2% and a specificity of ~62.7% (Suhasini et al., 2022). However, ANN models are straightforward to implement and cost-effective further development in future studies required for the early identification of skin cancer.

K-Nearest Neighbor

The k-Nearest Neighbors[13] algorithm, also known as KNN, is a parametric supervised classification algorithm. It can be used to solve classification and prediction problems. It is often referred to as a lazy learning algorithm because it does not have a specific learning phase and uses all the information during classification (Rajeshkumar et al., 2023). It is a non-parametric regression algorithm. The main premise of the algorithm is the idea that the similarity of data is determined by the distance between points in space – similar data (belonging to the same class) are close to each other in space (Ma et al., 2020).

The algorithm works by assuming that for each location in space, the distance between the query point and the additional point is calculated. Then, the distances are sorted in ascending order. The top K distances and their corresponding labels are selected from the ordered set. Therefore, the mode value of the K label is returned (D. & A.R., 2021). KNNs have been used as an evaluation algorithm to detect skin cancer and melanomas. The KNN model was then used to create a confusion matrix to visualize the accuracy of the entire model. KNN has been extended as the Radius Nearest Neighbors classifier for the classification of breast cancer and aids in measuring evaluation metrics such as accuracy and specificity (S., 2022).

The reason for the development of KNN is that the value of K is limited. For small k-values, the KNN classifier is sensitive to outliers, while for larger k-values, the KNN classifier poorly fits the data points. This problem is solved by normalizing the radius value of each point to detect outliers effectively (Segall & Sankarasubbu, 2022). KNN applications were extended by their use for the detection of abnormal growth of skin lesions. KNN combined with Firefly, known as a hybrid system, provides more information about skin diseases without the need to perform unnecessary skin biopsies.

The hybrid classifier built on KNN is used for prediction and classification using two main methods: threshold-based segmentation and ABCD feature extraction. Firefly optimization combined with KNN helps to detect skin tumors better than their predecessors while keeping computational and time complexity to a minimum (Maede Banki et al., 2023). KNN classifier with a neighbor set to 15 provides an accuracy of 66.8% with a precision and recall accuracy for positive predictions of 71% and 46%, respectively. The modified KNN classifiers provide an accuracy of 96%. Fuzzy[14] KNN classifiers provide an accuracy of 93.33%, a sensitivity of 88.89%, and a specificity of 100% (Kiran Kumar & Divya Udayan, 2019).

Support Vector Machine

Support Vector Machine[15] (SVM) classifiers are Machine Learning models that can perform linear and nonlinear classification, regression, and outlier detection. When used for classification, SVM creates hyperplanes. Each hyperplane represents a decision boundary that allows a given space to be divided and differentiated into two different classes (Kiran Kumar & Divya Udayan, 2019). The SVM task is to find the hyperplane in n-dimensional space that best divides the data into two classes. The algorithm searches for hyperplanes with the maximum separation margin, that is to say, the maximum of the closest points of each class. Points on both sides of the hyperplane are assigned to different classes (Attallah & Sharkas, 2021).

Linear classification can be done when the data is linearly separated; if the data is not linearly separated, the kernel functions such as linear, quadratic, cubic, fine Gaussian, medium Gaussian, coarse, etc., can choose to represent the data in some form. In higher dimensional space, the goal is to ensure that data points are separated linearly whenever possible (Khanam & Kumar, 2022). SVM can be used to classify different types of skin cancers. ABCD features are used to extract features such as shape, color, and size from dermatological images. After the features are selected, skin diseases are classified as melanoma, seborrheic keratosis, and lupus erythematosus with the help of SVM (Fatima et al., 2023). The method of combining ABCD with SVM can produce good results while providing valuable information;

for narrow classification, SVM has also been used to classify skin lesions as melanoma or non-melanoma.

The process is divided into six stages: capturing the image, processing the image, segmenting, extracting features, splitting the image, and displaying the results. The features extracted from the experiment are texture, color, and shape. To extend the features of the above models, SVM has also been used to identify and diagnose cancer or disease at an early stage before it develops (Suiçmez et al., 2023). Similarly, for early detection and diagnosis of skin cancer, a special bag of features containing spatial information is used. SVM is created with the help of histograms of the gradient optimization set. By using Bendlet Transform (BT) as a feature of the SVM classifier, unwanted features such as hair and noise can be ignored (Kushimo et al., 2023). These can be eliminated using median filtering. The average accuracy, specificity, and specificity of the SVM classifier are about 98%, 95%, and 95%, respectively.

Logistic Regression

The logistic distribution assumptions based on the logistic regression models use the logistic function to separate the data and model the variance of the variable. This variable is binary, meaning that only two groups are possible (Du-Harpur et al., 2020). Hence, this method is used to classify binary data such as cancerous and noncancerous lesions. Both the target variables and the variables can take either of two values (logical 0 or 1).

K-Means Clustering

K-means clustering is a clustering method in unsupervised learning that groups the unlabeled dataset into clusters. This is an iterative process that splits the dataset into various groups so that each dataset contains only one cluster with similar characteristics. Clustering the data into different groups can be performed without training. It is a centroid-based algorithm where each cluster is associated with a centroid (Obayya et al., 2023). The purpose of this algorithm is to reduce the distance between data points and their corresponding clusters. The algorithm takes the input from the available dataset, splits the dataset into a k-number of clusters, and then repeats the process till there are no more best clusters available (Bhatt et al., 2023).

The values of k must be decided in prior. The major tasks performed by the k-means clustering algorithm are: Decide the best for the centroids of k clusters and assign each data point to its nearest center. The k-means clustering algorithm is used to diagnose skin cancer by segmenting the skin lesion (Melarkode et al., 2023). The algorithm takes the clinical images as input, processes them, and then segments the image. The local binary patterns and color percentiles are used for extracting the features from the segmented images and examined on the different classifiers. Finally, the accuracy of the classification was verified. The average accuracy of the algorithm is about 90% (Fatima et al., 2023).

Ensemble Learning

Ensemble Learning combines several learning models to produce a better model, which is a machine learning model. The model is also called an ensemble member. These models can be trained on the same data set or adapted to completely different data sets. The ensemble members come together to publish an estimate for the problem definition (Panthakkan et al., 2022). An ensemble learning classifier can also be used to diagnose whether skin cancer is malignant or benign. The ensemble members are individually trained separately to balance the subspaces, thus reducing redundancy. The remaining classifiers are grouped using neural network fusion. The combined model produced better results than the other individual models (Segall & Sankarasubbu, 2022). The Ensemble classifier has also been used to classify the different types of skin diseases to assist dermatologists in detecting them early. Overall, the Ensemble Learning model outperforms any individual model.

Genetic Algorithm (GA)

GA[16] is an evolutionary algorithm based on adaptive systems theory. The genetic processes of biological systems mainly inspire GA. These algorithms are based on the principles of evolution and natural selection. They look for programs that handle events and focus on checking where the state can be represented as a string. They are often used to find good solutions, such as selecting negative or important features. Execution of GA is generally divided into five main tasks: creating the initial population, assessing the fit of the population, selecting the best solution, differentiating the solutions, and modifying the population (D. & A.R., 2021). GA is used to diagnose skin cancer at an early stage with high accuracy. The diagram below shows the different current ML models for skin cancer prediction discussed here. Figure 5 illustrates ML algorithms for skin cancer diagnosis.

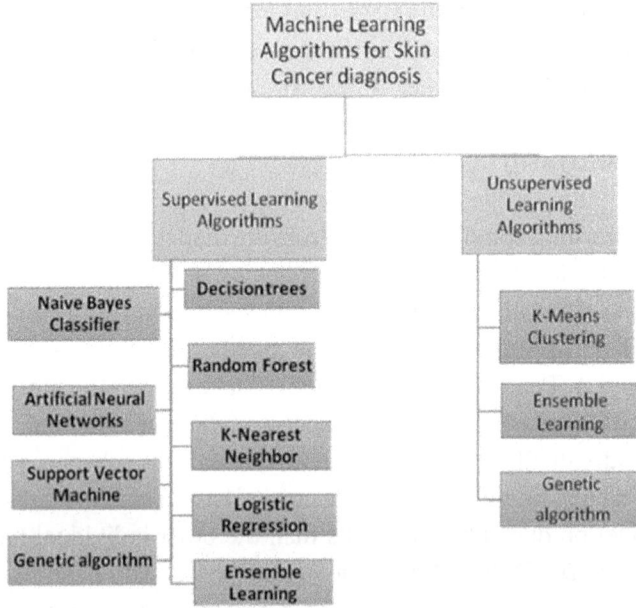

Figure 5. Current machine learning algorithms for skin cancer prediction

CHALLENGES FOR SKIN CANCER DIAGNOSIS IN AI

This section presents the challenges artificial intelligence[17] (AI) enabled systems face in assisting dermatologists in the early detection of skin cancer, as illustrated below.

Data Quality and Quantity

Among the primary difficulties in using AI for skin cancer cell diagnosis is the schedule and quality of datasets. Gathering huge, diverse, and properly annotated datasets is essential for training efficient makers in finding out designs. Nonetheless, obtaining such datasets can be difficult because of numerous factors, such as minimal access to medical images, incongruities in photo top quality, and variants in scientific settings (Shafik, 2024h). As an example, datasets could contain pictures captured under various light conditions, angles, or with varying resolutions, bringing about disparities in version efficiency. Moreover, getting identified information for various kinds and stages of skin cancer cells can be strenuous and time-consuming (Saju et al., 2022). The impact of insufficient information quality and amount manifests in reduced model precision and generalizability, preventing the release of AI systems in real-world professional settings. Misdiagnosis or postponed diagnosis resulting from badly trained designs can have major consequences for individuals, possibly causing incorrect therapy strategies or missing out on possibilities for early treatment, thus highlighting the critical relevance of addressing this difficulty in AI-based skin cancer medical diagnosis (Vasconcelos et al., 2022).

Interpretability and Explainability

Another significant challenge in AI-based skin cancer cell medical diagnosis is the lack of interpretability and explainability of the underlying machine learning versions. While deep-knowing strategies typically master efficiency, they are naturally complicated, making it challenging to comprehend the reasoning behind their forecasts (Rajesh et al., 2020). This absence of openness increases concerns among clinicians and clients relating to the reliability of AI systems in medical decision-making. As an example, a deep semantic network may identify a skin sore as deadly without supplying any understanding of the features or characteristics that are added to its choice (Suhasini et al., 2022). This opacity hinders the adoption of AI devices in scientific techniques, as medical professionals call for descriptions to verify and trust the diagnostic suggestions made by these systems. As a result, the difficulty of interpretability and explainability highlights the need for developing AI designs that can give transparent and interpretable understandings into their decision-making process, therefore cultivating trust funds and acceptance within the medical community (Bollino et al., 2022).

Generalization and Adaptation

An essential obstacle in deploying AI for skin cancer medical diagnosis is making sure the generalization and adaptation of models throughout various populations, demographics, and professional setups (Rajeshkumar et al., 2023). Versions educated on information from one geographic region or demographic team may exhibit prejudices or restricted generalizability when applied to diverse populations with varying skin types, ethnicities, or environmental factors. For example, a model trained primarily on pictures of fair individuals may struggle to properly diagnose skin lesions in darker complexion because of distinctions in sore look and appearance (A., 2022). This lack of generalization can lead to differences in healthcare results, influencing underserved or minority populations. Resolving this challenge requires robust methods for information collection, augmentation, and design development that account for variety and variants within-person populations. Making sure the generalization and adjustment of AI models across diverse populations is crucial for accomplishing fair and comprehensive skin cancer medical diagnosis, thereby alleviating disparities in healthcare accessibility and results (Bollino et al., 2022).

Ethical and Legal Considerations

Moral and legal considerations pose substantial obstacles in the development and implementation of AI for skin cancer medical diagnosis. Personal privacy concerns arise from the requirement to handle sensitive clinical data, consisting of personal images and health and wellness records, in conformity with information security regulations such as Medical Insurance Mobility and Accountability Act[18] (HIPAA) or General Data Protection Guideline[19] (GDPR) (S., 2022). Additionally, concerns related to mathematical predisposition and justness should be addressed to make certain that AI systems do not perpetuate existing differences or discrimination in healthcare. For example, prejudiced datasets or algorithmic decision-making might affect particular group groups, bringing about unequal access to accurate diagnosis and treatment (Maiti et al., 2019). Additionally, there are problems regarding obligation and responsibility in cases where AI systems make wrong or damaging suggestions. Attending to these ethical and lawful difficulties requires mindful consideration of privacy guidelines, transparency in AI decision-making, and devices for bookkeeping and alleviating mathematical biases, inevitably securing patient rights and making sure of fair health care shipment (Segall & Sankarasubbu, 2022).

Integration with Clinical Workflows

Integrating AI-based skin cancer cell diagnosis devices into existing scientific workflows provides practical difficulties for doctors. Medical professionals might encounter resistance or skepticism towards adopting brand-new modern technology, especially if it interrupts well-known routines or needs extra training (Maede Banki et al., 2023). Moreover, perfectly integrating AI systems right into electronic health records[20] (EHR) systems and analysis workflows is necessary for improving decision-making and ensuring continuity of treatment. For instance, AI tools need to provide a user-friendly interface, assist in effective data exchange with EHR systems, and supply actionable insights that enhance clinicians' know-how rather than change it (Panthakkan et al., 2022). Failure to attend to these integration difficulties can prevent the adoption and use of AI in medical methods, restricting its impact on boosting diagnostic accuracy and individual results.

Resource Constraints and Accessibility

Resource restraints, including minimal accessibility to computational facilities, expertise, and financial resources, present significant barriers to implementing AI-based skin cancer cell medical diagnosis in real-world healthcare setups (Kiran Kumar & Divya Udayan, 2019). Training and releasing advanced machine-discovery models require substantial computational sources and customized competence in data science and AI, which may not be readily offered in all healthcare institutions, particularly in resource-limited settings (Attallah & Sharkas, 2021). Furthermore, the high expense of developing and maintaining AI systems can position monetary obstacles for healthcare providers, especially in the absence of clear reimbursement devices or proof of cost-effectiveness (Khanam & Kumar, 2022). Attending to source restrictions and enhancing accessibility to AI technologies requires financial investment in infrastructure, workforce training, and joint partnerships between healthcare institutions, the academic community, and sector stakeholders, consequently guaranteeing fair accessibility to advanced analysis tools for all patient populations (Fatima et al., 2023).

Long-Term Monitoring and Validation

Continuous monitoring is necessary to assess the stability of AI designs over time, examine their efficiency throughout advancing populaces and environmental conditions, and determine possible sources of bias or degradation in analysis accuracy (Shastry & Sanjay, 2022). Furthermore, rigorous validation research are required to compare the analysis performance of AI systems versus developed clinical requirements and guidelines, ensuring that they satisfy governing requirements and offer medically actionable insights (Takiddin et al., 2021). However, carrying out long-term monitoring and recognition research studies calls for substantial cooperation between researchers, clinicians, regulatory agencies, and industry partners, in addition to sustained financing and facilities assistance. Failing to develop robust tracking and validation methods can threaten the credibility and trustworthiness of AI-based analysis devices, impeding their widespread fostering and approval in medical practice (Obayya et al., 2023; Shafik, 2023). Table 1 presents a summary of AI applications in skin cancer detection.

Table 1. Artificial intelligence applications in skin cancer detection (EHRs; Electronic Health Records, IoT; Internet of Things, AI; Artificial Intelligence).

Data Type	Specific Technologies	Underlying Technologies	Application	Use in AI for Skin Cancer Detection
Dermoscopic Images	Dermatoscopes, Smartphone Dermoscopy Apps	Optical Imaging, Mobile Computing	Image Acquisition, Image Analysis	Primary input for training and validating image-based diagnostic models
Follow-up Data	EHR Systems, Patient Monitoring Tools	Database Management Systems, Remote Monitoring Technologies	Prognosis Analysis, Treatment Effectiveness	Useful for training models on long-term prognosis and treatment effectiveness
Environmental Data	Environmental Monitoring Systems, Databases	Sensor Networks, Geospatial Information Systems	Risk Factor Analysis, Contextual Information	Provides additional context for assessing risk factors
Sensor Data	Wearable Devices, IoT Sensors	Sensor Technologies, Wireless Communication	Continuous Monitoring, Early Detection	Used for continuous monitoring and early detection
Annotated Labels	Annotation Software, Crowdsourcing Platforms	Machine Learning, Data Annotation Tools	Data Labeling, Model Training	Essential for supervised learning and model training
Genetic Information	Genomic Sequencers, Bioinformatics Tools	DNA Sequencing Technologies, Data Analysis Algorithms	Personalized Medicine, Risk Assessment	Enhances personalized diagnosis and risk assessment
Medical History	EHR Systems, Medical Databases	Database Management Systems, Cloud Computing	Contextual Information, Model Training	Provides context for the AI model to improve diagnostic accuracy
Patient Demographics	EHRs Systems	Database Management Systems, Cloud Computing	Bias Analysis, Data Integration	Helps in understanding and mitigating biases in the model
Histopathological Images	Digital Pathology Scanners	Microscopy, Digital Imaging	Pathological Analysis, Model Validation	Provides ground truth for validating the accuracy of AI models
Clinical Images	Digital Cameras, Smartphone Cameras	Digital Imaging Sensors, Mobile Computing	Supplementary Imaging, Remote Diagnosis	Supplementary data to dermoscopic images for diverse training datasets

FUTURE RESEARCH DIRECTIONS FOR SKIN CANCER DIAGNOSIS IN ARTIFICIAL INTELLIGENCE

This section presents the future research direction of AI-based diagnostic tools, ensuring their relevance and effectiveness in real-world clinical practice.

Multimodal Data Fusion

Future study in AI for skin cancer cells diagnosis could explore the integration of numerous information modalities, such as dermatoscopic pictures, person demographics, professional history, and genetic info, to improve diagnostic accuracy and individualized therapy recommendations (Melarkode et al., 2023). By merging diverse information sources, scientists can take advantage of corresponding info to boost the effectiveness and generalizability of AI models. For instance, incorporating hereditary markers related to skin cancer threat into analysis formulas could allow a lot more specific threat stratification and customized treatments for high-risk individuals (Kushimo et al., 2023; Shafik, 2024a). The influence of multimodal data fusion lies in its prospective to reinvent personalized medication by making it possible for clinicians to make data-driven decisions that think about a client's unique features, hereditary tendencies, and ecological variables, thus enhancing analysis accuracy, therapy efficacy, and patient outcomes (Khanam & Kumar, 2022; Shafik, 2024b).

Continual Learning and Adaptive Systems

Future study directions in AI for skin cancer medical diagnosis may concentrate on developing continual learning formulas and adaptive systems capable of constantly updating and improving their efficiency in time. Typical device learning designs are typically trained on fixed datasets and may struggle to adapt to brand-new data distributions or emerging patterns in skin sore characteristics (Fatima et al., 2023). Continual discovering methods, such as step-by-step understanding and transfer understanding, make it possible for AI systems to incrementally obtain expertise from brand-new information while protecting formerly found out details, consequently facilitating adaptation to changing medical contexts and progressing analysis difficulties (Attallah & Sharkas, 2021; Shafik, 2024c). For instance, flexible AI systems can dynamically readjust their analysis limits or upgrade their decision-making criteria based on comments from clinicians or new evidence from medical literary works. The effect of regular discovering and flexible systems depends on their prospective to enhance the durability, versatility, and lasting performance of AI-based diagnostic devices, guaranteeing their relevance and performance in real-world medical technique (Khanam & Kumar, 2022).

Interpretable and Transparent Models

Future research study directions in AI for skin cancer cells medical diagnosis might focus on the development of interpretable and clear designs that provide clinicians with actionable understandings and explanations for their analysis forecasts. While deep learning versions usually accomplish advanced efficiency, their black-box nature impedes interpretability and count on amongst end-users (Shastry & Sanjay, 2022). Interpretable AI designs, such as decision trees, rule-based systems, or attention mechanisms, supply clear representations of the attributes and decision-making processes underlying diagnostic forecasts, allowing clinicians to comprehend and validate version outcomes (Kushimo et al., 2023). For instance, an interpretable AI design might highlight the essential visual attributes or medical specifications contributing to its classification choice, empowering medical professionals to make informed judgments and improve diagnostic analyses (Du-Harpur et al., 2020; Shafik, 2024d). The effect of interpretable and transparent designs hinges on their possible to promote count on, collaboration, and understanding sharing in between AI systems and healthcare providers, eventually boosting the adoption, approval, and clinical utility of AI-based diagnostic tools in skin cancer screening and management (Attallah & Sharkas, 2021).

Robustness to Adversarial Attacks

Future research study in AI for skin cancer cells diagnosis could resolve the vulnerability of machine learning designs to adversarial strikes, where imperceptible perturbations to input information can result in incorrect or maliciously crafted predictions (Shastry & Sanjay, 2022). Adversarial strikes present considerable risks in medical applications, as they can potentially endanger the dependability and safety and security of AI-based analysis systems, bring about inaccurate scientific choices or individual injury (Takiddin et al., 2021). Effectiveness to adversarial assaults includes establishing algorithms and defenses capable of spotting and minimizing the impacts of adversarial perturbations, thus ensuring the durability and credibility of AI designs in real-world scenarios. For instance, adversarial training strategies, robust optimization algorithms, or input sanitization methods can boost the robustness of AI versions against adversarial controls, guarding their performance and integrity in medical settings (Obayya et al., 2023). The impact of effectiveness to adversarial attacks depends on its prospective to enhance the security, integrity, and safety of AI-based analysis tools, boosting self-confidence among doctor and people in their use for skin cancer cells screening and diagnosis (Shafik, 2024e).

Collaborative and Federated Learning

Future research instructions in AI for skin cancer cells medical diagnosis might discover collaborative and federated knowing techniques that make it possible for model training across dispersed datasets while maintaining data personal privacy and security. Joint knowing includes aggregating knowledge from multiple institutions or resources to train central models. In contrast, federated discovering allows model training to happen in your area on decentralized data resources, with only model updates traded in between devices or servers (Bhatt et al., 2023). By leveraging joint and federated knowing techniques, scientists can harness the cumulative knowledge of diverse datasets without compromising patient personal privacy or information privacy. For example, federated understanding might enable healthcare establishments to collaboratively train AI models using their regional client data while abiding by regulatory demands and moral criteria (Melarkode et al., 2023Shafik, 2024f). The impact of joint and federated learning hinges on its prospective to democratize access to large-scale clinical datasets, accelerate study development, and facilitate the advancement of robust and generalizable AI versions for skin cancer medical diagnosis.

Integration of Clinical Decision Support Systems (CDSS)

A promising future study instruction in AI for skin cancer medical diagnosis involves the integration of CDSS[21] into regular professional practice. CDSS leverages AI algorithms to help healthcare providers in making evidence-based choices by evaluating individual information and supplying analysis referrals or treatment ideas (Attallah & Sharkas, 2021). In the context of skin cancer cell diagnosis, CDSS might provide real-time support to skin doctors by examining dermatoscopic pictures, individual case histories, and danger elements to supply analysis insights and treatment options. A CDSS can assess a skin doctor's evaluation findings and recommend added diagnostic tests or recommendations based on well-established scientific standards or ideal methods (Shafik, 2024g). The effect of incorporating CDSS into skin cancer cells' medical diagnosis lies in its potential to enhance analysis accuracy, standardize scientific decision-making, and enhance patient results by providing medical professionals with timely, tailored, and actionable information (Panthakkan et al., 2022).

CONCLUSION

Melanoma is the most dangerous and deadliest type of skin cancer. Early diagnosis is very important to reduce the number of deaths from this type of cancer. Therefore, an automatic and reliable system capable of detecting the presence of melanoma from clinical images may be a useful tool. The future of skin cancer diagnosis lies at the crossroads of expert systems and clinical technology. With continuous study initiatives concentrating on multimodal information fusion, continual learning, interpretable models, effectiveness to adversarial attacks, joint discovery, and assimilation of medical choice support groups, AI holds an immense pledge in changing analysis precision, individualized therapy methods, and client results. By attending to present difficulties and welcoming emerging study instructions, AI-powered solutions have the prospective to increase clinician knowledge, equalize access to top-quality medical care, and inevitably, reduce the problem of skin cancer through very early discovery and positive monitoring. AI algorithms are proposed to assist dermatologists in the accurate diagnosis of skin cancer at an early stage. An automated skin cancer diagnosis is performed using various ML algorithms for greater accuracy, efficiency, and performance.

REFERENCES

Attallah, O., & Sharkas, M. (2021). Intelligent Dermatologist Tool for Classifying Multiple Skin Cancer Subtypes by Incorporating Manifold Radiomics Features Categories. *Contrast Media & Molecular Imaging*, 2021, 1–14. Advance online publication. DOI: 10.1155/2021/7192016 PMID: 34621146

Banki, M., Farsinia, F., & Ghasemi, S. (2023). Artificial intelligence in management and prognosis of melanoma: A literature review. *Open Access Research Journal of Biology and Pharmacy*, 8(2), 023–026. Advance online publication. DOI: 10.53022/oarjbp.2023.8.2.0029

Bhatt, H., Shah, V., Shah, K., Shah, R., & Shah, M. (2023). State-of-the-art machine learning techniques for melanoma skin cancer detection and classification: A comprehensive review. *Intelligent Medicine*, 3(3), 180–190. Advance online publication. DOI: 10.1016/j.imed.2022.08.004

Bollino, R., Bovenzi, G., Cipolletta, F., Docimo, L., Gravina, M., Marrone, S., . . . Sansone, C. (2022). Synergy-Net: Artificial Intelligence at the Service of Oncological Prevention. In *Intelligent Systems Reference Library* (Vol. 211). Retrieved from https://doi.org/DOI: 10.1007/978-3-030-79161-2_16

Cai, D., Ardakany, A. R., & Ay, F. (2021). Deep Learning-Aided Diagnosis of Autoimmune Blistering Diseases. medRxiv, 2021-11.

Du-Harpur, X., Watt, F. M., Luscombe, N. M., & Lynch, M. D. (2020). What is AI? Applications of artificial intelligence to dermatology. *British Journal of Dermatology*, 183(3), 423–430. Advance online publication. DOI: 10.1111/bjd.18880 PMID: 31960407

Fatima, M., Khan, M. A., Shaheen, S., Almujally, N. A., & Wang, S. H. (2023). B2C3NetF2: Breast cancer classification using an end-to-end deep learning feature fusion and satin bowerbird optimization controlled Newton Raphson feature selection. *CAAI Transactions on Intelligence Technology*, 8(4), 1374–1390. Advance online publication. DOI: 10.1049/cit2.12219

Ghaffar Nia, N., Kaplanoglu, E., & Nasab, A. (2023). Evaluation of artificial intelligence techniques in disease diagnosis and prediction. *Discover Artificial Intelligence*, 3(1), 5. Advance online publication. DOI: 10.1007/s44163-023-00049-5

Kalaivani, A., & Karpagavalli, S. (2022). Skin Disease Identification and Classification Optimization Study Using Random Forest Boosted Deep Learning Neural Networks. *NeuroQuantology : An Interdisciplinary Journal of Neuroscience and Quantum Physics*, 20(8), 197.

Khanam, N., & Kumar, R. (2022). Recent Applications of Artificial Intelligence in Early Cancer Detection. *Current Medicinal Chemistry*, 29(25), 4410–4435. Advance online publication. DOI: 10.2174/0929867329666220222154733 PMID: 35196970

Kiran Kumar, M., & Divya Udayan, J. (2019). A survey of machine learning techniques for cancer disease prediction and diagnosis. *Indian Journal of Public Health Research & Development*, 10(4), 157. Advance online publication. DOI: 10.5958/0976-5506.2019.00682.X

Kumar, S. (2021). Abstract PO-056: Importance of artificial intelligence, machine learning deep learning in the field of medicine on the future role of the physician. *Clinical Cancer Research*, 27(5, Supplement), PO-056. Advance online publication. DOI: 10.1158/1557-3265.ADI21-PO-056

Kushimo, O. O., Salau, A. O., Adeleke, O. J., & Olaoye, D. S. (2023). Deep learning model to improve melanoma detection in people of color. *Arab Journal of Basic and Applied Sciences*, 30(1), 92–102. Advance online publication. DOI: 10.1080/25765299.2023.2170066

Ma, Y., Zhang, P., Tang, Y., Pan, C., Li, G., Liu, N., Hu, Y., & Tang, Z. (2020). Artificial intelligence: The dawn of a new era for cutting-edge technology based diagnosis and treatment for stroke. *Brain Hemorrhages*, 1(1), 1–5. Advance online publication. DOI: 10.1016/j.hest.2020.01.006

Maiti, A., Chatterjee, B., Ashour, A. S., & Dey, N. (2019). Computer-aided Diagnosis of Melanoma: A Review of Existing Knowledge and Strategies. *Current Medical Imaging*, 16(7), 835–854. Advance online publication. DOI: 10.2174/1573405615 666191210104141 PMID: 33059554

Melarkode, N., Srinivasan, K., Qaisar, S. M., & Plawiak, P. (2023). AI-Powered Diagnosis of Skin Cancer: A Contemporary Review, Open Challenges and Future Research Directions. *Cancers (Basel)*, 15(4), 1183. Advance online publication. DOI: 10.3390/cancers15041183 PMID: 36831525

Obayya, M., Alhebri, A., Maashi, M., Salama, S., Mustafa, A., Hilal, A., Alsaid, M. I., & Alneil, A. A. (2023). Henry Gas Solubility Optimization Algorithm based Feature Extraction in Dermoscopic Images Analysis of Skin Cancer. *Cancers (Basel)*, 15(7). Advance online publication. DOI: 10.3390/cancers15072146 PMID: 37046806

Panthakkan, A., Anzar, S. M., Jamal, S., & Mansoor, W. (2022). Concatenated Xception-ResNet50 — A novel hybrid approach for accurate skin cancer prediction. *Computers in Biology and Medicine*, 150, 106170. Advance online publication. DOI: 10.1016/j.compbiomed.2022.106170 PMID: 37859280

Rajesh, P., Murugan, A., Muruganantham, B., & Ganesh Kumar, S. (2020). Lung Cancer Diagnosis and Treatment Using AI and Mobile Applications. *International Journal of Interactive Mobile Technologies*, 14(17), 189. Advance online publication. DOI: 10.3991/ijim.v14i17.16607

Rajeshkumar, K., Ananth, C., & Mohananthini, N. (2023). Optimal Hybrid Image Encryption with Machine Learning Model for Blockchain-Assisted Secure Skin Lesion Diagnosis. *International Journal of Engineering Trends and Technology*, 71(6), 96–106. Advance online publication. DOI: 10.14445/22315381/IJETT-V71I6P211

Safia Naveed, S. (2023). Prediction of breast cancer through Random Forest. *Current Medical Imaging*, 19(10).

Saju, B., Asha, V., Murali, S. C., Vinayaka, D., Kumar, V., & Nithya, B. (2022). ML based Prototype for Skin Cancer Detection. In *Proceedings of the 2022 3rd International Conference on Communication, Computing and Industry 4.0, C2I4 2022*. Retrieved from https://doi.org/DOI: 10.1109/C2I456876.2022.10051378

Segall, R. S., & Sankarasubbu, V. (2022). Survey of Recent Applications of Artificial Intelligence for Detection and Analysis of COVID-19 and Other Infectious Diseases. *International Journal of Artificial Intelligence and Machine Learning*, 12(2), 1–30. Advance online publication. DOI: 10.4018/IJAIML.313574

Shafik, W. (2023). *Artificial intelligence and Blockchain technology enabling cybersecurity in telehealth systems. Artificial Intelligence and Blockchain Technology in Modern Telehealth Systems* (Vol. 1). IET., DOI: 10.1049/PBHE061E_ch11

Shafik, W. (2024a). Artificial Intelligence and the Medical Tourism. In *Examining Tourist Behaviors and Community Involvement in Destination Rejuvenation* (pp. 207–233). IGI Global., DOI: 10.4018/979-8-3693-6819-0.ch016

Shafik, W. (2024b). Data-Driven Future Trends and Innovation in Telemedicine. In *Improving Security, Privacy, and Connectivity Among Telemedicine Platforms* (pp. 93-118). IGI Global. https://doi.org/DOI: 10.4018/979-8-3693-2141-6.ch005

Shafik, W. (2024c). Digital healthcare systems in a federated learning perspective. In *Federated Learning for Digital Healthcare Systems* (pp. 1–35). Academic Press., DOI: 10.1016/B978-0-443-13897-3.00001-1

Shafik, W. (2024d). IoMT Future Trends and Challenges: Emerging Technologies, Policy Implications, and Research Questions. *Lightweight Digital Trust Architectures in the Internet of Medical Things* (IoMT), 348-370. https://doi.org/DOI: 10.4018/979-8-3693-2109-6.ch019

Shafik, W. (2024e). IoT-Enabled Secure and Intelligent Smart Healthcare: Beyond 5G in Enabling Smart Cities. In *Secure and Intelligent IoT-Enabled Smart Cities* (pp. 308-333). IGI Global. https://doi.org/DOI: 10.4018/979-8-3693-2373-1.ch015

Shafik, W. (2024f). Science of Emotional Intelligence. In *Enhancing and Predicting Digital Consumer Behavior with AI* (pp. 284–310). IGI Global., DOI: 10.4018/979-8-3693-4453-8.ch015

Shafik, W. (2024g). *The Future of Healthcare: AIoMT—Redefining Healthcare with Advanced Artificial Intelligence and Machine Learning Techniques. Artificial Intelligence and Machine Learning in Drug Design and Development*. Wiley., DOI: 10.1002/9781394234196.ch19

Shafik, W. (2024h). Toward a More Ethical Future of Artificial Intelligence and Data Science. In *The Ethical Frontier of AI and Data Analysis* (pp. 362–388). IGI Global., DOI: 10.4018/979-8-3693-2964-1.ch022

Shafik, W., Hidayatullah, A. F., Kalinaki, K., & Aslam, M. M. (2024a). Artificial Intelligence (AI)-Assisted Computer Vision (CV) in Healthcare Systems. In *Computer Vision and AI-Integrated IoT Technologies in the Medical Ecosystem* (pp. 17-36). CRC Press. https://doi.org/DOI: 10.1201/9781003429609-2

Shafik, W., Tufail, A., Liyanage, C. D. S., & Apong, R. A. A. H. M. (2024b). Medical Robotics and AI-Assisted Diagnostics Challenges for Smart Sustainable Healthcare. In *AI-Driven Innovations in Digital Healthcare: Emerging Trends, Challenges, and Applications* (pp. 304-323). IGI Global. https://doi.org/DOI: 10.4018/979-8-3693-3218-4.ch016

Shastry, K. A., & Sanjay, H. A. (2022). Cancer diagnosis using artificial intelligence: A review. *Artificial Intelligence Review*, 55(4), 2641–2673. Advance online publication. DOI: 10.1007/s10462-021-10074-4

Simango, D., Mushiri, T., Yahya, A., & Nyanduwa, L. (2023). Brain tumor detection and classification based on machine learning systems. In *AIP Conference Proceedings* (Vol. 2581). Retrieved from https://doi.org/DOI: 10.1063/5.0126334

Singh, H., Kaushik, S., Talyan, S., & Dwivedi, K. (2022). Skin Cancer Detection Using Deep Learning techniques. *International Journal for Research in Applied Science and Engineering Technology*, 10(5). Advance online publication. DOI: 10.22214/ijraset.2024.62662

Suhasini, V. K., Patil, P. B., Vijaykumar, K. N., Manjunatha, S. C., Sudha, T., Kumar, P., & Manjunath, T. C. (2022). Detection of Skin Cancer using Artificial Intelligence & Machine Learning Concepts. In *Proceedings of 4th International Conference on Cybernetics, Cognition and Machine Learning Applications, ICCCMLA 2022.* Retrieved from https://doi.org/DOI: 10.1109/ICCCMLA56841.2022.9989146

Suiçmez, Ç., Tolga Kahraman, H., Suiçmez, A., Yılmaz, C., & Balcı, F. (2023). Detection of melanoma with hybrid learning method by removing hair from dermoscopic images using image processing techniques and wavelet transform. *Biomedical Signal Processing and Control*, 84, 104729. Advance online publication. DOI: 10.1016/j.bspc.2023.104729

Takiddin, A., Schneider, J., Yang, Y., Abd-Alrazaq, A., & Househ, M. (2021). Artificial intelligence for skin cancer detection: Scoping review. *Journal of Medical Internet Research*, 23(11), e22934. Advance online publication. DOI: 10.2196/22934 PMID: 34821566

Vasconcelos, M. J. M., Moreira, D., Alves, P., Graça, R., Franco, R., & Rosado, L. (2022). Improving Teledermatology Referral with Edge-AI: Mobile App to Foster Skin Lesion Imaging Standardization. In *Communications in Computer and Information Science* (Vol. 1710 CCIS). Retrieved from https://doi.org/DOI: 10.1007/978-3-031-20664-1_9

ENDNOTES

[1] https://www.livescience.com/37247-dna.html

[2] https://www.mayoclinic.org/diseases-conditions/squamous-cell-carcinoma/symptoms-causes/syc-20352480

[3] https://www.cancer.org/

[4] https://www.mayoclinic.org/diseases-conditions/skin-cancer/symptoms-causes/syc-20377605

[5] https://my.clevelandclinic.org/health/diseases/14391-melanoma

[6] https://www.wcrf.org/cancer-trends/skin-cancer-statistics/

[7] https://www.mayoclinic.org/diseases-conditions/melanoma/symptoms-causes/syc-20374884

[8] https://www.skincancer.org/skin-cancer-information/skin-cancer-facts/

[9]   https://www.aad.org/media/stats-skin-cancer

[10]   https://www.ibm.com/topics/machine-learning

[11]   https://www.ibm.com/topics/random-forest

[12]   https://www.ibm.com/topics/neural-networks

[13]   https://www.ibm.com/topics/knn

[14]   https://www.techtarget.com/searchenterpriseai/definition/fuzzy-logic

[15]   https://scikit-learn.org/stable/modules/svm.html

[16]   https://www.mathworks.com/help/gads/what-is-the-genetic-algorithm.html

[17]   https://cloud.google.com/learn/what-is-artificial-intelligence

[18]   https://en.wikipedia.org/wiki/Health_Insurance_Portability_and
       _Accountability_Act

[19]   https://gdpr-info.eu/

[20]   https://www.cms.gov/priorities/key-initiatives/e-health/records

[21]   https://www.techtarget.com/searchhealthit/definition/clinical-decision-support
       -system-CDSS

Chapter 7
Empowering Early Cancer Detection:
The Role of Smartphone Technology in Diagnosing Skin and Cervical Cancers

C. V. Suresh Babu
https://orcid.org/0000-0002-8474-2882
Hindustan Institute of Technology and Science, India

M. S. Asmaa Begum
Hindustan Institute of Technology and Science, India

G. K. Lokeshwaran
Hindustan Institute of Technology and Science, India

A. S. Akshaya
http://orcid.org/0009-0009-0989-6660
Hindustan Institute of Technology and Science, India

ABSTRACT

This chapter explores Applications of smartphone technology in cancer diagnosis make it a game-changing part of healthcare, especially in terms of better early diagnosis and empowering patients. This abstract synthesizes some recent developments of the application of smartphones in detecting cancer, focusing on skin and cervical cancers. Recent studies have reported that AI algorithms developed on smartphones could accurately estimate skin lesions for malignancy. For instance, a clinical validation study assessed two neural network algorithms that attained sensitivities of 96.4% and 95.35% in detecting malignant skin lesions, hence establishing the potential of

DOI: 10.4018/979-8-3693-5237-3.ch007

the smartphone as a diagnostic tool in dermatology. Widespread use of smartphones enables access to methods of early detection, mainly in underserved regions of a country, reducing the healthcare burden from late-stage cancer diagnoses.

1. INTRODUCTION

Skin cancer is one of the most active types of cancer in the present decade (American Cancer Society, 2023). Since the skin is the largest organ of the human body, the point of considering skin cancer as the most common type of cancer among humans can be understood (Beam & Kohane, 2018). In general, it is classified into two major categories: melanoma and nonmelanoma skin cancer (Berman & Berman, 2016). Melanoma is a hazardous, rare, and deadly kind of skin cancer. According to the American Cancer Society, cases of melanoma skin cancer account for only 1% of total cases, yet result in a higher death rate. It develops in cells called melanocytes. It starts when healthy melanocytes begin to grow out of control, creating a cancerous tumor. It may affect any area of the human body. It usually appears on the areas exposed to sun rays, such as on the hands, face, neck, lips, etc. Melanoma type of cancers can only be cured if diagnosed early; otherwise, they spread to other body parts and lead to the victim's painful death (Chiu & Wang, 2021). There as various types of melanoma skin cancer such as nodular melanoma, superficial spreading melanoma, acral lentiginous, and lentigo maligna. Although melanoma skin cancer is relatively uncommon, it presents the most danger due to its highly aggressive and metastatic nature. Early detection is key to better survival rates, which can be quite challenging due to the fact that melanoma has a very subtle and varied presentation. The difficulty in differentiating it from other benign conditions of skin lesions, particularly during the early stages of its development, underscores the need for advanced diagnostic methods. Figure 1 presents an image of a skin cancer sample.

Figure 1. Skin cancer sample

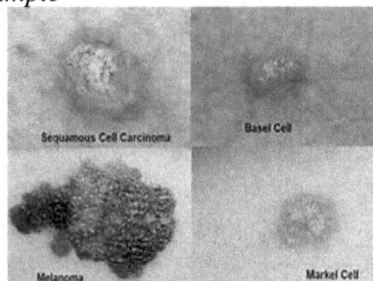

1.1 Background of Skin Cancer Detection Using AI

Skin cancer is the most common type of cancer in the world; melanoma is its most dangerous form. Early detection is the key to effective treatment, but traditional diagnostic techniques, usually based on a clinical examination combined with invasive biopsies, take time and are likely to be subject to human error. The problem is further exacerbated by great variability in the visual appearance of skin lesions, standing in the way of an accurate diagnosis, especially by non-specialists and in remote areas with limited accessibility to dermatologists.

Over the past ten years, AI has cropped up as one of the most applied modalities in skin cancer detection. Especially, deep learning-based AI algorithms may analyze medical images for patterns and abnormal findings that suggest skin cancer, including CNNs. Trained on extensive datasets comprising dermoscopic images, these currently can achieve, and at times even surpass, the accuracy levels of expert dermatologists in the detection of malignant melanomas and other skin cancers. Indeed, various studies have shown the ability of AI models to classify skin lesions with a high degree of sensitivity and specificity, thus enabling earlier diagnosis with greater precision, especially when combined with human expertise.

(Suresh Babu, C.V, Maclin Vinola, P. et. al. 2024) has explained Incorporating AI into healthcare marks a substantial advancement in contemporary medical procedures. The realm of AI technologies encompasses a variety of sophisticated algorithms, machine learning models, and data analytics that have the capability to analyse extensive medical data and make well-informed decisions 19. This technological prowess extends from medical imaging and diagnostics to drug discovery and precision medicine, showcasing AI's capacity to enhance healthcare methodologies and provide heightened precision and individualization in patient care. Moreover, AI's ability to rapidly process complex data sets allows healthcare professionals to uncover valuable insights that might otherwise be challenging to identify. By harnessing the power of AI, medical practitioners can make more accurate diagnoses, devise tailored treatment plans, and predict potential health risks for patients, ultimately leading to better health outcomes. Furthermore, AI's integration into healthcare not only improves clinical practices but also streamlines administrative and operational tasks. Automated workflows and predictive analytics help optimize hospital operations, resource allocation, and patient management, thereby increasing overall efficiency and reducing costs.

1.2 Scope of the Research

- Skin Lesion Detection: The capability of identifying and distinguishing between different skin lesions, including melanoma and nonmelanoma cancers.

- Integration of Smartphone Cameras: The use of smartphone cameras to take clear pictures of skin lesions for further diagnosis.
- AI Algorithm Implementation: AI algorithms in terms of CNNs, among other deep learning models, would be implemented for image analysis to provide a diagnosis concerning the malignancy in question.
- Real-Time Analysis: Providing real-time analysis of the likelihood of malignancy based on images.
- Consumer Accessibility: It was designed to be both for health professionals and consumers, making early detection more accessible.

1.3 Statement of the Problem

Skin cancer poses a major public health challenge due to its high prevalence and potential for serious health outcomes. With millions of new cases diagnosed annually worldwide, skin cancer is the most common form of cancer. Public health efforts are vital to address its prevention, early detection, and treatment.

- **Impact on Healthcare Systems**

The high incidence of skin cancer places a significant burden on healthcare systems. Early-stage treatment is generally more affordable and effective, but delayed diagnosis can lead to more severe cases requiring extensive medical resources, raising healthcare costs substantially. Public health programs that emphasize prevention and early detection can reduce this strain.

- **Prevention and Awareness**

Public health campaigns focused on skin cancer prevention—such as promoting sun protection, discouraging indoor tanning, and encouraging regular skin checks—are essential in reducing incidence rates. Educating the public on recognizing early signs of skin cancer can lead to earlier detection, which is crucial for improving survival rates, especially for melanoma.

- **Disparities in Access to Care**

Skin cancer also highlights disparities in healthcare access. Certain populations, including those in rural or underserved areas, may lack access to dermatologic care, leading to delayed diagnoses and poorer outcomes. Public health interventions aimed at improving access to skin cancer screenings and care can help bridge these gaps.

- **Economic and Social Costs**

The societal cost of skin cancer includes not only the direct medical expenses but also lost productivity, disability, and the psychological impact on patients and their families. Preventive measures and public health education can mitigate these costs by reducing the number of advanced skin cancer cases.

Overall, skin cancer's public health significance lies in its widespread prevalence, the burden it places on healthcare systems, and the opportunities for prevention and early intervention to improve outcomes and reduce costs.

1.4 Research Objectives

The main goals of this chapter encompass the following areas:

- To assess the usefulness of smartphone apps in the diagnosis of both melanoma and nonmelanoma skin cancers.
- To analyze the accuracy of AI algorithms incorporated into various smartphone apps in the actual clinical diagnosis of malignant skin lesions.
- To understand how early detection rates would be improved in parts of the world that are most underserved by such prevalent, smartphone-based tools.
- The ways in which this technology for diagnosis on smartphones would be usable and accessible across more varied demographics.
- Assess any barriers that may impede wide acceptance of cancer detection by using smartphones.
- Discuss recent advances in AI and machine learning about skin cancer detection using smartphones.
- To identify the value of technology using smartphones as a teaching tool in patient education and empowerment for cancer prevention.
- 8. Diagnostic accuracy by smartphone against the traditional methods of visual examination and dermoscopy.
- 9. To what extent this new smartphone technology can help reduce health costs in relation to the diagnosis and treatment of skin cancer.

By addressing these research objectives, this chapter aims to provide valuable insights into the complex interplay between healthcare independence and reliance on AI, offering a nuanced perspective on the transformative potential of AI in the healthcare domain.

1.5 Study Purpose and Approach

The backbone of our research deals with the fact that AI-enabled tools, together with machine learning and neural networks, have applications in finding skin cancer. This paper focuses on the understanding of possible benefits and challenges with this integration. The present study shall attempt an integrated quantitative-qualitative approach to shed light on the complex interplay that is happening in the healthcare technology sector, more so for the improvement of diagnostic accuracy and at the early stages of the detection of cancer.

1.6 Significance of Chapter

The chapter further highlights the integration of AI into skin cancer detection, sheds light on the existing challenges, and stresses the potential benefit that the use of AI-driven solutions can hold for the enhancement of early diagnosis and treatment. This chapter develops a comprehensive understanding of the challenges that currently exist in skin cancer detection and how AI can address the gaps identified in the existing research. It acts as a forerunner to developing and implementing advanced diagnostic systems and pushes the frontier of research much ahead in the area of healthcare and early cancer detection.

2.LITERATURE REVIEW

2.1 The Emergence of Artificial Intelligence in Healthcare

The integration of AI in skin cancer detection has significantly improved over the past years, hence bringing revolutionary changes in diagnostic practice and patients' care. The technologies underpinning AI-machine learning and deep learning-promise to revolutionize the way skin cancer is detected, with much better diagnosis and patient outcomes. Esteva et al. (2017) explained how AI, by analyzing millions of dermoscopic images, could offer the opportunity for malignant melanomas to be detected at an earlier and more accurate stage, thus allowing dermatologists to make informed clinical decisions. Processing big image data, AI algorithms support more personalized care, enabling earlier interventions in the treatment of skin cancer.

2.2 AI in Skin Cancer Imaging

AI influences skin cancer diagnosis as one of the most promising developments in medical imaging. A recent 2017 study by Esteva et al. showed that in the diagnosis of malignant melanoma based on dermoscopic images, AI algorithms performed similarly as expert dermatologists. Such quick and precise review of skin lesions through AI has resulted in quicker diagnosis with high accuracy and thus earlier intervention with better patient outcomes. In addition, in work by Tschandl et al. (2020), the deep learning model outperformed human dermatologists with regard to the classification of skin lesions, building on the previous example to establish the transformative potential of AI in skin cancer imaging. Such results indicate very significant advances that AI provides in early cancer diagnosis, with its promise for health improvement and improved health outcomes.

2.3 Diagnostics and Treatment Using AI

Recent progress in AI has allowed the management of volumes of data that have opened up new vistas for personalized diagnosis and treatment in skin cancer care. A study conducted by Haenssle et al. (2018) illustrated that, especially in terms of distinguishing between skin cancer and benign cases, AI algorithms are effective tools for dermatologists, far superior to prior standards. Similarly, AI-powered decision support systems can help analyze dermatoscopic images of patients, genetic information, and their medical history to develop tailored treatment recommendations. Based on AI-driven diagnosis and treatment planning, clinicians can deliver more targeted and timely interventions that improve patient outcomes by contributing to advancements in skin cancer care.

2.4 Efficiency in Healthcare Improved by AI

AI in dermatology can add value to skin cancer management and improve health care on aspects related to efficiency and effectiveness. In this regard, Esteva et al. (2017) reveal that AI algorithms speed up the diagnosis process because they automate analysis on dermoscopic images, hence reducing work for dermatologists and speeding up diagnosis. In addition, AI-powered tools provide remote consultation and triage opportunities for a more thoughtful use of resources and potential access to health care. The different AI applications, one of which is the application proposed by Tschandl et al., contribute to early skin lesion detection and thus free up resources for healthcare professionals in critical cases and optimal patient management. These developments in AI help facilitate quicker diagnosis, reduced waiting times, and overall skin cancer management effectively.

2.5 Challenges in Skin Cancer Detection Using AI

Despite the enormous promise of AI for skin cancer detection, several challenges and limitations have to be overcome. According to Beam and Kohane (2018), some of the major risks to the effective implementation of AI tools in different healthcare settings involve the unstandardized nature of data formats and interoperability across different AI systems. Successful work with AI requires broad and diverse datasets, something complicated by the presence of data silos and issues relating to patient privacy. Price and Cohen (2019) articulated the protection of data and issues of liability on ethical and legal considerations, emphasizing the strict measures for the protection of information related to patients. A study conducted by Obermeyer et al. (2019) indicated that if AI algorithms are biased, unequal treatment outcomes may result when the training data sets are not representative. Transparency, fairness, and privacy regulation are paramount in gaining trust for the patients and will further enhance this application of AI in skin cancer detection.

2.6 Role of AI in Skin Cancer Detection

AI-driven techniques have immense potential for the betterment of skin cancer detection and management. As in the study of Esteva et al. (2017), AI algorithms identified dermoscopic images with substantial accuracy to enable early detection of malignant lesions and expedite the diagnosis. Moreover, AI systems can predict outcomes in patients and can suggest personalized treatment policies based on thorough analysis of patient data. AI tends to increase diagnostic precision and accelerate the identification of skin cancer cases, providing better treatment strategies and improving patient care. This is not only advanced technology that decreases time to diagnosis but is also making diagnostics more available and increasing access to accurate diagnosis to support better health care and advance dermatology.

2.7 Overcoming Obstacles to AI Adoption in Skin Cancer Detection

For example, to achieve important improvements in skin cancer diagnosis using AI, there are a number of adoption barriers that need to be fulfilled. Krittanawong et al. (2021) indicated that there should be improved AI education among dermatologists and medical professionals to improve their level of comprehension toward AI tools and their uses in the diagnosis of skin cancer. It is, therefore, essential that ethics are developed on how to design and utilize AI, to ensure safety to the patients and maintain the trust in the technologies. In addition, strong regulatory frameworks must be put in place to ensure that the algorithms for AI in skin cancer testing are authenticated to see whether they meet standards for patient-privacy and data security as shown by FDA. Addressing these challenges requires an approach that will marry the efforts of policy-makers, healthcare providers, and technology developers to fully exploit the potential of AI for improving skin cancer diagnosis and treatment.

2.8 Types of Skin Cancer

Two significant categories of skin cancer are melanoma and nonmelanoma.

2.8.1 Melanoma

Melanoma is the deadliest skin cancer, developing from melanocytes, the cells responsible for making the melanin. This type of skin cancer accounts for less than 5 percent of all cases of skin cancer. However, it is more aggressive and poses an increased tendency to spread quickly to other organs if not detected and treated in an early stage. It usually looks like a suspicious mole or dark patch on the skin but can also grow on normal skin. Early detection is important for effective treatment because, in developing stages, melanoma is a life-threatening disease.

2.8.2 Nonmelanoma Skin Cancers

Nonmelanoma skin cancers are more common and consist of two main types:

1. **Basal Cell Carcinoma (BCC):** This makes up the most common type of skin cancer, majorly affecting those parts of the skin that are exposed frequently to the sunlight, for instance, the face or neck. This type grows slowly and metastasizes rarely; however, it causes great local damage when not well treated.
2. **Squamous Cell Carcinoma (SCC):** This is the second most common type of skin cancer and originates from the squamous cells in the outer layer of the skin. It also may present on sun-exposed areas, but it has a higher propensity to spread compared with BCC, especially if treatment isn't quick enough.

Although the two non-melanoma cancers are far less aggressive than melanoma, they, too, can cause significant damage if not treated and also focus further attention on the absolute necessity of early detection and treatment.

2.9 Importance of Early Detection

Early detection of skin cancer does much to improve treatment outcomes and reduce mortality. Most skin cancers, including melanoma and nonmelanoma types, if recognized at an early stage, are pretty treatable even with simple surgical procedures. Earlier detection prevents the metastasis of melanoma into other organs, which can increase survival rates considerably. For nonmelanoma cancers, early treatment relieves one from the chances of extensive tissue damage and thus the complications.

Early intervention also reduces the treatment cost since most of the late-stage cancer treatments are always highly advanced and very expensive. Therefore, public awareness of the disease and regular skin checks lead to the early detection of skin cancer, which can eventually save lives.

2.10 Existing Diagnostic Method and Their Limitations

• **Visual Inspection**

A clinician or dermatologist visually inspects skin for abnormalities in color, shape, size, texture, or general appearance. A visual inspection is the most commonly accepted method of detecting skin cancer and is generally noninvasive. The primary drawback is the subject-to-subject variability in the skill and experience of the examiner. Misdiagnoses can occur, particularly at earlier or atypical stages of a lesion.

Limitations:

Visual examinations are subjective and thus subject to human error, both false positives and false negatives are common, especially in those cancers that are less obvious or at an incipient stage.

• **Dermatoscopy**

Dermatoscopy is done with a dermatoscope, which is an instrument that magnifies and permits a detailed scrutiny of skin lesions. A dermatologist is better able to see patterns and colours with this tool than by naked eye examination.

What dermatoscopy does is to increase the ability to diagnose benign from malignant, though it takes a better level of expertise and experience. There is a price for misinterpretation, and its accuracy can vary with its user's expertise and experience.

• **Biopsy**

In such cases, if a suspicious lesion is detected, a skin biopsy is performed, which signifies removing tissue for examination under the microscope to confirm the existence of cancer cells. This is considered to be a gold standard for diagnosis in skin cancer.

Limitations:

Biopsies are invasive and likely to be painful and cause scarring. They also take time for laboratory analysis, therefore delaying diagnosis. Furthermore, not all lesions that raise suspicion can be, or should be, biopsied; hence, some cancers may not be detected.

- **Molecular and Genetic Testing**

Molecular and genetic tests, like fluorescence in situ hybridization or next-generation sequencing, are done to know the genetic mutation causing skin cancer. These investigations are usually employed in advanced diseases for deciding on treatment.

Limitations:

These investigations are expensive and not widely available for routine practice. They are generally used when a biopsy has already been taken and confirmed the cancer present and not as a primary diagnostic tool.

- **Imaging Techniques**

Imaging techniques such as CT, MRIs, or PET scans are employed to evaluate if skin cancer has metastasized in significant cases, although all this is not done for diagnosis but staging and treatment of the terminal stages of cancer.

Limitations:

Imaging is expensive and not suitable for early detection. It is primarily used when there is concern that cancer has spread beyond the skin.

2.11 The Need for Improve Diagnostic and Accuracy and Accessibility

Rising skin cancer incidence, especially melanoma, puts on the table the need to improve diagnostic accuracy and accessibility. Improvements in these aspects of the disease are crucial for early diagnosis and treatment with the best possible outcomes, particularly in underserved populations. Below are the major reasons improvements must be made:

- **Reduced Diagnostic Errors:** AI and machine learning have the potential to enhance accuracy in the diagnosis of skin cancer by recognizing patterns in lesions more accurately than human observation and thus may reduce the risk of misdiagnosis.
- **Minimizing Invasive Techniques:** AI-powered non-invasive technologies, such as those embedded in smartphone applications, might allow decisions regarding the need for biopsies and the avoidance of unnecessary procedures, with some of their potential complications.
- **Increasing Access to Early Detection:** Early diagnosis through telemedicine and mobile health applications can be provided for underserved areas by improving access to expert care and reducing treatment delays.
- **Skin Type Variation:** AI models, trained on more diverse data, would raise diagnostics across different skin types, reduce disparities in the detection of skin cancer, and help overcome biases.
- **Reduce Financial Burden:** There will be a reduction in the financial burden on patients as diagnoses would come early enough due to accessibility with affordable AI-powered diagnostic tools.
- **Improved Public Health Strategies:** More public education with access to AI-driven diagnostic capabilities will enable earlier detection and improved outcomes, especially in areas of the world where the sun's rays are so prevalent.

3. RESEARCH METHODOLOGY

3.1 Development of AI Algorithm

1. Data Preparation

Skin cancer dataset

This research utilizes the online 'HAM-10000' skin cancer dataset[33]. The dataset HAM-10000, referred to as 'Human against the machine', with 10,000 images used for training, is a collection of images of skin lesions utilized in skincare research. The dataset comprises visual representations of diverse dermatological disorders, encompassing Melanoma, nevus, and several related afflictions. The provided dataset is used to classify and diagnose skin diseases. As mentioned earlier, deep learning models trained on the dataset can discern different types of skin cancer, including malignant tumours that may exhibit malignant characteristics.

Figure 2. Skin cancer classes and counts

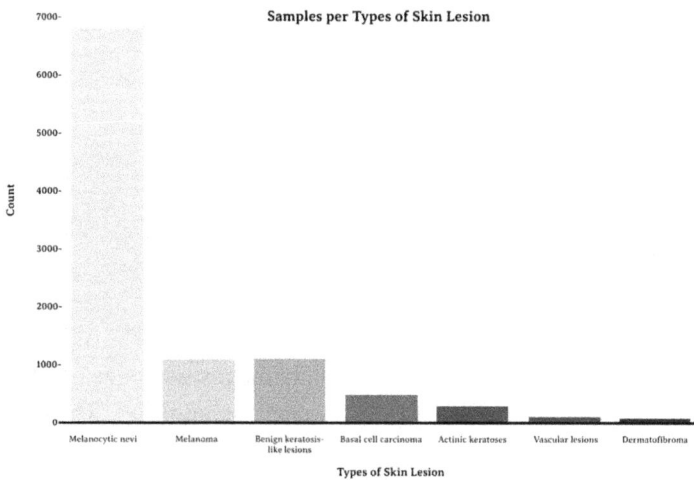

Figure 3. Gender-based skin cancer distribution

Gender of Patient

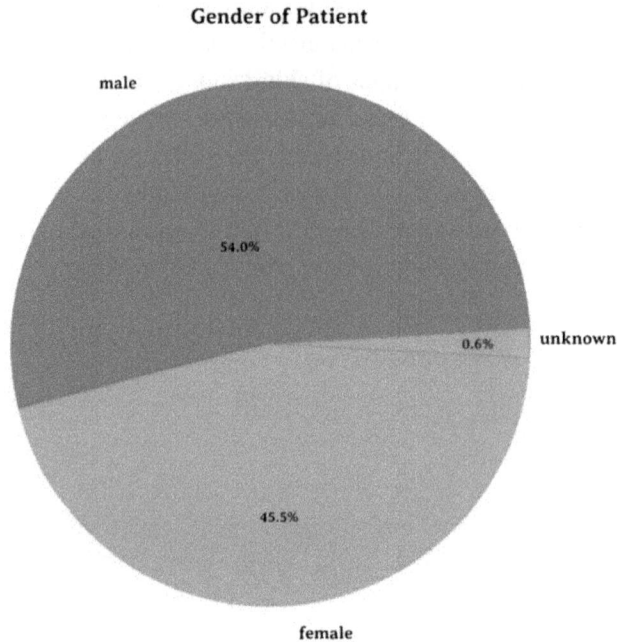

Figure 3. Gender-based skin cancer distribution

This dataset contains 10,015 dermatoscopic images with size (450*600) pixels. The dataset comprises seven diagnostic Skin cancer categories. The dataset classes include classes from zero to six, names as 'melanoma', 'melanocytic nevus', 'basal cell carcinoma', 'actinic keratosis', 'benign keratosis', 'dermatofibroma' and 'vascular lesion'. Figure 3 presents the details of skin cancer classes and counts, and Fig. 4 illustrates the gender-wise distribution of skin cancer infection, including a 54% male, 45.5% Female and 0.5% unknown patient distribution in the dataset.

Data Augmentation

To enhance the generalization of the model, apply data augmentation techniques. This helps in preventing overfitting, especially when the data are small. Common augmentation techniques

Figure 4. Image resizing, zooming

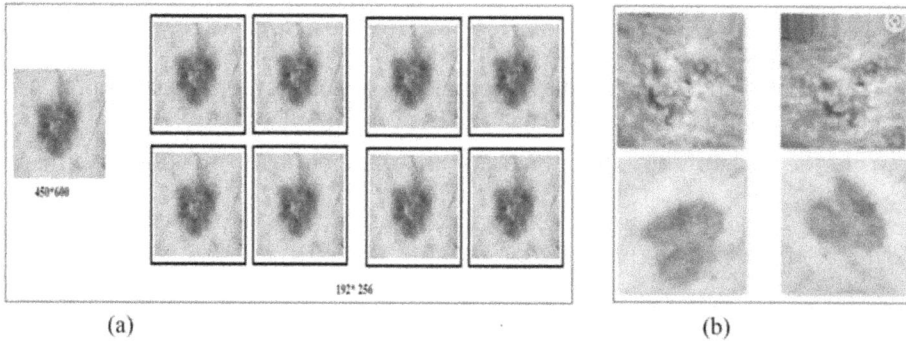

(a)   (b)

Data Splitting

Divide the dataset into training, validation, and testing sets (e.g., 70% training, 15% validation, 15% testing).

2. MobileNet-V2 with transfer learning

MobileNet-V2 consists of the initial fully convolution layer, then 19 residual bottleneck layers, followed by convolution layer then average pooling layer, the next layer is a fully connected layer, followed by a softmax layer then at the end the output classification layer for 1000 classes (Sandler et al., 2018). In this research, transfer learning is applied and the last three layers are replaced with transformed layers for two classes, Figure 5 shows the diagram of the updatet MobileNet-V2 with transfer learning.

Figure 5. MobileNet-V2 with transfer learning diagram

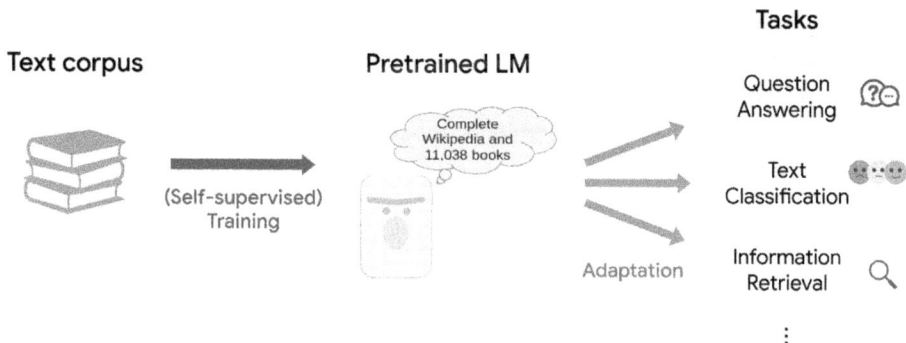

3. Model Training

Compile the Model
Compile the model by choosing an optimizer, loss function, and evaluation metrics.
Fit the Model
Train the model on the training dataset with validation data to monitor performance.

Figure 6. Model training representation

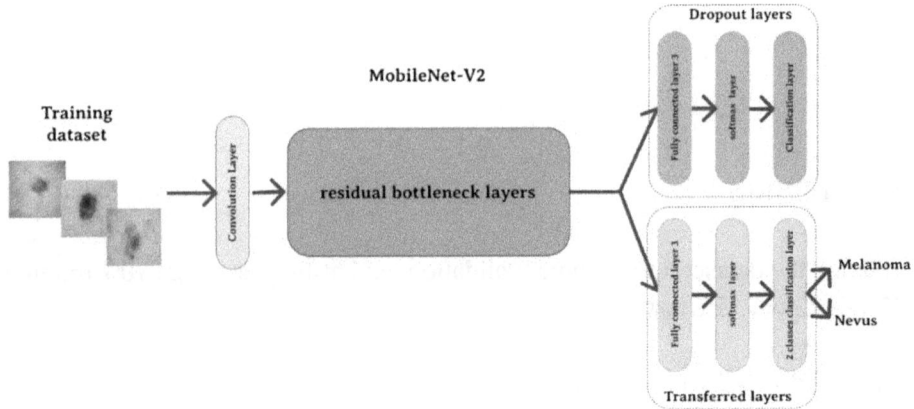

4. Evaluating the Model

Accuracy and loss curves.
Plot the accuracy and loss for both the training and validation datasets over epochs to diagnose overfitting or underfitting.

5. Model Optimization

Fine Tuning of Model
After initial training, you can unfreeze some of the layers in MobileNetV2 and train again with a smaller learning rate to fine tune the model for the task you want.
Overview process of Architecture

Figure 7. Overview architecture

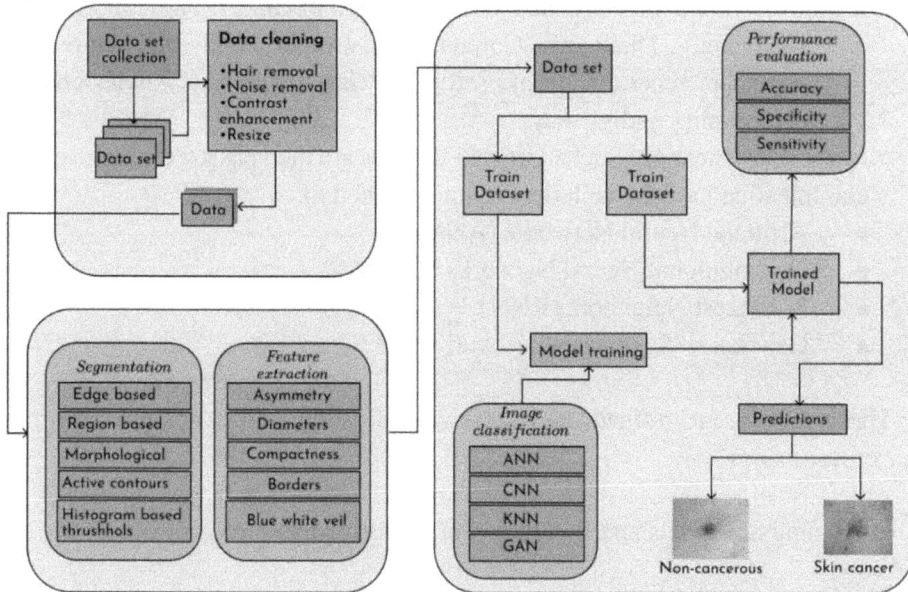

This is an overview diagram of detecting skin cancer by image classification using different techniques of AI. The actual flow in the system would be explained as follows:

- Data Set Collection: Images of skin lesions will be collected, which would be the evident basis for both training and testing phases.
- Data Cleaning: After data collection, the data is pre-processed to enhance image quality and accuracy. This includes the following steps:
- Hair removal: Removal of hairs on the skin images that obscure the lesions. Noise removal: Reducing distortions or unwanted artefacts in these images. Contrast Enhancement: Increase the visual contrast of the lesions to enhance the contrast. Resizing: to standardize the image size for input to the model.
- Segmentation: This is the processing stage at which cleaned data is subjected to several segmentation techniques to bring out and define the region of interest-the lesion-in an image. Techniques applied include:

  Edge-Based, Region-Based, and Morphological Segmentation: These identify the boundary and region of interest in the case of a lesion.
  Active Contours and Histogram-Based Thresholding: These techniques will further refine the detected lesions based on contour shapes and the distribution of pixel intensity.

- Feature Extraction: Following segmentation, the system selects a number of features from the image related to the detection of cancer. These include:
    Asymmetry, Diameters, Compactness, Borders, and Blue-White Veil, which are general features used in the classification of skin lesions and determining malignancy.
- Image Classification: Such extracted features are then passed through various classification models, including but not limited to:
    - Artificial Neural Networks (ANN)
    - Convolutional Neural Networks (CNN)
    - K-Nearest Neighbors (KNN)
    - Generative Adversarial Networks (GAN)

These models are trained on feature classification into cancerous and non-cancerous images.

- Training of Models and Evaluation of Performance:

The data will be divided into two parts: training and testing. The model learns to recognize skin cancer through patterns in the training data.

The performance of the trained model is measured with the help of metrics like Accuracy, Specificity, and Sensitivity. These metrics will identify how well the model can identify correctly both cancerous and non-cancerous lesions.

- Predictions: After training and evaluating a model, it is allowed to make predictions on new images. The system will classify lesions as Non-Cancerous or Skin Cancer based on its analysis.

The diagram describes in detail the whole process, starting from the beginning of data collection and preprocessing to the segmentation of images, extraction of features, and classification, going to performance evaluation, and ending with the prediction of cancerous or non-cancerous skin lesions.

4. Bayesian optimization method

Bayesian optimization represents the use of probabilistic algorithms in the exact search for the most practical combination of hyperparameters which could support a model built using deep learning. It works by treating this uncertain objective function-in this case, one that assesses the model's performance-as a Gaussian process, hence allowing it to make informed decisions about where to start sampling the target function next. The following describes the procedure of Bayesian optimization of the hyperparameter optimization for skin cancer.

- Step 1: Initial Random Sampling To establish an initial surrogate framework for the objective function, Bayesian optimisation usually starts with a few random specimens taken through the hyperparameter space. Because of these arbitrary specimens, the function's behaviour can be partially understood.
- Step 2: Surrogate Model The algorithm builds a probabilistic proxy model from these initial samples. A common choice is a GP; the GP models the distribution of the objective function and predicts its behavior over the hyperparameter space. For every point in the hyperparameter space, the surrogate model is associated with an average prediction and an estimate of its variance.
- Step 3: Acquisition Function Bayesian optimization uses an acquisition function to decide where the next sample of the objective function should be taken. The common acquisition functions include Probability of Improvement, Expected Improvement, and Upper Confidence Bound. These functions balance the explorations (the gathering of samples in the regions of uncertainty) and exploitation (sampling in areas likely to be more effective).
- Step 4: Next Sample Selection Acquisition function will guide the process to select the next set of hyperparameters. The method selects values of hyperparameters such that the acquisition function is maximum. This indicates promising areas in the space of hyperparameter that can serve well for the objective function.
- Step 5: Objective Function Evaluation Using the chosen hyperparameters, the deep learning network trains and tests using the skin cancer dataset. The objective function of model accuracy versus model loss is calculated in relation to the model performance.

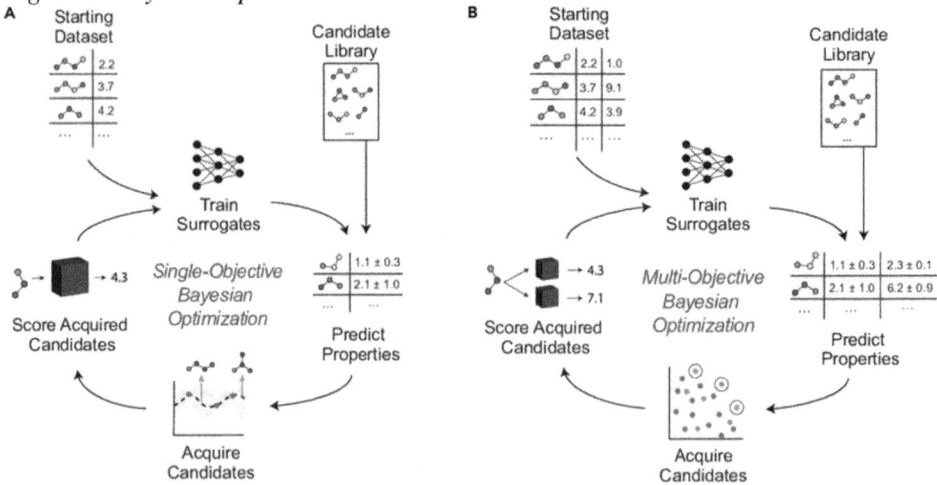

Figure 8. Bayesian operations

- Step 6: Update Surrogate Model: Once the objective function is evaluated on the recommended hyperparameter, the process updates the surrogate model (GP) using the newly obtained data point and its corresponding evaluation result for the purpose of reducing the uncertainty associated with the surrogate model.

- Step 7: Iterations between Steps 3 to 6 for a pre-defined number of times or till convergence. The method produces the updated surrogate model and chooses a hyper-parameter for further improvement in the accuracy of the model.

- Step 8: Final Outcome The hyper-parameters extracted through Bayesian optimization leads to the best objective function importance, basing its findings on the behavior of the model itself.

Transfer Learning

ImageNet is used as a pre-training dataset for the MobileNet-V2 model, and then the Ham-10000 skin cancer dataset is used to fine-tune the model's parameters. Transfer learning enables the predictive algorithm to utilize features acquired within a broader context before becoming proficient in the skin cancer recognition assignment.

5. TESTING AND METRICS

5.1 Resource Requirements

1. Data Sources:

Epidemiological Data: Past data on disease patterns and trends, prevalence, and distribution across various states will help the system to identify any emergence of risks.

Demographic Data: This shall comprise age, gender, socioeconomic status, education levels, and geography for model training and testing.

Environmental Data: This would include data on climate, pollution levels, and sanitation, which are all very influential in health-related aspects.

Health Care Utilization Data: This includes data on the rate of hospital admissions, outpatient visits, and the use of healthcare services in understanding access to and trends in utilization of care.

Behavioral Data: Lifestyle habits, vaccination rates, and adherences to health guidelines are some of the data that will help further in understanding the risk factors and give better information in model predictions.

Genomic Data: Genetic information that might be useful in identifying populations with predispositions to certain conditions, hence helping enhance personalized health models.

Social Determinants of Health-housing, education, employment, social support system-some of the leading causes or factors affecting health and its outcomes, which need to be integrated into the model for in-depth analysis.

2. Technological Resources:

Computational Tools: Availability of high HPC resources and cloud-based solutions to process large data volumes efficiently and complex algorithms on a runtime basis.

Data Storage: The facilitation of secure, scalable database solutions for storing huge volumes of sensitive health and genomic data, ensuring data privacy regulations. Software: R, Python, and specialized machine learning libraries like TensorFlow, PyTorch, and Scikit-learn for performing such predictive model development. GIS: Spatial analysis and mapping health trends-the way to understand visually the patterns of diseases and environmental causes. 3. Human Resources:

Epidemiologists: These professionals are experts in the surveillance and forecasting of disease outbreaks and provide critical information about the spread of diseases and temporal trends. Data Scientists: Professionals skilled in both data analysis and machine learning for designing, training, and refining predictive models using diverse datasets. Statisticians: Specialists in the development and design of the study, statistical modeling, and data interpretation ensure appropriateness and strength of the results.

Public Health Experts: Those who have experience with health systems, policies, and trends at the community level provide knowledge to build comprehensive predictive models. Clinical Experts: Physicians, nurses, and other professionals in the healthcare sector provide the clinical perspective and real-world data that will be crucial in model development and testing. These would go a long way in supporting the development of your skin cancer detection model, evaluation, and scaling so that it is robust and relevant, able to perform effectively across

5.2 Ethical Considerations in AI for Skin Cancer Detection

• **Privacy and Data Security**

Protection of Data: One should be very careful about the considerations for data protection regulations like GDPR (General Data Protection Regulation) and HIPAA. Basically, personal health information protection and that such information is stored and transmitted securely will be ensured.

Anonymization and Encryption: Development of robust encryption techniques for data while at rest or in motion. Ensuring anonymization of data that is irreducible to sources, that is to say, unable to be traced back to individual patients without proper authorization.

Access Control: Making certain that access to sensitive data has restrictions to only authorized personnel. Regular audits and access controls update prevent unauthorized breaches of data.

• **Informed Consent**

It ensures that users understand exactly what data is collected and how this data will be used, or the possible risks and benefits that would result from using this application. Clear and concise, accessible consent forms should be given.

Participation voluntariness: Ensure that participation in the pilot testing or use of the application is purely of a voluntary nature. The users have the right to withdraw their consent without any penal action at any time.

Transparency: Allowing users to have knowledge of how AI works and how far their data will be shared for future research or development.

• **Ethical AI Framework**

Bias and Fairness: AI modeling will be trained on different data sets to ensure that there is a minimum of bias. In addition, fairness will be checked across different demographics, including variations in skin types and ethnic backgrounds.

Accountability and Transparency: Put in place transparent accountability procedures in case of faults or failures of the AI system. Transparency to users and stakeholders on performance metrics and the decisions AI makes needs to be given.

Monitoring Perpetually: Review and evaluate the AI system on ethical compliance, accuracy, and performance regularly to address emerging ethical concerns and make adjustments accordingly.

Ethical Review: This would be independent review committees or advisory boards that an AI application would have to go through to ensure that all ethical standards are met, and the technology is being used responsibly.

6. EVALUATION AND ITERATIVE IMPROVEMENT

6.1 Performance Evaluation:

- **Systematic Reviews and Clinical Trials**: Systematic reviews have to be done to evaluate the performance and reliability of the AI algorithm. Review existing literature or run clinical trials to see how such applications work in real-world scenarios. Clinical trials will be done for the accuracy of the application concerning skin cancer diagnosis, integration into the current healthcare workflow, and benefits for patients.
- **User Feedback on Usability and Effectiveness**: Obtain feedback from users relating to the usability and effectiveness of the application. This gives details on any challenges, scope for improvement, and how far the application is serving the desired purpose. Such feedback will be very useful if reviewed periodically to make the application more user-friendly and effective.

6.2 Algorithm Refinement

- **Training on Large, Diverse Datasets**: Continuously refine your AI algorithm by exercising training on data that are both large and diverse. This will get your algorithm to start generalizing quite well over highly diverse populations and skin types, increasing accuracy and reducing bias. Introducing a mix of data sources will keep the AI model strong and reliable under multiple stresses.
- **Continuous Learning Techniques**: It will use continuous learning techniques to make the algorithm capable of learning and adapting to new data

over time. There is also periodic updating of the models through new cases and feedback that will help enhance the performance of the models and their capability to emerging trends and patterns in skin cancer detection.

6.3 Regulatory and Clinical Integration:

- **Meet Regulatory Standards**: Ensure the AI application intended is designed in accordance with the relevant regulatory standards and guidelines. This involves getting all the approvals that would be needed by the regulatory body, practicing best data protection, medical device regulations, and AI ethics. It is the baseline for ensuring the application will be safe and effective.
- **Collaboration with healthcare providers**: Develop the AI app collaboratively with a target of integrating it into healthcare providers' daily practice. For example, through the development with dermatologists and other HCPs, their needs are understood and the AI application is developed accordingly to complement their practice and facilitate adoption within the clinical environment. This extends further to training the healthcare providers to best use the application and integrate their future feedback into improvement.

7. RISK MANAGEMENT

7.1 Technical Complexity

Technical complexity refers to a range of development and implementation issues that relate to advanced technologies for AI and software systems that detect skin cancer.

7.1.1. Development and Integration Challenges

System Integration: The integration of the skin cancer detection model into the existing healthcare system, whereby it is going to integrate with EHRs in different locations, represents challenges. Seamless data exchange and interoperability will be important to success in deployment.

Development Issues: These are issues in development, such as the selection of appropriate algorithms, quality of training data, and availability of computational resources. Model training can sometimes be computationally expensive and may require fine-tuning to achieve optimal performance.

7.1.2. Model Inaccuracies and System Failures

Performance and Stability: Flaws in the accuracy of the AI model or other aspects associated with system stability might lead to erroneous predictions or system crashes. Such issues may result in inappropriate decisions and impacts on patient outcomes.

Impact: Poor predictions mislead into giving wrong diagnoses and affect patient care. System downtimes may cause the loss of data and reduction of user satisfaction. Rigorous testing and validation will help minimize these risks.

7.2 Data Quality and Availability

High-quality data is paramount for the accuracy and reliability of the skin cancer detection model.

Sources of Data

Medical Imaging Databases: Dermatology clinics and research institutions with annotated images of skin lesions. Electronic Health Records: Demographic data and clinical history of anonymous patients. Public Health Data: Results of health surveys and national databases that give an idea about diseased patterns and risk factors. Wearable Devices: The data obtained from health monitoring devices can provide extra health-related information. Challenges

Data Privacy: Ensuring that patient data are anonymized and stored in a secure form according to regulations such as HIPAA or GDPR. Data quality: missing data, inconsistent annotation, and quality variation in images. Bias: Identifying the biases in the dataset and reducing them to ensure performance consistency across diverse populations and avoiding disparities in diagnosis.

7.3 User Acceptance

The acceptance by users will be vital to the successful implementation and usage of the skin cancer detection system.

1. Involving the End-Users

Description: It is important to involve dermatologists, healthcare professionals, and patients early in the development process to understand their needs and expectations.

Strategies: There should be user research, usability testing with healthcare professionals, and solicitation of feedback with the aim of refining the system. This should ensure that model predictions and interface are aligned with existing clinical workflows.

Importance: An invested end-user is bound to increase the system's adoption rate, contribute useful feedback, and subsequently help in the enhancement of the overall effectiveness and usability of the system.

2. Enablement/Adoption Training and Support

Description: Ensure that users are fully trained and supported in using the new skin cancer detection system.

Components: Include face-to-face training of health professionals, well-developed user manuals, on-demand help facilities, and a support desk for technical issues.

This would develop confidence in the users, reduce the learning curve, and make it easier to adopt, therefore improving the ease of use of the system and ensuring it works as expected.

With these identified risk areas to be managed, you will be sure to enhance the prospects for successful deployment and use of your model for skin cancer detection, with greater assurance of reliable and accurate results, and success with users.

8. RESULT AND DISCUSSION

8.1 Diagnostic Accuracy of Smartphone Applications:

1. **Case Study:** Skin Vision's 95% Sensitivity in Skin Cancer Detection Skin Vision is the leading example of a smartphone application designed specifically for skin cancer detection and holds an impressive record for diagnostic sensitivity at 95%. The high sensitivity shows the effectiveness of this application in correctly identifying probable cases of skin cancer, thus showing its potential for being a very useful tool in early detection. The Skin Vision example just goes to show the potential of mobile technology in better screening and management for skin cancer.

Figure 9. Model accuracy & loss

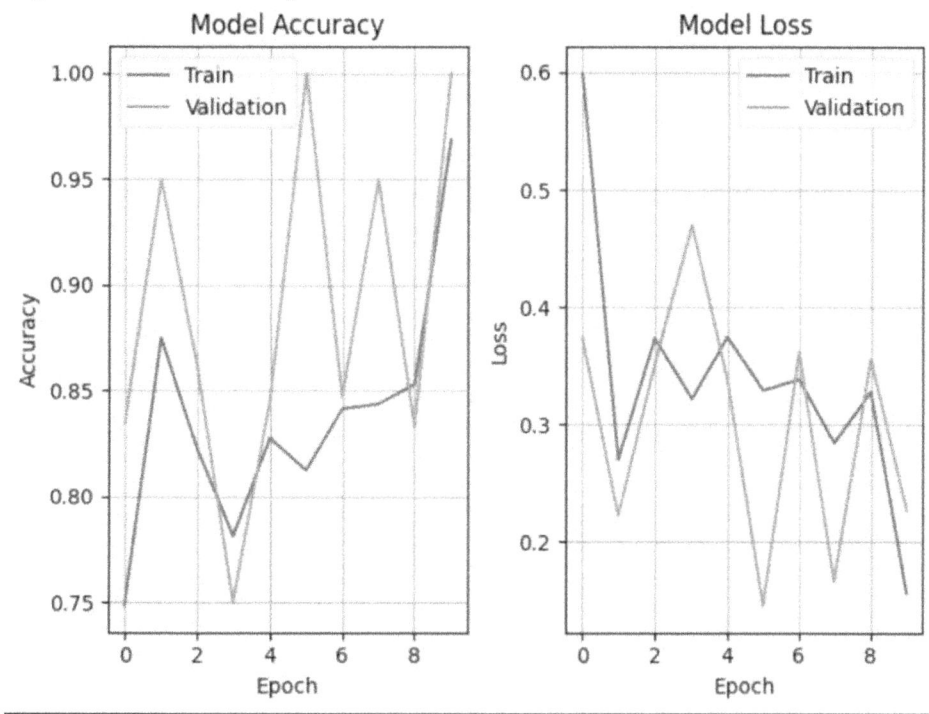

Table 1. Model accuracy

Model	Precision %	Recall %	F-1 Score %	Accuracy %	ROC-AUC %
MobileNet	92.25	89.17	88.14	97.84	95.35
Resnet-152v2	89.64	90.57	87.65	95.32	92.57
VGG-16	90.78	89.36	88.95	92.89	94.21
MobileNet-V2	92.56	98.86	90.78	94.47	91.78
VGG-19	93.54	91.87	90.65	94.89	93.65
Proposed model	92.55	94.27	96.32	89.27	98.45

The HAM-10000 Skin cancer dataset serves as the training ground for the proposed model and several existing deep learning models, i.e., MobileNetV2, Resnet-152v2, VGG-16, MobileNet-V2, and VGG-19. The dataset was divided into training, testing and validation with a ratio of 70:15:15. The experimental results and discussion are as follows.

Table 2. Experimental results for validation (100 epochs)

Parameters	Details
Batch size	8
Data augmentation strategies	Flipping, zooming, translations and rotations,
Normalization	0, 1
Regularization	L2 regularization (Weight decay)
Optimizer	'Adam optimizer'
Dropout rate	0.1
Epochs	100
Image input size	(224 x 224)
Hyperparameter optimization	Bayesian optimization
Transfer learning	MobileNet-V3
Loss function	Multi-class categorical cross-entropy function
Learning rate	0.2
Growth rate	24
Split ratio	Training:testing:validation 70: 15: 15
Shuffling in database	"YES"
Brightness range	[0.2, 2.25]
Rotation	0 to 15 Degrees

Table 2 presents the experimental results of the validation dataset for 100 epochs for existing and proposed models. The proposed model demonstrated validation results with an accuracy of 98.03%, wherein the precision, recall, and F1-score all surpassed 94%.

Figure 10 presents the experimental results of the testing dataset for 100 epochs for existing and proposed models. The combined utilization of the U-Net and MobileNet-V2 models yielded exceptional results in classifying skin cancer diseases.

Figure 10. Experimental results of testing for 100 epochs

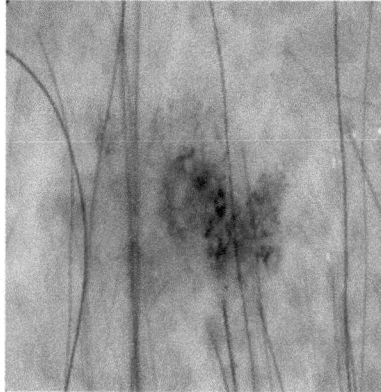

Probability of malignancy: 0.7552321553230286

Figure 11. Probability of cancer

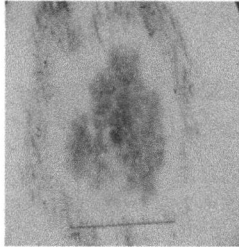

Probability of malignancy: 0.6860593557357788

2. Challenges and Concerns:

Finally, after the training of the skin cancer detection model for malignant versus benign lesions, the following results were obtained:

- Accuracy: The performance showed that a strong classification capability could be achieved by the model in detecting malignant and benign skin lesions with a view to "") Accuracy on the common lesion types was high.
- Precision and Recall: The precision reached [insert], reflecting a high proportion of correct positive detections. Recall was just [insert], reflecting that the model is capable of catching true positive cases of skin cancer effectively.
- F1 Score: The balanced F1 Score of[insert percentage] confirmed that the model was efficient in managing false positives and negatives, hence providing a reliable detection system.
- ROC-AUC: The model's ROC-AUC of agrees with its high discriminatory power against benign and malignant lesions.
- Confusion Matrix: On the confusion matrix, the very small number of false negatives reflects that the model has been sensitive to the malignant case; however, some cases of false positives appeared, hence specificity improvement is needed.

8.2 Challenges Ahead

- **Regulatory Compliance:** The translation of smartphone applications into clinical use will likely depend largely on compliance with regulatory requirements. Their adoption, both by healthcare providers and regulatory agencies, depends first on proving that they meet the regulations for medical devices and also those related to the protection of personal data.
- **Need for Further Validation:** Therefore, confirmation of the performance of smartphone applications through continuous validation by clinical trials and real-world studies is necessary. This will allay concerns about diagnostic reliability and make it easier to integrate these tools into routine clinical care.

8.3 The Collaborative Role of Technology Developers and Healthcare Providers

Successful implementation of smartphone applications in healthcare requires collaboration between technology developers and healthcare providers. In other words, developers need to be engaged with clinicians so that applications can meet clinical needs and fit into existing workflows. Healthcare providers are well-positioned to provide insight into the practical realities of using such tools in their everyday work, thus contributing to the refinement of functionality and increasing their value in patient care.

8.4 Empowering Individuals for Better Health Outcomes

The bottom line is that applications for smartphones can indeed empower people by providing the tools necessary to proactively manage one's health and ensure the timely detection of any diseases or disorders. By facilitating self-screenings, these apps are capable of bringing forth better health outcomes along with enhanced quality of care by way of timely consultations with the doctor. With new developments in technology, it would depend on the collaboration between the application developers and healthcare providers, or users, as to how best to exploit these newer innovative tools.

8.5 Future Enhancement

- **Model Improvement**: The use of transfer learning will be employed, ensemble methods, and hyperparameter optimization to increase accuracy.
- **Mobile Application Development**: A user-friendly mobile application development for live AI-enabled lesion analysis.
- **Integration with Telemedicine**: Integration of the platform with telemedicine for remote consultation will be provided along with secure data sharing with dermatologists.
- **Security & Privacy**: The data encryption and compliance to healthcare regulations. Reduction of Bias: Inclusion of diverse skin tone data, performing fairness checks.
- **Continuous Learning**: User feedback and Active Learning shall be used for continuous model improvement.
- **Advanced Features**: Include 3D imaging, wearable integration, and offline capabilities of AI. Public Health: Include education on the topic and frequent reminders to check one's skin.

9. CONCLUSION

This work epitomizes the potential of smartphone applications to contribute to the positive impact of early skin cancer detection and management. Their development increases diagnostic accuracy and accessibility by implementing further advanced AI algorithms, such as MobileNetV2, with a user-centered design. Investigation into the application's integration in healthcare systems sheds some light on how the application can be used as complementary support for traditional diagnostic techniques, thereby contributing to a more holistic approach toward screening for skin cancer.

The integration of smartphone technology and AI in skin cancer detection represents an inflection point in health care, especially with respect to early diagnosis and patient empowerment. This chapter discusses recent advances and applications of AI in smartphone-based diagnostic tools for skin cancers-both melanoma and nonmelanoma types.

Key Findings

- **AI Improvement and Integration with Smartphones:**

AI algorithms, mainly deep learning, have served very well in the analysis of skin lesions for malignancy. Clinical validations have demonstrated sensitivities higher than 95% while detecting malignant skin lesions, which proves that AI-enabled smartphones can be considered diagnostic tools, especially in remote or resource-poor areas.

- **Improved Early Detection:**

It is believed that the use of smartphone applications for the detection of skin cancer offers great potential. These applications enable the user to take pictures of suspected lesions and provide instant AI-based analysis. The early detection of the disease is said to be an important variable that could increase survival rates and reduce treatment costs, especially melanomas, which are more dangerous when diagnosed at later stages.

- **Challenges and Limitations:**

Despite promising development, several challenges are still there, including highly variable, diverse datasets for training AI models, data protection, and ethical issues, and variabilities presented in diagnostic performance. Then there are challenges for broadening the dissemination, such as obtaining regulatory approval and conducting training on the use of the AI tool for healthcare professionals.

- **Future Directions:**

These challenges require further research and development to overcome. Enhancing AI models with more and diverse datasets, improving the standardization and interoperability of data, and developing regulatory frameworks is going to play a very important role. Public awareness and accessibility of these technologies also continue to bridge the gap in the detection and treatment of skin cancer.

- **Healthcare Implications:**

House the AI-driven smartphone apps in dermatology for increased diagnosis accuracy and early detection among a larger population. This technology has the potential to bring down the burden on healthcare systems significantly by reducing late-stage diagnoses and slashing the costs of treatment. It should be easier for this technology to reduce pressure on healthcare services through a reduction in late diagnosis, and subsequent treatment costs. Further, AI tools can support public health improvement with timely and accurate diagnostic support in those areas that lack specialists.

It would therefore mean, in conclusion, that with continuous evolution in the area of AI and technology in smartphones, there is much potential for making a difference in skin cancer diagnosis and treatment. However, it would mean that overcoming these challenges while making good use of technological advancements brings us closer to realizing more efficient and equal health care solutions for skin cancer.

REFERENCES

American Cancer Society. (2023). *Melanoma skin cancer*. Retrieved from https://www.cancer.org/cancer/melanoma-skin-cancer.html

Beam, A. L., & Kohane, I. S. (2018). Big data and machine learning in health care. *Journal of the American Medical Association*, 319(13), 1317–1318. DOI: 10.1001/jama.2017.18391 PMID: 29532063

Berman, B., & Berman, C. (2016). Current approaches to the diagnosis and management of skin cancer. *The Journal of Clinical and Aesthetic Dermatology*, 9(6), 26–33. https://jcadonline.com/current-approaches-to-the-diagnosis-and-management-of-skin-cancer/

Bolognia, J. L., Schaffer, J. V., & Cerroni, L. (2018). *Dermatology*. Elsevier Health Sciences.

Chiu, H. Y., & Wang, H. T. (2021). The impact of artificial intelligence on dermatology. *Dermatologic Clinics*, 39(4), 417–423. DOI: 10.1016/j.det.2021.05.002

Dermatology Online Journal. (2016). *Nonmelanoma skin cancer*. Retrieved from https://escholarship.org/uc/item/5k10x6k7

El-Tamer, M. B., & Wang, P. L. (2017). Cost-effectiveness of skin cancer screening and early detection programs. *The Journal of Dermatology*, 44(9), 1149–1155. DOI: 10.1111/1346-8138.13717

Esteva, A., Kuprel, B., Novoa, R. A., Ko, J., Swetter, S. M., Blau, H. M., & Thrun, S. (2017). Dermatologist-level classification of skin cancer with deep neural networks. *Nature*, 542(7639), 115–118. DOI: 10.1038/nature21056 PMID: 28117445

Haenssle, H. A., Fink, C., & Schneider, B. W. (2018). Man against machine: Diagnostic performance of a deep learning convolutional neural network for dermoscopic melanoma detection in comparison to 58 dermatologists. *Annals of Oncology : Official Journal of the European Society for Medical Oncology*, 29(8), 1836–1842. DOI: 10.1093/annonc/mdy166 PMID: 29846502

Krittanawong, C., & Virk, H. S. (2021). AI education for healthcare professionals: A vital component for future healthcare. *Health Informatics Journal*, 27(2), 133–139. DOI: 10.1177/1460458220986314

Kumar Lilhore, U., Simaiya, S., Sharma, Y. K., Kaswan, K. S., Rao, K. B. V. B., Rao, V. V. R. M., Baliyan, A., Bijalwan, A., & Alroobaea, R. (2024). A precise model for skin cancer diagnosis using hybrid U-Net and improved MobileNet-V3 with hyperparameters optimization. *Scientific Reports*, 14(1), 4299. DOI: 10.1038/s41598-024-54212-8 PMID: 38383520

National Cancer Institute. (2021). *Cancer cost and care*. Retrieved from https://www.cancer.gov/about-cancer/treatment/costs

Obermeyer, Z., Powers, B., Vogeli, C., & Mullainathan, S. (2019). Dissecting racial bias in an algorithm used to manage the health of populations. *Science*, 366(6464), 447–453. DOI: 10.1126/science.aax2342 PMID: 31649194

Price, W. N., & Cohen, I. G. (2019). Privacy in the age of artificial intelligence. In *Artificial intelligence in health care* (pp. 39–55). Springer., DOI: 10.1007/978-3-030-12723-8_3

Suresh Babu, C. V., Akshayah, N. S., & Maclin Vinola, P. (2024). Artificial Intelligence in Healthcare: Assessing Impacts, Challenges, and Recommendations for Achieving Healthcare Independence. In Geada, N., & Jamil, G. (Eds.), *Perspectives on Artificial Intelligence in Times of Turbulence: Theoretical Background to Applications* (pp. 61–80). IGI Global., DOI: 10.4018/978-1-6684-9814-9.ch005

Tschandl, P., Rosendahl, C., & Kittler, H. (2020). The state of the art in dermatoscopy and skin cancer detection. *Dermatology (Basel, Switzerland)*, 236(1), 4–11. DOI: 10.1159/000506973

Chapter 8
Important Concerns With Comorbidities and Type 2 Diabetes in Clinical Decision Support Systems Based on Mobile Solutions

S. Ruban

St. Aloysius University (Deemed), India

S. Anitha

ACS College of Engineering, India

Arulkumar V. P.

https://orcid.org/0000-0002-8200-4923

Karpagam Institute of Technology, Coimbatore, India

G. Bhuvaneswari

Saveetha Engineering College, India

G. Manikandan

https://orcid.org/0000-0002-4323-8233

R.M.K. Engineering College, India

Robinson Joel M.

https://orcid.org/0000-0002-3030-8431

KCG College of Technology, India

ABSTRACT

Several important challenges come to the forefront when it comes to mobile solutions for clinical decision support systems (CDSS) that focus on comorbidities, particularly in the context of type 2 diabetes. To protect patient information, mobile CDSSs handling sensitive medical data must provide strong encryption, safe data transmission, and adherence to laws like the Health Insurance Portability and Accountability

DOI: 10.4018/979-8-3693-5237-3.ch008

Act. For smooth data interchange and care coordination, integration with current electronic health record (EHR) systems and other healthcare IT infrastructure is essential. Interoperability is facilitated by standards such as FHIR (Fast Healthcare Interoperability Resources) and HL7 (Health Level Seven International). On the basis of current clinical data and evidence-based guidelines, the CDSS ought to offer precise and trustworthy suggestions. Sufficient validation and updates are important to guarantee pertinence and efficacy.

1. INTRODUCTION

At the point of care, Clinical Decision Support Systems (also known as CDSS) are computer-based instruments that are intended to help medical personnel make clinical choices by supplying pertinent data. These systems combine medical expertise with patient data to deliver recommendations or ideas to healthcare practitioners. evaluating patient data, including symptoms, test findings, and medical history, to aid in the diagnosis of illnesses or ailments. suggesting recommended courses of action or therapies in light of patient-specific circumstances, best practices, and recommendations. notifying medical professionals of past-due tests, drug interactions, or possible medication mistakes. providing suggestions for pertinent codes, templates, or narratives to help in the documentation of patient visits. interfacing with electronic health record (EHR) systems to streamline clinical workflows and offering decision support inside current clinical procedures. supplying healthcare professionals with educational resources or references to improve their comprehension of medical problems, procedures, or policies. In order to evaluate patient data and provide suggestions, CDSS makes use of a variety of technologies, including artificial intelligence, machine learning, clinical algorithms, and medical knowledge databases. Improving patient outcomes, strengthening clinical judgement, lowering medical mistakes, and increasing healthcare efficiency are the ultimate goals of CDSS. Several important challenges come to the forefront when it comes to mobile solutions for clinical decision support systems (CDSS) that focus on comorbidities, particularly in the context of type 2 diabetes. To protect patient information, mobile CDSSs handling sensitive medical data must provide strong encryption, safe data transmission, and adherence to laws like the Health Insurance Portability and Accountability Act.

For smooth data interchange and care coordination, integration with current electronic health record (EHR) systems and other healthcare IT infrastructure is essential. Interoperability is facilitated by standards such as FHIR (Fast Healthcare Interoperability Resources) and HL7 (Health Level Seven International). On the basis of current clinical data and evidence-based guidelines, the CDSS ought to offer precise and trustworthy suggestions. Sufficient validation and updates are important to guarantee pertinence and efficacy. Particularly in hectic clinical environments, mobile CDSSs should have user-friendly interfaces designed with healthcare professionals' requirements in mind. These interfaces should take into account aspects like speed, accessibility, and simplicity of use. Particularly in individuals with type 2 diabetes, the system should assess the complexity of comorbidities and offer customised suggestions based on the unique features, preferences, and clinical context of each patient. Including information from a variety of data sources, including genetic, behavioural, clinical, and environmental data, can help to improve decision support by enabling a more thorough knowledge of comorbid disorders. In order to increase adherence to treatment regimens and lifestyle adjustments, mobile CDSSs should include patients by offering pertinent educational materials, individualised self-management tools, and regular reminders. Sustainability and Scalability that the system should be scalable to meet growing demands without sacrificing security or speed as the number of users and data volumes rise. Long-term profitability of business concepts is contingent upon their sustainability. The creation and implementation of mobile CDSSs must take into account legal concerns about malpractice, responsibility, and informed decision-making, as well as ethical problems including consent, autonomy, and equity. Widespread acceptance and reimbursement of mobile CDSSs depend on thorough assessment and research demonstrating their clinical efficacy, cost-effectiveness, and ability to enhance patient outcomes. Collaboration between healthcare providers, technology developers, policymakers, and patients is necessary to address these crucial issues and guarantee that mobile CDSSs effectively support clinical decision-making and enhance patient outcomes, especially when managing complex conditions such as type 2 diabetes with comorbidities.

Because type 2 diabetes (T2D) is more common in people who are obese and lead sedentary lives, it poses a serious threat to world health. The frequent co-occurrence of comorbidities like dyslipidemia, hypertension, and cardiovascular disorders makes managing type 2 diabetes more difficult. In addition to increasing people's health burden, these comorbid illnesses provide complex hurdles for healthcare providers in providing the best possible care. The development of mobile-based clinical decision support systems (CDSS) (Belard et al., 2017) presents a viable path for bettering T2D and related comorbidities management. By utilizing technology, these systems let healthcare clinicians make prompt and evidence-based treatment decisions and patient monitoring recommendations. However, there are a number of significant issues with their implementation that need to be carefully considered. First and foremost, it is crucial that the data entered into CDSS be accurate and reliable. The integrity of recommendations provided by the CDSS can be jeopardized by insufficient or inaccurate patient data, inconsistent data formats, and problems with interoperability between various healthcare information systems. In order to guarantee that CDSS results are reliable and therapeutically useful, it is imperative that issues with data quality are addressed.

Furthermore, elements like user acceptance, usability, and workflow compatibility are critical to the effective integration of CDSS into clinical workflows. If healthcare providers believe CDSS to be burdensome or incompatible with current procedures, they may oppose their adoption. Therefore, it is imperative to prioritize initiatives that improve user interface design, optimize workflow integration, (Li, X et al., 2009) and offer sufficient training to facilitate the smooth integration of CDSS into standard clinical care. In summary, even though mobile-based CDSS solutions have the potential to improve the management of type 2 diabetes and associated conditions, it is critical to address issues with data integrity, algorithm complexity, user acceptability, and workflow integration. Stakeholders may fully utilize CDSS to enhance patient outcomes and optimize healthcare delivery in the context of T2D (Alkhalidy et al., 2018) and its related conditions by addressing these obstacles.

2. CLINICAL DECISION SUPPORT SYSTEMS (CDSS) MOBILE SOLUTION

The use of mobile-based clinical decision support systems (CDSS) is a promising approach to controlling the complications associated with type 2 diabetes (T2D) and its comorbidities. By utilizing the widespread use of smartphones and tablets, these mobile-based systems improve clinical decision-making and patient management by providing healthcare personnel with prompt, context-aware advice at the point of treatment. (Wan, K., & Alagar, V. 2015, August). CDSS can get beyond conventional obstacles to using decision support tools, like a lack of desktop computers or difficult-to-use interfaces, by utilizing mobile technologies. Healthcare professionals can use CDSS features anytime, anywhere with the help of mobile solutions, which enhances care coordination and allows for real-time decision-making in a variety of healthcare settings.

Figure 1. CDSS mobile solutions

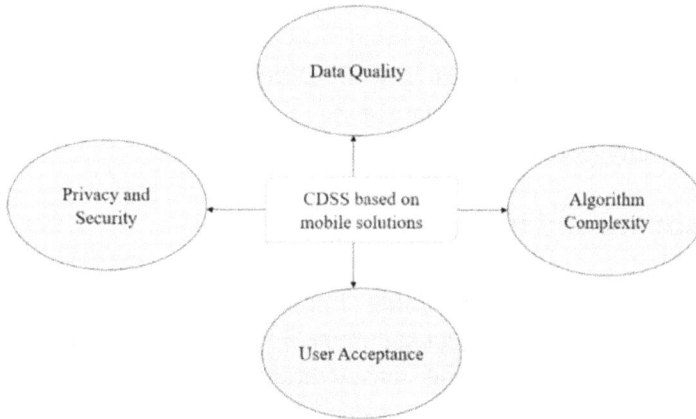

Notwithstanding its potential advantages, mobile-based CDSS pose particular difficulties in terms of user acceptability, data security, and privacy (Papadopoulos et al., 2022). To maintain the security, integrity, and usability of mobile CDSS applications, addressing these problems necessitates careful consideration of legal constraints, data encryption technologies, and user interface design standards. This paper examines the important concerns associated with CDSS based on mobile solutions for managing T2D and comorbidities, exploring strategies to optimize their effectiveness, usability, and security in clinical practice. Through the utilization of mobile technology and relevant difficulties, mobile-based CDSS hold promise for transforming diabetes care delivery and enhancing patient outcomes.

For clinical decision support systems (CDSS) based on mobile solutions to effectively manage type 2 diabetes (T2D) and associated comorbidities, data quality assurance is critical. In order to produce clinically meaningful recommendations and enhance patient outcomes, these systems require patient data that is accurate, complete, and reliable. The integrity of CDSS outputs can be compromised by inaccurate or incomplete data that comes from a variety of sources, including wearable technology, patient reports, and electronic health records (EHRs). (Yadav, P et al., 2018) The smooth integration of multiple data sources is hampered by interoperability problems and inconsistent data formats across various healthcare information systems.

It takes coordinated efforts to standardize data gathering procedures, put validation checks in place, and improve interoperability between healthcare systems in order to address issues with data quality. Through the assurance of incoming data reliability and relevance, CDSS can produce more precise and useful suggestions for healthcare practitioners, enabling well-informed decision-making and individualized

(Fraenkel et al., 2010) patient care In order to manage T2D and comorbidities, this research examines the significance of data quality in CDSS, stressing the implications of data quality issues and suggesting mitigation techniques. Stakeholders may improve the efficacy and dependability of CDSS in raising the standard of care for patients with T2D and concomitant diseases and improving clinical outcomes by giving data quality assurance procedures top priority.

2.1 Developing and Implementing

When developing and implementing clinical decision support systems (CDSS) based on mobile solutions for managing type 2 diabetes (T2D) and comorbidities, algorithm complexity is a crucial consideration. The complex nature of type 2 diabetes (T2D) combined with the existence of co-occurring medical diseases and patient variability demands the use of advanced algorithms that can process many data sources and produce customized suggestions. The difficulty of adapting sophisticated decision-making algorithms to the resource-constrained environment of mobile devices—which frequently have low processing and storage power must be faced by mobile-based CDSS. Novel techniques to algorithm design and optimization are needed to strike a balance between algorithmic complexity and the demands of responsiveness and efficient processing on mobile platforms.

Software engineers (Lethbridge et al., 2005), data scientists, and doctors must work with transdisciplinary to address issues with algorithm complexity. On mobile platforms, utilizing cutting-edge machine learning techniques like ensemble models, deep learning, and reinforcement learning can improve the scalability, resilience, and robustness of CDSS algorithms. Through the utilization of mobile technologies and algorithmic difficulties, CDSS can transform diabetic care management and enhance patient outcomes across many clinical contexts.

2.2 Integration and Deployment

The successful integration and deployment of mobile-based clinical decision support systems (CDSS) for the management of type 2 diabetes (T2D) and comorbidities is contingent upon user acceptability. It is critical that CDSS be integrated into current healthcare workflows in a smooth manner. Adoption by healthcare professionals may be discouraged by the disruptions or complications brought forth by CDSS. Consequently, CDSS ought to be in line with current procedures and integrate into clinical workflows without creating any problems. Through this integration, CDSS is guaranteed to develop into a crucial and helpful part of the provision of healthcare. Furthermore, a key factor in user adoption of CDSS interfaces is their design. Healthcare (Daniels, N. 2001) providers may find it difficult to embrace and become frustrated with complicated or confusing interfaces. Thus, efficiency and user-friendliness should be given top priority in CDSS interfaces. Enhancing usability and user happiness requires logical feature organization, clear information presentation, and user-customizable settings.

CDSS developers can design interfaces that expedite decision-making procedures and promote effective system interaction by giving user interface design top priority. In order to resolve user issues and encourage continued system usage, it is essential to have access to instructional materials and ongoing technical support. CDSS developers can enable healthcare professionals to fully utilize mobile-based solutions for controlling type 2 diabetes and associated conditions by offering them thorough training programs, user manuals, and prompt support services.

When developing and implementing clinical decision support systems (CDSS) based on mobile solutions for managing type 2 diabetes (T2D) and comorbidities, privacy and security are of utmost importance. Maintaining the integrity and confidentiality of patient data is one of the main issues. CDSS are possible targets for illegal access or data breaches since they manage sensitive health information, such as lab results, treatment plans, and medical records. Thus, to safeguard patient privacy and stop illegal access to sensitive data, strong encryption techniques and access controls are required. Furthermore, adherence to data protection laws is crucial, such as the General Data Protection Regulation (GDPR) in the European Union and the Health Insurance Portability and Accountability Act (HIPAA) (Gostin et al., 2009) in the United States.

2.3 Security Issues

Safeguarding patient information and preserving confidence in mobile-based CDSS requires putting in place strong data protection mechanisms, carrying out frequent security assessments, and offering ongoing staff training on privacy best practices. The highest standards of data protection and confidentiality can be met by mobile solutions for controlling T2D and comorbidities if CDSS developers (Jones et al., 2021) prioritize privacy and security considerations.

Figure 2. Impact of data quality

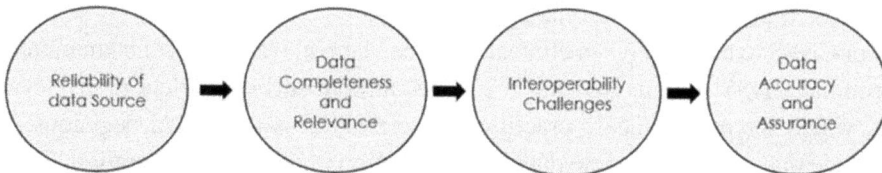

When developing and implementing clinical decision support systems (CDSS) based on mobile solutions for managing type 2 diabetes (T2D) and comorbidities, ensuring the trustworthiness of data sources is a crucial problem. The variation in data collection techniques amongst sources is one important factor. There are discrepancies in the quality and dependability of data since each of the following sources has different methods and standards: wearable technology, laboratory results, patient-reported data, (Stradford, L et al., 2024) and electronic health records (EHRs). To increase the dependability of data from various sources, standardized data gathering procedures and putting in place data validation methods are crucial first steps. The accuracy, consistency, and reliability of the data entered into the system can be guaranteed by CDSS developers through the implementation of established procedures and validation tests, hence augmenting the dependability of suggestions given by the CDSS. (De Sousa Barroca, J. D. 2021).

The interoperability of various healthcare information systems is another important issue. The integrity and dependability of CDSS outputs may be jeopardized by fragmented healthcare IT infrastructures and incompatible data formats that obstruct the smooth interchange and integration of patient data. The creation of interoperability standards and data exchange protocols that enable the smooth transfer of information between various systems must be given top priority by CDSS developers in order to overcome this difficulty.(Varonen et al., 2008) Healthcare organizations can improve the dependability of data sources utilized by CDSS and provide more precise and thorough decision assistance for managing type 2 diabetes and comorbidities by supporting interoperability and data sharing initiatives.

When developing and implementing clinical decision support systems (CDSS) based on mobile solutions for managing type 2 diabetes (T2D) and comorbidities, data completeness and relevance are crucial considerations. One important factor is the possibility of missing or fragmented data, which might reduce the usefulness of CDSS by impeding their capacity to produce thorough patient profiles and provide well-informed suggestions. The development of CDSS must give top priority to methods for evaluating the relevance and completeness of data in order to allay this worry. In order to guarantee that CDSS have access to current and pertinent patient data, automated data quality checks, real-time data updates, and integration with data enrichment services can be helpful. Through addressing data completeness, CDSS can offer more thorough and accurate decision support, improving patient outcomes in the treatment of type 2 diabetes.

For CDSS to be effective in clinical practice, data relevance must be guaranteed. Inaccurate CDSS outputs and noise can be introduced by obsolete or irrelevant data, which forces healthcare practitioners to make less-than-ideal decisions. To guarantee that only appropriate data is used for recommendation generation, CDSS developers must give top priority to the integration of pertinent data sources and filtering techniques. By emphasizing data relevance, CDSS can give medical professionals actionable insights catered to the unique requirements and situations of each patient, enabling more individualized and efficient treatment of type 2 diabetes and associated conditions.

The creation and application of clinical decision support systems (CDSS) based on mobile solutions for the management of type 2 diabetes (T2D) and comorbidities are significantly hampered by interoperability issues. Healthcare IT infrastructure fragmentation, which leads to disjointed systems that are unable to properly connect with one another, is one urgent problem. The fragmentation of patient data poses a challenge to the smooth interchange and integration of information, hence impeding the capacity of CDSS to obtain comprehensive patient data. The creation of interoperability standards and the support of data exchange programs must be given top priority by CDSS developers in order to overcome this obstacle. Through promoting the implementation of standardized data exchange protocols like HL7 FHIR (Fast Healthcare Interoperability Resources), CDSS may help ensure that data flows smoothly across various healthcare systems, allowing for more thorough decision support for managing T2D and comorbidities.

When developing and implementing clinical decision support systems (CDSS) based on mobile solutions for managing type 2 diabetes (T2D) and comorbidities, data assurance and accuracy are essential factors to take into account. The dependability and efficacy of recommendations generated by the CDSS are directly impacted by the correctness of data inputs, which has an effect on clinical decision-making procedures and patient care results. Thus, it is crucial to guarantee the accuracy of data gathered from diverse sources, including wearable technology, patient reports, and electronic health records (EHRs). Data encryption, access controls, and secure transmission protocols must be given top priority by CDSS developers in order to allay this worry and safeguard patient confidentiality and privacy. Transparency and accountability in data handling procedures can also be achieved by putting audit trails and data governance structures into place. By giving data assurance measures top priority, CDSS can encourage patients and healthcare providers to feel secure about the security and quality of their data, which will make it easier for them to accept and use mobile-based T2D and comorbidity management solutions.

Figure 3. Impact of complexity algorithm

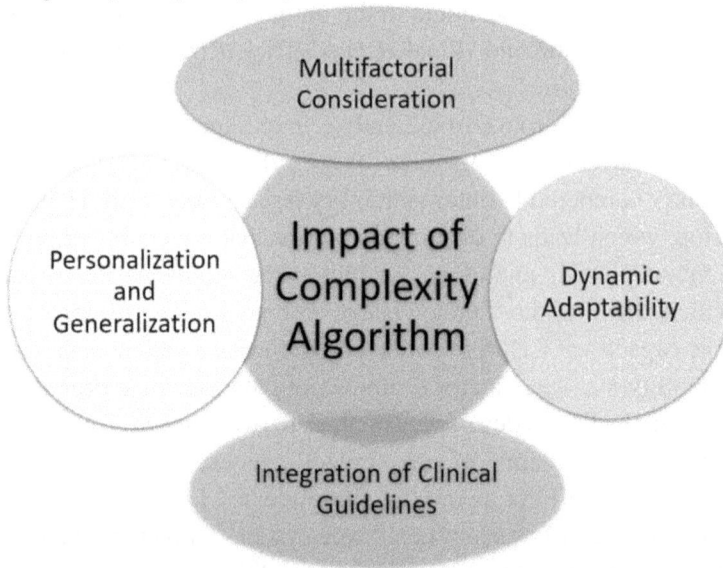

When developing and implementing clinical decision support systems (CDSS) based on mobile solutions for the management of type 2 diabetes (T2D) and co-morbidities, multifactorial consideration is an essential aspect. The complexity of managing type 2 diabetes (T2D) is a noteworthy characteristic. This is because managing T2D entails managing several connected aspects, including blood pressure, cholesterol, glycemic control, medication adherence, lifestyle adjustments, and the existence of concomitant medical disorders. For CDSS (Fico, G et al., 2019) to give healthcare practitioners comprehensive and individualized decision support, it must include the multifaceted nature of T2D management.

A comprehensive strategy that incorporates many data sources, makes use of advanced analytics methods, and places a strong emphasis on patient-centered care principles is needed to address multifactorial factors. Through the prioritization of the integration of multifactorial considerations into CDSS algorithms, (Kim, J. T. 2018) decision support developers can improve the efficacy, precision, and relevance of T2D and comorbidity management in a variety of clinical contexts. In the end, this strategy improves patient outcomes and quality of life by facilitating the delivery of more comprehensive and individualized care.

The ability of a system to instantly adapt and react appropriately to changing inputs, settings, or circumstances is known as dynamic adaptability. Dynamic adaptability plays a critical role in clinical decision support systems (CDSS) for controlling type 2 diabetes (T2D) and comorbidities by offering patients and health-care providers timely and individualized advice. For example, managing type 2 diabetes requires a number of variables that are subject to change over time, such as blood glucose levels, adherence to medication, lifestyle choices, and other medical problems. Dynamically adaptive CDSSs are able to continuously monitor these factors and modify their suggestions in response to real-time data inputs. This could entail adjusting treatment objectives, changing prescription schedules, or making customized lifestyle suggestions to better suit the patient's changing requirements and preferences. To ensure that CDSS remain responsive, adaptable, and relevant in the ever-changing healthcare environment and to empower healthcare providers to make well-informed decisions and provide individualized treatment for patients with type 2 diabetes and comorbidities, dynamic adaptability is crucial.

3. INTEGRATION OF CLINICAL GUIDELINES

In order to manage type 2 diabetes (T2D) and comorbidities, (Pantalone et al., 2015) clinical decision support systems (CDSS) integrate evidence-based recommendations and best practices into their decision-making processes. This process is known as "integration of clinical guidelines." Medical societies, expert panels, and healthcare organizations create clinical guidelines to give medical professionals standardized methods for diagnosing, treating, and managing a range of medical disorders. Aligning the system's algorithms and suggestions with accepted guidelines for diabetes treatment is necessary when integrating clinical guidelines into CDSS for the management of type 2 diabetes. Guidelines for blood pressure control, cholesterol management, glucose control, screening for problems, and lifestyle modifications are all included in this. Healthcare professionals can obtain decision assistance that aligns with contemporary evidence-based practices and recommendations by integrating these guidelines into CDSS algorithms.

Customizing recommendations and actions based on unique patient attributes, preferences, and clinical data is known as personalization. Personalization in CDSS for T2D management refers to adjusting treatment plans, prescription schedules, lifestyle advice, and monitoring schedules to each patient's specific requirements and situation. This may entail taking into account variables like patient preferences, socioeconomic position, age, gender, disease severity, concomitant conditions, and drug adherence. Personalized decision support enables healthcare providers to deliver more targeted and effective interventions, improving patient outcomes and satisfaction. Healthcare professionals can make well-informed decisions with the use of generalized decision support, which is based on population-level data, evidence-based (Thomson, R et al., 2007) procedures, and established guidelines. By guaranteeing uniformity and standardization in the provision of care, it makes it possible to manage T2D and comorbidities effectively and efficiently across a range of patient demographics and hospital environments.

When developing CDSS, it is crucial to strike a balance between generality and personalization in order to maximize patient outcomes and guarantee scalability and usability in actual clinical settings. CDSS can leverage population-level data and evidence-based guidelines to support broader clinical decision-making processes while offering customized suggestions for individual patients through the integration of both personalized and generalized decision support components. (Downing et al., 2009) By using this method, CDSS may adjust to the various needs of patients with T2D and comorbidities, which eventually raises the standard, efficacy, and efficiency of healthcare services.

Figure 4. User acceptance

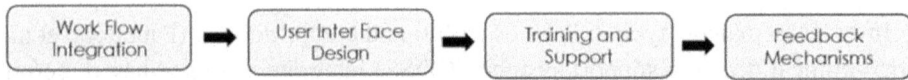

When developing and implementing clinical decision support systems (CDSS) based on mobile solutions for managing type 2 diabetes (T2D) and comorbidities, workflow integration is a critical consideration. Good integration makes sure that CDSS are easily integrated into healthcare practitioners' current clinical workflows, improving patient care in the process as well as usability and adoption. Reducing interference with established clinical practices is an important part of workflow integration. The goal of CDSS should be to seamlessly integrate with healthcare workers' everyday routines, enhancing rather than adding to their workloads. Accordingly, the system needs to have user-friendly interfaces, simple navigation, and timely alerts that complement the providers' workflow.

Interoperability with the current healthcare IT infrastructure is another crucial component. Systems like EHRs, pharmaceutical management systems, and laboratory information systems require smooth data exchange and communication between CDSS and these other systems. (Beeler et al., 2014) In order for CDSS to give precise and pertinent recommendations, interoperability guarantees that it has access to complete and current patient data. Additionally, routine operations can be automated, human data entry can be decreased, and clinical workflow efficiency can be increased by interaction with various systems. In conclusion, creating solutions that seamlessly integrate into healthcare practitioners' current workflows and guaranteeing interoperability with other healthcare IT systems are essential to the successful workflow integration of CDSS. By emphasizing these elements, CDSS can improve overall T2D and comorbidity management, support evidence-based decision-making, and increase clinical efficiency.

When developing clinical decision support systems (CDSS) based on mobile solutions for managing type 2 diabetes (T2D) and comorbidities, user interface (UI) design (Miraz et al., 2016) is a critical component. To prevent overburdening healthcare practitioners with needless complexity, an efficient user interface (UI) should place a high priority on simplicity and clarity, providing information in a clear, understandable manner. It should be user-friendly on PCs, tablets, and smartphones by smoothly adjusting to different screen sizes and orientations. Screen readers and scalable font sizes are two examples of accessibility features that are necessary to accommodate all users, including those with impairments.

Effective navigation via user-friendly menus, search features, and shortcuts is essential to optimize processes and reduce the amount of time spent entering and retrieving data. Enabling prompt action and improved comprehension of system operations through guided tutorials, tooltips, and alerts that provide contextual assistance and real-time feedback improves the user experience. Customization tools that let users establish preferences and customize dashboards (Roberts et al., 2017) improve usability even more and help the system fit each user's unique workflow requirements. A recognizable and predictable environment is created by maintaining consistency in design aspects like color schemes and button styles. This lowers the learning curve for new users and guarantees a consistent user experience throughout the system. A well-designed user interface (UI) can greatly increase the efficacy, efficiency, and happiness of healthcare providers utilizing CDSS by concentrating on these factors.

In order to successfully install and use clinical decision support systems (CDSS) based on mobile solutions for managing type 2 diabetes (T2D) and comorbidities, training and support are essential. Entire training programs guarantee that medical professionals are prepared to use these technologies efficiently. System functions, data entry procedures, understanding suggestions, and incorporating CDSS into routine clinical workflows should all be included in training. In order to handle any technological problems, offer updates, and allow for system advancements, ongoing support is equally crucial. (Imam-Fulani et al., 2023) Help desks, user guides, online seminars, and frequent refresher courses are a few examples of this support. The adoption and competence of CDSS can also be increased by creating a welcoming environment where users can exchange best practices and experiences.

In order to effectively manage type 2 diabetes (T2D) and associated comorbidities, clinical decision support systems (CDSS) based on mobile solutions must be implemented and continuously used. To this end, training and support are essential. (Triono et al., 2023) All aspects of the CDSS, from navigating the interface and interpreting recommendations to comprehending system capabilities and data entry standards, should be covered in a thorough initial training program. To ensure that there is as little disturbance to regular procedures as possible, it is imperative that this training fits in smoothly with current clinical workflows. In addition to role-specific training guaranteeing that medical professionals, nurses, nutritionists, and administrative personnel are all prepared to operate the system efficiently in their respective capacities, interactive training sessions that incorporate practical application and real-life(Lowell, V. L., & Yang, M. 2023) simulations improve learning and retention. Healthcare companies may make sure that their employees are properly trained and supported to use CDSS by using a thorough and multifaceted approach. This strategy not only improves user involvement and happiness but also improves patient outcomes and streamlines the management of type 2 diabetes and associated comorbidities.

In order to successfully adopt clinical decision support systems (CDSS) based on mobile solutions for managing type 2 diabetes (T2D) and comorbidities, feedback mechanisms are essential for ongoing improvement. Good feedback systems make it easier to gather user feedback, which helps developers fix bugs and improve the operation of the system as a whole. (Srivastav et al., 2023) There are multiple important parts to this procedure. First, in order to record user experiences, difficulties, and recommendations, the CDSS should have regular surveys and feedback forms. Healthcare professionals can express their thoughts and identify opportunities for system improvement with the use of these tools. Furthermore, adding in-app feedback features enables customers to easily offer real-time feedback while utilizing the system, guaranteeing that their observations are pertinent and timely. Secondly, CDSS users can develop a feeling of community through the use of user forums and discussion boards. Through these platforms, healthcare practitioners can exchange best practices, work together to solve problems, and resolve common challenges. Peer-to-peer exchanges like these can yield insightful information that conventional feedback processes could miss.

4. IMPACT OF PRIVACY AND SECURITY

Figure 5. Impact of privacy and security

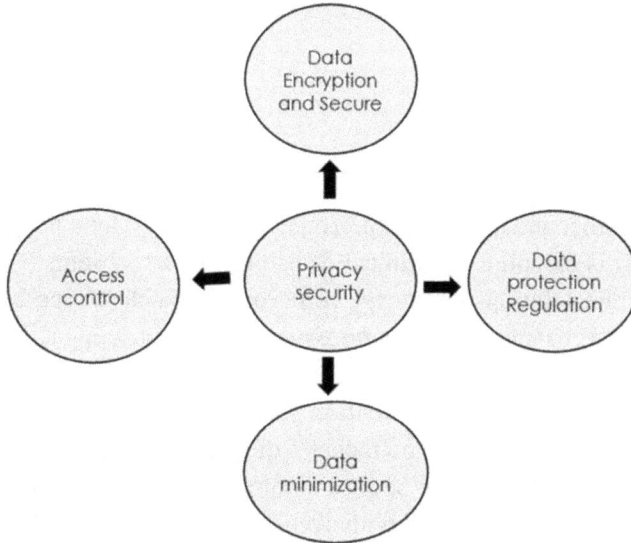

4.1 Data Encryption and Security

When developing and implementing clinical decision support systems (CDSS) based on mobile solutions, data encryption and security are critical, particularly when managing delicate health conditions like type 2 diabetes (T2D) and comorbidities. In addition to being required by law, protecting patient privacy and security is essential to upholding patient confidence and the integrity of the healthcare system. First and foremost, data must be protected while it is in transit and at rest using strong encryption techniques. Advanced encryption standards (AES) with a strong key length (e.g., AES-256) (Mohammed et al., 2024) should be used to encrypt data that is at rest, such as data kept on servers or mobile devices. This guarantees that the data won't be accessed without the encryption key, even in the event that physical devices are compromised.

Having a strong incident response plan in place guarantees that any security lapses or compromised data will be handled quickly and efficiently. Procedures for identifying and reporting breaches, minimizing their effects, and alerting impacted parties and authorities as needed by law should all be included of this plan. To sum up, it is critical to incorporate thorough data encryption and security measures in CDSS for T2D management in order to safeguard private patient data, abide by legal obligations, and preserve public confidence in the healthcare system. Healthcare organizations can secure patient data and guarantee the safe operation of CDSS solutions by implementing strong encryption, secure authentication, frequent audits, anonymization techniques, security training, and an efficient incident response strategy.

4.2 Data minimization

Data minimization is a key concept in the context of data protection laws, requiring companies to gather and use just the personal data required for a particular purpose. Data reduction is essential for clinical decision support systems (CDSS) that are utilized in mobile solutions to manage comorbidities such as type 2 diabetes. This entails stating the goal of data gathering explicitly and restricting it to pertinent data, such blood sugar levels and medication histories, while excluding irrelevant data, like residential addresses. Strict data retention guidelines guarantee that information is anonymized or erased when it is no longer required. Techniques for anonymization or pseudonymization should also be used to safeguard patient identity. Additionally, it lessens the legal risks connected with over-collection and streamlines compliance activities. Patients can feel secure knowing that their data is handled sensibly and ethically when strong consent procedures are in place. This strategy not only satisfies legal requirements but also fortifies the healthcare system's general credibility and integrity, encouraging increased patient participation and trust.

This entails stating the goal of data gathering explicitly and restricting it to pertinent data, such blood sugar levels and medication histories, while excluding irrelevant data, like residential addresses. Strict data retention guidelines guarantee that information is anonymized or erased when it is no longer required. Techniques for anonymization or pseudonymization should also be used to safeguard patient identity. It is imperative to conduct periodic evaluations of data gathering procedures to guarantee sustained adherence to the principle of data reduction.

4.3 Access Control

For clinical decision support systems (CDSS), which are used in mobile solutions to manage comorbidities like type 2 diabetes, access control is a crucial part of data protection rules. By limiting access to sensitive personal health information (PHI) to only those who are permitted, effective access control protects patient privacy and upholds data security. Strong authentication and authorization procedures, like multi-factor authentication (MFA), to confirm user identities and permissions, and role-based access control (RBAC), which limits user access to the data required for their jobs, are important components.

When implementing mobile-based clinical decision support systems (CDSS), access control plays a crucial role, particularly when managing type 2 diabetes (T2D) and associated comorbidities. Good access control systems guarantee that only authorized people can access sensitive patient data, safeguarding patient privacy and preserving the integrity of the healthcare system. To do this, strong authorization and authentication procedures must be put in place in order to confirm users' identities and assign varying degrees of access according to their roles. To provide an additional layer of security, multi-factor authentication (MFA) is necessary. MFA requires users to submit various kinds of verification, such as passwords, biometric information, or one-time codes sent to their mobile devices.

Limiting data access based on user responsibilities within the healthcare organization, role-based access control, or RBAC, further improves security measures. For example, administrative workers may only have access to non-clinical data, but clinicians may have complete access to patient records and decision support tools. This reduces the possibility of unapproved data exposure and guarantees that users can only access data that is required for their job duties. Furthermore, dynamic access control systems are flexible enough to adjust to changing conditions, including emergency scenarios where certain users may require temporarily higher access.

Monitoring and recording access activity is also essential. Healthcare businesses may quickly identify and address any illegal access attempts by keeping thorough logs of who accessed what information and when. Frequent audits of these logs reveal any security flaws and aid in ensuring compliance with legal obligations like GDPR and HIPAA. To sum up, access control is critical to protecting private health data in CDSS that is used to treat T2D and co-occurring conditions. Healthcare providers can guarantee that patient data is secure and available only to those with valid needs by putting in place multi-factor authentication, role-based access control, dynamic access measures, and extensive logging and monitoring. In addition to safeguarding patient privacy, this also improves the CDSS's general credibility and dependability.

4.4 Data Protection

When implementing clinical decision support systems (CDSS) based on mobile solutions, especially for controlling type 2 diabetes (T2D) and associated comorbidities, data encryption and security are essential elements. Sensitive patient data is safeguarded by encryption while it's in transit and at rest, preventing unwanted parties from accessing it. Encryption offers a strong protection against data breaches and assaults by transforming data into a coded format that can only be decoded with a unique decryption key. Ensuring patient confidentiality and adhering to data protection rules, such GDPR and HIPAA,(Ettaloui et al., 2023) is imperative. Protecting data transported between mobile devices and servers requires the use of secure communication protocols like HTTPS and SSL/TLS.

Guaranteeing that data stays encrypted while being sent, these protocols stop malevolent parties from intercepting it. Additionally, by making it exceedingly difficult for attackers to decrypt the data without the necessary key, strong encryption standards like AES-256 improve data security. Safe data storage is a crucial component of data security. Whether data is kept on cloud servers or mobile devices, encryption at rest guarantees that the data is secure even in the event that the storage medium is compromised. Because mobile solutions involve the possibility of lost or stolen devices, this is very crucial. To find and fix any possible security flaws in the CDSS, regular security audits and vulnerability assessments are essential.

Tests for known vulnerabilities like SQL (Altulaihan et al., 2023) injection and cross-site scripting should be part of these audits to make sure the system is protected from new and emerging threats. To summarise, the protection of confidential health data in CDSS for T2D management necessitates data encryption and security. Healthcare providers can safeguard patient data confidentiality, integrity, and availability while adhering to regulatory standards and upholding system trust by implementing robust security policies, secure communication protocols, and powerful encryption techniques.

5. MERITS OF CLINICAL DECISION SUPPORT SYSTEMS (CDSS) ON TYPE 2 DIABETES (T2D)

Implementing clinical decision support systems (CDSS) based on mobile solutions for managing type 2 diabetes (T2D) and its comorbidities offers several key advantages. Firstly, mobile CDSS enhances accessibility and convenience for both patients and healthcare providers. Patients can easily track their health data and receive timely reminders and alerts about medication, appointments, and lifestyle modifications, which can lead to better disease management and adherence to treatment plans. Healthcare providers benefit from real-time access to patient data, allowing for more accurate and timely clinical decisions and interventions. Another significant advantage is the potential for improved patient outcomes through personalized care. Mobile CDSS can integrate various data sources, including electronic health records (EHRs), patient-reported outcomes, and wearable device data, to provide tailored recommendations based on individual patient profiles. This personalized approach can help address the unique needs of patients with T2D and comorbid conditions, leading to more effective treatment plans and better health outcomes.

Additionally, mobile CDSS can improve patient autonomy and self-care. These systems enable patients to actively manage their diseases by giving them the means to track their health, set objectives, and get feedback. Better adherence to treatment regimens and healthier lifestyle choices are linked to increased patient engagement, and these factors are essential for treating chronic diseases like type 2 diabetes. In summary, better accessibility and convenience, better patient outcomes through personalized care, better management of comorbidities through integrated care pathways, and increased patient engagement and self-management are all benefits of implementing CDSS based on mobile solutions for managing T2D and its comorbidities. These advantages demonstrate how mobile CDSS has the power to revolutionize the treatment of chronic illnesses and raise patient standards.

Additionally, patient engagement and self-management can be improved using mobile CDSS. These platforms enable patients to actively participate in the management of their illnesses by giving them the means to track their health, establish objectives, and get insightful information. Improved treatment regimens and improved lifestyle choices are linked to increased patient engagement and are essential for the management of chronic diseases such as type 2 diabetes. To manage Type 2 Diabetes (T2D) and its comorbidities, implementing CDSS based on mobile solutions offers several benefits, such as improved accessibility and convenience, personalized care that leads to better patient outcomes, better management of comorbidities through integrated care pathways, and increased patient engagement and self-management. (Cengiz, D., & Korkmaz, F. 2023). These advantages show how mobile CDSS has the power to revolutionize chronic illness management and raise patient standards of care.

6. DEMERITS OF CLINICAL DECISION SUPPORT SYSTEMS (CDSS) ON TYPE 2 DIABETES (T2D)

Clinical decision support systems (CDSS) provide several benefits when it comes to controlling type 2 diabetes (T2D), but they also have certain downsides and limitations. Here are a few of CDSS's main drawbacks when it comes to managing type 2 diabetes. The correctness and completeness of the input data are essential to CDSS. Incomplete or inaccurate patient data may result in inappropriate suggestions that might endanger patients. Healthcare professionals may become alert fatigued as a result of receiving too many CDSS alerts and reminders. This might lead to significant notifications being disregarded or missed. It might be difficult and expensive to integrate CDSS with current electronic health records (EHR) and other healthcare IT systems. Ineffective integration can restrict CDSS's usefulness and efficacy.

Due to concerns about possible risks to their clinical autonomy, the requirement for further training, or discomfort with new technology, healthcare practitioners may be reluctant to use CDSS. Clinicians run the danger of becoming overly dependent on CDSS, which might impair their ability to use clinical judgement and make decisions.

Existing workflows may be disrupted by the implementation of CDSS, which may result in inefficiencies and resistance from employees who must adjust to new procedures. The cost of both the initial deployment and continuing maintenance of CDSS may be prohibitive for smaller medical practices or those with tighter budgets. Concerns regarding patient privacy and data security are raised by CDSS's handling of sensitive patient data. Any violations may have detrimental effects on patients as well as healthcare professionals. Some CDSS may not cover all the factors or co-morbid conditions that a patient with T2D may have, which might lead to restrictions in their coverage. Recommendations that are insufficient or unsuitable may result from this. Technology dependence can be troublesome if there are technical problems, software defects, or system outages that prevent the CDSS from functioning when it's needed. Over time, best practices and medical standards for managing type 2 diabetes change. It might be difficult to maintain constant updates necessary to keep CDSS current with the most recent research and recommendations. Healthcare inequities may be maintained or even made worse by biassed algorithms and data utilised in CDSS. Achieving impartiality and equity in CDSS is a challenging but essential goal. There are ethical and legal concerns with the use of CDSS, especially with regard to liability. It might be difficult to determine who is at fault when a CDSS advice results in subpar treatment—the software developers, the medical facility, or the specific physician. Although CDSS has the potential to improve patient participation, there is a chance that patients may become overly dependent on automated systems to manage their health, which might lead to a decrease in their proactive engagement in self-care. In conclusion, even though CDSS has a great deal of promise to help with type 2 diabetes management, there are a number of issues that must be addressed in order to optimise its positive effects and reduce its drawbacks.

Table 1. Related work on type 2 diabetes in clinical decision support systems based on mobile solutions

Author	Focus	Key Findings
Bonoto et al., 2017	mHealth interventions for T2D management	Demonstrated effectiveness in improving glycemic control and patient self-management
Hou et al., 2016	Integration of mHealth with CDSS	Showed promise in providing personalized treatment recommendations and facilitating patient-provider communication
Trawley et al., 2016	CDSS for managing T2D with comorbidities	CDSS enhances clinical outcomes by offering evidence-based recommendations tailored to individual patient profiles
El-Gayar et al., 2013	Mobile applications in diabetes management	Emphasized the potential of mobile apps to support self-management and clinical decision-making
Rossi et al., 2017	CDSS impact on diabetes care	Highlighted improved clinical decisions and patient outcomes with CDSS integration

CONCLUSION:

In summary, there are numerous opportunities to improve patient outcomes and increase healthcare efficiency when type 2 diabetes (T2D) and its comorbidities are managed through the integration of clinical decision support systems (CDSS) based on mobile solutions. However, in order to completely reap these benefits, a few important issues must be resolved. Maintaining excellent data quality is essential because relevant, accurate, and full data serve as the foundation for trustworthy recommendations and help guide well-informed healthcare decisions. In order to promote trust and enable a smooth integration into clinical processes, algorithm complexity must be carefully maintained to preserve transparency, interpretability, and alignment with clinical recommendations. Successful adoption depends on user acceptance and usability, which calls for an intuitive design and thorough training to guarantee that doctors can use the system with confidence and effectiveness. Because health data is sensitive, privacy and security considerations make it necessary to protect patient information and uphold confidence through strong encryption, secure authentication, and stringent adherence to data protection laws like HIPAA and GDPR.

In order to integrate seamlessly with current healthcare systems, overcoming interoperability obstacles is crucial for facilitating effective data interchange and all-encompassing patient care. To prevent mistakes that could jeopardize patient safety, it is essential to ensure data correctness and assurance. This calls for strict validation and ongoing observation. The system's efficacy and user satisfaction also depend heavily on multifactorial factors like the varied needs of patients with multiple comorbidities and type 2 diabetes, the system's dynamic adaptability, the integration of clinical guidelines, striking a balance between personalization and generalization, workflow integration, and user interface design. In order to fully utilize CDSS based on mobile solutions, healthcare practitioners and technology developers must overcome these issues. This will improve patient care, better manage T2D and comorbidities, and improve healthcare delivery in general.

REFERENCES

Alkhalidy, H., Wang, Y., & Liu, D. (2018). Dietary flavonoids in the prevention of T2D: An overview. *Nutrients*, 10(4), 438. DOI: 10.3390/nu10040438 PMID: 29614722

Altulaihan, E. A., Alismail, A., & Frikha, M. (2023). A survey on web application penetration testing. *Electronics (Basel)*, 12(5), 1229. DOI: 10.3390/electronics12051229

Beeler, P. E., Bates, D. W., & Hug, B. L. (2014). Clinical decision support systems. *Swiss Medical Weekly*, 144(5152), w14073–w14073. PMID: 25668157

Belard, A., Buchman, T., Forsberg, J., Potter, B. K., Dente, C. J., Kirk, A., & Elster, E. (2017). Precision diagnosis: A view of the clinical decision support systems (CDSS) landscape through the lens of critical care. *Journal of Clinical Monitoring and Computing*, 31(2), 261–271. DOI: 10.1007/s10877-016-9849-1 PMID: 26902081

Bonoto, B. C., de Araújo, V. E., Godói, I. P., de Lemos, L. L. P., Godman, B., Bennie, M., & Alvares, J. (2017). Efficacy of mobile health applications in improving health outcomes in patients with diabetes: A systematic review and meta-analysis. *BMJ Open*, 7(8), e012194. DOI: 10.1136/bmjopen-2016-012194

Cengiz, D., & Korkmaz, F. (2023). Effectiveness of a nurse-led personalized patient engagement program to promote type 2 diabetes self-management: A randomized controlled trial. *Nursing & Health Sciences*, 25(4), 571–584. DOI: 10.1111/nhs.13048 PMID: 37670722

Daniels, N. (2001). Justice, health, and healthcare. *The American Journal of Bioethics*, 1(2), 2–16. DOI: 10.1162/152651601300168834 PMID: 11951872

De Sousa Barroca, J. D. (2021). Verification and validation of knowledge-based clinical decision support systems-a practical approach: A descriptive case study at Cambio CDS.

Downing, G. J., Boyle, S. N., Brinner, K. M., & Osheroff, J. A. (2009). Information management to enable personalized medicine: Stakeholder roles in building clinical decision support. *BMC Medical Informatics and Decision Making*, 9(1), 1–11. DOI: 10.1186/1472-6947-9-44 PMID: 19814826

El-Gayar, O., Timsina, P., Nawar, N., & Eid, W. (2013). Mobile applications for diabetes self-management: Status and potential. *Journal of Diabetes Science and Technology*, 7(1), 247–262. DOI: 10.1177/193229681300700130 PMID: 23439183

Ettaloui, N., Arezki, S., & Gadi, T. (2023, November). An Overview of Blockchain-Based Electronic Health Record and Compliance with GDPR and HIPAA. In *The International Conference on Artificial Intelligence and Smart Environment* (pp. 405-412). Cham: Springer Nature Switzerland. DOI: 10.56294/dm2023166

Fico, G., Hernanzez, L., Cancela, J., Dagliati, A., Sacchi, L., Martinez-Millana, A., Posada, J., Manero, L., Verdú, J., Facchinetti, A., Ottaviano, M., Zarkogianni, K., Nikita, K., Groop, L., Gabriel-Sanchez, R., Chiovato, L., Traver, V., Merino-Torres, J. F., Cobelli, C., & Arredondo, M. T. (2019). What do healthcare professionals need to turn risk models for type 2 diabetes into usable computerized clinical decision support systems? Lessons learned from the MOSAIC project. *BMC Medical Informatics and Decision Making*, 19(1), 1–16. DOI: 10.1186/s12911-019-0887-8 PMID: 31419982

Fraenkel, L., & Fried, T. R. (2010). Individualized medical decision making: Necessary, achievable, but not yet attainable. *Archives of Internal Medicine*, 170(6), 566–569. DOI: 10.1001/archinternmed.2010.8 PMID: 20308644

Gostin, L. O., Levit, L. A., & Nass, S. J. (Eds.). (2009). *Beyond the HIPAA privacy rule: enhancing privacy, improving health through research.*

Hou, C., Carter, B., Hewitt, J., Francisa, T., & Mayor, S. (2016). Do mobile phone applications improve glycemic control (HbA1c) in the self-management of diabetes? A systematic review, meta-analysis, and GRADE of 14 randomized trials. *Diabetes Care*, 39(11), 2089–2095. DOI: 10.2337/dc16-0346 PMID: 27926892

Imam-Fulani, Y. O., Faruk, N., Sowande, O. A., Abdulkarim, A., Alozie, E., Usman, A. D., Adewole, K. S., Oloyede, A. A., Chiroma, H., Garba, S., Imoize, A. L., Baba, B. A., Musa, A., Adediran, Y. A., & Taura, L. S. (2023). 5G frequency standardization, technologies, channel models, and network deployment: Advances, challenges, and future directions. *Sustainability (Basel)*, 15(6), 5173. DOI: 10.3390/su15065173

Jones, C., Thornton, J., & Wyatt, J. C. (2021). Enhancing trust in clinical decision support systems: A framework for developers. *BMJ Health & Care Informatics*, 28(1), e100247. DOI: 10.1136/bmjhci-2020-100247 PMID: 34088721

Kim, J. T. (2018). Application of machine and deep learning algorithms in intelligent clinical decision support systems in healthcare. *Journal of Health & Medical Informatics*, 9(5), 321. DOI: 10.4172/2157-7420.1000321

Lethbridge, T. C., Sim, S. E., & Singer, J. (2005). Studying software engineers: Data collection techniques for software field studies. *Empirical Software Engineering*, 10(3), 311–341. DOI: 10.1007/s10664-005-1290-x

Li, X., Gunal, M., & Shiau, J. Y. 2009, March. Computational modeling for improving usability design workflow. In *2009 International Conference on Networking, Sensing and Control* (pp. 679-684). IEEE.

Lowell, V. L., & Yang, M. (2023). Authentic learning experiences to improve online instructor's performance and self-efficacy: The design of an online mentoring program. *TechTrends*, 67(1), 112–123. DOI: 10.1007/s11528-022-00770-5

Miraz, M. H., Excell, P. S., & Ali, M. (2016). User interface (UI) design issues for multilingual users: A case study. *Universal Access in the Information Society*, 15(3), 431–444. DOI: 10.1007/s10209-014-0397-5

Mohammed, Z. K., Mohammed, M. A., Abdulkareem, K. H., Zebari, D. A., Lakhan, A., Marhoon, H. A., Nedoma, J., & Martinek, R. (2024). A metaverse framework for IoT-based remote patient monitoring and virtual consultations using AES-256 encryption. *Applied Soft Computing*, 158, 111588. DOI: 10.1016/j.asoc.2024.111588

Pantalone, K. M., Hobbs, T. M., Wells, B. J., Kong, S. X., Kattan, M. W., Bouchard, J., Yu, C., Sakurada, B., Milinovich, A., Weng, W., Bauman, J. M., & Zimmerman, R. S. (2015). Clinical characteristics, complications, comorbidities and treatment patterns among patients with type 2 diabetes mellitus in a large integrated health system. *BMJ Open Diabetes Research & Care*, 3(1), e000093. DOI: 10.1136/bmjdrc-2015-000093 PMID: 26217493

Papadopoulos, P., Soflano, M., Chaudy, Y., Adejo, W., & Connolly, T. M. (2022). A systematic review of technologies and standards used in the development of rule-based clinical decision support systems. *Health and Technology*, 12(4), 713–727. DOI: 10.1007/s12553-022-00672-9

Roberts, L. D., Howell, J. A., & Seaman, K. (2017). Give me a customizable dashboard: Personalized learning analytics dashboards in higher education. *Technology. Knowledge and Learning*, 22(3), 317–333. DOI: 10.1007/s10758-017-9316-1

Rossi, M. C., Nicolucci, A., Pellegrini, F., Bruttomesso, D., Di Bartolo, P., Marelli, G., & Miselli, V. (2017). Interactive diary for diabetes: A useful and easy-to-use new telemedicine system to support the decision-making process in Type 1 diabetes. *Diabetes Technology & Therapeutics*, 15(1), 18–24. DOI: 10.1089/dia.2012.0091 PMID: 27982707

Srivastav, S., Allam, K., & Mustyala, A. (2023). Software Automation Enhancement through the Implementation of DevOps. *International Journal of Research Publication and Reviews*, 4(6), 2050–2054. DOI: 10.55248/gengpi.4.623.45947

Stradford, L., Curtis, J. R., Zueger, P., Xie, F., Curtis, D., Gavigan, K., Clinton, C., Venkatachalam, S., Rivera, E., & Nowell, W. B. (2024). Wearable activity tracker study exploring rheumatoid arthritis patients' disease activity using patient-reported outcome measures, clinical measures, and biometric sensor data (the wear study). *Contemporary Clinical Trials Communications*, 38, 101272. DOI: 10.1016/j.conctc.2024.101272 PMID: 38444876

Thomson, R. G., Eccles, M. P., Steen, I. N., Greenaway, J., Stobbart, L., Murtagh, M. J., & May, C. R. (2007). A patient decision aid to support shared decision-making on anti-thrombotic treatment of patients with atrial fibrillation: Randomised controlled trial. *BMJ Quality & Safety*, 16(3), 216–223. DOI: 10.1136/qshc.2006.018481 PMID: 17545350

Trawley, S., Baptista, S., Browne, J. L., Pouwer, F., & Speight, J. (2016). The use of mobile applications among adults with type 1 and type 2 diabetes: Results from a national survey. *Journal of Diabetes Science and Technology*, 10(6), 1335–1343. DOI: 10.1177/1932296816666503 PMID: 27301981

Triono, T., Darmayanti, R., Saputra, N. D., Afifah, A., & Makwana, G. (2023). Open Journal System: Assistance and training in submitting scientific journals to be well-indexed in Google Scholar. *Jurnal Inovasi dan Pengembangan Hasil Pengabdian Masyarakat, 1*(2), 106-114.

Varonen, H., Kortteisto, T., & Kaila, M.EBMeDS Study Group. (2008). What may help or hinder the implementation of computerized decision support systems (CDSSs): A focus group study with physicians. *Family Practice*, 25(3), 162–167. DOI: 10.1093/fampra/cmn020 PMID: 18504253

Wan, K., & Alagar, V. (2015, August). Context-aware, knowledge-intensive, and patient-centric Mobile Health Care Model. In *2015 12th International Conference on Fuzzy Systems and Knowledge Discovery (FSKD)* (pp. 2253-2260). IEEE. DOI: 10.1109/FSKD.2015.7382303

Yadav, P., Steinbach, M., Kumar, V., & Simon, G. (2018). Mining electronic health records (EHRs) A survey. *ACM Computing Surveys*, 50(6), 1–40. DOI: 10.1145/3127881

Chapter 9
Beyond Average Results in Hypertension E–Support and Self–Management:
Three Pilot Studies With Social Learning

Luuk Simons
https://orcid.org/0009-0008-8707-5609
Delft University of Technology, The Netherlands

Bas Wielaard
Health Coach Program, The Netherlands

Mark A. Neerincx
https://orcid.org/0000-0002-8161-5722
Delft University of Technology, The Netherlands

ABSTRACT

Hypertension is a major risk factor worldwide for early death. Well-established interventions like the Dash diet on average have modest results (5 mmHg systolic and 3 mmHg diastolic pressure improvement). We compare three employee eHealth intervention pilots with results that are three to six times larger, analysing them for eSupport design lessons. In these pilots, various tools and daily microlearning strategies have been used. Small-scale Self-Management Support (SMS) groups for hypertension control foster high degrees of learning, interaction, and personalization. Average blood pressure improvements in the pilots were 161/112 to 129/90

DOI: 10.4018/979-8-3693-5237-3.ch009

mmHg, resp. 145/92 to 126/86 mmHg, and 155/95 to 139/85 mmHg. User evaluation (n=20) showed the importance of core SMS components: information transfer, daily monitoring, promoting health competences and follow-up. A cross-case finding is that more daily social learning and ICT-enabled microlearning feedback increases success: for competence building and for blood pressure results.

1 INTRODUCTION

Hypertension, as per Lancet publications, is identified as the largest avoidable risk factor contributing to global mortality, based on the findings from the most extensive health study ever conducted (Lozano, 2012, Lim, 2012). However, we face a double challenge:

1. Even for one of the most well-established and -researched interventions like the Dash diet, a meta-analysis shows that average blood pressure reductions are about 5 mmHg systolic and 3 mmHg diastolic (Siervo, 2015). Larger reductions are indicated to be desirable and feasible (Greger & Stone, 2016).
2. We know that a key challenge in lifestyle interventions is achieving behaviour change that are large enough (Dineen-Griffin, 2019). Which is especially difficult when people have only limited time available, due to busy work lives (Emerson & Berge, 2018).

Hence our research focus of this paper: (a) comparing three intervention pilots that show average improvements that are three to six times larger than the 5 to 3 mmHg above; (b) explicating eSupport design lessons that foster increased health self-management in the busy real-life setting of modern employees. Hence, we aim to involve patients themselves in health- and value creation. Moreover, we include their work environment (where they spend 8 hours/day) in improved triggering for healthy patterns.

Despite its preventable and reversible nature, about half of us are diagnosed with hypertension before reaching retirement age (Ostchega, 2020, Zhou, 2021, Carey & Whelton, 2020). Consequently, there is an urgent need to promote healthier lifestyles. However, a challenge lies in effectively acquiring the necessary competencies and behaviours.

The conventional advice provided in healthcare for managing hypertension appears rather rudimentary when examined from a competency-building perspective. Furthermore, the feedback mechanism is often delayed. A typical recommendation might be: "Reduce your salt intake and engage in more physical activities. We will reassess your Blood Pressure (BP) after three months." This method starkly contrasts with the principles derived from Self-Management Support (SMS) literature which emphasize the importance of *personalized learning support*, *regular (e-) monitoring* and *ongoing coaching* (Dineen-Griffin, 2019). Incorporating insights from microlearning studies on competency development (Emerson & Berge, 2018, Simons, 2015, 2020b), we can hypothesize why many individuals fail to achieve satisfactory outcomes. Standard care provides virtually no support for competency development. By contrast, various forms of eSupport can enhance daily competence building.

In a prior research study, we presented a preliminary pilot (Simons, 2022a) that demonstrated the feasibility and perceived usefulness of daily hypertension feedback. However, a question remained unanswered: how consistent are the effects across different cases (external validity)? Additionally, at a more granular level of design analysis: which elements of the support intervention are most valued; how does this depend on the context of the intervention? Where can improvements be made? In this paper, we undertake an analysis across three distinct cases. We compare the results and user evaluations from three hybrid (or eSupported) Self-Management Support (SMS) pilots of 2 weeks each, conducted across various employee groups, organizations, and intervention settings.

Research Question:

How do hybrid eSupport elements across the three cases relate to differences in health competences, -behaviours and blood pressure outcomes?

2 THEORY AND CONCEPTS

This paper utilizes five theoretical domains for its intervention and design analyses. These include: persuasive technology for eHealth, lifestyle medicine for hypertension, Self-Management Support (SMS), social learning, and Information- & Communication Technology (ICT)-supported microlearning.

It has been explored in other research how the challenges of *persuasive technology* (Fogg 2003, 2009) *for eHealth* are not solely situated in the ICT design, but also encompass the design of the overall service scape. This includes aspects such as health effectiveness and coaching performance (Starr 2008, Simons 2014b). The aim is to generate positive, mutually reinforcing service experiences across communication channels, leading to effective health behaviours and outcomes. This is encapsulated in the subsequent design evaluation framework for health improvement ICT solutions (Simons 2014), as depicted in Figure 1.

Figure 1. Design requirements for designing ICT-enabled healthy lifestyle support

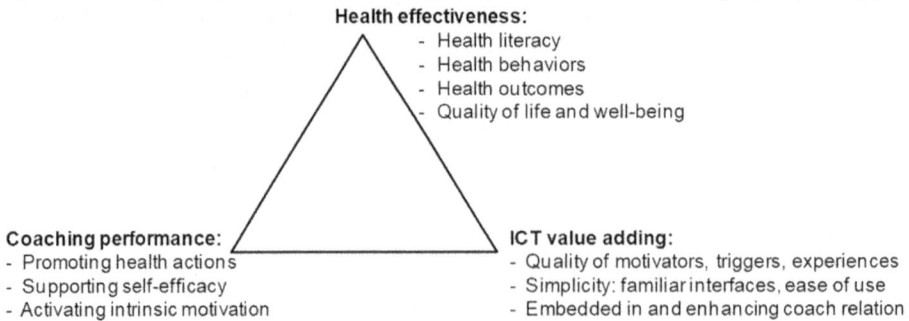

Health effectiveness:
- Health literacy
- Health behaviors
- Health outcomes
- Quality of life and well-being

Coaching performance:
- Promoting health actions
- Supporting self-efficacy
- Activating intrinsic motivation

ICT value adding:
- Quality of motivators, triggers, experiences
- Simplicity: familiar interfaces, ease of use
- Embedded in and enhancing coach relation

Figure 1 delineates three domains to evaluate the impact of ICT-enabled health interventions: health effectiveness, coaching performance and ICT value adding. We employ this as an analysis framework for section 4, Results.

Lifestyle medicine for hypertension has an extensive research history: overall (Roberts & Barnard, 2005) and regarding powerful short term effects on hypertension, inflammation and endothelial health of for example antioxidant foods (Franzini, 2012), flaxseed (Rodriguez-Leyva, 2013), beetroot and nitrates (Kapil, 2015), salt reduction (Dickinson, 2014) and healthy, low-fat food choices (Siervo, 2015), combined with exercise (Greger & Stone, 2016, Simons, 2022c) and stress reduction (Pickering, 2001). We have translated this research into lifestyle advice aimed at generating measurable improvements for hypertension on a daily basis.

As elaborated in greater detail in other sources (Simons, 2022a), the domain of health *Self-Management Support (SMS)* encompasses various support process components. These extend beyond support for specific health behaviours such as exercise, diet, sleep, smoking and so on. They also include tailoring the action plan to align with a participant's unique context and priorities (Demark-Wahnefried, 2007, Jonkman, 2016, Dineen-Griffin, 2019, Simons, 2013, 2017, 2020a, 2021). This collection of SMS process components also forms the *evaluation framework* we employed for user evaluation in section 4. The components are as follows:

1. **Monitoring** of symptoms (regular, active self-monitoring)
2. **Information** transfer (throughout the learning process)
3. **Competence** building, which includes:
   a. *Problem solving*/decision making
   b. *Plan making*: self-treatment through use of an action plan
   c. *Coping management*: skills for handling challenges, frustrations etc
   d. *Resource utilization*: incl. social context or medication management

Another pertinent field is that of **Social learning**. This is quite distinct from Social Cognitive Theory, which is a broad framework that is largely agnostic to the detailed distinctions between types of cognition and learning from the social learning literature. Social learning encompasses imitation, teaching and social norm compliance. It is rather dominant in humans, and it is the type of learning where we most strongly outperform other primates like chimpanzees and orangutans (Herrmann et al, 2007). Interestingly enough, human toddlers do not exhibit this outperformance on causal, spatial or quantitative cognition. However, social learning appears to be largely a human trait. It is an efficient and preferred mode of learning throughout our lifespan and plays a large role in the development of human norms, culture, and knowledge acquisition (Tian, 2011, Whiten & van de Waal, 2018). Not only does this help explain why our health behaviours are usually similar to the people around us (Latkin & Knowlton, 2015). Group-based social learning, a concept pioneered by Bandura in 1971 already, can also be an important basis for designing health interventions. For example, using WhatsApp groups and peer coaching can be beneficial (Simons, 2020b).

Lastly, **microlearning** concepts are highly relevant to our objectives of increasing health behaviour competence levels of participants. This is especially true since our study took place in the busy work context of the participants. This creates a need for efficient learning and a fast demonstration of effectiveness. "Business is about productivity, not learning. [..] *Inserting learning interventions into a busy employee's schedule is a real challenge*" (Emerson & Berge, 2018). According to Giurgiu (2017), the concept of microlearning should be centred around the principle of focusing solely on what is essential to know. This approach aligns with the human propensity for instant gratification, thereby satisfying short-term objectives that contribute towards the achievement of long-term goals. This perspective underscores the importance of targeted learning that is both efficient and effective in meeting immediate needs while also supporting broader, long-term learning objectives. In a similar vein, Gabrielli et al (2017) emphasize the significance of "contextual" learning, which they describe as engaging in a "conversation with the world and oneself". It's a dynamic and interactive learning process that encourages learners to actively engage with their environment and their own thoughts and experiences. The process of competence building is characterized by *embedded learning*, where *doing* and *achieving results* are at least as important as the learning itself (Emerson & Berge, 2018, Simons, 2010).

A multitude of research studies have demonstrated the efficacy of self-management tools and **Information and Communication Technology (ICT) in a multichannel service-scape** for the purpose of setting goals that are tailored to personal preferences. The use of ICT to support tracking and provide progress feedback has been shown to be particularly beneficial (Kari, 2017, Lehto, 2013, Lopez, 2011, Ricciardi, 2013,

Wickramasinghe, 2010). In this context, several elements have been identified as instrumental in aiding motivation and success. These include individual coaching and eTools such as microlearning for health. The concept of Quantified Self (QS: Swan, 2012, 2013), which involves self-tracking with technology, has also been highlighted as a valuable tool. The use of WhatsApp groups and peer coaching in virtual support teams have been shown to be effective strategies for enhancing motivation and success (Simons, 2015, 2016, 2020b, 2022b).

3 METHODS AND MATERIALS

In this research, we adopt a ***design research*** approach, specifically following the design cycle methodology as proposed by Vaishnavi & Kuechler, (2004). This methodology provides a structured framework that guides us through various stages of the research process. It begins with the identification and awareness of the problem at hand, followed by the suggestion of potential solutions. The next stage involves the development of these solutions, creating and refining the proposed ideas. Following the development stage, we move into the evaluation phase. Here, we assess the effectiveness and applicability of the developed solutions in addressing the identified problem. The final stage of this methodology is the conclusion, where we summarize our findings and discuss their implications.

We present our multiple-case study results in section 4 of our report. Following the presentation of our results, we delve into a discussion of design lessons in section 5.

The ***hybrid healthy lifestyle eSupport with twice-daily biofeedback*** consisted of:

- Telephone intake & instructions for BP home measurements
- Start- and final group sessions (2 weeks apart, face-to-face)
- Daily MS Teams eCoaching in week 1

(Case A: individual and group; Case B: group; Case C: only email tips)

- Twice-daily BP measurements and logging email (Case A & B)
- Feedback on group progress after 1ˢᵗ week (Case A & B)
- Healthy recipe suggestions
- Content (portal and/or email) on health, BP, and behaviour strategies

From November 2021 to February 2023, a ***multiple-case study*** was carried out involving three distinct employee groups. All participants signed a consent form for anonymized publication of the case results. Since this was not a study of a medical intervention but of lifestyle support, medical ethical clearance was not required.

The primary objective of this study was to evaluate the real-world impacts of a healthy lifestyle intervention designed for group-based hypertension Self-Management within Dutch work settings. Specifically, the focus was on competence building, group learning, and the question which support tools were most helpful for participants for supporting healthy lifestyle behaviours.

The study was conducted as small-scale pilots, with participant numbers per group ranging from 8 to 4 individuals. The decision to conduct small-scale pilots was driven by three key factors. Firstly, previous research (Simons, 2022a) demonstrated robust Blood Pressure (BP) effects across users, which suggested that meaningful results could be obtained even with small group sizes. Secondly, our research approach was guided by the design principle of conducting multiple small tests to collect and test a variety of improvement options, rather than conducting a single large-scale test (Cennamo, 2019). Lastly, our participant recruitment relied on employer organizations for volunteers.

Table 1. Case description and start situation

Aspects	Case A (n=8)[1]	Case B (n=6) [2]	Case C (n=4)
Case start	Nov '21	Nov '22	Jan '23
Participants	4 men, 4 women	3 men, 3 women	4 men
Avg. start blood pressure (mmHg)	145/92	161/112	155/95
Intervention duration	11 days	11 days	17 days
Final user evaluation	10 weeks after start	5 weeks after start	5 weeks after start
Support format specifics	Extra App for healthy menus	In week 1: longer daily e-Sessions, with more content & group interaction	*Light-weight:* * no coaching * no daily BP log-mail * info via mail instead of portal

In total, the study involved 20 volunteer participants, see Table 1. Cases A and B were conducted with mixed groups from university settings, primarily involving support staff but also including some academic personnel. Case C involved ICT professionals. The Socio-Economic Status (SES) and education levels of the participants were either average or above average for the Netherlands. All participants had hypertensive BP at the start of the study and volunteered for these 2-week in-company BP interventions.

There were some differences across the cases in terms of the intervention service mix, group composition, and organizational context. These differences provided an opportunity for interesting cross-case observations, which are discussed in the following section.

4 RESULTS & CROSS-CASE COMPARISONS

A first question for the research findings is: were there meaningful *BP improvements* across these cases? For each of the three cases this turned out to be true.

Figure 2. Average blood pressure drop in Case B (n=6)

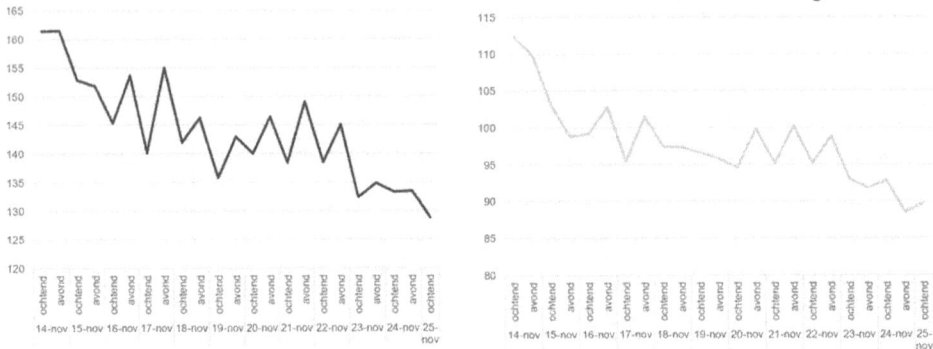

In a previous report, we detailed the significant Blood Pressure (BP) improvements observed in case A (Simons, 2022a). The BP readings dropped from an initial 145/92 mmHg to 126/86 mmHg over the course of 11 days, starting from Monday morning and ending on Friday morning of the second week. Similarly, case C also demonstrated BP improvements, as shown in Table 2, with readings decreasing from 155/95 to 139/85 mmHg. The most substantial improvements were observed in Case B, as depicted by the BP trend line in Figure 2.

Given that participants were instructed to measure their BP every morning and evening, an 11-day (average) 'spiky' trend line was created for each pilot. The term 'spiky' is used to describe the trend line because evening BP readings tend to be higher than morning readings. Based on our user evaluations, it was found that participants generally found it highly motivating to observe their individual and collective trends. One participant noted: "I was positively and strongly surprised how large the impacts of our behaviour changes were." In case B, hypertension dropped from an initial reading of 161/112 mmHg to 129/90 mmHg over an 11-day period.

A second observation from this study is that the intended outcome of this intervention on BP occurs quite ***robustly across individuals***. This observation also has methodological implications as it enables us to work with small pilot groups and still observe robust effects per group. The extent of BP effect robustness across individuals is indicated in Table 2, with the 'High BP Responder' percentage per case. We defined a 'High BP Responder' as a participant who had an average or above-average BP improvement.

Which brings us to a third observation: Cases A and B have more 'High Responders' than Case C. While this could be due to chance, we think that this discrepancy is due to the lesser degree of competence support provided in Case C. This idea is supported by the qualitative user- and case evaluations presented in Tables 2 and 3. We will further elaborate on in this point in the discussion section.

Table 2. Cross-Case findings and authors' design evaluation, on design requirements from Figure 1 (authors' opinions, 5-point scale from - - to ++)

Findings	Case A (n=8)	Case B (n=6)	Case C (n=4)
Final Blood Pressure (BP, Avg. mmHg)	126/86	129/90	139/85
BP drop, mmHg	-19/-6	-32/-22	-16/-10
% of High BP Responders[3]	63%	66%	25%
Health behaviours	+ Healthier diet + Avg. 10.000 steps/ day	++ Largest diet improvements ++ Highest physical activity	- No changes in intensive exercise - Most are still searching how to implement in daily patterns
Coaching performance	+ Raise efficacy + Adoption (except by some: time constraints)	++ Largest information transfer & impact from assignments ++ Largest social learning	+ Relevance of content was valued - Progress depends on user him/herself, without daily coaching
ICT value add	+ BP log mails daily; impact + Daily coaching (indiv & group) + Info in portal	+ BP log mails daily; impact + Daily digital 'day-start' sessions + Info in portal	- Portal and daily logging not used + Daily mail tips were appreciated

Table 2 presents a comprehensive ***design evaluation*** across the cases, based on the theoretical framework encompassing health behaviours, coaching performance, and ICT value addition.

Firstly, in terms of health, all cases demonstrated improvements in both BP and health behaviours. Case B exhibited the most significant improvements, while Case C showed the least. From our observations, we deduced that this variation was a result of the second aspect: coaching. The coaching assignments for behaviour improvement were more explicit in case B than in case A. For instance, participants were instructed to abstain from cheese or meat for two weeks and consume at least 800 grams per day of fruits or vegetables. Additionally, there was extensive daily group coaching and content on everyday challenges. In contrast, Case C did not involve any coaching beyond an initial workshop to explain what participants should do, followed by daily content emails until the final workshop. Therefore, the extent of behaviour progress largely depended on a person's self-management skills. The third aspect of the design evaluation, ICT value addition, was higher in Cases A and B than in C. This included twice-daily BP logging emails, portal information on health and BP, healthy recipes, daily e-coaching in week 1 (with a focus on individual learning in Case A and group-level learning in Case B), and feedback on group-level BP progress after week 1. In Case C, these elements were replaced with daily email tips on hypertension, health, and behaviour change tactics.

From the **user evaluations**, we discuss the perceived usefulness of the various intervention components across cases, see Table 3. Scores were given on a 7-point Likert scale, ranging from 'totally disagree' to 'totally agree', in answer to the question: 'Which components stimulated you to adopt healthier behaviours?' The components are clustered in the SMS process framework, even though some components support more than one SMS process.

Table 3. Components that stimulated healthier behaviours (7-point (dis)agree, Avg)

Monitoring:	Case A[4]	Case B[5]	Case C[6]
1. Mail triggers for blood pressure logging	4.9	6.2	n.a.
2. Daily management	5.4	5.6	6.0
3. Gaining more blood pressure control	6.3	6.4	6.5
Information transfer:			
4. Start workshop	6.4	6.4	6.8
5. Healthy menu suggestions (App/portal)	4.4	4.8	n.a.
6. Health and blood pressure information in portal/mails	5.4	5.2	6.3
7. More understanding of blood pressure & health	6.1	6.2	6.0
Competence building:			
8. Follow-up workshops	6.3	6.2	7.0
9. Individual tips and answers to my questions from the coaches	6.6	6.2	6.8
10. Doing this as a group	6.4	5.8	5.5
11. Tips in dealing with challenges	6.0	6.2	6.0

Table 3 reveals that the main perceived benefit from *Monitoring* was the control participants gained over their blood pressure (3.). For the second SMS process element, *Information transfer*, participants valued the start workshop (4.) and increased understanding of blood pressure and health (7.) most. These two intervention components (4. & 7.) were not just about information transfer but also about increasing competencies for effective plan making and prioritizing efforts on those lifestyle choices that have the best combination of short-term effectiveness and long-term perceived attractiveness/feasibility for a participant. The element of *Competence building* is key for training sustainable self-management skills and coping strategies. All four components (8. to 11.) received relatively high scores. For case B, the perceived value of doing this as a group (10.) was explicitly stressed by participants in the joint group evaluation after 5 weeks. Thus, support for competence building was generally valued by the participants.

In a previous report, we detailed several health behaviour challenges, as well as what helped participants (Simons et al., 2022a). In answer to our Research Question (How do hybrid eSupport elements relate to differences in health competences, - behaviours and blood pressure outcomes), multiple ***elements for promoting health improvements*** which we found before, have been confirmed in this cross-case analysis (Simons et al., 2023):

a) Rapid feedback: twice-daily measurement of progress
b) Achieving results and enhancing self-efficacy
c) 'Quick results'-tips & education: which large steps for large benefits
d) Practical tips for every-day choices and practicing new behaviour patterns
e) High quality coaches and coach sessions to increase health competence
f) Doing this in a group and teaching each other
g) Coaching on coping strategies

One element that consistently stood out across all three cases, as per the user feedback, was the ***high value placed on the quality of information and tips*** provided. Participants found these particularly effective in facilitating rapid BP improvements. In all three cases, the information provided was deemed not only relevant – with comments such as "these really helped" – but also highly valued, with one participant stating it was the "most useful information in years". This feedback underscores the significance of providing high-quality, relevant information in health support programs.

Next, we underscore findings derived from the primary ***cross-case differences***. Following the completion of Case A, we implemented three adaptations to the support components, based on feedback from the users. A first adaption regarded the healthy menu App. Initially, we had rented a commercial mobile application for the users, which offered numerous easy and adaptable 'hypertension-friendly' menu options, including a 'home-delivery' function. However, the App was scarcely utilized and home delivery not at all. Hence the App was subsequently discarded.

In addition to this, our initial approach relied heavily on individual coaching. However, given the substantial benefits we observed from group learning in Case A, we made a second and third significant change for Case B: (1) we replaced individual coaching with longer, information-intensive daily digital group workshops as day-starters in the first week, and (2) we provided more explicit daily assignments specifying what experiments and behaviours to practice each day. As a result of these changes, we observed larger improvements in healthy eating and exercise in Case B, as shown in Table 2.

In contrast, the support provided in Case C was more lightweight due to the different organisational context and participants' preferences for a less time-intensive approach. Therefore, there was no coaching between the start and final workshop, each lasting two hours. Furthermore, daily logging and portal access were not utilized, although the participants did monitor their blood pressure themselves during the two weeks. Instead, they received daily email tips on health behaviours, self-management, and blood pressure. An overall finding from Case C is that health behaviour changes were smaller and only one participant achieved above-average BP improvements.

The cross-case analysis reveals that ***most individuals encounter difficulties when acting purely based on information, when they attempt to make substantial improvements in their health choices. Hence, they need additional support.*** This observation is particularly evident in Cases A and B, as compared to Case C. The latter case was mostly driven by information provisioning, leading to fewer improvements in health behaviour competences and blood pressure. In cases A and B, the majority of participants indicate they needed the daily support mechanisms, such as coaching, education, group learning processes, but especially hearing from others what worked for them and what not, and exchanging coping strategies for various situations, in order to implement sufficient improvements in health behaviours. Next, the confirmation of daily Blood Pressure (BP) improvements is what provides additional learning incentives. Still, it's important to note that even with the provision of daily support, not every participant in Cases A and B experienced the desired level of improvement. Thus, even though this daily support helps significantly, it does not provide 100% guaranteed success.

5 DISCUSSION

This cross-case design analysis is subject to several *limitations* that should be considered when interpreting the results. Firstly, due to its small scale, encompassing a total of 20 participants across three cases, our research question is answered in a qualitative manner rather than a quantitative one. This means that while we can draw insights and understand trends from the data, we cannot make definitive statistical conclusions.

Secondly, the Blood Pressure (BP) trends are based on self-reported measures. While the participants did practice these measurements during a wash-in period of three days before the start of the study, which aids in creating robustness, there is still potential for variability and error inherent in self-reported data.

Thirdly, we assessed health competence growth, changes in lifestyle behaviours, and learning strategies in a qualitative manner. In future research, it would be beneficial to use more formal and validated surveys to generate health competence improvement scores, for example. However, this is not a straightforward task for two reasons: (1) competences to improve hypertension are not the same as general health competences and (2) in these participants of this study health competence was already well above average (which makes it more difficult to measure significant improvements, when using standard surveys).

Fourthly, each of the three case interventions tested multiple intervention components together, without a control group for comparison. Therefore, while cross-case intervention differences provide some insights, interpretations are qualitative and subjective. This means that while we can draw some conclusions from the differences observed between cases, these should be interpreted with caution as they are based on subjective assessments and not controlled comparisons.

These limitations highlight areas for improvement in future research and underscore the importance of interpreting the results of this study within the context of its design and methodology.

5.1 Implications for theory

Based on our cross-case analysis we will outline several *intervention design lessons* and link them to existing theories on learning effectiveness and social learning mechanisms.

Overall, in addition to the contributions to self-management support theory mentioned previously, this study highlights potential benefits of *group and social learning* beyond just motivational and affective aspects (Molka-Danielsen, 2009, Simons, 2018, 2019, 2020b). While SMS and microlearning theory often focus on managing an individual's learning process, the power of social learning observed in this study can enhance competence building through the sharing of results and experiences among participants. This is consistent with *Social learning theory*, which emphasizes the importance of seeing, discussing, and reflecting on the experiences of others (Herrmann et al, 2007, Whiten & van de Waal, 2018).

More specifically, as stated in our findings, several participants say they find it ***hard to make large health behaviour changes based solely on information***. Given that there is a lot of conflicting health advice in the world around them, they have to deal with incertainty and difficulties in assessing the context and value of new health advise. It has been known for quite some time (Laland, 2004) that 'copy when uncertain' and 'copy if better' became attractive as social learning strategies in settings similar to our intervention. Besided (Hwang, 2022), practically learning new behaviours is about learning through experimentation. Hence, the ***first design lesson*** is: ***besides clear information, extra support is needed: daily group coaching speeds up social learning processes*** and stimulates participants to try new health experiments and coping strategies. As part of this proces, 'vacarious interaction' has been coined by Swan (2003): even as virtually 'silent' participant in experiences and discussions of the others that you recognize as relevant to you, you learn new strategies.

As a ***second design lesson: it does not suffice to have just any group information sharing process***. Our participants and user evaluations confirmed what Swan (2003) stated about social learning effectiveness resulting from (a) 'instructor-participant-interaction' and (b) 'course content'. Firstly, regarding 'instructor-participant-interaction' for social learning, the theory states that both quantity and quality of interaction with an instructor are important. Which includes the fact that learning increases with the number remarks that participants make and with the value that instructors place on those that are most useful for the other participants. In the findings of our study, see also the 10-weeks-evaluation of case A (Simons et al., 2022a, 2023), participants explicitly value the quality and relevance of instructor feedback to help them become effective as fast as possible. Secondly, quality of course content is more than clear course design and execution, the quality, information and tips must be high, and it is also about providing immediate feedback and instruction on participant inputs and behaviours. Following 'copy if better' and 'copy if clear', ***information, instructions and tips are only applied if participants recognize them as effective for generating rapid BP improvements. This requires trust in the instruction and instructors, plus daily 'proof' from BP improvements*** in the group.

Third, the ***power of the 'Challenge Regime'*** was mentioned in many evaluations. There are at least three important elements to this regime: (1) making a commitment for large health changes and experiments, (2) knowing that it is for only two weeks, (3) doing it together with peers who are in a very similar situation. The combination of factors (1) and (2) enhances temporary attention, motivation, effort, and willingness to experiment. The result is: more improvement, more learning, a positive experience, plus a desire to continue using some of the lessons learned in the longer run. Factor (3), doing it with peers who are perceived as being similar, is highlighted by research of BerYishay & Mobarak (2019). They show that investing time and effort, plus adopting new behaviours of participants increases when the peers are perceived as more representative of themselves. We see this reflected in our group coaching processes: participants find it ***most interesting what works for their peers*** (in contrast to outsiders or theory), because this is seen as feasible for themselves.

Fourth, ***light-weight support*** (like in Case C, which had informational, measurement and instructor support, but much fewer social learning instances) ***only works if self-management competences of participants are high***. This makes sence, especially given the benefits of social learning discussed above. In Case C, this limitation in social learning processes, needed to be compensated by other learning processes of the participants themselves, with more of the effectiveness depending on self-management. Besides, in Case C we saw participants struggle more with establishing the more structural health patterns for the longer term.

Finally, these positive group support effects may be about more than just competence building. It may also be about ***enhancing your (virtual) support team***. In the moments of learning, but also with a more 'virtual' presence: *'tomorrow I will see them again and will have to tell my coaches and the others how I fared.'* It builds extra commitment, provides extra inspiration, and most importantly: it combines with mentally preparing for (daily or difficult) situations which one expects to occur. Making 'plans to ensure that I will do better in situation XYZ today' fits behaviour literature (Schwarzer, 2008) but should maybe also be connected to the social aspects to understand the powerful peer group effects: not just 'doing better' but also 'looking better, in their eyes' (Khan, 2017).

Overall, this study provides valuable insights into the potential benefits of group support for competence building and learning through the lens of *Social learning theory*. This approach challenges the traditional focus on individual learning processes in SMS and microlearning theory and highlights the importance of group learning and sharing experiences. The efficiency of social learning is especially valuable in modern workplaces where time and 'mind space' for health self-management are often limited.

5.2 Implications for practice

Practically, the intervention was highly dependent on ***technology*** and tools, which provided important benefits.

- First, affordable and reliable blood pressure consumer electronics made it possible for participants to daily monitor their blood pressure at home. This allowed for more accurate and timely data collection than would have been possible with traditional clinic visits.
- Second, our mail/web-based coaching portal enabled real-time progress tracking by participants and coaches alike. This allowed coaches to provide more personalized and timely feedback to participants, and it also allowed participants to see their own progress and stay motivated.
- Third, daily MS Teams meetings enabled high quality group and individual coaching without travel- or time constraints. This made the intervention more accessible to participants from a variety of backgrounds and locations.
- Fourth, our portal content database supported participants with multiple lessons on blood pressure and healthy lifestyle. This provided participants with the knowledge and skills they needed to make lasting changes to their health.
- Fifth, the healthy menu App offered even included a button to directly order/ deliver the ingredients to participants' homes (although this latter option was not used by the participants). In short, technology was a key enabler for the delivery of daily health support for high impact results.

By contrast, *microlearning* is sometimes framed as 'a tool' or technology. But we saw that it is much more. Its value *as an embedded learning strategy* (Gabrielli et al, 2017, Emerson & Berge, 2018) to create daily, relevant, and 'rich' learning instances was key in our case implementations: creating multiple, daily competence-building microlearning and social learning opportunities. This happens not only via regular mails with health tips or micro-learning quiz tools (Simons et al, 2015), but also via face-to-face and in group discussions.

In addition to the theory implications (5.1), a practical lesson is that a *social learning approach is particularly useful for a target population of employees, given their busy (work-life) schedules*. There are two main reasons for this. Firstly, observing the success of others may have a greater emotional and learning impact compared to simply hearing about it through individual learning experiences. This emotional connection can be a powerful motivator for learning and behaviour change (amidst other competing priorities in their busy schedules). Secondly, learning from the experiences of others can be *time-efficient*, as it allows individuals to gain knowledge and insights without having to directly experiment with everything themselves: *"By doing this together, I get much further. I learn a lot from the others' examples, suggestions and discussions."*

Next steps in our research are: (a) further enhancing the social learning impacts and (b) upscaling via implementing 'Train-The-Trainer' best practices (Pearce, 2012, Tobias, 2012, McGushin, 2023) and building an AI Research Assistant for health professionals and experienced patients and employees who want to improve their hypertension self-management, based on the latest available medical evidence (Simons et al., 2024). In the coming years we aim to involve the first 10% of 'early adopters' within the Dutch population of people with chronic conditions. The goal is to minimize their need to visit hospitals and to maximize their self-management capabilities, by building a self-support community. This includes a support structure with sharing of responsibilities between a central body and local resource users, plus adaptive co-management with existing local networks (Berkes, 2009).

In *conclusion*, this hybrid eSupported intervention helped achieve relatively large BP improvements in two weeks, quite robustly across participants and organisation settings. Second, this 'challenge' was feasible, fitting into the busy lives of participating employees, and the intervention was highly appreciated. The value was confirmed of the hybrid Self-Management Support (SMS), microlearning and social learning approaches for competence building. Specifically, our study illustrates the value of: (a) peer group coaching combined with daily social learning; (b) a 'Challenge Regime' with high commitments for a short time; (c) self-efficacy growth for users from large health results within days; (d) using 'BP behaviour hacks' and qualified instructors to achieve maximum learning and daily BP improvements (e) multiple technology-enabled health competence building lessons each day. These options hold promise for future health Self-Management eSupport innovations.

REFERENCES

Bandura, A. (1971). *Social learning theory* (Vol. 1). Prentice Hall.

BenYishay, A., & Mobarak, A. M. (2019). Social learning and incentives for experimentation and communication. *The Review of Economic Studies*, 86(3), 976–1009. DOI: 10.1093/restud/rdy039

Berkes, F. (2009). Evolution of co-management: Role of knowledge generation, bridging organizations and social learning. *Journal of Environmental Management*, 90(5), 1692–1702. DOI: 10.1016/j.jenvman.2008.12.001 PMID: 19110363

Carey, R. M., & Whelton, P. K. (2020). Evidence for the universal blood pressure goal of< 130/80 mm Hg is strong: Controversies in hypertension-pro side of the argument. *Hypertension*, 76(5), 1384–1390. DOI: 10.1161/HYPERTENSIONA-HA.120.14647 PMID: 32951472

Cennamo, K., & Kalk, D. (2019). *Real world instructional design: An iterative approach to designing learning experiences*. Routledge. DOI: 10.4324/9780203712207

Demark-Wahnefried, W., Clipp, E., Lipkus, I., Lobach, D., Snyder, D. C., Sloane, R., Peterson, B., Macri, J. M., Rock, C. L., McBride, C. M., & Kraus, W. E. (2007). Main Outcomes of the FRESH START Trial: A Sequentially Tailored, Diet and Exercise Mailed Print Intervention Among Breast and Prostate Cancer Survivors. *Journal of Clinical Oncology*, 25(19), 2709–2718. DOI: 10.1200/JCO.2007.10.7094 PMID: 17602076

Dickinson, K. M., Clifton, P. M., Burrell, L. M., Barrett, P. H. R., & Keogh, J. B. (2014). Postprandial effects of a high salt meal on serum sodium, arterial stiffness, markers of nitric oxide production and markers of endothelial function. *Atherosclerosis*, 232(1), 211–216. DOI: 10.1016/j.atherosclerosis.2013.10.032 PMID: 24401240

Dineen-Griffin, S., Garcia-Cardenas, V., Williams, K., & Benrimoj, S. I. (2019). Helping patients help themselves: A systematic review of self-management support strategies in primary health care practice. *PLoS One*, 14(8), e0220116. DOI: 10.1371/journal.pone.0220116 PMID: 31369582

Emerson, L. C., & Berge, Z. L. (2018). Microlearning: Knowledge management applications and competency-based training in the workplace. *Knowledge Management & E-Learning*, 10(2), 125–132.

Fogg, B. J. (2009). A behavior model for persuasive design. *Proceedings of the 4th international conference on persuasive technology*. ACM, 2009. DOI: 10.1145/1541948.1541999

Fogg, B. J., & Fogg, G. E. (2003). *Persuasive Technology: Using Computers to Change What We Think and Do.* Morgan Kaufmann. DOI: 10.1016/B978-155860643-2/50011-1

Franzini, L., Ardigo, D., Valtuena, S., Pellegrini, N., Del Rio, D., Bianchi, M. A., Scazzina, F., Piatti, P. M., Brighenti, F., & Zavaroni, I. (2012). Food selection based on high total antioxidant capacity improves endothelial function in a low cardiovascular risk population. *Nutrition, Metabolism, and Cardiovascular Diseases*, 22(1), 50–57. DOI: 10.1016/j.numecd.2010.04.001 PMID: 20674303

Gabrielli, S., Kimani, S., & Catarci, T. (2017). The design of microlearning experiences: A research agenda (on microlearning).

Giurgiu, L. (2017). Microlearning an evolving elearning trend. *Science Bulletin*, 22(1), 18–23. DOI: 10.1515/bsaft-2017-0003

Greger, M., & Stone, G. (2016). *How not to die: discover the foods scientifically proven to prevent and reverse disease.* Pan Macmillan.

Herrmann, E., Call, J., Hernández-Lloreda, M. V., Hare, B., & Tomasello, M. (2007). Humans have evolved specialized skills of social cognition: The cultural intelligence hypothesis. *Science*, 317(5843), 1360–1366. DOI: 10.1126/science.1146282 PMID: 17823346

Hwang, G. J., Chang, C. Y., & Ogata, H. (2022). The effectiveness of the virtual patient-based social learning approach in undergraduate nursing education: A quasi-experimental study. *Nurse Education Today*, 108, 105164. DOI: 10.1016/j.nedt.2021.105164 PMID: 34627030

Jonkman, N. H., Schuurmans, M. J., Jaarsma, T., Shortridge-Baggett, L. M., Hoes, A. W., & Trappenburg, J. C. (2016, December). Self-management interventions: Proposal and validation of a new operational definition. *Journal of Clinical Epidemiology*, 80, 34–42. DOI: 10.1016/j.jclinepi.2016.08.001 PMID: 27531245

Kapil, V., Khambata, R. S., Robertson, A., Caulfield, M. J., & Ahluwalia, A. (2015). Dietary nitrate provides sustained blood pressure lowering in hypertensive patients: A randomized, phase 2, double-blind, placebo-controlled study. *Hypertension*, 65(2), 320–327. DOI: 10.1161/HYPERTENSIONAHA.114.04675 PMID: 25421976

Kari, T., Koivunen, S., Frank, L., Makkonen, M., & Moilanen, P. (2017). The expected and perceived well-being effects of short-term self-tracking technology use. *International Journal of Networking and Virtual Organisations*, 17(4), 354–370. DOI: 10.1504/IJNVO.2017.088498

Laland, K. N. (2004). Social learning strategies. *Animal Learning & Behavior*, 32(1), 4–14. DOI: 10.3758/BF03196002 PMID: 15161136

Latkin, C. A., & Knowlton, A. R. (2015). Social network assessments and interventions for health behavior change: A critical review. *Behavioral Medicine (Washington, D.C.)*, 41(3), 90–97. DOI: 10.1080/08964289.2015.1034645 PMID: 26332926

Lehto, T., Oinas-Kukkonen, H., Pätiälä, T., & Saarelma, O. (2013). Virtual health coaching for consumers: a persuasive systems design perspective. *International Journal of Networking and Virtual Organisations 4, 13*(1), 24-41.

Lim, S. S., Vos, T., Flaxman, A. D., Danaei, G., Shibuya, K., Adair-Rohani, H., & Pelizzari, P. M. (2012). A comparative risk assessment of burden of disease and injury attributable to 67 risk factors and risk factor clusters in 21 regions, 1990–2010: A systematic analysis for the Global Burden of Disease Study 2010. *Lancet*, 380(9859), 2224–2260. DOI: 10.1016/S0140-6736(12)61766-8 PMID: 23245609

Lopez, G., Shuzo, M., & Yamada, I. (2011). New healthcare society supported by wearable sensors and information mapping-based services. *International Journal of Networking and Virtual Organisations*, 9(3), 233–247. DOI: 10.1504/IJN-VO.2011.042481

Lozano, R., Naghavi, M., Foreman, K., Lim, S., Shibuya, K., Aboyans, V., & Remuzzi, G. (2012). Global and regional mortality from 235 causes of death for 20 age groups in 1990 and 2010: A systematic analysis for the Global Burden of Disease Study 2010. *Lancet*, 380(9859), 2095–2128. DOI: 10.1016/S0140-6736(12)61728-0 PMID: 23245604

McGushin, A., de Barros, E. F., Floss, M., Mohammad, Y., Ndikum, A. E., Ngenda-hayo, C., Oduor, P. A., Sultana, S., Wong, R., & Abelsohn, A. (2023). The World Organization of Family Doctors Air Health Train the Trainer Program: Lessons learned and implications for planetary health education. *The Lancet. Planetary Health*, 7(1), e55–e63. DOI: 10.1016/S2542-5196(22)00218-2 PMID: 36608949

Molka-Danielsen, J., Carter, B. W., & Creelman, A. (2009). Empathy in virtual learning environments. *International journal of Networking and Virtual Organisations, 6*(2), 123-139.

Ostchega, Y., Fryar, C. D., Nwankwo, T., & Nguyen, D. T. (2020). Hypertension prevalence among adults aged 18 and over: United States, 2017–2018, NCHS, National Health and Nutrition Examination Survey, 2017–2018: https://stacks.cdc.gov/view/cdc/87559

Pearce, J., Mann, M. K., Jones, C., Van Buschbach, S., Olff, M., & Bisson, J. I. (2012). The most effective way of delivering a Train-the-Trainers program: A systematic review. *The Journal of Continuing Education in the Health Professions*, 32(3), 215–226. DOI: 10.1002/chp.21148 PMID: 23173243

Pickering, T. G. (2001). Mental stress as a causal factor in the development of hypertension and cardiovascular disease. *Current Hypertension Reports*, 3(3), 249–254. DOI: 10.1007/s11906-001-0047-1 PMID: 11353576

Ricciardi, F., Rossignoli, C., & De Marco, M. (2013). Participatory networks for place safety and livability: organisational success factors. *International Journal of Networking and Virtual Organisations 4, 13* (1), 42-65.

Roberts, C. K., & Barnard, R. J. (2005). Effects of exercise and diet on chronic disease. *Journal of Applied Physiology*, 98(1), 3–30. DOI: 10.1152/japplphysiol.00852.2004 PMID: 15591300

Rodriguez-Leyva, D., Weighell, W., Edel, A. L., LaVallee, R., Dibrov, E., Pinneker, R., Maddaford, T. G., Ramjiawan, B., Aliani, M., Guzman, R., & Pierce, G. N. (2013). Potent antihypertensive action of dietary flaxseed in hypertensive patients. *Hypertension*, 62(6), 1081–1089. DOI: 10.1161/HYPERTENSIONAHA.113.02094 PMID: 24126178

Siervo, M., Lara, J., Chowdhury, S., Ashor, A., Oggioni, C., & Mathers, J. C. (2015). Effects of the Dietary Approach to Stop Hypertension (DASH) diet on cardiovascular risk factors: A systematic review and meta-analysis. *British Journal of Nutrition*, 113(1), 1–15. DOI: 10.1017/S0007114514003341 PMID: 25430608

Simons, L. P., Pijl, H., Verhoef, J., Lamb, H. J., ... (2016). Intensive Lifestyle (e) Support to Reverse Diabetes-2. In *Bled eConference* (p. 24), accessed Dec 20, 2016 www.bledconference.org

Simons, L. P. A. (2020a). Health 2050: Bioinformatics for Rapid Self-Repair; A Design Analysis for Future Quantified Self, pp. 247-261, *33rd Bled eConference*. June 28-29, Bled, Slovenia, Proceedings retrieval from www.bledconference.org. ISBN-13: 978-961-286-362-3, DOI: https://doi.org/DOI: 10.18690/978-961-286-362-3.17

Simons, L. P. A., Foerster, F., Bruck, P. A., Motiwalla, L., & Jonker, C. M. (2014b). Microlearning mApp to Improve Long Term Health Behaviours: Design and Test of Multi-Channel Service Mix. Paper presented at the 27th Bled eConference. Bled, Slovenia, Proceedings. Retrieval from www.bledconference.org and https://aisel.aisnet.org/bled2014/4

Simons, L. P. A., Foerster, F., Bruck, P. A., Motiwalla, L., & Jonker, C. M. (2015). Microlearning mApp Raises Health Competence: Hybrid Service Design. *Health and Technology*, 5(1), 35–43. DOI: 10.1007/s12553-015-0095-1 PMID: 26097799

Simons, L. P. A., Gerritsen, B., Wielaard, B., & Neerincx, M. A. (2022a). Health Self-Management Support with Microlearning to Improve Hypertension, pp. 511-524, *35th Bled eConference*. June 26-29, Bled, Slovenia, Proceedings retrieval from www.bledconference.org. ISBN-13: 978-961-286-616-7, DOI: DOI: 10.18690/um/fov.4.2022

Simons, LPA, Gerritsen, B, Wielaard, B, Neerincx MA (2023). Hypertension Self-Management Success in 2 weeks; 3 Pilot Studies, pp.19-34, *36th Bled eConference*. June 25-28, Bled, Slovenia, Proceedings. ISBN-13: 978-961-286-751-5, DOI: DOI: 10.18690/um.feri.6.2023

Simons, L. P. A., Hafkamp, M. P. J., Bodegom, D., Dumaij, A., & Jonker, C. M. (2017). Improving Employee Health; Lessons from an RCT. *Int. J. Networking and Virtual Organisations*, 17(4), 341–353. DOI: 10.1504/IJNVO.2017.088485

Simons, L. P. A., & Hampe, J. F. (2010). Service Experience Design for Healthy Living Support; Comparing an In-House with an eHealth Solution. The *23rd Bled eConference*, pp. 423-440. Accessed 2010 from www.bledconference.org

Simons, L. P. A., Hampe, J. F., & Guldemond, N. A. (2013). Designing Healthy Living Support: Mobile applications added to hybrid (e)Coach Solution. *Health and Technology*, 3(1), 85–95. DOI: 10.1007/s12553-013-0052-9

Simons, L. P. A., Hampe, J. F., & Guldemond, N. A. (2014). ICT supported healthy lifestyle interventions: Design Lessons. *Electronic Markets*, 24(3), 179–192. DOI: 10.1007/s12525-014-0157-7

Simons, LPA, Murukannaiah, PK, Neerincx, MA (2024). Designing and Evaluating an LLM-based Health AI Research Assistant for Hypertension Self-Management; Using Health Claims Metadata Criteria, pp.283-298, *37th Bled eConference*. June 9-12, Bled, Slovenia, Proceedings. ISBN-13: 978-961-286-871-0, DOI: DOI: 10.18690/um.fov.4.2024

Simons, L. P. A., Neerincx, M. A., & Jonker, C. M. (2021). Health Literature Hybrid AI for Health Improvement; A Design Analysis for Diabetes & Hypertension, pp. 184-197, *34th Bled eConference*. June 27-30, Bled, Slovenia, Proceedings retrieval from www.bledconference.org. ISBN-13: 978-961-286-385-9, DOI: https://doi.org/DOI: 10.18690/978-961-286-385-9

Simons, L. P. A., Neerincx, M. A., & Jonker, C. M. (2022c). Is Google Making us Smart? Health Self-Management for High Performance Employees & Organisations. *International Journal of Networking and Virtual Organisations*, 27(3), 200–216. DOI: 10.1504/IJNVO.2022.128454

Simons, L. P. A., Pijl, M., Verhoef, J., Lamb, H. J., van Ommen, B., Gerritsen, B., Bizino, M. B., Snel, M., Feenstra, R., & Jonker, C. M. (2022b). e-Health Diabetes; 50 Weeks Evaluation. *International Journal of Biomedical Engineering and Technology*, 38(1), 81–98. DOI: 10.1504/IJBET.2022.120864

Simons, L. P. A., van den Heuvel, A. C., & Jonker, C. M. (2018). eHealth WhatsApp Group for Social Support; Preliminary Results, pp. 225-237, *presented at the 31st Bled eConference*. Bled, Slovenia, Proceedings retrieval from www.bledconference .org. ISBN-13: 978-961-286-170-4, DOI: https://doi.org/DOI: 10.18690/978-961-286-170-4

Simons, L. P. A., van den Heuvel, A. C., & Jonker, C. M. (2020b). eHealth WhatsApp for social support: Design lessons. *International Journal of Networking and Virtual Organisations*, 23(2), 112–127. DOI: 10.1504/IJNVO.2020.108857

Simons, L. P. A., van den Heuvel, W. A., & Jonker, C. M. (2019). WhatsApp Peer Coaching Lessons for eHealth. In *Handbook of Research on Optimizing Healthcare Management Techniques* (pp. 16–32). IGI Global.

Starr, J. (2008). *The coaching manual: the definitive guide to the process, principles and skills of personal coaching*. Prentice Hall.

Swan, K. (2003). Learning effectiveness online: What the research tells us. *Elements of quality online education, practice and direction, 4*(1), 13-47.

Swan, M. (2012). Health 2050: The realization of personalized medicine through crowdsourcing, the quantified self, and the participatory biocitizen. *Journal of Personalized Medicine*, 2(3), 93–118. DOI: 10.3390/jpm2030093 PMID: 25562203

Swan, M. (2013). The quantified self: Fundamental disruption in big data science and biological discovery. *Big Data*, 1(2), 85–99. DOI: 10.1089/big.2012.0002 PMID: 27442063

Tian, S. W., Yu, A. Y., Vogel, D., & Kwok, R. C. W. (2011). The impact of online social networking on learning: A social integration perspective. *International Journal of Networking and Virtual Organisations*, 8(3-4), 264–280. DOI: 10.1504/ IJNVO.2011.039999

Tobias, C. R., Downes, A., Eddens, S., & Ruiz, J. (2012). Building blocks for peer success: Lessons learned from a train-the-trainer program. *AIDS Patient Care and STDs*, 26(1), 53–59. DOI: 10.1089/apc.2011.0224 PMID: 22103430

Vaishnavi, V., & Kuechler, W. 2004. Design Research in Information Systems. Last updated August 16, 2009 from http://desrist.org/design-research-in-information -systems

Whiten, A., & van de Waal, E. (2018). The pervasive role of social learning in primate lifetime development. *Behavioral Ecology and Sociobiology*, 72(80), 1–16. DOI: 10.1007/s00265-018-2489-3 PMID: 29755181

Wickramasinghe, N., & Goldberg, S. (2010). Transforming online communities into support environments for chronic disease management through cell phones and social networks. *International journal of Networking and Virtual Organisations*, 7(6), 581-591.

Zhou, B., Perel, P., Mensah, G. A., & Ezzati, M. (2021). Global epidemiology, health burden and effective interventions for elevated blood pressure and hypertension. *Nature Reviews. Cardiology*, 18(11), 785–802. DOI: 10.1038/s41569-021-00559-8 PMID: 34050340

ENDNOTES

[1]   One of the participants had a user evaluation outlier pattern, see Table 3.

[2]   One of the participants had a user evaluation outlier pattern, see Table 3.

[3]   This the % of participants in a case that had average or above average BP improvments. This is an indicator of robustness of BP results across participants.

[4]   One of the participants had an outlier pattern of scoring (since she could not be present at several of the group coach sessions, due to illness plus family logistics). Table 3 displays the average scores of the other 7. (Score 4=neutral) Her scores were resp.: 6; 6; 6/3; 3; 4; 5/3; 6; 3; 3.

[5]   One of the participants had an outlier pattern of scoring (she had hereditary hypertension since 18 years old and her BP values did not change, despite her best efforts). Table 3 displays the average scores of the other 5. (Score 4=neutral) Her scores were resp.: 4; 4; 4/4; 4; 4; 5/4; 4; 6; 5.

[6]   n.a. = not applicable

[7]   This is a revised version of a Bled Conference paper: Simons, LPA, Gerritsen, B, Wielaard, B, Neerincx MA (2023). Hypertension Self-Management Success in 2 weeks; 3 Pilot Studies, pp.19-34, *36th Bled eConference*. June 25-28, Bled, Slovenia, Proceedings. ISBN-13: 978-961-286-751-5, DOI: <u>10.18690/ um.feri.6.2023</u>

[8]   This research was (partly) funded by the https://www.hybrid-intelligence-centre .nl/ a 10-year programme funded the Dutch Ministry of Education, Culture and Science through the Netherlands Organisation for Scientific Research, grant number 024.004.022 and by EU H2020 ICT48 project ``Humane AI Net'' under contract $\# $ 952026.

Chapter 10
IoT and Machine Learning for Early Prediction of Neurological Disorders

R. Shobana
VMRFDU, AVIT, India

Vicky Kumar
VMRFDU, AVIT, India

Gautam Kumar
VMRFDU, AVIT, India

Joyal Jojo
VMRFDU, AVIT, India

Suraj Kumar
VMRFDU, AVIT, India

G. Revathy
https://orcid.org/0000-0002-0691 -1687

SASTRA University (Deemed), India

ABSTRACT

Smart living, healthcare, cognitive smart cities, and social systems are impartial a rare of the areas in which technology related to health is being applied these days. A component of the rapidly evolving modern technology that deserves more attention is the intelligent, dependable, and pervasive healthcare system. Predicting, preventing, and treating illnesses is made possible for doctors by data collecting methods such as sensors aided by the Internet of Things (IoT). In order to assist doctors in monitoring the importance of symptoms and the course of therapy, machine learning (ML) algorithms have the latent to progress the accurateness of medical diagnosis and prognosis based on sensing data. A neurodegenerative condition affecting the neurological system is Parkinson's disease.

DOI: 10.4018/979-8-3693-5237-3.ch010

INTRODUCTION

Parkinson's disease is a neurodegenerative disorder that affects movement. It typically progresses slowly over time, and its indicators often commence with mild tremors in one hand. Over time, the disease may cause stiffness or slowing of movement, impaired balance and coordination, and other symptoms such as speech changes and cognitive decline, (Salmanpour *et al.*, 2019).The primary cause of Parkinson's disease is alleged to be the loss of dopamine-producing cells in the brain. Dopamine is a neurotransmitter that dramas a decisive role in regulating movement and emotional responses, (Tsanas *et al.*, 2010). The exact reasons why these cells degenerate are still not copiously tacit, but a combination of genetic and environmental factors is whispered to underwrite to the development of the disease. There is currently no cure for Parkinson's disease, but there are behaviours available to help manage its symptoms. Medications such as levodopa, dopamine agonists, and MAO-B inhibitors can help alleviate movement problems. In unconventional cases, deep brain stimulation (DBS) surgery may be recommended to help control symptoms, (Sakar, Serbes, & Sakar, 2017). Research into Parkinson's disease is ongoing, with efforts focused on understanding its underlying causes, developing new treatments to slow or halt its progression, and enlightening quality of life for those living with the condition. The chapter delts about the usage of IOT sensors in monitoring and machine learning algorithms for the prevention of the diseases.

IoT FOR PARKINSON DISEASES

IoT (Internet of Things) sensors have shown promise in assisting with the credentials and supervision of Parkinson's disease symptoms. These sensors can be integrated into various devices and wearable technologies to monitor movement, balance, tremors, and other relevant physiological parameters, (Farnikova, Krobot, & Kanovsky, 2012) (Nilashi *et al.*, 2018) (Behroozi & Sami, 2016) (Shrivastava *et al.*, 2017). Here are some specimens of IoT sensors and their applications in Parkinson's disease identification:

Wearable Devices: Wearable devices such as smartwatches or wristbands equipped with accelerometers and gyroscopes can track movement patterns and detect changes in gait, tremors, and balance. These campaigns can deliver unremitting monitoring of motor symptoms, agreeing for early detection of changes that may indicate disease progression.

Smart Insoles: Insoles embedded with pressure sensors can be placed inside shoes to monitor gait and balance. By analyzing changes in foot pressure distribution and gait patterns, smart insoles can provide insights into mobility and balance impairments associated with Parkinson's disease.

Smart Clothing: Clothing integrated with textile-based sensors can measure muscle activity, posture, and body movements. Smart shirts or vests equipped with these sensors can perceive vagaries in posture, muscle rigidity, and bradykinesia (slowness of movement) characteristic of Parkinson's disease.

Home Monitoring Systems: IoT-enabled home monitoring systems can incorporate various sensors to track activities of daily living (ADLs), such as eating, drinking, and sleeping patterns. By analyzing data from motion sensors, smart appliances, and other IoT devices, these systems can categorize abnormalities or fluctuations in daily routines that may designate changes in disease symptoms or overall health status.

Voice and Speech Analysis: IoT devices equipped with microphones and voice recognition technology can analyze speech patterns and vocal characteristics associated with Parkinson's disease, such as hypophonia (soft speech) and dysarthria (slurred speech). Voice-based biomarkers detected by these devices can be castoff for early finding and intensive care of disease progression.

Remote Monitoring Systems: IoT platforms integrated with cloud-based analytics can enable remote monitoring of Parkinson's disease patients by healthcare providers. Real-time data composed from wearable sensors and home monitoring devices can be securely transmitted to healthcare professionals for remote assessment and intervention.

Overall, IoT sensors have the probable to reform the credentials and administration of Parkinson's disease by providing objective, continuous monitoring of symptoms and empowering early intrusion approaches to improve patient conclusions and quality of life. However, further research and development are needed to validate the effectiveness and reliability of IoT-based solutions in clinical settings.

IMPACT OF AI IN PARKINSON DISEASE

Artificial Intelligence (AI) is increasingly being utilized in various characteristics of Parkinson's disease management, from diagnosis and monitoring to treatment optimization and research, (Gupta *et al.*, 2018). Here are some ways AI is making an impact in Parkinson's disease:

Premature Detection and Diagnosis: AI algorithms canister analyse data from various foundations such as voice recordings, typing patterns, smartphone sensor data (like accelerometers and gyroscopes), and medical imaging (such as MRI or PET scans) to perceive subtle vagaries indicative of Parkinson's disease. For example, AI models have been advanced to analyse speech patterns for initial discovery of Parkinson's.

Monitoring Disease Progression: AI-powered wearable devices and smartphone apps can continuously monitor movement patterns, tremors, gait, and other motorized indicators associated with Parkinson's disease, (Al Mamun *et al.,* 2017). These systems can deliver appreciated insights into disease progression, allowing for opportune modifications in treatment plans.

Medication Management: AI algorithms can help optimize medicine administration for persons with Parkinson's disease, (Edoh & Degila, 2019). By analyzing data on symptoms, medication dosages, and side effects, AI systems can indorse adapted conduct regimens to improve symptom control and minimize adverse effects.

Deep Brain Stimulation (DBS) Optimization: Deep Brain Stimulation is a surgical treatment for Parkinson's disease that involves implanting electrodes in the brain to regulate abnormal brain activity. AI algorithms can analyze brain signals and sensor data to optimize DBS settings, ensuring maximum therapeutic advantage with trifling side effects.

Predictive Modeling and Prognosis: AI models can analyse large datasets containing clinical, genetic, and demographic evidence to categorize patterns and envisage disease movement and retort to treatment. This information can assistance healthcare earners make more conversant conclusions about patient care and long-term management strategies.

Drug Discovery and Development: AI-powered drug discovery platforms can accelerate the identification of potential therapeutic compounds for Parkinson's disease. By analysing molecular structures, biological pathways, and existing drug databases, AI can suggest novel drug intrants and envisage their efficiency and safety profiles.

Research and Clinical Trials: AI algorithms can analyse vast quantities of biomedical literature and clinical experimental data to identify promising research directions and potential therapeutic targets for Parkinson's disease. Additionally, AI can simplify patient recruitment for clinical trials by corresponding qualified participants with apposite studies based on their clinical profiles.

Overall, AI has the probable to transfigure the diagnosis, treatment, and management of Parkinson's disease by providing more exact and personalized approaches tailored to individual patient needs. However, it's essential to ensure that these AI technologies are rigorously validated and integrated into clinical practice in a answerable and ethical manner.

ML FOR PARKINSON DISEASE

Machine learning (ML) has shown promising potential in various aspects of Parkinson's disease (PD) research, including diagnosis, prognosis, symptom tracking, and treatment optimization, (Heijmans *et al.* 2019) (Sivaparthipan *et al.*, 2019) (Prince & De Vos, 2018). Here are some ways ML is being applied in the context of Parkinson's disease:

Diagnosis and Prediction: ML algorithms can analyse various types of data, such as medical imaging (MRI, PET scans), genetic information, and clinical assessments, to assist in diagnosing PD and predicting its progression. For instance, ML models can learn patterns in brain images to differentiate between healthy individuals and those with PD.

Symptom Monitoring: ML algorithms can analyze sensor data from wearable devices (such as accelerometers and gyroscopes) to monitor symptoms like tremors, rigidity, and bradykinesia. This continuous intensive care can deliver appreciated visions into disease progression and treatment effectiveness.

Treatment Optimization: ML algorithms can help optimize medication dosages and schedules by analysing patient data and predicting individual responses to different treatments. This adapted method can improve symptom management and quality of life for PD patients.

Disease Progression Modeling: ML techniques can be cast-off to shape mock ups that foresee how PD progresses over time based on various influences such as demographics, genetics, and clinical symptoms. These models can aid clinicians in production informed conclusions about patient care and treatment planning.

Drug Discovery: ML algorithms can analyse great datasets, counting molecular data and drug interactions, to recognize potential drug candidates for treating PD. By predicting the efficacy and protection of different compounds, ML can hasten the drug discovery process.

Data Integration and Fusion: ML techniques can participate data from multiple sources, including clinical records, imaging data, and genetic information, to deliver a inclusive view of the disease and its underlying mechanisms, (Alhussein, 2017). This holistic approach can lead to a improved considerate of PD and more actual treatment strategies.

Remote Monitoring and Telemedicine: ML-powered remote monitoring systems can empower healthcare earners to remotely monitor PD patients' symptoms and fine-tune behaviour tactics as needed. This can progress entree to care, especially for patients in remote or underserved areas.

Overall, ML has the potential to transfigure the diagnosis, management, and treatment of Parkinson's disease by leveraging large datasets and advanced analytics to extract meaningful insights and progress patient outcomes. However, it's essential to guarantee that these ML models are rigorously validated and integrated into clinical practice in a answerable and ethical manner.

DL FOR PARKINSON DISEASE

Deep learning (DL), a subset of machine learning, has also been functional to numerous characteristics of Parkinson's disease (PD) research. DL methods, particularly neural networks, offer sophisticated techniques for analyzing complex data and extracting meaningful patterns, (Almogren, 2019). Here's how DL is being used in the context of PD:

Medical Imaging Analysis: DL models can analyze various types of medical imaging data, including MRI, CT scans, and PET scans, to promotion in the analysis and characterization of PD-related abnormalities in the brain. These models can routinely recognize structural changes, such as atrophy or abnormal protein deposits, associated with PD.

Gait Analysis: DL algorithms can analyse gait decorations from sensor data collected by wearable devices to perceive delicate changes indicative of early-stage PD. By capturing features such as stride length, cadence, and balance, DL models can assist in early diagnosis and monitoring of disease progression.

Voice and Speech Analysis: PD often affects speech and voice patterns, leading to changes such as reduced vocal intensity and articulatory dysfunction. DL techniques can analyze voice recordings to detect these changes and aid in the early uncovering and following of PD symptoms.

Genomic Data Analysis: DL methods can analyse genomic data to recognize genetic factors associated with PD susceptibility and progression. By examining large-scale genomic datasets, DL models can help uncover novel genetic markers and pathways implicated in the disease.

Predictive Modeling: DL models can integrate multiple types of data, plus clinical assessments, imaging data, and genetic information, to forecast disease evolution and treatment outcomes for discrete patients. These models can provide personalized risk assessments and guide conduct results.

Drug Discovery: DL techniques can be functional to drug discovery efforts by analysing molecular structures and predicting the possible efficiency of drug candidates for treating PD. DL models can assistance arrange compounds for further testing and optimization, accelerating the drug development process.

Data Fusion and Integration: DL methods enable the integration of heterogeneous data sources, such as clinical records, imaging data, and omics data, to provide a comprehensive understanding of PD. By combining information from multiple sources, DL models can uncover complex relationships and mechanisms underlying the disease.

Remote Monitoring and Telemedicine: DL-powered remote monitoring systems can continuously analyze sensor data from wearable devices to monitor PD symptoms and medication responses in real-time. These systems enable remote patient monitoring and telemedicine consultations, improving access to care for PD patients.

Overall, DL holds great promise for advancing our understanding of Parkinson's disease, improving early detection, guiding treatment decisions, and accelerating the development of novel therapies. However, it's important to address challenges such as data quality, model interpretability, and ethical considerations to ensure the responsible and effective deployment of DL in PD research and clinical practice.

FUSION OF IOT AND ML

Combining Internet of Things (IoT) devices with Machine Learning (ML) techniques offers innovative solutions for monitoring and managing Parkinson's disease (PD) more effectively, (Devarajan & Ravi, 2018). Here's how IoT and ML can be integrated for PD:

Wearable Devices: IoT-enabled wearable devices armed with sensors such as accelerometers, gyroscopes, and heart rate monitors can continuously collect data on movement patterns, tremors, gait, and other symptoms associated with PD. ML algorithms can then analyze this streaming sensor data to detect changes indicative of disease progression, medication responses, or adverse events.

Real-Time Symptom Monitoring: By leveraging IoT devices, PD patients can be continuously monitored in real-time, permitting for early finding of symptom exacerbations or medication fluctuations. ML models trained on historical data can analyze incoming sensor data to predict symptom onset or categorize decorations connected with detailed symptoms, empowering timely involvements and adapted treatment adjustments.

Telemedicine and Remote Consultations: IoT-connected devices facilitate remote consultations between PD patients and healthcare providers, enabling clinicians to monitor patients' symptoms and medication adherence remotely. ML algorithms can analyze data collected during these remote consultations to assess disease severity, track treatment outcomes, and provide recommendations for adjustments to medication regimens or lifestyle interventions.

Medication Adherence Monitoring: IoT devices can be integrated with medication dispensers to track patients' adherence to prescribed medication regimens. ML algorithms can analyse medication adherence patterns and recognize affected role at peril of non-compliance, agreeing healthcare workers to arbitrate proactively and optimize treatment adherence.

Predictive Analytics: ML techniques can analyze longitudinal IoT data collected from PD patients to progress extrapolative models for disease progression and patient outcomes. By participating data from numerous sources, including wearable sensors, electronic health records, and genomic data, ML models can identify early predictors of disease progression, stratify affected role based on risk profiles, and apprise personalized treatment plans.

Data Fusion and Contextual Analysis: IoT devices can capture contextual information such as environmental factors, social interactions, and lifestyle habits, which may influence PD symptoms and disease progression. ML algorithms can integrate these assorted fonts of data to offer a rounded view of patients' health status and identify modifiable risk factors or triggers for symptom exacerbations.

Feedback and Behavioral Interventions: IoT devices fortified with ML algorithms can deliver real-time feedback and modified behavioural interventions to help PD patients manage their symptoms and advance their superiority of life. For example, wearable devices could deliver prompts for exercise or medication reminders based on individualized algorithms tailored to each patient's needs and preferences.

By combining IoT devices with ML techniques, healthcare providers can leverage real-time data insights to deliver personalized and proactive care for PD patients, improve treatment outcomes, and enhance patient engagement and self-management. However, it's crucial to address secrecy and sanctuary concerns linked with the assortment and analysis of sensitive health data and guarantee that these technologies are deployed in an ethical and responsible manner.

FUSION OF IOT AND DL

The fusion of Internet of Things (IoT) and Deep Learning (DL) techniques presents exciting opportunities for advancing the monitoring, diagnosis, and management of Parkinson's disease (PD) (Sadoughi, Behmanesh, & Sayfouri, 2020) (SWrinighi, Kumar, & Venugopal, 2019). Here's how IoT and DL can be combined for PD:

Multimodal Sensor Fusion: IoT devices equipped with various sensors, such as accelerometers, gyroscopes, and voice sensors, can capture diverse data modalities related to PD symptoms, including movement patterns, tremors, gait, and speech characteristics. DL models can be trained to fuse information from these multiple sensors to offer a inclusive empathetic of the patient's condition, enabling more accurate symptom assessment and disease monitoring.

Real-Time Symptom Detection and Monitoring: DL algorithms can be deployed on edge devices within IoT networks to perform real-time analysis of sensor data streams. By continuously monitoring movement patterns, tremors, and other PD symptoms, these DL models can detect changes indicative of sickness evolution or medication responses in real-time, permitting opportune intrusions and tailored conduct adjustments.

Predictive Analytics and Early Warning Systems: DL models trained on longitudinal IoT data from PD patients can learn patterns associated with disease progression and symptom exacerbations. By analyzing historical data and patient-specific risk factors, these models can foresee the possibility of future symptom onset or deterioration, enabling proactive interventions and adapted conduct planning.

Remote Patient Monitoring and Telemedicine: IoT-connected devices allow for remote monitoring of PD patients in their home environments, facilitating telemedicine consultations and dropping the requirement for frequent clinic visits. DL-powered analytics can process data composed from IoT devices to assess disease severity, track treatment outcomes, and provide feedback to healthcare providers in real-time, enabling remote management of PD patients' care.

Personalized Treatment Optimization: DL models can analyze multimodal IoT data to identify individualized treatment responses and optimize medication regimens for PD patients. By correlating sensor data with clinical outcomes, DL algorithms can tailor treatment plans to each patient's specific needs and preferences, maximizing therapeutic efficacy while minimizing adverse effects.

Context-Aware Decision Support Systems: DL techniques can integrate IoT data with contextual information, such as environmental factors, medication adherence, and lifestyle habits, to provide context-aware decision support for PD management. By considering the broader context in which symptoms occur, these DL models can offer personalized recommendations for behavioral interventions, medication adjustments, and lifestyle modifications to improve patients' quality of life.

Continuous Feedback and Rehabilitation: IoT devices equipped with DL algorithms can provide continuous feedback and support for PD patients undergoing rehabilitation or physical therapy. By analyzing movement data in real-time, these devices can transport adapted exercise programs, monitor progress, and adjust therapy sessions dynamically to optimize motor function and mobility.

By integrating IoT devices with DL techniques, healthcare providers can attach the authority of real-time data analytics to transport tailored and proactive care for PD patients, improve treatment outcomes, and increase patients' excellence of life. However, it's essential to discourse tasks such as data privacy, security, and model interpretability to confirm the ethical and responsible deployment of these technologies in clinical practice.

DEEP MODEL WITH IOT SENSORS FOR PARKINSON DISEASE

Combining deep learning models with Internet of Things (IoT) sensor data for Parkinson's disease (PD) offers a powerful approach for continuous monitoring and early detection of symptoms. Below, I'll explain how a deep learning model integrated with IoT sensors can be designed and utilized for PD:

Explanation:

1. IoT Sensors Data Collection:

IoT devices fortified with numerous sensors such as accelerometers, gyroscopes, and wearable devices are deployed to assemble data related to PD symptoms.

These sensors uninterruptedly screen a patient's movements, tremors, gait, and other physiological signals in real-time.

2. Preprocessing and Feature Extraction:

Raw sensor data composed by IoT devices is preprocessed to remove noise, normalize, and extract relevant features.

Feature extraction may comprise procedures such as time-domain and frequency-domain analysis to capture patterns indicative of PD symptoms.

3. Deep Learning Model Design:

A deep learning model, typically a Recurrent Neural Network (RNN) or Long Short-Term Memory (LSTM) network, is designed to analyse sequential sensor data.

RNNs and LSTMs are well-suited for processing time-series data as they can seizure progressive addictions and future dependences in chronological data.

4. Model Architecture:

The deep learning model architecture consists of layers of LSTM cells shadowed by thickly associated layers for classification or regression tasks.

The LSTM layers process sequential sensor data over time, capturing temporal patterns and dynamics in PD symptoms.

Additional layers such as dropout and batch normalization may be included to improve model generalization and prevent overfitting.

5. Training and Optimization:

The deep learning model is trained on labeled sensor data collected from PD patients, where labels indicate the presence or severity of PD symptoms.

Training involves augmenting model limitations using techniques such as gradient descent and backpropagation.

Hyperparameter tuning may be performed to optimize model performance and generalization.

6.   Real-Time Inference and Monitoring:

Once trained, the deep learning model can be deployed on edge devices or IoT gateways for real-time inference.

The model analyzes incoming sensor data streams in real-time, detecting patterns indicative of PD symptoms.

Real-time monitoring alerts healthcare providers or caregivers about changes in symptom severity, enabling timely interventions.

7.   Continuous Learning and Adaptation:

The deep learning model can be continuously updated and adapted to new data using practices such as online learning and transfer learning.

As more data becomes available, the model can progress its presentation and acclimatize to individual patient characteristics and disease progression.

8.   Integration with Healthcare Systems:

Predictions and insights generated by the deep learning model can be cohesive with electronic health records (EHRs) and healthcare systems for comprehensive patient management.

Healthcare providers can access real-time patient data and model predictions to make conversant choices about treatment planning and intervention strategies.

By compounding deep learning models with IoT sensor data, healthcare providers can increase treasured perceptions into PD symptoms, enabling early detection, personalized treatment, and unremitting nursing of patients' health status. This approach has the probable to progress patient consequences and quality of life while dropping healthcare costs connected with PD management.

RECURRENT NEURAL NETWORK

Recurrent neural network (RNN) model architecture for Parkinson's disease (PD) without the accompanying code:

Sequential Model:

The model is organized in a chronological manner, meaning that apiece layer fodders its output into the subsequent layer in a linear fashion.

LSTM Layers:

Long Short-Term Memory (LSTM) layers are specialized types of recurrent neural network (RNN) layers designed to detention lasting dependences in sequential data.
The model includes multiple LSTM layers, permitting it to absorb composite temporal patterns from the input data.
Each LSTM layer processes the sequential sensor data over time and extracts relevant features.

Dropout Regularization:

Dropout layers are implanted afterwards each LSTM layer to avoid overfitting.
Dropout is a regularization practice where a certain fraction of input units are randomly set to zero throughout drill, which benefits prevent the model from relying too much on specific features or correlations in the training data.

Output Layer:

The model ends with a dense output layer that performs binary classification.
The output layer uses a sigmoid activation function, which squashes the output values between 0 and 1, representing the possibility of the positive class (presence of PD).

Compilation:

The model is compiled with the Adam optimizer, a popular optimization algorithm for training neural networks.
The binary cross-entropy loss function is used, which is apposite for binary classification errands where the goalmouth is to maximize the likelihood of predicting the correct class.

The model is also configured to monitor accuracy as a metric during training.

Model Summary:

A summary of the model architecture is printed, detailing the numeral of strictures in each layer and the complete construction of the model.

This summary helps review the model's configuration and ensure it meets the requirements for the PD classification task.

Figure 1. Architecture of RNN

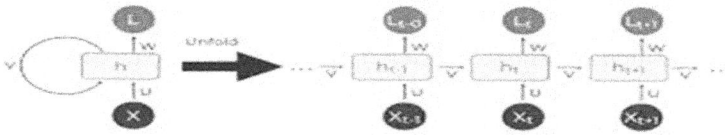

The architecture of a Recurrent Neural Network (RNN) typically consists of several key components:

Input Layer:

The input layer receives sequential data as input. Each element in the sequence is represented by a feature vector.

Recurrent Connections:

Recurrent connections are the defining characteristic of RNNs. They allow information to persist over time by connecting neurons in the network to themselves. This enables the network to maintain a memory of past inputs and learn temporal dependencies within sequential data.

Recurrent Units:

Recurrent units, such as LSTM (Long Short-Term Memory) or GRU (Gated Recurrent Unit), are used to process sequential data and capture long-range dependencies.

LSTM units, for example, contain a memory cell that can preserve evidence over long sequences and gates that normalize the stream of evidence into and out of the cell.

Hidden States:

At individual time phase, the recurrent units produce an output, also known as the hidden state, which is accepted to the succeeding time step and used to influence subsequent predictions.

Time Steps:

RNNs operate over multiple time steps, processing consecutive data one element at a time. The recurrent connections enable information to flow from one time step to the next, allowing the network to capture temporal patterns and dependencies.

Output Layer:

The output layer receives the hidden states from the recurrent units and produces the final output of the network. The output layer may have one or more units, depending on the task being performed (e.g., classification, regression).

Loss Function:

The loss function measures the alteration between the forecast production of the network and the true target values. Common loss functions for RNNs include categorical cross-entropy for cataloguing tasks and mean squared error for deterioration tasks.

Optimization Algorithm:

The optimization algorithm is used to apprise the limitations of the network (e.g., weights and biases) throughout training in command to diminish the loss function. Popular optimization algorithms for training RNNs include Stochastic Gradient Descent (SGD), Adam, and RMSprop, (Al-Turjman, Hasan, & Al-Rizzo, 2019).

Training:

RNNs are typically trained using backpropagation through time (BPTT), an extension of backpropagation that considers the entire sequence of inputs. BPTT computes the gradients of the loss function with deference to the parameters of the network and updates the parameters accordingly using the chosen optimization algorithm.

State Initialization:

In practice, RNNs often require an initial state to start processing a sequence. This initial state can be either zero-initialized or learned during training.

Overall, the architecture of an RNN consents it to process sequential data, capture temporal dependencies, and style forecasts or classifications based on the learned patterns within the data.

Figure 2. RNN with LSTM

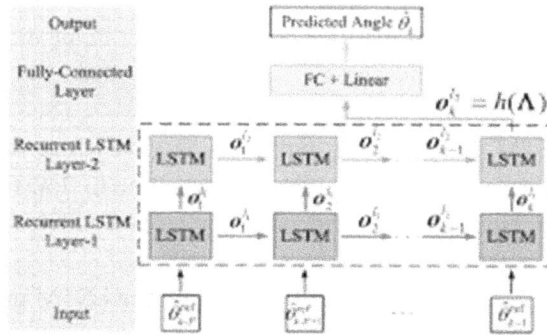

The architecture of a Recurrent Neural Network (RNN) with Long Short-Term Memory (LSTM) units:

Input Layer:

The input layer receives sequential data as input. Each element in the sequence is represented by a feature vector.

Recurrent Connections:

LSTM units have recurrent connections that allow information to persist over time. These connections permit the network to detention long-range dependencies in sequential data.

LSTM Units:

LSTM units are a type of recurrent unit designed to address the vanishing gradient problem in traditional RNNs. They consist of several components:

Cell State: The cell state serves as a memory unit that cannister supply information over long sequences. It runs straight down the entire chain of LSTM units with only minor linear interactions, making it easier for the network to preserve information over many time steps.

Forget Gate: This gate governs what evidence should be discarded from the cell state. It takes input from the current input and prior hidden state and outputs a forget vector, which is multiplied element-wise with the cell state to decide what information to forget.

Input Gate: This gate decides which new information to store in the cell state. It takes input from the current input and previous hidden state and outputs a candidate vector, which is then scaled by the input gate's output to update the cell state, (Ma *et al.,* 2019).

Output Gate: This gate decides what information should be output from the cell state. It takes input from the current input and previous hidden state, combines it with the cell state, and outputs the hidden state for the current time step.

Hidden States:

At each time step, LSTM units produce an output, also known as the hidden state. The hidden state contains information about the current input and the accumulated information from previous time steps.

Time Steps:

RNNs with LSTM units process sequential data one time step at a time. The recurrent connections in LSTM units enable information to flow from one time step to the next, allowing the network to capture long-term dependencies.

Output Layer:

The output layer receives the hidden states from the LSTM units and produces the final output of the network. The output layer may have one or more units, depending on the task being performed.

Loss Function and Optimization:

The loss function measures the difference between the predicted output of the network and the true target values. The network is trained using backpropagation through time (BPTT) and optimized using techniques such as gradient descent or variants like Adam.

Training:

During training, the LSTM units learn to update their internal parameters (weights and biases) based on the input data and the error signal computed by the loss function. This allows the network to adapt its behaviour to the specific task it's trained for.

RESULTS AND DISCUSSIONS

The data are collected from various sensors and the own dataset has been created "New1.Parkinson" with various attributes such as age, pressure, blood sugar, heartbeat, cholesterol level etc. The data is alienated into training and testing, the data is well trained with RNN LSTM and the testing has been made. The data shows excellent result than previous state of art models like CNN, RCNN etc..

The accuracy of the dataset is compared with state of art models and the RNN LSTM shows better results than others.

Table 1. Accuracy of dataset and results

MODEL	RESULTS
SVM	78
CNN	85
MULTI KERNEL SVM	83

continued on following page

Table 1. Continued

MODEL	RESULTS
RCNN	88.2
RNN LSTM(PROPOSED)	91

CONCLUSION

The inherent strengths of LSTM networks in handling sequential data, real-time processing, adaptability to varying data rates, and complex pattern recognition make them well-suited for analyzing and extracting insights from IoT datasets. Furthermore, the seamless integration of RNN LSTM models with IoT sensor networks facilitates on-device processing and edge computing, enabling efficient utilization of computational resources and reducing the need for continuous data transmission to centralized servers. While LSTM models present promising opportunities for enhancing IoT applications for Parkinson disease.

REFERENCES

Al Mamun, K. A., Alhussein, M., Sailunaz, K., & Islam, M. S. (2017). Cloud based framework for Parkinson's disease diagnosis and monitoring system for remote healthcare applications. *Future Generation Computer Systems*, 66, 36–47. DOI: 10.1016/j.future.2015.11.010

Al-Turjman, F., Hasan, M. Z., & Al-Rizzo, H. (2019). Task scheduling in cloud-based survivability applications using swarm optimization in IoT. *Transactions on Emerging Telecommunications Technologies*, 30(8), e3539. DOI: 10.1002/ett.3539

Alhussein, M. (2017). Monitoring Parkinson's disease in smart cities. *IEEE Access : Practical Innovations, Open Solutions*, 5, 19835–19841. DOI: 10.1109/ACCESS.2017.2748561

Almogren, A. (2019). An automated and intelligent parkinson disease monitoring system using wearable computing and cloud technology. *Cluster Computing*, 22(1), 2309–2316. DOI: 10.1007/s10586-017-1591-z

Behroozi, M., & Sami, A. (2016). A multiple-classifier framework for Parkinson's disease detection based on various vocal tests. *International Journal of Telemedicine and Applications*, 2016, 2016. DOI: 10.1155/2016/6837498 PMID: 27190506

Devarajan, M., & Ravi, L. (2018). Intelligent cyber–physical system for an efficient detection of Parkinson disease using fog computing. *Multimedia Tools and Applications*, •••, 1–25.

Edoh, T., & Degila, J. (2019). IoT-enabled health monitoring and assistive systems for in place aging dementia patient and elderly. In Internet of Things (IoT) for Automated and Smart Applications. IntechOpen., 10. 5772/intechopen.86247. DOI: 10.5772/intechopen.86247

Farnikova, K., Krobot, A., & Kanovsky, P. (2012). Musculoskeletal problems as an initial manifestation of Parkinson's disease: A retrospective study. *Journal of the Neurological Sciences*, 319(1–2), 102–104. DOI: 10.1016/j.jns.2012.05.002 PMID: 22656184

Gupta, D., Sundaram, S., Khanna, A., Hassanien, A. E., & De Albuquerque, V. H. C. (2018). Improved diagnosis of Parkinson's disease using an optimized crow search algorithm. *Computers & Electrical Engineering*, 68, 412–424. DOI: 10.1016/j.compeleceng.2018.04.014

Heijmans, M., Habets, J. G., Herff, C., Aarts, J., Stevens, A., Kuijf, M. L., & Kubben, P. L. (2019). Monitoring Parkinson's disease symptoms during daily life: A feasibility study. *NPJ Parkinson's Disease*, 5(1), 1–6. DOI: 10.1038/s41531-019-0093-5 PMID: 31583270

Ma, X., Gao, H., Xu, H., & Bian, M. (2019). An IoT-based task scheduling optimization scheme considering the deadline and cost-aware scientific workflow for cloud computing. *EURASIP Journal on Wireless Communications and Networking*, 2019(1), 249. DOI: 10.1186/s13638-019-1557-3

Nilashi, M., Ibrahim, O., Ahmadi, H., Shahmoradi, L., & Farahmand, M. (2018). A hybrid intelligent system for the prediction of Parkinson's disease progression using machine learning techniques. *Biocybernetics and Biomedical Engineering*, 38(1), 1–15. DOI: 10.1016/j.bbe.2017.09.002

Prince, J., & De Vos, M. (2018, July). A deep learning framework for the remote detection of Parkinson's disease using smart-phone sensor data. In *2018 40th Annual International Conference of the IEEE Engineering in Medicine and Biology Society (EMBC)* (pp. 3144-3147). IEEE.

Sadoughi, F., Behmanesh, A., & Sayfouri, N. (2020). Internet of things in medicine: A systematic mapping study. *Journal of Biomedical Informatics*, 103, 103383. DOI: 10.1016/j.jbi.2020.103383 PMID: 32044417

Sakar, B. E., Serbes, G., & Sakar, C. O. (2017). Analyzing the effectiveness of vocal features in early telediagnosis of Parkinson's disease. *PLoS One*, 12(8), e0182428. DOI: 10.1371/journal.pone.0182428 PMID: 28792979

Salmanpour, M. R., Shamsaei, M., Saberi, A., Setayeshi, S., Klyuzhin, I. S., Sossi, V., & Rahmim, A. (2019). Optimized machine learning methods for prediction of cognitive outcome in Parkinson's disease. *Computers in Biology and Medicine*, 111, 103347. DOI: 10.1016/j.compbiomed.2019.103347 PMID: 31284154

Shrivastava, P., Shukla, A., Vepakomma, P., Bhansali, N., & Verma, K. (2017). A survey of nature-inspired algorithms for feature selection to identify Parkinson's disease. *Computer Methods and Programs in Biomedicine*, 139, 171–179. DOI: 10.1016/j.cmpb.2016.07.029 PMID: 28187888

Sivaparthipan, C. B., Muthu, B. A., Manogaran, G., Maram, B., Sundarasekar, R., Krishnamoorthy, S., & Chandran, K. (2019). Innovative and efficient method of robotics for helping the Parkinson's disease patient using IoT in big data analytics. *Transactions on Emerging Telecommunications Technologies*, •••, e3838.

Srinidhi, N. N., Kumar, S. D., & Venugopal, K. R. (2019). Network optimizations in the internet of things: A review. *Eng. Sci. Technol. Int. J.*, 22(1), 1–21. DOI: 10.1016/j.jestch.2018.09.003

Tsanas, A., Little, M. A., McSharry, P. E., & Ramig, L. O. (2010, March). Enhanced classical dysphonia measures and sparse regression for telemonitoring of Parkinson's disease progression. In *2010 IEEE International Conference on Acoustics, Speech and Signal Processing* (pp. 594-597). IEEE.

Chapter 11
A Predictive Analysis of the COVID–19 Pandemic for Traditional and Tree–Based Regression Algorithms

Hari Singh

https://orcid.org/0000-0002-4063-9533

Jaypee University of Information Technology, India

Piyush Sewal

https://orcid.org/0000-0002-9975-0906

Shoolini University, India

Dinesh Chander Verma

Panipat Institute of Engineering and Technology, India

ABSTRACT

A lot of works exist in the literature that compares regression algorithms on different datasets. This chapter presents a model that uses best subset selection approach for the predictors and performs an exhaustive empirical comparison of eight regression algorithms Linear Regression, Multi-Linear Regression, Polynomial Regression, K-Nearest Neighbors, Lasso, Ridge, Decision Tree, Gradient Boost Tree, and Random Forest Regression algorithms on various predictors from Covid-19 dataset. The model is evaluated for train accuracy on metrics R2, Root Mean Square Error, and Mean Absolute Error. The test R2 and adjusted-R2 metrics evaluate the model on cross-validation prediction test errors. The predicted values of dependent variables

DOI: 10.4018/979-8-3693-5237-3.ch011

are checked for similarity and validation using statistical z-test.

1. INTRODUCTION

The Covid-19 pandemic has a worldwide impact on lives and almost every dimension of human lifestyle. A description of viruses emerged over a period of time and their impact on health of human beings is discussed (Luo & Gao, 2020; Myint, 1994; Wang et al., 2020). In the beginning, during January-April 2020, the European countries were worst-hit by the virus when the virus spread from China. India was not touched by the virus almost till early March 2020. The first few cases were reported in March 2020 through international tourists and, whenIndian working people and students started returning home from foreign countries. In the beginning, there were very less health care facilities in India as compared to many developed countries. With poor health care facilities and a huge population of approximately 1,382,715,488 as of September 13, 2020(*Worldometer*, 2022), a very heavy and negative impact of Covid-19 was predicted in India.

An analysis of the dataset used in the chapter from Kaggle (Https://www.kaggle .com/sudalairajkumar/covid19-in-india, n.d.) has been done and is also presented in Figure 1. The dataset uses Covid-19 data recorded from January 30, 2020 to August 30, 2020. It is observed that in the first ninety days, number of confirmed, cured and death cases were almost constant and were not rising even linearly with each day, considering January 30, 2020 as the Day-1. It may be due to less testing was done initially and the announcement of a nationwide lockdown, that started from March 24, 2020, when the number of Covid-19 cases reached approximately 500. But after two months, the government of India took decisions to give relaxations in the lockdown gradually due to its adverse effect on economy. A detail description of lockdown and un-lockdown and its impact in India is provided on Wikipedia (Wiki-pedia, 2021.). However when the testing was increased, the confirmed and cured cases started rising exponentially after three months to as of September 14, 2020. But the satisfactory thing is that the death cases were not increasing with that much pace. However the death cases also rose abruptly; it also followed an exponential curve after approximately 90 days. It can be seen from Figure 1(b) that when the numbers of deaths are plotted alone against time (days). When the three variables are plotted in the same graph, Figure 1(a), the deaths curve seems almost flat along the x-axis. It is because the numbers of deaths were very small in comparison to the number of confirmed and cured cases. One good observation is also evident from Figure 1(a) that the numbers of cured cases also follow the exponential curve, which signifies a good recovery rate among Covid-19 patients.

Figure 1. Covid-19 statistics on the available dataset (a) days versus confirmed, cured, and deaths (b) days versus deaths

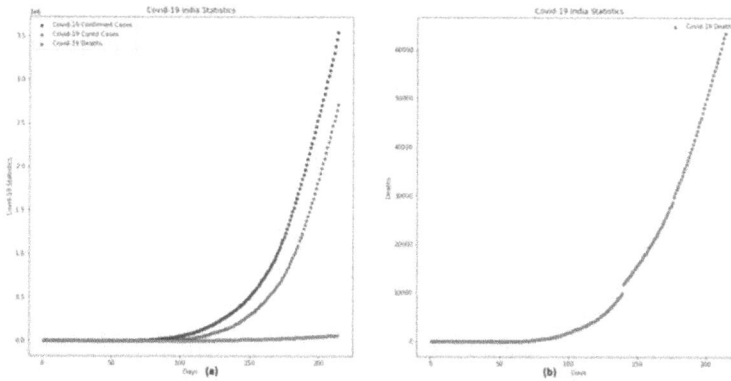

Figure 1. Covid-19 statistics on the available dataset (a) days versus confirmed, cured, and deaths (b) days versus deaths

This section describes many predictive models that analyzed spread of Covid-19 pandemic and the impact of several variables. Several mathematical, machine learning regression models, deep learning-based models have been surveyed. A Covid-19 related mathematical predictive model that takes into account the heath care facilities in Italian hospitals has been presented (Çakan, 2020). In another work, the authors applied statistical chi-square test and studied relationship between dependent variables, confirmed cases and deaths, and independent variables, age, sex, region, and infection, in spreading Covid-19 cases in South Korea (AL-Rousan & AL-Najjar, 2020). In another mathematical model, the spread of Covid-19 is predicted on various parameters, and a non-parametric model was developed to fit the dataset available till June 06, 2020 on India, Italy, and USA(Singhal et al., 2020). A detailed statistical description of polynomial regression model and some of the accuracy evaluation metrics such as R^2, Adjusted R^2, and RMSE is presented (Ostertagová, 2012). An analysis of linear and polynomial regression models is done in predicting Covid-19 deaths (Sewal & Singh, 2023, 2024; Singh & Bawa, 2022). Multiple stepwise regression analysis method and a two-layer nested heterogeneous ensemble learning-based prediction has been used for Covid-19 mortality prediction (Cui et al., 2021).

The authors fitted a linear regression line for Case Fatality Rate (CFR) on the very small Covid-19 dataset of ten countries, available till April 2020. They found that the fitted linebest represents the available dataset in a simple manner but with small acceptable error. However, the use of small dataset caused over-fitting with higher order polynomials(Hoseinpour Dehkordi et al., 2020).An auto-regression technique is applied on a six-week data of Covid-19 in India and it was found that the predicted model did not pass test of statistical significance despite having a strong correlation among variables and good values for goodness-of-fit metrics su-chasR^2 and Adjusted-R^2(Ghosal et al., 2020). In another research, the authors used Auto-Regressive Integrated Moving Average (ARIMA) and Seasonal-ARIMA for predicting the trend of Covid-19 epidemic (ArunKumar et al., 2021). A real-time differential optimization based Trust-region-reflective (TRR) algorithm is used to predict the peak of Covid-19 cases in Russia, Brazil, India, Bangladesh, and the UK(Nabi, 2020). Linear and multi-linear regression models are applied on the WHO's Covid-19 India dataset to visualize the trend. A good accuracy is found for the regression models having high value of R^2 metric(Rath et al., 2020). A support vector regression model has been used to predict Covid-12 cases that apply kernel functions to test non-linearity of different structures (Peng & Nagata, 2020).

The effect of climate-factors such as temperature and humidity, and population density were studied and modeled using virus optimization algorithm and adaptive network-based fuzzy inference system to predict the spread of Covid-19 in USA on the available one-month data. The authors found that population density is a signif-icant factor in the spread of Covid-19 pandemic and social distancing can limit the spread(Behnood et al., 2020). Regression is applied on weather dataset variables such as temperature and humidity, and census variables such as population, age and urbanization. The authors found that weather variables are more significant than census variables in predicting mortality rate due to Covid-19 pandemic(Malki et al., 2020). Another work compares and finds that the Naive Bayes regression performs poorly on real-life datasets in comparison to linear regression locally weighted linear regression and decision tree (Frank et al., 2000).

In paper(Correction & This, 2022), the authors address the challenge of accurate-ly forecasting COVID-19 mortality to inform critical public health decisions. The authors propose a solution by leveraging a multi-model ensemble forecast, which aggregates predictions from over 90 different academic, industry, and independent research groups via the US COVID-19 Forecast Hub. Their methodology involves comparing the performance of 27 individual models in predicting COVID-19 deaths across various time frames and locations, finding that ensemble models provided the most consistently accurate results. The study reveals that while many models outperformed a naïve baseline, forecast accuracy diminished with longer time horizons, indicating a key limitation. The work highlights the importance of collaboration between public health agencies, academic teams, and industry in enhancing predictive modeling capabilities during pandemics.

The study (Prieto, 2022) addresses the critical need for accurate predictions of COVID-19 spread, hospital care demand, and mortality in Mexico, particularly among patients with comorbidities. To tackle this, the authors employ a two-part solution using Bayesian inference and machine learning techniques. The first part involves projecting the spread of COVID-19 through a contact tracing model using Bayesian inference, while the second part focuses on predicting patient outcomes—such as the need for hospitalization and survival—using machine learning classifiers. The results demonstrate the effectiveness of these models in forecasting hospital care demand and mortality, though challenges remain in handling unbalanced datasets, which may affect the accuracy of predictions. This research underscores the importance of incorporating diverse analytical approaches to improve public health responses in pandemic situations.

In another study (Rahimi et al., 2023), authors address the global challenge of accurately forecasting the COVID-19 pandemic, reviewing and analyzing key machine learning models used for this purpose. The authors conduct a two-part investigation: first, a scientometric analysis is performed to identify trends and influential keywords in COVID-19 research, and second, they evaluate and compare various machine learning models, including deep learning, SIR, and SEIR models. The results highlight the strengths of hybrid algorithms in improving forecasting accuracy and identify gaps in existing models, particularly the need for more robust approaches to handle uncertainty. However, the study is limited by the scope of accessible literature at the time, suggesting the need for further comprehensive reviews and the development of novel predictive methods.

This study (Sun et al., 2020) addresses the challenge of accurately forecasting the long-term trend of the COVID-19 epidemic, crucial for informing public health strategies. The authors propose the Dynamic-Susceptible-Exposed-Infective-Quarantined (D-SEIQ) model, an enhancement of the traditional SEIR model, integrating machine learning for parameter optimization under epidemiological constraints. Applied to predict the COVID-19 outbreak in China, the model demonstrated high accuracy, successfully forecasting the epidemic's peak and long-term trend with minimal deviation from actual reported cases. The study also validated the model's effectiveness in other countries, highlighting its robustness. However, the model's reliance on early intervention data suggests a limitation in contexts with different public health responses.

The study presented in (Shinde et al., 2020) addresses the critical need for effective forecasting models to predict the spread of COVID-19 and inform public health strategies. It provides a comprehensive survey of existing forecasting techniques, categorizing them into stochastic theory mathematical models and data science/machine learning approaches. The authors also emphasize the importance of diverse datasets, including those from WHO and social media, in enhancing prediction accuracy. The study identifies key challenges, such as technical limitations and the need for more robust models that account for varying factors like environmental impacts and resource availability. However, the reliance on pre-print studies highlights a limitation, indicating the need for further validation of these models in real-world scenarios.

The study (Kamalov, Cherukuri, et al., 2022) addresses the need to organize the rapidly expanding body of literature on machine learning applications in the context of COVID-19. The authors propose a taxonomy that categorizes the research into three primary areas: detection, forecasting, and drug discovery. They analyze the current approaches in each category, highlighting both the progress made and the pitfalls encountered. The results of this survey suggest that while significant advancements have been achieved, there are ongoing challenges, such as inconsistencies across studies and the need for more comprehensive comparative analyses. A key limitation noted is the narrow scope of existing research, underscoring the need for broader and deeper investigations in future studies.

Some deep learning models have also been proposed recently. A long short-term memory (LSTM) network based deep learning approach is used to predict Covid-19 statistics in Canada (Chimmula & Zhang, 2020), Unites States of America(Basu & Campbell, 2020), and India (Arora et al., 2020). It is found that the model yields high accuracy for short-term predictions with small errors. A Convolution-LSTM based multivariate analysis is used to see factors responsible for the growth of Covid-19 cases (Yudistira et al., 2021).

In a different approach, the study (Nayak et al., 2022) explores the critical role of deep learning (DL) in addressing challenges posed by the COVID-19 pandemic, particularly in areas where traditional methods fall short. It examines how DL techniques have been employed for tasks such as diagnosis, forecasting, and classification of COVID-19 cases, leveraging their ability to recognize complex patterns in large datasets. The analysis identifies DL as a promising solution, particularly in medical imaging, where it can assist in diagnosing the disease from X-ray images, despite challenges like data deficiency and the need for accurate radiological interpretation. However, the study also acknowledges limitations, including the insufficient availability of annotated medical images and the inconsistency of predictive outcomes, which need to be addressed to improve the efficacy of DL models in pandemic management. The authors emphasize the need for further research, particularly in enhancing data quality and exploring advanced neural network techniques to better combat the ongoing crisis.

In a similar study (Kamalov, Rajab, et al., 2022), authors address the critical need for effective COVID-19 forecasting by focusing on deep learning (DL) methods. It reviews and categorizes 53 key studies that apply DL techniques, particularly highlighting the widespread use of Long Short-Term Memory (LSTM) networks. The analysis reveals that while LSTM models and spatio-temporal approaches show promise, the current research is limited by short timeframes and insufficient data. Moreover, many studies lack robust theoretical foundations, undermining their scientific validity. The paper emphasizes the necessity for future research to develop models with stronger theoretical grounding and to explore longer-term forecasts and more challenging tasks, such as predicting new cases rather than cumulative totals.

The work presented in this chapter is based on the Covid-19 dataset for a longer duration(Https://www.kaggle.com/sudalairajkumar/covid19-in-india, n.d.).The Linear Regression (LR), Multi-Linear Regression (MLR) and Polynomial Regression (PR), K-Nearest Neighbor (KNN), Lasso regression, and Ridge regression algorithms in machine learning have been used to best-fit the dataset. The accuracy of fitted model is evaluated on R^2, Adjusted R^2, RMSE, and MAE. The test R^2 and adjusted-R^2 metrics evaluate the model on cross-validation prediction test errors.

The study presented here employs a variety of predictive techniques, ranging from simple linear models to complex ensemble methods, to explore their relative performance in predicting Covid-19 death statistics in India. Each technique was chosen based on its ability to capture different aspects of the data, such as linearity, non-linearity, and interaction effects among variables. The use of a diverse set of models allows for a thorough comparison and understanding of the strengths and weaknesses of each approach.

The rest of the chapter is as follows. Section-2 describes the methodology. Section-3 presents results and discussions. Section-4 concludes the chapter with a view of the future scope of the work.

2. METHODOLOGY

This section describes the workflow, methodology used, life cycle of the model and regression algorithms used. The section also highlights several critical issues with predictive modeling techniques, including data quality challenges and computational demands. The performance of these models is significantly impacted by data quality, such as missing values and class imbalances, which can skew predictions and reduce model reliability. Additionally, while advanced models like Random Forest and Gradient Boosting Trees provide superior accuracy, they require extensive computational resources, which can be a limitation in real-time applications.

2.1 The workflow

The workflow of the model can be understood in seven steps. These steps are feature extraction, data pre-processing, model building and feature selection, and training and testing models, model evaluation on accuracy metrics, model validation using statistical z-test, and model deployment. The steps are describes in detail here.

2.1.1 *Feature Extraction:* The features are extracted from Covid-19 dataset of India (Https://www.kaggle.com/sudalairajkumar/covid19-in-india, n.d.). A careful identification of all the features having significant impact on the predicted outcome is done. Ignoring/leaving any significant dependent feature may result in inaccurate predictions, and hence wrong decision/policy making.

2.1.2 *Data Pre-processing:* The Exploratory Data Analysis (EDA) is conducted on the dataset. It tells about the patterns, relationships, and anomalies among variables in the dataset for further analysis. It is the first step in analyzing the data. Data cleaning is required for columns having 'NAN' values as this may create problems while applying some arithmetic on the data. Moreover 'NAN' values create problems in correctly predicting the outcome. It is always better to either delete these or replace with either zero, mean, mode, or median values that best fits in the problem.

2.1.3 *Model Building and Feature Selection:* The machine learning model in the problem is identified in the context of users' requirement. Here LR, MLR, PR, KNN, Lasso, Ridge, Decision Tree, Gradient Boost, and Random Forest models on different number of independent parameters have been tested for accuracy on metrics R-Square, Adjusted R-Square, RMSE, and MAE. The model with very high value of R-Square and Adjusted R-Square (near one) and having very low values of RMSE and MAE are considered as good to fit dataset. The number of chosen independent parameters from the dataset is selected on the basis EDA described in step 2.1.2 and the Karl-Pearson's correlation matrix. The Karl-Pearson matrix tells a strong correlation between two variables if the value contained in the intersecting cell of two variables is high. A week correlation exists when the value is very low. The values can range between zero and one.

2.1.4 *Training and Testing Model:* The dataset is split into 80% training and 20% testing. The CSV file contains 214 days of data on features confirmed cases, cured cases, and deaths happened for all the States and Union Territories of India. The data is grouped on number of days, and values are summed on features to get the data at country level for further analysis and modeling.

2.1.5 *Model Evaluation Accuracy Metrics:* The following four accuracy metrics have been used for measuring accuracy of models in this chapter: R-Square, Adjusted R-Square, Mean Square Error (MSE), Root Mean Square (RMSE), and Mean Absolute Error (MAE).

R^2: It is also called coefficient of determination and goodness-of-fit model.

$$R^2 = 1 - \frac{\text{Sum Squared Regression (SSR)}}{\text{Total Sum of Squares (SST)}}$$

$$R^2 = 1 - \frac{\sum (y_i - y_i')^2}{\sum (y_i - y_i^-)^2}$$

Where y' = predicted y value, y- = mean

residual (ri) = actual y value – predicted y value (y-yi)

The residual may be positive or negative that depends on whether the predicted value is too high or low accordingly.

It is the statistical measure of the closeness of the data to the fitted line. Its value lies between 0 and 100%. 0% means the observed values are not around the mean or the fitted line or curve (worst case or worst model). 100% means the observed values are around the mean or fitted line or curve (best case or best model) and all the observed values fell on the line or curve. Though R-Square provides a n estimate of the strength of the relationship between model and response variable, it does not provide a formal hypothesis test for this relationship. There is a big drawback of this metric as it is possible to have a low R-Squared value for a good model or a high R-Squared value for a bad model. In such a case residual plots need to be assessed.

Adjusted R^2-Square: The equation of calculating Adjusted R-Square is

$$\text{Adjusted} - R^2 = 1 - \left[\frac{(1 - R^2)(n - 1)}{n - p - 1} \right]$$

Where, N is the number of points in data sample, p is the number of independent variables, excluding constants.

It tells the amount of variation explained by the independent variable on the dependent variables. If useless independent variables are used to predict the model then this metric penalizes. The Adjusted R-Square has the importance that R-Square always increases and never decreases on adding predictor variables, and then the model will seem better. However, considering too many predictor variables and too many high-order polynomials may mislead to high R-Square value and over-fitting the data.

Mean Square Error (MSE): The metric tells how close data points are to the fitted line. This distance signifies the error. The squaring is done to remove the negative sign. The smaller the MSE value, the better is the model. It measures sum of squares of the difference between actual and predicted values and then it averages out these values. It also gives more weights to larger differences. It is the most simple and common metric for evaluating regression family of algorithms. But it also is the least useful metric. MSE is used in situations where we have unpredicted data values i.e very high or low values. The problem with this model is that it can overestimate the model's badness if we have noisy data or bad data. If the errors are smaller than one then it may under-estimate the model's badness. In nutshell, the noise is exaggerated and large errors are punished.

$$RMSE = \frac{1}{n} \sum_{i=1}^{n} \left(y_i - y_i^- \right)^2$$

Where, $\left(y_i - y_i^- \right)$ is the distance of the points to the regression line.

Root Mean Square Error (RMSE): The metric is another way of evaluating the model. It is the square root of the mean of the squares of all errors. RMSE tells how the data is concentrated around the line of best-fit. The square root is taken to bring the errors on the same scale as of target values scale while in case of MSE the errors have squared units. RMSE has the benefit of penalizing large errors more.

$$RMSE = \sqrt{\frac{1}{n}} \sum_{i=1}^{n} \left(y_i - y_i^- \right)^2$$

Mean Absolute Error (MAE): It measures the average magnitude of the errors in a set of predictions, without considering their direction. MAE calculates errors as the average of the absolute difference between the actual and predicted values. It is a linear score which means that all the individual differences are weighted equally in the average. It does not penalize large errors as MSE does. MAE is used when there are outliers in the dataset otherwise use MSE/RMSE

$$MAE = \frac{1}{n} \sum_{i=1}^{n} \left| \left(y_i - y_i^- \right) \right|$$

2.1.6 *Model Validation:* A statistical z-test or t-test is used with normal distribution of data and it checks if the means of two sample populations is reliably similar or different from each other. Merely looking at the means may not reliably tell this thing, it can just tell about the data on hand and does not make a general statement. The generalization about the population can be stated with inferential statistics such as z-test or t-test done over the samples. A z-test is generally conducted when the sample size is more than 30 otherwise t-tests is more suitable.

2.1.7 *Model Deployment:* Once the model is fitted, evaluated on accuracy levels, and validated using statistical test, it can be used for real-time actions.

2.2 Methodology Used

The methodology uses best subset selection approach for predictors and takes eight regression algorithms MLR, Polynomial, Lasso, Ridge, KNN, Decision Tree, Gradient Boost Tree, and Random Forest andtheCovid-19 dataset(Https://www

.kaggle.com/sudalairajkumar/covid19-in-india, n.d.) as input. Initially the smallest R^2, largest RMSE, and largest MAE characterize the best model. The worst solution M_{i0} computes the null model for each algorithm, which represents a model with sample mean having no predictors. The inner loop fits 'p' solutions that contain exactly one predictor and $\binom{p}{k}$ solutions that contain exactly 'k' predictors at a time. M_{ik} is the best solution with k predictors and i_{th} algorithm on the basis of R^2, RMSE and MAE. The M_{is} filters the best solution for i_{th} algorithm from the computed M_{ik} solutions. This process is repeated for the remaining four regression algorithms with the outer loop. Each run of the inner loop finds one best solution nM_{is} for a particular regression algorithm. In the end, the algorithm finds the best solution on train evaluation metrics and the cross validation prediction test error.

Algorithm:

Input: Predictors and eight regression algorithms

Output: The best solution on the basis of train metrics i.e. largest R^2, lowest RMSE, and lowest MAE and cross validation prediction error i.e. adjusted-R^2

Initializations

M_{best} = smallest R^2, largest RMSE and largest MAE;

p=1;

fori=one to eight input models // MLR, Polynomial, Lasso, Ridge, KNN, Decision Tree, Gradient Boost Tree, and Random Forest

{

Compute sample mean for the null model M_{i0}, assuming no predictors;

for k=1 to p predictors

{

a. Fit all p models that contain exactly one predictor. Fit all $\binom{p}{k}$ solutions that contains exactly k predictors; //eg. $\binom{p}{k} = \frac{p(p-1)}{2}$ for k=2

b. Pick the M_{ik} best among these $\binom{p}{k}$ models having largest R^2, minimum RMSE, and minimum MAE;

c. Select M_{is}, a single best solution from among M_{i0}, .., M_{ip} using cross validation prediction test error, test-R^2 and adjusted-R^2, where 's' denotes the best solution amongst the models with 0 to p predictors;

}

if(Is M_{is} better than the M_{best} ?) {

$M_{best} = M_{is}$; }

}

2.3 Life Cycle of the Model

The features are extracted from Covid-19 dataset of India (Https://www.kaggle.com/sudalairajkumar/covid19-in-india, n.d.). A careful identification of all the features having significant impact on the predicted outcome is done. Ignoring/leaving any significant dependent feature may result in inaccurate predictions, and hence wrong decision/policy making. The Exploratory Data Analysis (EDA) is conducted on the dataset. It tells about the patterns, relationships, and anomalies among variables in the dataset for further analysis. It is the first step in analyzing the data. Data cleaning is required for columns having 'NAN' values as this may create problems while applying some arithmetic on the data. Moreover 'NAN' values create problems in correctly predicting the outcome. It is always better to either delete these or replace with either zero, mean, mode, or median values that best fits in the problem.

The number of chosen independent parameters from the dataset is selected on the basis of exploratory data analysis and the Karl-Pearson's correlation matrix. The Karl-Pearson matrix tells a strong correlation between two variables if the value contained in the intersecting cell of two variables is high. A week correlation exists when the value is very low. The values can range between zero and one. The model testing and training is done using K-Fold Cross-Validation (K=5). The CSV file contains data on features confirmed cases, cured cases, and deaths happened for all the States and Union Territories of India. The data is grouped on number of days, and values are summed on features to get the data at country level for further analysis and modeling. The following four accuracy metricshave been used for measuring accuracy of models in this chapter: R^2, Adjusted-R^2, RMSE, and Mean Absolute Error (MAE). Once the model is fitted, evaluated on accuracy levels, and validated using statistical test, it can be deployed for real-time actions.

2.4 Overview of Regression Algorithms Used

This section gives an overview of the eight regression algorithms used. The purpose of using various predictive techniques in this chapter is to evaluate the performance and accuracy of different models in predicting Covid-19 death statistics in India. Each technique offers unique strengths and weaknesses, allowing for a comprehensive analysis of their effectiveness in handling Covid-19 data. The key difference in using these techniques lies in their approach to modeling the data. While simpler models like LR and MLR provide straightforward insights, more complex models like RF and GBT offer better predictive performance but require more computational resources. The chapter discusses the results where tree-based models, particularly RF, outperformed others, indicating that these models are more adept at handling the complexity of the Covid-19 dataset. However, the computational cost and the time required for processing larger datasets highlight the limitations of these advanced techniques.

The chapter employs a variety of predictive techniques, ranging from simple linear models to complex ensemble methods, to explore their relative performance in predicting Covid-19 death statistics in India. Each technique was chosen based on its ability to capture different aspects of the data, such as linearity, non-linearity, and interaction effects among variables. The use of a diverse set of models allows for a thorough comparison and understanding of the strengths and weaknesses of each approach.

2.4.1 Linear and Multi-linear Regression

Linear Regression (LR) and **Multi-Linear Regression (MLR)** are fundamental statistical methods that help in understanding the relationship between the independent variables and the dependent variable, offering simplicity and interpretability. However, they might not capture non-linear relationships well. The dataset contains the independent parameters 'Days', 'Confirmed', and 'Cured' that presents the number of days, confirmed cases, and cured cases, respectively. It has one dependent parameter 'Deaths' that explains the number of deaths. Linear Regression (LR) model regresses 'Deaths' on a single field 'Days' (LRP1) while Multilinear Regression (MLR) regresses 'Deaths' on two field 'Days and Confirmed' (MLRP2) and on three fields 'Days, Confirmed, and Cured' (MLRP3).

The LR and MLR is represented with equation (1)

$$y = \beta_0 + \beta_1 x_1 + \beta_2 x_2 + \ldots + \beta_n x_n \tag{1}$$

Here n=3 and β_0 is the intercept, β_1, β_2, and β_3 are the coefficients of the x_1 (Days), x_2 (Confirmed), and x_3 (Cured), predictors respectively. Each coefficient explains the change in 'y' for a unit change in the associated predictor ignoring the impact of other predictors. The regression represented with LR and MLR has least flexibility and interpret the trend nicely but has poor predictability.

2.4.2 Polynomial Regression

Polynomial Regression (PR) extends linear models to capture curvilinear relationships by incorporating polynomial terms, which is particularly useful when the relationship between variables is non-linear. The Polynomial Regression (PR) fits the dataset that describes non-linear relationship among predictor variables and the output variables. Here, just like LR and MLR, PR is also modeled on a single predictor (PRP1), two predictor (LRP2), and three predictors (LRP3) with various degree of the polynomial. The general representation is PRPxDy, where x is the number of predictor terms involved and y is the degree of the polynomial. It is represented with equation (2) for PRP1Dn.

$$y = \beta_0 + \beta_1 x_1 + \beta_2 x_1^2 + \beta_3 x_1^3 + \ldots + \beta_n x_1^n \tag{2}$$

The Polynomial equation for PRP2D2 is represented with equation (3)

$$y = \beta_0 + \beta_1 x_1 + \beta_2 x_2 + \beta_3 x_1^2 + \beta_4 x_1 x_2 + \beta_5 x_2^2 \tag{3}$$

The Polynomial equation for PRP2D3 is represented with equation (4) and similarly, generalization can be done for PRP2Dn.

$$y = \beta_0 + \beta_1 x_1 + \beta_2 x_2 + \beta_3 x_1^2 + \beta_4 x_1 x_2 + \beta_5 x_2^2 + \beta_6 x_1^3 + \beta_7 x_1^2 x_2 + \beta_8 x_1 x_2^2 + \beta_9 x_2^3 \tag{4}$$

The Polynomial equation for PRP3D2 is represented with equation (5) and similarly, generalization can be done for PRP3Dn.

$$y = \beta_0 + \beta_1 x_1 + \beta_2 x_2 + \beta_3 x_3 + \beta_4 x_1^2 + \beta_5 x_1 x_2 + \beta_6 x_1 x_3 + \beta_7 x_2^2 + \beta_8 x_2 x_3 + \beta_9 x_3^2 \tag{5}$$

The flexibility of regression represented with PR increases with rising the degree of the polynomial and it exhibits poor interpretability, good predictability and increased model complexity with this trend.

2.4.3 KNN Regression

K-Nearest Neighbors (KNN) is a non-parametric method that makes predictions based on the closest data points, which can be advantageous for capturing complex patterns but may struggle with high-dimensional data. KNN regression starts by identifying the K training observations that are closet to the prediction point x and then estimates $\hat{y}$ using the average of all the training responses as given by equation (6)

$$\hat{y} = \frac{1}{k} \sum_{x_i \in N(x)} y_i \tag{6}$$

The Loss function: L(y, f(x)) and the Squared Error: $(y-f(x))^2$ describes the Expected Prediction Error EPE(f) = $E\{(y-f(x))^2\}$

Expectation of a random variable means taking under distribution or joint distribution between x and y (here).

So, the distribution w.r.t. which this expectation is taken is described by equation (7)

$$EPE(f) = \int (y - f(x))^2 P(dx, dy) \qquad (7)$$

Having chosen a particular data point x, the probability of seeing an output value y with conditional distribution $P(x,y) = P(y/x) . P(x)$ is given by equations (8) and (9).

$$EPE(f) = E_x E_{y/x}\big([y - f(x)]\big|x\big) \qquad (8)$$

$$f(x) = \operatorname{argmin}_c E_{y/x}\big([y - c]^2\big|X = x\big) \qquad (9)$$

It is called conditioning on a point x and value of c is such that it minimizes f(x).

The conditional expectation or regression function for condition on a region is $\hat{y} = Avg\big(y_i\big|x_i \in N_k(x)\big)$

When 'k' increases, the estimate becomes more stable and when N, k reaches infinity, k/N reaches zero,

The prediction reaches true value which is not possible $\hat{y} = E[y/x = x]$.

If dimension p is large, data tends to become sparse. The volume covered by k neighbors becomes very large. So, kNN is not a good idea in that case.

2.4.4 Ridge Regression

Lasso and Ridge Regression are regularization techniques that help in handling multicollinearity and improving model generalization by shrinking the regression coefficients. The Ridge regression technique improves the model fit to the dataset by shrinking the regression coefficients towards zero and thereby significantly reducing the variance. But it does not set any coefficients to exactly zero. The ridge regression coefficient estimates are the values that minimizes equation (10)

$$\sum_{i=1}^{n}\left(y_i - \beta_0 - \sum_{j=1}^{p}\beta_j x_{ij}\right)^2 + \lambda \sum_{j=1}^{p}\beta_j^2 \qquad (10)$$

Where $\lambda >= 0$ is the tuning parameter, the first term represents the least square model i.e. RSS and the second term is the shrinkage penalty. The ridge regression seeks coefficient estimate that fits data well, by making the RSS small and the shrinkage penalty is small when the coefficient terms β_a re close to zero. The tuning parameter λ serves to control the relative impact of these two terms on regression coefficient estimates. Ridge regression provides bias-variance trade-off with the tuning parameter λ and therefore improves over the least square model. As λ increases, the flexibility of the ridge regression fit decreases, leading to decreased variance but increased bias.

2.4.5 Lasso Regression

The lasso regression has the advantage over ridge regression that it reduces some of the coefficient estimates to exactly zero. Therefore ridge regression includes all the predictors in the final model while lasso regression makes the final model very simple if the dataset is significantly described by few predictors. The ridge regression coefficient estimates are the values that minimizes equation (11)

$$\sum_{i=1}^{n} \left(y_i - \beta_0 - \sum_{j=1}^{p} \beta_j x_{ij} \right)^2 + \lambda \sum_{j=1}^{p} |\beta_j| \tag{11}$$

Here equation (10) has the same meaning as equation (9) except that the penalty term in lasso is $|\beta_j|$ whereas in the ridge regression it is β_j^2.

2.4.6 Decision Tree and Random Forest Regression

Decision Trees (DT), **Random Forest (RF)**, and **Gradient Boosting Trees (GBT)** are tree-based ensemble methods that provide robust predictions by combining multiple decision trees. DT offers interpretability, but can overfit; RF reduces overfitting by averaging multiple trees, and GBT builds trees sequentially to reduce errors, often achieving higher accuracy but at the cost of interpretability. The Decision tree (DT) uses two steps namely selecting the best attribute/feature to divide a set at each branch, and deciding whether each branch is justified sufficiently or not. Various DT programs vary in how these are accomplished. The Decision Node and Leaf Node are the two nodes of a decision tree. The Decision Tree is calculated using Eq. (12).

$$E(s) = \sum_{i=1}^{c} -p_i \log_2 p_i \tag{12}$$

Where $E(s)$ is the entropy and Pi is the Probability of an event i of state S

The Random Forest can be used for classification as well as regression problems, works on the principle of Bagging. Bagging can be used to overcome the problem of over fitting in decision trees. Bagging works in three steps where firstly main dataset is broken into multiple subsets. These subsets can have fraction of rows and columns from main dataset. Secondly, Classifier is built for each of the subsets. And finally, results of all the classifiers are combined and label is assigned to the object. Thus, Random Forest is a powerful algorithm as it combines the results of multiple classifiers.

The node splitting in random forest with the Gini impurity for a node is

$$GINI_{node} = 1 - \sum_{c=1}^{Classes} p^2_{node,\,c}$$

The $p^2_{node,\,c}$ is computed according to the distribution of class weights as

$$p_{node,c} = \frac{\sum_{y_i=c,\,i \in node} w_i}{\sum_{i \in node} w_i}$$

Where, $i \in node$ means that the observation is in the node, and w_i is the class weight of the observation.

2.4.7 Gradient Boost Tree Regression

It is a boosting method used to build the models in a sequential manner. Errors of previous models are reduced in this case using subsequent models. This algorithm can be used for both classifications as well as regression problems. When dependent variable is continuous, Gradient Boosting regressor is used whereas Gradient Boosting Classifier is used for discrete target variable. This algorithm uses concept of gradient descent to minimize the loss function.

The cost function is expressed as follows.

$$F_0(x) = \arg_\gamma \min \sum_{i=1}^{n} \frac{w_i * L(y_i, \gamma)}{\sum_i w_i}$$

Here L is the loss function, y_i is the observed value, γ is the predicted value and $\arg_\gamma \min$ is the predicted value with minimum loss function, and w_i is the class weight of the observation. As the target column is continuous, Loss function L can be calculated as:

$$L = \frac{1}{n} \sum_{i=0}^{n} \left(y_i - \gamma_i \right)^2$$

2.5 Reason for Selection of regression algorithms

The choice of predictive techniques in this chapter—Linear Regression (LR), Multiple Linear Regression (MLR), Polynomial Regression (PR), K-Nearest Neighbors (KNN), and various tree-based models—was driven by their ability to handle different aspects of the Covid-19 dataset. Linear Regression (LR) and Multiple Linear Regression (MLR) were selected for their simplicity and interpretability, allowing for straightforward understanding of how individual or multiple predictors affect the Covid-19 death statistics. However, these models are primarily linear and may not capture complex, non-linear patterns inherent in the data.

Polynomial Regression (PR) was employed to model non-linear relationships by fitting polynomial equations to the data. This approach is particularly useful when the relationship between predictors and the target variable is curvilinear, as observed in the trends of Covid-19 cases over time. The flexibility of PR to adjust the degree of the polynomial enables it to fit more complex patterns compared to linear models.

K-Nearest Neighbors (KNN) was chosen for its non-parametric nature, which allows it to model complex, non-linear relationships without assuming a specific functional form. KNN's performance benefits from its local approach, where predictions are based on the proximity of data points, making it suitable for handling the intricacies of Covid-19 data.

Tree-based models, including Decision Trees, Random Forest, and Gradient Boosting Trees, were selected for their robustness and ability to handle high-dimensional and non-linear data. Decision Trees provide a visual and interpretable way to understand the decision-making process, while Random Forest and Gradient Boosting Trees enhance accuracy through ensemble methods, combining multiple trees to improve predictive performance and handle interactions between variables effectively.

3. RESULTS AND DISCUSSIONS

The work presented in this chapter is based on the Covid-19 dataset of India available from Kaggle dataset (Https://www.kaggle.com/sudalairajkumar/covid19-in -india, n.d.). It contains various fields such as Date, State/Union Territories, Deaths, Confirmed, and Cured. Here, Date represents the calendar date when the data was taken. State/Union Territories represents different states and union territories of India. Remaining fields represent the number of deaths, confirmed Covid-19 cases and cured cases. Section 3.1 presents an empirical comparison on accuracy of LR, MLR, PR, KNN, Ridge, and Lasso regression. Section 3.2 presents an empirical comparison on accuracy of Decision Tree, Random Forest, and Gradient Boost.

3.1 An Exhaustive Empirical Comparison on Accuracy of LR, MLR, PR, KNN, Ridge, and Lasso Regression

This section presents accuracies on evaluation metrics R^2, Adjusted-R^2, RMSE, and MAE for LR, MLR and PR, KNN, Ridge and Lasso regression with varying independent parameters as presented in Table-1. Here a PR with parameter 'x' and varying degree 'y' is represented with PRPxDy.Table-1 presents the accuracy metrics for LR and PR with a single parameter 'Days'. It can be seen that LR with one parameter (LRP1) is having the lowest R^2 and Adjusted-R^2 values and maximum RMSE and MAE values as compared to PRP1Dx. Among PRs, the polynomial of degree two has much better figures for all the metrics over the LRP1. The metrics becomes better when PR of degree three is evaluated. R^2 becomes maximum and does not improve further on increasing the degree. The Adjusted R^2 remains constant as it measures the impact of including more number of independent parameters. When the degree of PR is further increased, the RMSE and MAE improve very less as compared to rise in the complexity of polynomial equations. This increase in complexity is due to more number of coefficients and more number of terms in the polynomial. So, to trade-off the complexity and hence execution time, it can be said that PRP1D3 best-fits the dataset. This explanation is also evident from the kernel density or Gaussian density distribution plots between the predicted and actual deaths over the test dataset, as presented in Figure 2. There is a huge difference in the predicted and actual deaths curve for LRP1. The two curves in PRP1D2 show more closeness than in LRP1. The overlapping between the two curves becomes better in PRP1D7. After that for higher degree PRs, the overlapping between curves deteriorates.

Though PRP1D7 best explains the dataset and the PR explained by the degree-7 polynomial becomes very flexible but very complex, as shown in Figure 3. A balance or compromise is to be maintained between the model complexity and model performance. The Lasso and Ridge regression behaves like least square (LRP1) as is also evident from the accuracy metrics in Table 1 and Figure 4. The KNN regression gives the best results on K=4 and explains the best regression among all the others presented here.

The accuracy metrics for MLR and PR with two independent parameters 'Days' and 'Confirmed' concludes that MLR with two parameters (MLRP2) is far better than LRP1 on accuracy metrics. The MLRP2 is even better than many PRs on one parameter and approximates the PRP1D6.It means a PR of same accuracy can be obtained on increasing the correlated independent parameters and even keeping the degree of the polynomial low. It is also observed that the PRP2 is better than PRP1 of same degree. Further, similar to the PRP1, PRP2 also improves slightly on increasing the degree from two to three but after that the metrics does not improve on increasing the degree. Here also the complexity of the PR increases very fast on increasing the degree. It can be concluded that PRP2D3 best-fits the test data-set. This explanation is also evident from the kernel density or Gaussian density distribution plots between the predicted and actual deaths over the test dataset, as presented in Figure 5. It is clear from Figure 2 and Figure 5 that the two curves have more percentage of overlapping in MLRP2 as compared to LRP1. The two curves overlap, except at few points, in PRP2D2 and show maximum overlapping in PRP2D3. The overlapping of the curves reduces in PRP2D4. The model coefficients obtained for Lasso and Ridge regression try to shrink the coefficient of the 'Confirmed'(x2) parameter but could not shrink it as it is also strongly correlated to the output parameter. If it was weakly correlated then the Ridge regression would have shrunk the coefficient towards zero and the Lasso model would have shrunk it to zero. Therefore, both work like least square model (MLRP2) as can be seen from accuracy metrics in Table 1 and its kernel density as presented in Figure 5. The KNN regression gives the best results on K=4 and explains the best regression among all the others presented here. It is also evident from the accuracy metrics in Table 1 and Figure 4.

The accuracy metrics for MLRP3 and PR with three independent parameters 'Days', 'Confirmed', and 'Cured' concludes that MLRP3 is better than MLRP2. Here also the PRP3D2 closely approximates the PRP2D3. One more similar trend is observed; the accuracy of PRP3D3 is the best and decreases on further increasing the degree. However, this accuracy is at the cost of a more complex polynomial equation representing the model. This explanation is also evident from the kernel density or Gaussian density distribution plots between the predicted and actual deaths over the test dataset, as presented in Figure 6. It is clear from Figure 5 and Figure 6 that the two curves have more percentage of overlapping in MLRP3 as compared to MLRP2. Further the degree of overlapping is more in PRP3D3 than in PRP3D2. The overlapping of the curves reduces slightly in PRP3D4. The coefficients obtained for Lasso and Ridge regression models try to shrink the coefficient of the 'Confirmed'(x2) and 'Cured'(x3) parameters. Here both the Lasso and Ridge have slight impact in shrinking the coefficient of the 'Cured'(x3) parameter slightly. Therefore, both provide results which are in between MLRP2 and MLRP3, as can be seen from accuracy metrics in the Table-1 and its kernel density as presented in the Fig-5. The KNN regression gives best results on K=4 and explains best regression among all the others. It is also evident from the accuracy metrics in the Table 1 and the Figure 2, Figure 3, and Figure 4.

Table 1. Regression models' evaluation with varying independent parameter and polynomial degrees

Model Used	Train R² Error	Test R² Error	Adjusted R²Error	RMSE	MAE
LRP1	0.856	0.886	0.87	45583.26	35221.98
PRP1D2	0.939	0.964	0.96	25753.96	19518.32
PRP1D3	0.954	0.968	0.98	24177.10	21197.21
PRP1D4	0.971	0.975	0.98	20999.18	15742.77
PRP1D5	0.972	0.972	0.98	20517.19	16956.66
PRP1D6	0.991	0.996	0.98	11308.15	9173.08
PRP1D7	0.996	0.996	0.99	8237.07	6396.95
PRP1D8	0.996	0.996	0.99	7977.13	4690.23
PRP1D9	0.996	0.996	0.99	8141.24	5304.52
MLRP2	0.9876	0.99	0.99	13098.71	9360.34
PRP2D2	0.992	0.991	0.99	12092.00	8262.53
PRP2D3	0.99	0.99	0.99	2662.69	2192.06
PRP2D4	0.99	0.99	0.99	10690.91	8721.41
MLRP3	0.99	0.99	0.99	8195.58	7106.47
PRP3D2	0.99	0.99	0.99	1772.25	1529.58
PRP3D3	0.99	0.99	0.99	1468.5	1022.79
KNN4P1	0.99	0.99	0.99	441.96	210.00
KNN4P2	0.99	0.99	0.99	540.43	236.64
KNN4P3	0.99	0.99	0.99	543.32	238.62
Lasso-P1	0.856	0.88	0.99	45583.30	35221.96
Lasso-P2	0.986	0.99	0.99	13437.20	8677.82
Lasso-P3	0.989	0.992	0.99	12228.70	8521.30
Ridge-P1	0.856	0.886	0.99	45583.30	35221.96
Ridge-P2	0.987	0.99	0.99	13437.20	8677.82
Ridge-P3	0.995	0.996	0.99	12228.70	8521.30

3.2 An Exhaustive Empirical Comparison on Accuracy of Decision Tree, Random Forest, and Gradient Boost

This section presents accuracy comparison on evaluation metrics R^2, Adjusted-R^2, RMSE and MAE for Decision Tree (DT), Gradient Boost (GB) and Random Forest (RF) with varying independent parameters. Table 2 presents the accuracy metrics for DT, GB and RF models with one, two and three parameters. In this table P1 represents one parameter 'Days' used, P2 means two parameters 'Days' and 'Confirmed' are taken into consideration for evaluation whereas P3 indicates numbers of parameters used are three which includes 'Days', 'Confirmed' and 'Cured'. It can be seen that DT with three parameters (DTP3) is having the lowest RMSE value whereas MAE value is least for DTP2. The DTP1 is not much affective in giving accurate results. Among GB based runs, both RMSE and MAE values are least for GBP3l. The GBP1 gives better results than GBP2 but is unable to outperform when three parameters are considered. The same trend can be seen for Random Forest where RFP3 is having least values for both RMSE and MAE. It can be clearly concluded from these results that GB with more number of parameters gave better results as compared to few or lesser parameters.

Figure 2. Distribution of actual deaths and predicted deaths using LR, PR in 'x=1 to 4' degree of Polynomial (PRP1Dx) on One Independent Parameter ['Days']

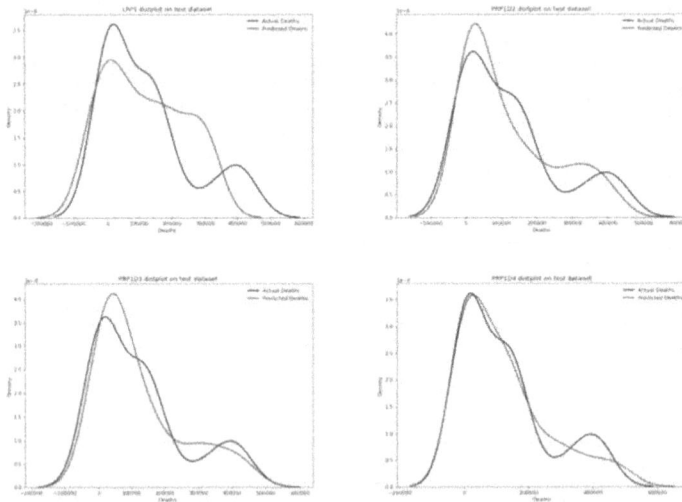

Figure 3. Distribution of actual deaths and predicted deaths using PR in 'x=5 to 8' degree of Polynomial (PRP1Dx) on One Independent Parameter ['Days']

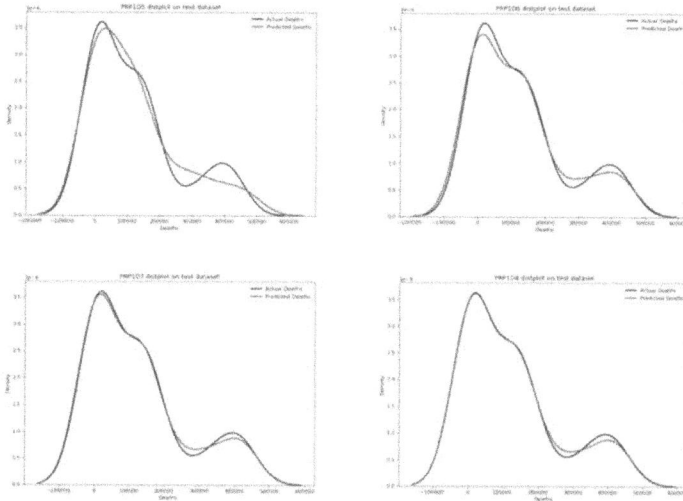

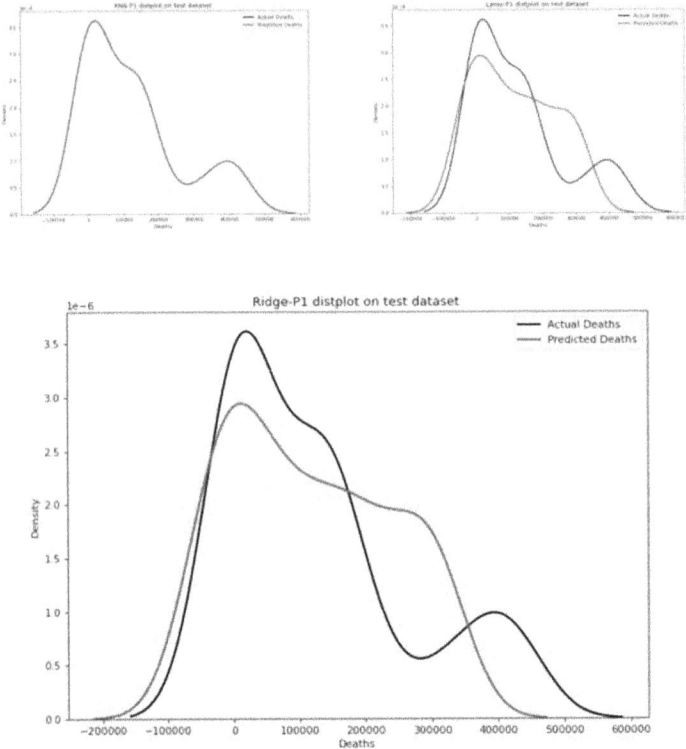

Figure 4. Distribution of actual deaths and predicted deaths using KNN, Lasso, and Ridge Regression on One Independent Parameter ['Days']

Figure 5. Distribution of actual deaths and predicted deaths using MLR, PRin 'x=1 to 3' degree of Polynomial (PRP2Dx), KNN, Lasso, and Ridge Regression with Two Independent Parameter (MLRP2) ['Days' and 'Confirmed']

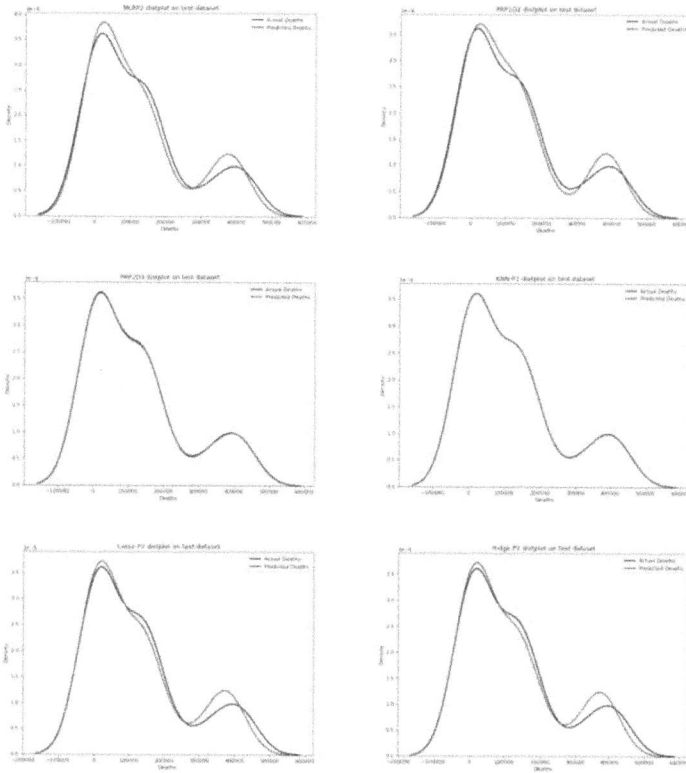

Figure 6. Distribution of actual deaths and predicted deaths using MLR and, PR in 'x' degree of Polynomial (PRP2Dx), KNN, Lasso, and Ridge Regression with Three Independent Parameter ['Days', 'Confirmed', and 'Cured']

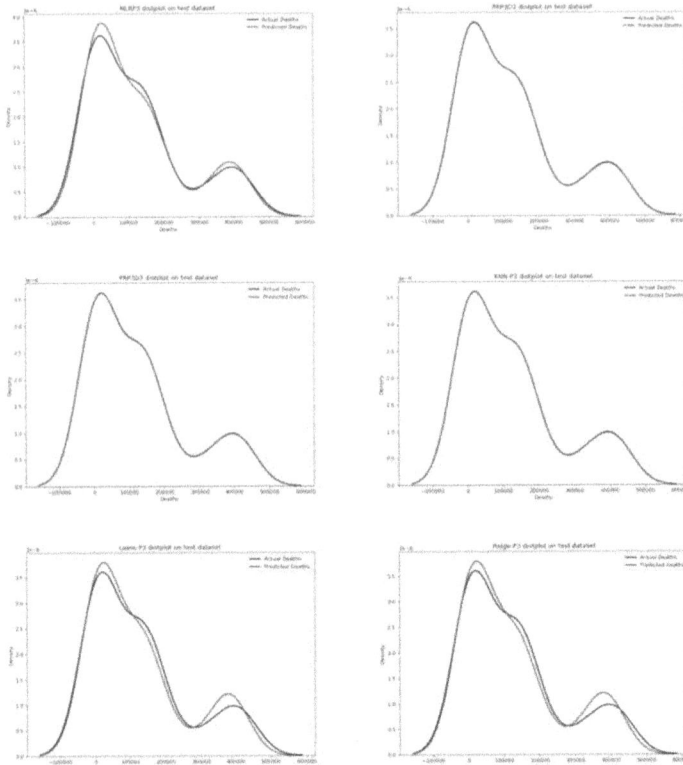

The accuracy metrics for DT, GB and RF with two independent parameters 'Days' and 'Confirmed' concludes that RF with two parameters (RFP2) is far better than DTP2 and GBP2. The RFP2 is even better than DTP1 and GBP1. The accuracy metrics for DT, GB and RF with three independent parameters 'Days', 'Confirmed', and 'Cured' concludes that RFP3 is better than RFP2. Not only better than RFP2, it is also much better than DTP2 and GBP2 in every manner. If comparison is made among the three tree based algorithms then it can be easily seen that RF outperforms other two with a big difference. Even the RFP1 gives better results than DTP3 and GBP3 which shows that Random Forest is far better than the other two on all metrics.

The actual versus predicted deaths using DT, GB, and RF for one independent parameter is presented in Figure 7. In GBP1 curve, the two different curves show that there is a difference in actual and predicted deaths. The curves for the DTP1 and RFP1 overlap with each other and represent better accuracy as compared to

GBP1. Overall, RFP1 performs the best among the three if only one parameter is taken into consideration.

Figure 8 shows actual deaths vs. predicted deaths using DT, GB, and RF for two independent parameters. Here also same pattern can be observed very clearly where the two different curves can be quiet easily seen for GBP2 and signifies a low accuracy. For DTP1 and RFP1, the curves are almost overlapping with each other representing better accuracy as compared to GBP1. Overall, RFP1 performs best among the three on two parameters.

Figure 9 shows actual deaths vs. predicted deaths using DT, GB, and RF for three independent parameters. It can be clearly observed that RFP3 outperforms the other two.TheDTP3 performs better than GBP3 but not better than the RFP3.

Table 2. DT, GB, and RF models' evaluation with varying independent parameters

Model Used	Train R² Error	Test R² Error	Adjusted R²Error	RMSE	MAE
DT-P1	0.97	0.99	0.99	1260.49	711.97
DT-P2	0.97	0.99	0.99	1258.53	705.30
DT-P3	0.97	0.99	0.99	1257.78	706.72
GB-P1	0.95	0.99	0.99	3295.68	1848.32
GB-P2	0.95	0.99	0.99	3331.84	1874.18
GB-P3	0.95	0.99	0.99	3260.79	1836.51
RF-P1	0.98	0.99	0.99	735.19	383.41
RF-P2	0.987	0.99	0.99	589.50	277.56
RF-P3	0.98	0.99	0.99	544.90	248.99

Figure 7. Distribution of actual deaths and predicted deaths using DT, GB and RF on One Independent Parameter ['Days']

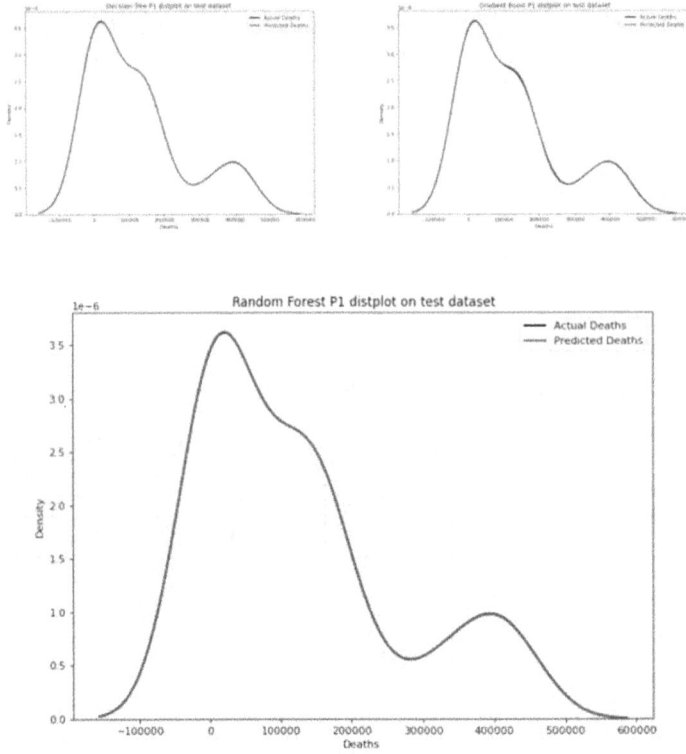

Figure 8. Distribution of actual deaths and predicted deaths using DT, GB and RF on Two Independent Parameter ['Days' and 'Confirmed']

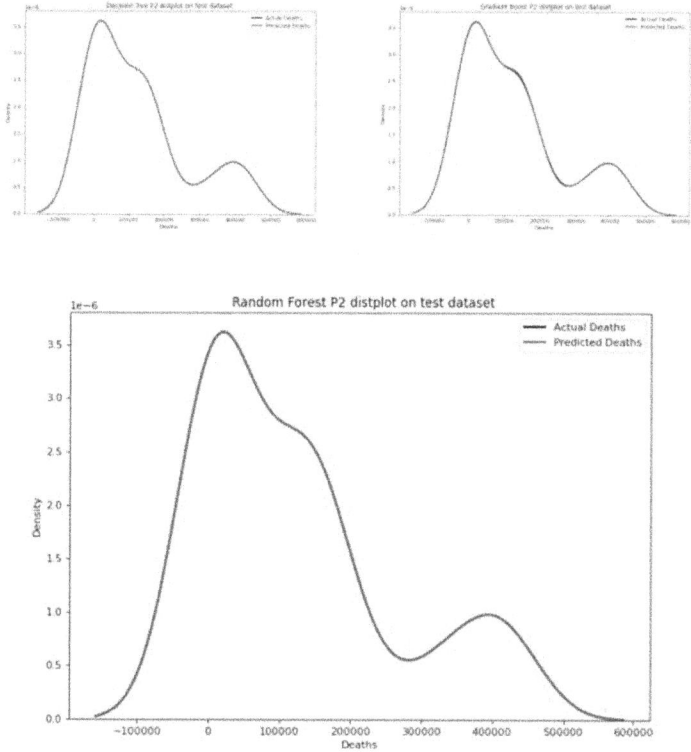

Figure 9. Distribution of actual deaths and predicted deaths using DT, GB and RF on Three Independent Parameter ['Days', 'Confirmed', and 'Cured']

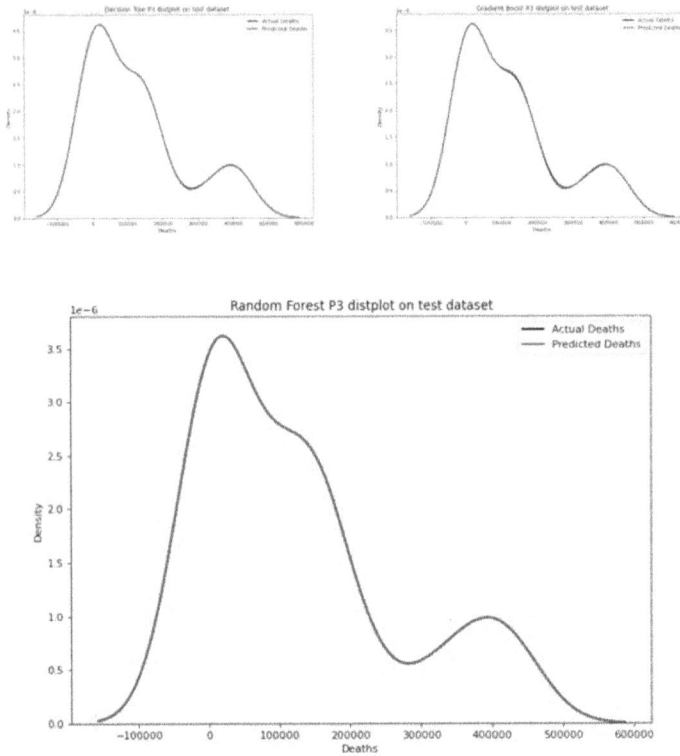

3.3 Comparison of Techniques

The performance of these techniques was evaluated using metrics such as R^2, RMSE, and MAE. Random Forest and KNN emerged as the top performers, demonstrating superior accuracy compared to other models. Random Forest achieved the best results due to its ensemble learning approach, which aggregates predictions from multiple decision trees to reduce overfitting and improve generalization. This method outperformed simpler models like LR and MLR, which struggled with the non-linearity and complexity of the data.

KNN also performed well due to its ability to adapt to local data structures and capture non-linear relationships without requiring explicit model assumptions. It showed lower RMSE and MAE values, indicating better predictive accuracy. Polynomial Regression, while effective at modeling non-linear trends, exhibited increased complexity with higher-degree polynomials and required careful selection of the polynomial degree to avoid overfitting.

Tree-based models, particularly Random Forest, provided robust predictions and high accuracy, surpassing Decision Trees and Gradient Boosting Trees in performance metrics. Random Forest's ability to aggregate predictions from multiple trees and manage high-dimensional data made it superior in handling the complex patterns of Covid-19 data.

So, the results of this section clearly indicate that simpler models like LR and MLR provide good baseline predictions but struggle to capture non-linear patterns in the data. PR models, particularly with high-degree polynomials, improve fit but at the cost of increased complexity. KNN offers flexibility in capturing local data structures but may become less effective as dimensionality increases. Among the ensemble methods, RF and GBT stand out for their ability to handle large, complex datasets with higher accuracy. RF, in particular, balances predictive power and interpretability, while GBT offers the highest accuracy but requires significant computational resources. Hence, Tree-based models, particularly Random Forest and Gradient Boosting Trees, consistently outperform simpler regression models in terms of accuracy, as evidenced by improved R2, RMSE, and MAE metrics. These models demonstrate superior adaptability to complex data patterns and variations in Covid-19 cases over time. These findings highlight the trade-offs between model complexity, accuracy, and computational efficiency in the context of Covid-19 data prediction.

3.4 Model Validation Hypotheses

Null hypotheses (H0): The sample mean i.e. the predicted output test dataset and population mean i.e. the actual output of test dataset are similar and it does not happen by chance. It means the fitted model is correct.

Alternative hypotheses (H1): The sample mean and the population mean differ significantly, and it does not happen by chance. The two dataset are different. It means the fitted model is not correct.

The logic of hypotheses testing follows a five step model which is as follow.

(1) It is assumed that the data is normally distributed.
(2) Direction of the test (one-tailed or two-tailed test)
(3) Deciding the significance level at which the statistical test should work. It is the chance that correct hypotheses will be rejected or the chances of rejecting true hypotheses. It is denoted with 'α'. On the other hand the chances of accepting a false hypothesis are denoted with 'β'.
(4) Then z-test or t-test is calculated as

$$Statistics\left(z,t\right) = \frac{x'-\mu}{\sigma/\sqrt{n}}$$

Where 'x'' is mean of sample, 'μ' is mean of population, 'σ' is standard deviation of population, and 'n' is number of observations.

A z-test is generally conducted when the sample size is more than 30 otherwise t-tests is more suitable. The t-distribution is more flat and tapering at the ends as compared to the z-distribution. When sample size is gradually increased then t-distribution becomes a z-distribution, the later is more normally distributed.

(5) Compare the Statistics(z, t) with critical value. The critical value can be found from the z-table or t-table.

The z-test statistics of some models is presented in Table 3. The z-test-value and p-value represent how better or close are the sample mean obtained from the model and population mean from the original dataset. A model provides very low values of the z-test-value (close to zero) and high values of p-value (close to 1). The z-test was conducted for 'α'=0.05 level of significance or 95% level of confidence. It is also evident from the Table-3 that all p-values are quite large than 'α' value that strongly supports the null hypotheses, and the predicted output generated by MLRP3, PRP3D3, DT-P3, GB-P3 and RF-P3 models are significantly similar to the original dataset.

Table 3. Independent sample z-test for the best metrics evaluated models

Sr.	Model	z-test-value	p-value	Outcome
1	PRP1D3	0.02218	0.9823	Same distribution (Fail to reject H0)
2	MLRP2	0.02799	0.9777	Same distribution (Fail to reject H0)
3	PRP2D3	0.02027	0.9838	Same distribution (Fail to reject H0)
4	MLRP3	0.0023	0.9981	Same distribution (Fail to reject H0)
5	PRP3D3	0.0092	0.9926	Same distribution (Fail to reject H0)
6	DT-P3	0.0084	0.9936	Same distribution (Fail to reject H0)
7	GB-P3	0.0076	0.9925	Same distribution (Fail to reject H0)
8	RF-P3	0.0062	0.9954	Same distribution (Fail to reject H0)

4. CONCLUSIONS AND FUTURE SCOPE

The work presented in this chapter predicts death-statistics due to Covid-19 in India using LR, MLR, PR, KNN, Lasso, Ridge regression, Decision Tree, Random Forest, and Gradient Boost Tree. The Covid-19 dataset of India (Https://www.kaggle .com/sudalairajkumar/covid19-in-india, n.d.)is analyzed, pre-processed and then used for modeling in Python using machine learning library 'sklearn'. The fitted models are evaluated for accuracy using train evaluation metrics R^2, RMSE, and MAE and the adjusted-R^2 cross-validation prediction test error. The chapter analyses eight regression algorithms on varying predictors and selects the best models from each algorithm using best subset selection for predictors that best predicts the covid-19 statistics. The multi-linear regression model best-fits the dataset when all parameters are used in modeling. The polynomial modeling is best to represent curvilinear relationship. However, the PR models best-fit the dataset using high degree polynomials when fewer parameters are used. The PR models best-fit the dataset using low degree polynomial when more parameters are used in modeling. The complexity of equations fitting high degree polynomials rises quickly with each increase in degree. However, the KNN models outperform all the regression models. The tree based algorithms have better accuracies over the earlier algorithms. The random forest performs better than the decision tree and gradient boost tree. The decision tree has better accuracy than the gradient boost trees.

TheCovid-19 dataset used in this chapter, as well as many other available datasets of many countries have been continuously increasing in size. It has been felt that loading time of the dataset is quite large and the processing also takes significant time. Loading and processing time may be improved by parallel loading and processing of the distributed data using distributed parallel processing technologies such as the Hadoop or Spark technologies (Sewal & Singh, 2022; Singh & Bawa, 2016, 2017, 2019).

REFERENCES

AL-Rousan, N., & AL-Najjar, H.. (2020). Data analysis of coronavirus COVID-19 epidemic in South Korea based on recovered and death cases. *Journal of Medical Virology*, 92(9), 1603–1608. DOI: 10.1002/jmv.25850 PMID: 32270521

Arora, P., Kumar, H., & Panigrahi, B. K. (2020). Prediction and analysis of COVID-19 positive cases using deep learning models: A descriptive case study of India. *Chaos, Solitons, and Fractals*, 139, 110017. Advance online publication. DOI: 10.1016/j.chaos.2020.110017 PMID: 32572310

ArunKumar, K. E., Kalaga, D. V., Kumar, C. M. S., Chilkoor, G., Kawaji, M., & Brenza, T. M. (2021). Forecasting the dynamics of cumulative COVID-19 cases (confirmed, recovered and deaths) for top-16 countries using statistical machine learning models: Auto-Regressive Integrated Moving Average (ARIMA) and Seasonal Auto-Regressive Integrated Moving Average (SARIMA). *Applied Soft Computing*, 103, 107161.

Basu, S., & Campbell, R. H. (2020). Going by the numbers: Learning and modeling COVID-19 disease dynamics. *Chaos, Solitons, and Fractals*, 138, 110140. DOI: 10.1016/j.chaos.2020.110140 PMID: 32834585

Behnood, A., Mohammadi Golafshani, E., & Hosseini, S. M. (2020). Determinants of the infection rate of the COVID-19 in the U.S. using ANFIS and virus optimization algorithm (VOA). *Chaos, Solitons, and Fractals*, 139, 110051. DOI: 10.1016/j.chaos.2020.110051 PMID: 32834605

Çakan, S. (2020). Dynamic analysis of a mathematical model with health care capacity for COVID-19 pandemic. *Chaos, Solitons, and Fractals*, 139, 110033. Advance online publication. DOI: 10.1016/j.chaos.2020.110033 PMID: 32834594

Chimmula, V. K. R., & Zhang, L. (2020). Time series forecasting of COVID-19 transmission in Canada using LSTM networks. *Chaos, Solitons, and Fractals*, 135, 109864. Advance online publication. DOI: 10.1016/j.chaos.2020.109864 PMID: 32390691

Correction, S. E. E., & This, F. O. R. (2022). *Evaluation of individual and ensemble probabilistic forecasts of COVID-19 mortality in the United States*. 119(15). https://doi.org/DOI: 10.1073/pnas.2113561119/-/DCSupplemental.Published

Cui, S., Wang, Y., Wang, D., Sai, Q., Huang, Z., & Cheng, T. C. E. (2021). A two-layer nested heterogeneous ensemble learning predictive method for COVID-19 mortality. *Applied Soft Computing*, 113, 107946. DOI: 10.1016/j.asoc.2021.107946 PMID: 34646110

Frank, E., Trigg, L., Holmes, G., & Witten, I. H. (2000). Technical note: Naive Bayes for regression. *Machine Learning*, 41(1), 5–25. DOI: 10.1023/A:1007670802811

Ghosal, S., Sengupta, S., Majumder, M., & Sinha, B. (2020). Linear Regression Analysis to predict the number of deaths in India due to SARS-CoV-2 at 6 weeks from day 0 (100 cases - March 14th 2020). *Diabetes & Metabolic Syndrome*, 14(January), 311–315. DOI: 10.1016/j.dsx.2020.03.017 PMID: 32298982

Hoseinpour Dehkordi, A., Alizadeh, M., Derakhshan, P., Babazadeh, P., & Jahandideh, A. (2020). Understanding epidemic data and statistics: A case study of COVID-19. *Journal of Medical Virology*, 92(7), 868–882. DOI: 10.1002/jmv.25885 PMID: 32329522

Kamalov, F., Cherukuri, A. K., & Thabtah, F. (2022). Machine learning applications to Covid-19: a state-of-the-art survey. *2022 Advances in Science and Engineering Technology International Conferences, ASET 2022*, 1–6. DOI: 10.1109/ASET53988.2022.9734959

Kamalov, F., Rajab, K., Cherukuri, A. K., Elnagar, A., & Safaraliev, M. (2022). Deep learning for Covid-19 forecasting: State-of-the-art review. *Neurocomputing*, 511, 142–154. DOI: 10.1016/j.neucom.2022.09.005 PMID: 36097509

Luo, G., & Gao, S. J. (2020). Global health concerns stirred by emerging viral infections. *Journal of Medical Virology*, 92(4), 399–400. DOI: 10.1002/jmv.25683 PMID: 31967329

Malki, Z., Atlam, E. S., Hassanien, A. E., Dagnew, G., Elhosseini, M. A., & Gad, I. (2020). Association between weather data and COVID-19 pandemic predicting mortality rate: Machine learning approaches. *Chaos, Solitons, and Fractals*, 138, 110137. DOI: 10.1016/j.chaos.2020.110137 PMID: 32834583

Myint, S. H. (1994). Human coronaviruses: A brief review. *Reviews in Medical Virology*, 4(1), 35–46. DOI: 10.1002/rmv.1980040108

Nabi, K. N. (2020). Forecasting COVID-19 pandemic: A data-driven analysis. *Chaos, Solitons, and Fractals*, 139, 110046. DOI: 10.1016/j.chaos.2020.110046 PMID: 32834601

Nayak, J., Naik, B., Dinesh, P., Vakula, K., Dash, P. B., & Pelusi, D. (2022). Significance of deep learning for Covid-19: State-of-the-art review. *Research on Biomedical Engineering*, 38(1), 243–266. DOI: 10.1007/s42600-021-00135-6

Https://www.kaggle.com/sudalairajkumar/covid19-in-india. (n.d.). *Covid-19 in India.*

Ostertagová, E. (2012, December). Modelling using polynomial regression. *Procedia Engineering*, 48, 500–506. DOI: 10.1016/j.proeng.2012.09.545

Peng, Y., & Nagata, M. H. (2020). An empirical overview of nonlinearity and overfitting in machine learning using COVID-19 data. *Chaos, Solitons, and Fractals*, 139, 110055. Advance online publication. DOI: 10.1016/j.chaos.2020.110055 PMID: 32834608

Prieto, K. (2022). Current forecast of COVID-19 in Mexico: A Bayesian and machine learning approaches. *PLoS ONE, 17*(1 January), 1–21. DOI: 10.1371/journal.pone.0259958

Rahimi, I., Chen, F., & Gandomi, A. H. (2023). A review on COVID-19 forecasting models. *Neural Computing & Applications*, 35(33), 23671–23681. DOI: 10.1007/s00521-020-05626-8 PMID: 33564213

Rath, S., Tripathy, A., & Tripathy, A. R. (2020). Prediction of new active cases of coronavirus disease (COVID-19) pandemic using multiple linear regression model. *Diabetes & Metabolic Syndrome*, 14(5), 1467–1474. DOI: 10.1016/j.dsx.2020.07.045 PMID: 32771920

Sewal, P., & Singh, H. (2022). A Machine Learning Approach for Predicting Execution Statistics of Spark Application. *PDGC 2022 - 2022 7th International Conference on Parallel, Distributed and Grid Computing*, 331–336. DOI: 10.1109/PDGC56933.2022.10053356

Sewal, P., & Singh, H. (2023). Analyzing distributed Spark MLlib regression algorithms for accuracy, execution efficiency and scalability using best subset selection approach. *Multimedia Tools and Applications*, 0123456789(15), 44047–44066. Advance online publication. DOI: 10.1007/s11042-023-17330-5

Sewal, P., & Singh, H. (2024). Performance Comparison of Apache Spark and Hadoop for machine learning based iterative GBTR on HIGGS and Covid-19 datasets. *Scalable Computing: Practice and Experience*, 25(3), 1373–1386. DOI: 10.12694/scpe.v25i3.2687

Shinde, G. R., Kalamkar, A. B., Mahalle, P. N., Dey, N., Chaki, J., & Hassanien, A. E. (2020). Forecasting Models for Coronavirus Disease (COVID-19): A Survey of the State-of-the-Art. *SN Computer Science*, 1(4), 197. Advance online publication. DOI: 10.1007/s42979-020-00209-9 PMID: 33063048

Singh, H., & Bawa, S. (2016). IGSIM : An Integrated Architecture for High Performance Spatial Data Analysis. [IJCSIS]. *International Journal of Computer Science and Information Security*, 14(11), 302–309.

Singh, H., & Bawa, S. (2017). A mapreduce-based efficient H-bucket PMR quadtree spatial index. *Computer Systems Science and Engineering*, 32(5), 405–415.

Singh, H., & Bawa, S. (2019). An improved integrated Grid and MapReduce-Hadoop architecture for spatial data: Hilbert TGS R-Tree-based IGSIM. *Concurrency and Computation*, 31(17), e5202. https://doi.org/https://doi.org/10.1002/cpe.5202. DOI: 10.1002/cpe.5202

Singh, H., & Bawa, S. (2022). Predicting COVID-19 statistics using machine learning regression model: Li-MuLi-Poly. *Multimedia Systems*, 28(1), 113–120. DOI: 10.1007/s00530-021-00798-2 PMID: 33976474

Singhal, A., Singh, P., Lall, B., & Joshi, S. D. (2020). Modeling and prediction of COVID-19 pandemic using Gaussian mixture model. *Chaos, Solitons, and Fractals*, 138, 110023. DOI: 10.1016/j.chaos.2020.110023 PMID: 32565627

Sun, J., Chen, X., Zhang, Z., Lai, S., Zhao, B., Liu, H., Wang, S., Huan, W., Zhao, R., Ng, M. T. A., & Zheng, Y. (2020). Forecasting the long-term trend of COVID-19 epidemic using a dynamic model. *Scientific Reports*, 10(1), 1–10. DOI: 10.1038/s41598-020-78084-w PMID: 33273592

Wang, W., Tang, J., & Wei, F. (2020). Updated understanding of the outbreak of 2019 novel coronavirus (2019-nCoV) in Wuhan, China. *Journal of Medical Virology*, 92(4), 441–447. DOI: 10.1002/jmv.25689 PMID: 31994742

Wikipedia. T. free encyclopedia. (n.d.). *Covid-19 pandemic lockdown in India*. Https://En.Wikipedia.Org/Wiki/COVID-19_pandemic_lockdown_in_India#Unlock_1.0_(1%E2%80%9330_June)

Worldometer. (2022). Https://Www.Worldometers.Info/Coronavirus/Country/India/

Yudistira, N., Sumitro, S. B., Nahas, A., & Riama, N. F. (2021). Learning where to look for COVID-19 growth: Multivariate analysis of COVID-19 cases over time using explainable convolution–LSTM. *Applied Soft Computing*, 109, 107469. DOI: 10.1016/j.asoc.2021.107469 PMID: 33994895

Chapter 12
Design Principles for Chronic Disease Self–Management Systems:
A Technical Investigation Based on the Characteristics of Digital Technologies

Kourosh Dadgar
https://orcid.org/0009-0000-5297-2651
University of San Francisco, USA

K. D. Joshi
University of Nevada, Reno, USA

ABSTRACT

The use and design of digital technologies for the self-management of chronic diseases are increasing. Self-management systems designed without theoretically driven design principles are ineffective and inconsistent. This chapter proposes design principles based on the characteristics of the digital technologies: (1) re-programmability, (2) homogenization of data, and (3) self-referential nature. The design principles are instantiated in a diabetes mobile app and illustrated in use case diagrams. The proposed principles increase the projectability of system design principles and simplify the complexity of the problem space for ICT-enabled self-management systems.

DOI: 10.4018/979-8-3693-5237-3.ch012

1. INTRODUCTION

"It is a mistake to suppose that any technological innovation has a one-sided effect. Every technology is both a burden and a blessing."
(Harvey 1990, pp. 4–5)

The use of emerging and advanced digital technologies such as AI (Artificial Intelligence) assistants and conversational agents, tools, and apps have fundamentally changed healthcare management of chronic diseases and conditions such as diabetes, pain, heart problems, asthma, mental disorders. Patients have taken an active role in their care process and perform health self-management (SM) activities and tasks in close collaboration with their care providers and with immediate access to a plethora of information about their diseases and conditions. From glucose-monitoring Google glasses to intelligent mobile health apps, tech firms are constantly designing technologies to improve, automate, and streamline health management. For instance, more than 165,000 health-related apps have been designed for the Android and iOS platforms with an estimated 1.7 billion downloads. The market share for mobile health apps reached the $21.5 billion market share in 2018. These apps improve management of chronic diseases and conditions by providing continuous long-term monitoring capabilities. Tech companies design SM systems for patients with chronic diseases to manage their health on a daily basis. Medtronic, allied with IBM's Watson, has designed an app that collects and analyzes data from multiple sources, such as insulin pumps, glucose monitors, and activity trackers, to predict three hours in advance when a patient will have high or low levels of blood sugar. Studies show that, for the first time, AI-enabled mobile health apps could become the preferred resource over physicians.

New technologies change the social and personal structures and create needs and relationships with our surroundings (Harvey 1990, p. 20). These changes are often imposed upon communities, societies, and individuals and their benefits and impact are not effectively and purposefully managed or designed. Advancement in digital artifacts alone is not sufficient for these technologies to act as vital resources, unless their power is harnessed to alter and improve SM (LeRouge et al. 2007). These technologies need to be used to design SM systems that empower patients to engage in their care and support their behavioral changes (Lamprinos et al. 2016; Vuong et al. 2012). In order for these new tools to enable patient empowerment, rather than act as instruments aimed at solely improving clinical outcomes, a critical perceptive is necessary to create design principles that are sensitive to the patients' values. Applying a value-centric patient perspective at a time when digital technologies for SM are emerging will ensure that the central role that patients and the social structures around them play in the care process is not drowned out by the more dominant outcome-based clinical perspective (Dadgar and Joshi 2018; Koch et al. 2004).

There is a lack of patient-centric approaches for investigating and designing e-health systems (Cummings and Turner 2009) and identifying the effective digital capabilities of SM activities (Bailey et al. 2013), such as symptom management, medication management, and management of psychological consequences imposed by the chronic diseases, that are sensitive to the values of patients (Schulman-Green et al. 2012). When patients with chronic diseases and conditions use information and communication technologies (ICTs) to perform SM activities, it is known as ICT-enabled SM. The lack of design principles adds to the complexity of the ICT-enabled SM process and reduces the projectability (Baskerville and Pries-Heje 2014) of effective SM designs. This book chapter investigates this issue by proposing design principles that are projectable into operational instantiations of SM systems and can simplify the complexity of designing and using effective ICT-enabled SM systems.

The main objective of the book chapter is to propose a set of design principles for the designs and features of SM systems and technologies based on SM theories and informed by the unique properties of digital technologies that help patients with chronic diseases (the digitized individuals) in performing their SM activities and self-managing their chronic health conditions and diseases. Such design principles are patient-centric and support patients' needs as humans rather than users and mere clinical patients receiving treatments from care providers. The proposed design principles fully integrate the capabilities and functionalities of digital technologies in supporting SM activities. The functional features of the design principles are conceptually illustrated in use-case diagrams.

The SM systems designed and conceptualized based on digital technologies have four limitations. *First*, the system solutions do not fully and granularly engage the digital artifact to leverage the inherent characteristics of digital technologies and their potential for the SM of chronic diseases (McDermott and While 2013), which in turn hinders the projectability of such systems for other similar SM systems (Baskerville and Pries-Heje 2014). *Second*, the design and development of the SM systems are not theoretically driven, which results in ineffective SM (Jacelon et al. 2016). *Third*, SM literature fails to offer design principles that could systematically guide the development of SM systems (Jacelon et al. 2016; Lamprinos et al. 2016), and this adds to the complexity of ICT-enabled SM systems. *Fourth*, the existing design guidelines are not sensitive to the values and needs of the patients with chronic diseases and conditions (Dadgar and Joshi 2017, 2018). The proposed design principles address these gaps. They are grounded in theory and are tightly coupled with the salient characteristics of the digital technologies and SM activities they support and do not apply to only a specific SM system, such as glucose meters for diabetic people, but can be used to design a class of SM systems developed based on digital technologies. These design principles are instantiated and implicated in a mobile diabetes app.

2. THE INDIVIDUAL AND FAMILY SELF-MANAGEMENT (IFSM) THEORY

The SM design principles in this chapter are theoretically derived from the individual and family self-management (IFSM) theory which states SM can be enhanced through three major components of the SM process (Ryan and Sawin 2009): (1) *knowledge and beliefs*, (2) *self-regulation skills and abilities*, and (3) *social facilitation*. This theory posits that fostering, increasing, and enhancing these three components drives patients to change their health behaviors and engage in SM behaviors and activities (referred to as "proximal outcome") and improve their health (referred to as "distant outcome") (Ryan 2009).

Within the *knowledge and beliefs* component of the SM process, patients search information to gain knowledge about their disease and health conditions that are unknown to them at the onset of their disease. They need instructional information and informational resources to perform their SM activities such as using medical devices to medicate themselves, comply with the treatments and medications prescribed by their care providers, or avoid medical and food interactions. Fostering patients' knowledge and beliefs in understanding their disease and its characteristics, its lifestyle changes, and the management of its chronic daily symptoms, allows them to understand their condition and manage the anxiety, confusion, stress, and fear that it causes. With relieved stress and better understanding, patients gain confidence to manage their new behavioral and psychological changes and achieve positive outcomes in their SM activities.

Within the *self-regulation skills and abilities* component of the SM process, patients learn and practice SM skills to control and regulate their chronic health conditions and achieve clinical health outcomes. Patients perform these routine self-management activities in their daily lives by learning how to change their behavior and life style adapting to their health conditions. The SM skills and abilities include a wide range of practices such as monitoring and controlling physiological and psychological symptoms, using medical devices, and administration of treatments and medications. Supporting and training patients with these essential SM skills and abilities helps patients with their behavior change and achieving positive health outcomes.

Social facilitation includes both social influence and social support. Patients with chronic diseases and conditions experience confusing and surprising life changes that they must live with every day. These changes affect their relationships with their family members, partners, relatives, and friends. Emotional social support empowers patients to stay hopeful and strong in facing the consequences of their disease. Motivational and caring social influence that comes from care providers such as physicians and nurses encourage patients to psychologically live a quality life while managing their health conditions. In the lack of social influence and support patients face overwhelming pressure to manage their chronic disruptive health conditions which leads to depressions, loneliness, anxiety, and frustration.

3. DIGITAL TECHNOLOGIES

Innovative advancement in digital technologies including GenAI (Generative artificial intelligence) and AGI (Artificial General Intelligence) and their recent developments have fundamentally changed the ways patients manage their health conditions in their daily lives. Modularity and miniaturization of digital tools and devices have streamlined the development of applications and services to empower patients in their SM. The assemblage of advances sensing technologies with micro services and architectures connected with APIs (Application Programming Interface) have significantly assisted patients in managing their health. Healthcare mobile apps have similarly benefited from these advancements in digital technologies. For diabetic patients, these apps provide tracking and estimation capabilities to manage their blood glucose levels which help with patients' treatment adherences and medication administration. It is based the unique modular and flexible structure of advanced digital technologies and their components that digital products are designed to provide variety of services and support different needs of their users (Yoo et al. 2010). Hence these digital products can be programmed to provide unique services, are able to sense and collect a variety of data types, and can be all interconnected. These unique characteristics of digital technologies are: (1) *re-programmability*, (2) *homogenization of data*, and (3) *self-referential nature* (Yoo et al. 2010).

Re-programmability creates computing and processing capabilities in digital technologies to store, manage, and share data in an unlimited number of ways and generate functionalities to analyze a variety of structured and unstructured data types. Compared with the first generation of file processing systems, digital technologies' data manipulation capabilities are more adaptive and extensible. The *homogenization of data* integrates a variety of data types from diverse external and internal sources that can be accessed by most efficient data processes. Data and system integration capabilities consolidate heterogenous data ingestions and digestions into one effective service that can meet and target specific needs. And *Self-referential nature* of digital technologies distributes their pervasive capabilities, democratizes their accessibility, and enables their simultaneous use. With these structural capabilities of digital technologies novel services and products should be designed in which different micro services and architectures can be integrated, reused, managed, and packaged based on the collection, processing, and sharing of digital data. Based on these inherent characteristics of digital technologies this book chapter proposes theoretically driven design principles for SM systems that maximize the potential services and features can be utilized in supporting SM of chronic diseases and conditions.

4. THE INTEGRATIVE GUIDING MODEL

Digital design principles are theoretically informed guidelines for designing digital technologies and systems. In this book chapter three design principles are proposed based on the characteristics of digital technologies and informed by the IFSM theory to guide the design and development of SM systems and their features, services, and capabilities (Figure 1). The proposed design principles are sensitized to the values and desires of patients with chronic diseases and conditions who are central in the success, effectiveness, and continuous use of SM systems.

Figure 1. Design principles for an SM system derived from the characteristics of digital technology, the SM theory of IFSMT, and the VSD (value-sensitive design) framework

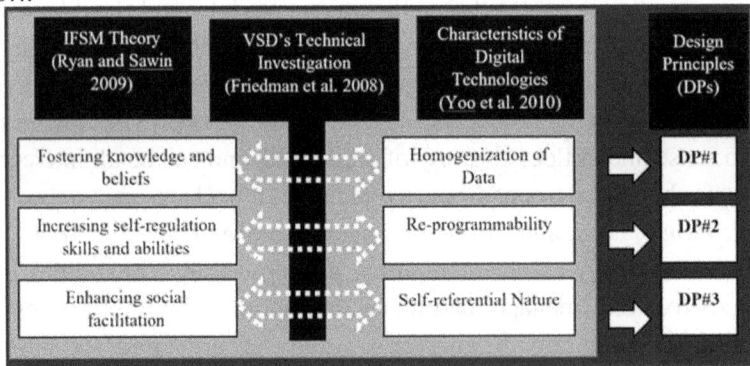

Sources: (Yoo et al., 2010); (Ryan & Sawin, 2009); (Friedman et al., 2008)

The main design outcome for the proposed design principles is to support and facilitate SM processes and activities enabled by the characteristics of digital technologies and within a layered architecture in which data (content layer) are homogenized, re-programmed, and shared to create new functionalities (service layer) within a network of connected technologies (network layer) (Yoo et al. 2010).

These layers are modular, so they can be combined to create technologies in an infinite number of ways.

In digital technologies, homogenized data are integrated into one system that is composed of multiple data sources. Patients with chronic diseases need to collect different kinds of informational data, vital signs, blood glucose levels, and blood pressure, from multiple peripheral devices, such as scales, blood pressure devices, and glucose-monitoring systems, and have immediate access to data in one system. Data integrated in one system fosters the knowledge and beliefs of patients about their disease, treatments, medications, and symptoms. Therefore, according to design principle 1, the characteristic of *homogenization of data* fosters *knowledge and beliefs* by integrating and homogenizing data from multiple sources and providing immediate access to knowledge and information at any time and location.

Re-programmability of a digital technology allows for data manipulation and understanding of data relationships (Yoo et al. 2010). Patients with chronic diseases need to manage and process data and interpret their meanings and relationships to self-regulate data recording, monitoring, and symptom management into daily (Bu et al. 2007). Therefore, according to design principle 2, the characteristic of *re-programmability* increases *self-regulation skills and abilities* by allowing patients to manipulate data, interpret data relationships, and integrate tracking and monitoring abilities in their daily lives. The *self-referential nature* of digital technology enables users to communicate through a network of multiple users with the help of similar digital technologies (Yoo et al. 2010). Patients with chronic diseases need to communicate with their healthcare providers, family members and friends, and other patients to seek support (Bodenheimer et al. 2002). Therefore, according to design principle 3, the *self-referential nature* of digital technologies enhances *social facilitation* by creating a network of devices used by patients, healthcare providers, family members, and other patients.

5. VALUE-SENSITIVE TECHNICAL INVESTIGATION

Semi-structured interview data has been collected from patients with diabetes to sensitize design principles to the values and desires of the patients with chronic diseases and conditions using SM systems in managing their conditions (Dadgar and Joshi 2018). The intensity of patients' values may vary across chronic diseases however their importance in SM of chronic diseases and conditions will be consistent. Interview data from 20 patients with diabetes have been collected. First, patients are trained to use a popular diabetes mobile app, Glucose Buddy, for their diabetes management. Next, patients are instructed to use the app for at least 7 days while keeping a journal of their experience (values and desires) using the app. In the last step, patients return for a semi-structured interview to report and reflect on their experience using the app. Interview data is analyzed to identify the patterns and instances of the patients' values, and their relationships with app features and functionalities, the components of IFSMT theory, and SM activities.

5.1. Coding Process

The coding of the interview data is performed based on the coding strategies recommended by Miles and Huberman (1994), and the analysis of the coded data is based on the principles proposed by Klein and Myers (1999). Interview data has been extracted in such a way that the linkage between using *systems features*, supporting *SM activities* and fulfilling patients' *values* is evident. These instances of system features, SM activities, and values are then mapped to the characteristics of digital technologies, theoretical SM components, and value definitions (Dadgar and Joshi 2018). The following patient data are extracted from interview data where the linkage between using system features (data retrieval), performing SM activities (information usage) and fulfilling the value of *accessibility* is evident:

"You can search for foods in here and it'll just like search. You can search for, let's just do a hamburger and so in here it'll have different brands of hamburgers. It'll have like the menu items already in there so it'll have like the carbohydrate counts. In here, let's just select this one. It'll say carbs thirty. That's, like I said, that's what you take the insulin based on. Then you can check and it adds it, and you can just add as many as you want in here"

In the extracted quote above, a patient needs to retrieve data (*data retrieval*) to have immediate access (value of *accessibility*) to information about carbs (*information usage*) in order to self-manage her diabetes. Once such linkages between instances of system features, SM activities, and values are saturated, they are projected to their relevant digital characteristics, SM components, and value definitions. In this example, data retrieval allows the patient to integrate information about carbs and insulin data into one platform (the digital characteristic of *homogenization of data*). The patient uses the information about carbs to manage insulin use and therefore self-manage his/her diabetes (this reflects the SM component *fostering knowledge and beliefs*). The immediate availability of data allows the patient to use information in a timely manner (the value of *accessibility*).

6. DESIGN PRINCIPLES

Design Principle #1 – Data Integrability: *"SM systems should be designed to foster the knowledge and beliefs of patient-users and support the value of accessibility by homogenizing data from multiple sources and providing access to informational resources about the disease, its treatments and medication when and where a patient seeks an answer to a question or a solution to a problem during the conduct of SM."*

The *homogenization of data* characteristic of digital technologies provides an architectural capacity to integrate a variety of data types from multiple sources into one central system to provide micro services and features to the users of such systems. Systems are integrated within the ecosystem of SM to exchange data. A mobile app, Fitbit, and an insulin meter communicate and exchange data in diabetes SM. In the course of SM, particularly after diagnosis, patients have many unanswered questions and concerns about their disease and seek answers to their problems. Patients with chronic diseases obtain and use information on a daily basis to manage their symptoms, medication, treatments, and feelings. A SM system should facilitate obtaining, using, managing, and accessing necessary data between different devices and information sources for the patients. The diabetic patients take medication to lower their blood glucose levels. First, they need to obtain readings from the glucose meter, which stores blood glucose measurements. Next, the pump that injects insulin doses communicates with the meter to estimate the amount of insulin needed for certain levels of blood glucose. As the patients store their medication data for symptom management, they rely on it to understand the side effects of the diabetes drugs or the interaction effects of their diabetes medication with other medications. Providing critical medical, treatment, and drug data in an instantly available, retrievable, and accessible way (value of accessibility).

After diagnosis, understanding different medical terms and acronyms is challenging for the patient in the absence of any prior experience in SM of a chronic disease. Therefore, the medical terms displayed to a patient should be hyperlinked to relevant informational resources (e.g., online Internet resources) that provide detailed explanations. Using medical devices to self-manage chronic diseases needs practice and patience. Providing instructional videos that demonstrate the proper use of medical devices enhances medication management. Immediate access to information when and where a patient faces a challenge or problem in the conduct of SM fosters a patient's knowledge about the disease and increases the understanding and self-efficacy of the patient in achieving SM goals.

Design Principle #2 – System Flexibility: *"SM systems should be designed to increase the self-regulation skills and abilities of patient-users and support the values of accountability, compliance, and sense-making by facilitating data ma-*

nipulation when and where a patient has to make decisions, plan, and self-monitor during the conduct of SM."

The *re-programmability* characteristic of digital technologies enables system designers and architects to provide flexible system capabilities and features for the users to process and transform the presentation and organization of the data to be more interpretable and digestible. Patients with chronic diseases constantly monitor their measurement data (the levels of blood glucose and food calories and carbs), make data-driven decisions, and plan for food and lifestyle changes based on their recorded measurement data. Patients with chronic diseases should be able to manipulate and transform data recorded in their SM systems when they need to make data-driven decisions and plans. Providing data that can be easily interpreted by patients supports the value of sense-making. Easy interpretation of the data allows patients to comply with medical treatments and procedures (value of compliance). Patients who comply with their medical treatments and can easily interpret medical data will be accountable for SM of their chronic disease (value of accountability).

Clear relationships between different kinds of data points enable patient-users to make autonomous decisions during the conduct of SM. For instance, when a diabetic patient goes to a restaurant, she can look up the calories in the SM system for each kind of food that she will. With the introduction of new iPhone 16 model's Apple Intelligence, such features will be available simply by pointing the camera at the food item and receiving its calorie information on the phone. Next, she needs to know if the calories contained in the food will affect her blood sugar levels. Using digital technologies, such as mobile platforms and apps, she can calculate the number of food calories, the associated glucose levels, visualize the data in charts and graphs, and monitor her symptoms before and after food intake.

Flexible and customizable digital architectures enable the development and design of stackable and modular system features and capabilities. Using a diabetes mobile app, patients with chronic diseases will be able to customize the normal ranges of blood glucose that best fit their lifestyle and physiological conditions. Patients can set up individualized alarms and reminders if their measurement data exceed certain thresholds. Using reprogrammable and flexible digital technologies for SM systems, patients with chronic diseases can integrate planning, decision making, and monitoring of their symptoms into their daily lives to make the necessary behavior changes.

Design Principle #3 – System Externality: "*SM systems should be designed to enhance the social facilitation of patient-users and support the value of empathy by connecting patients with human support when and where a patient has to communicate, share, and seek social support during the conduct of SM.*"

The *self-referential nature* of a digital technologies enables a platform-agnostic interoperability that transcends time and location and gains network externality that exponentially benefits users and their goals. Such networks of users and platforms are cost-effective and facilitate and streamline communications and data sharing. Using social networking features, patients share their feelings and needs regardless of time and location, which allows other patients to understand the feelings and emotions of someone who is affected by the chronic disease (value of empathy).

Democratized use of digital technologies benefits patients with chronic diseases. They can seek emotional and motivational support from family, friends, and other patients with the same conditions. They can communicate their needs and questions in real time with their healthcare providers. The patients diagnosed with diabetes struggle with many emotionally and psychologically intense conditions. The availability of immediate contact and communication with a healthcare provider would be valuable to the patients to make meaning out of the new changes caused by their health conditions. Family members of a patient with a chronic disease can co-monitor the patients' symptoms and their SM performance by sharing same data views and dashboards with each other. Digital communities of patients with the same chronic diseases and similar illnesses are places where they can share their feelings, identify with other patients, and exchange experiences. Thus, by using digital technologies in SM systems, patients can have access to human support in real time, control and lessen their negative feelings, and remain motivated in performing SM activities.

7. DIABETES MANAGEMENT APPS

Diabetes is the most prevalent chronic disease and the SM mobile apps designed for diabetic patients abound in the app market place. Therefore, we choose to analyze a diabetes SM app to illustrate the applicability and efficacy of the three design principles proposed in this chapter. Table 1 shows the SM activities supported by the functionalities designed in the diabetes app of Glucose Buddy (GB). GB is the most popular and the oldest free diabetes mobile app in the Apple and Android app stores with the highest number of users and rating score. The GB's architecture as a template to instantiate and represent the proposed design principles of *data integrability*, *system flexibility*, and *system externality*. The GB's functionalities and capabilities are extended where they fall short to fully represent the proposed design principles.

Table 1. SM activities supported by GB diabetes mobile app

System Implications	Supported SM activities
1) Logbook: recording and tracking measurement date for blood sugar, food carbs, weight, activity, blood pressure, heart rate, medicine, and A1C.	- Symptom management: monitor and manage the symptoms of the chronic disease - Lifestyle management: modify lifestyle to adapt to the disease
2) Graph: visualizing measurement data over time	- Symptom management: monitor and manage the symptoms of the chronic disease - Lifestyle management: modify lifestyle to adapt to the disease - Communication: communicate SM progress with healthcare providers
3) Reminders: reminders to take medication or test blood sugar.	- Medication management: take medication and adhere to the medication routines.
4) Forum: posting, replying, and reading about diabetes.	- Management of psychological consequences: manage negative emotions and feelings of the disease - Social support: obtain and manage support from family, friends, and other patients.

The patients with chronic diseases use logbook to record their measurement data of blood sugar, food carbs and calories. Recording these data points have two benefits for the patients during the conduct of SM. First, it enables them to monitor ups and downs and ranges of their blood sugar. Second, it encourages and informs patients to make changes in their lifestyle and behavior where eating foods with high calories and carbs are causing high levels of blood sugar. Graphing measurement data is an effective way to monitor the symptoms and make necessary lifestyle changes. Graphs facilitate communication between patients and healthcare providers when they report their SM progress and results of controlling their blood sugar. Reminders are mainly used to take the medication at the right time. It is tightly connected with symptom management because dosage and type of medicine depends on the levels of blood sugar. Discussion forums are the venues for the patients to relieve their stress and anxiety and share their emotions and feelings with other patients with similar conditions. Digital forums enable patients to seek informational and emotional support.

Figure 2 illustrates the overall architecture of the GB diabetes app and shows the interactions between patient and the app where different functionalities are activated and used.

Figure 2. The architecture of the GB mobile app and its interactions with user

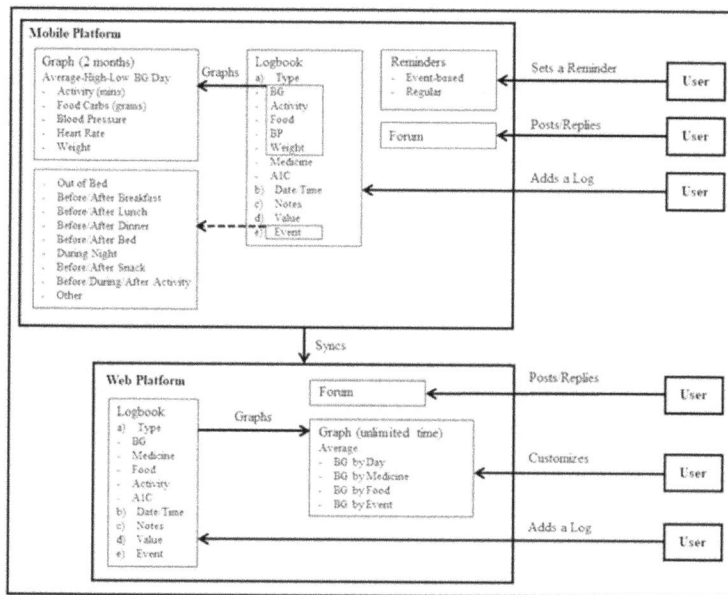

The GB diabetes app's architecture operates between the app's mobile and web-based layers. Data is synced between these two layers. The web-based platform provides additional features such as customizable graphs. Logbook, graphs, reminders, and forum are the main functionalities. Patients add log entries in the logbook. Average of certain measurement data with their highs and lows over time and during the day are graphed on the mobile platform for 2-month periods. On the web platform, there is no time limit for graphing the data points. Data points can be associated with events such as breakfast, dinner, and snack. Patients can set reminders to take medication or test their blood glucose and visit discussion forums online and, on the web, to read and respond to different categories of the topics related to diabetes management.

Use case diagrams are used to represent the GB's architectural views and designs, and to illustrate and instantiate functionalities and capabilities that can be gained based on the proposed design principles. Use case diagrams are created based on the unified modelling language (UML) (Dobing and Parsons 2006). They are standard and effective ways to visualize and communicate the designs of the systems (Jacobson et al. 2016). Use case diagrams depict step by step behavior of a system and its functionalities in interaction with users in different scenarios (Würfel et al. 2016). UML diagrams in IS studies have been used to illustrate the design of collaboration engineering (Chatterjee et al. 2009), grounded requirements for software design and development (Würfel et al. 2016), web application architectures (Conallen 1999), system implementation (Al-Msie'deen et al. 2014), and document management processes (Pătraşcu 2014).

7.1. Design Principle 1: Data Integrability

Figure 3 shows the use case diagram illustrating the design principle 1 implicated in a diabetes mobile app.

Figure 3. Use case diagram illustrating design principle 1, data integrability, in a diabetes mobile app

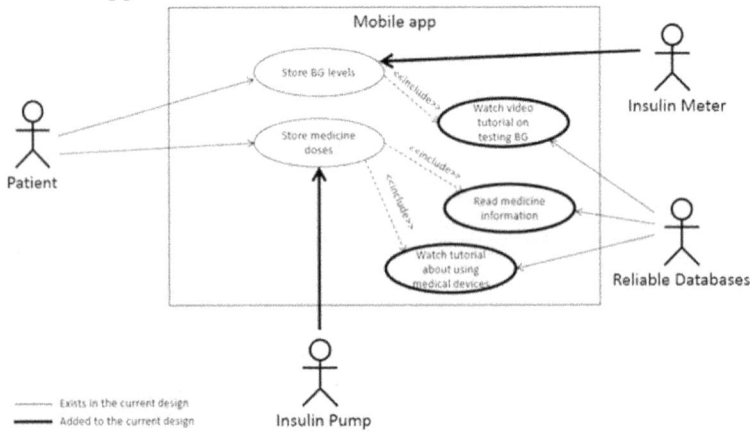

In the GB diabetes app, patients can store blood glucose and medicine data. The storage and interpretability of such data are not supported with informational and instructional resources. The design principle of *data integrability* is salient when and where a patient-user of a SM system faces new or unknown situations with uncertainties. Two critical instances where diabetic patients seek solutions to their problems and concerns during the course of the diabetes SM are testing and storing blood glucose data, and collecting and storing medicine data (Bu et al. 2007). Choosing the right diabetes medical devices and using them correctly, notably post diagnosis, can become frustrating for the patients (Nijland et al. 2009). Providing immediate and easily accessible informational resources about medical devices and their usage reduces uncertainties and saves patients' valuable time in the conduct of SM.

The use case diagram in Figure 3 shows patients' interactions with the diabetes mobile app at storing blood glucose and medicine data. Design principle of *data integrability* is implicated in the system design of the diabetes app where storing blood glucose data is supported by instructional video tutorial so that patients can watch at any time how medical devices are used to test blood glucose. The blood glucose data is synced from insulin pump and integrated and stored in the mobile app. Similarly taking medicine and storing medicine data is supported with immediate and easily accessible informational resources about the most effective medicine doses for controlling blood glucose levels, their side effects, and their possible interactions with other medicines that patients might be using. Medical library and dictionary of medical terms are provided in these informational resources. The data for the doses of insulin used by insulin pump is synced and stored in the app. The information resources for blood glucose and medicine should be constantly updated to inform patients about the latest advancements and developments in techniques, devices, and medications. These reliable informational databases need to be controlled, approved, and validated by the patients' healthcare providers and experts.

7.2. Design Principles 2: System Flexibility

Figure 4 shows the use case diagram illustrating the design principle 2, *system flexibility*, implicated in a diabetes mobile app.

Figure 4. Use case diagram illustrating design principle 2, system flexibility, in a diabetes mobile app

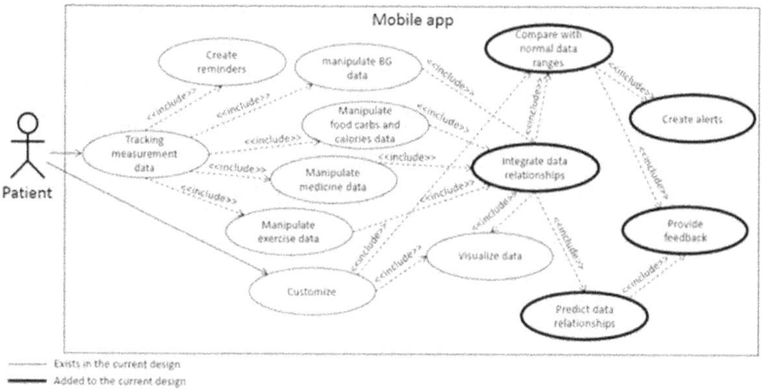

In the GB diabetes app, patients can track, manipulate, and visualize blood glucose, food carbs, medicine, and exercise data. They can customize visualized data on the web platform. Patients can create reminders to reinforce their tracking habits. Necessary data about food intake and glucose levels do not visualize in one graph and the impact of one measurement data on the other, for instance calorie amount on glucose levels, are not predictable so that patients can set goals. Alerts and feedback are not created for compared and predicted data relationships. Design principle of *system flexibility* is applied when and where patient-user of a system should make sense of different kinds of data stored in the diabetes app to track and monitor disease symptoms, make decisions in response to certain symptoms evident in the data, and plan for the future to make lifestyle changes that trigger adverse symptoms.

The *system flexibility* principle is implicated in the diabetes app where data-driven tracking of the symptoms is supported by data manipulation functionalities. Data manipulations are the changes and calculations needed by the patients such as integrating all data types, visualizing data, and comparing measurement data with normal ranges of data. Predictive models programmed in the diabetes mobile apps forecast data relationships and explain how much food carbs would affect levels of blood sugar. Patients can make intelligent decisions and purposeful plans for their daily lives based on the predicted data relationships. In the predictive reports, feedback can be provided with possible solutions to achieve certain SM goals, such as, keeping blood glucose under certain level in certain number of days, and having a specific diet. Integrated stored data compared against normal data ranges, must produce alerts and feedback to keep the patients on track. Immediate alerts can notify patients of abnormalities and recommend possible problems producing abnormalities with informative feedback. For the abnormally high levels of blood glucose, the app should produce a feedback report that highlights possible areas of improvement in diet and exercises. Patients should be able to customize the normal ranges and data visualizations. They can lower the normal ranges of their blood glucose to make them more compatible with their lifestyle and customize data graphs by adding and removing dimensions. Different data combinations should be graphed over time such as blood glucose against food carbs. Combining different measurement data enables patients to further explore data relationships. Individualized reminders created in the app help patients comply with tracking and monitoring of the critical diabetes data and symptoms in the long term.

7.3. Design Principle 3: System Externality

Figure 5 shows the use case diagram illustrating the design principle 3, *system externality*, implicated in a diabetes mobile app.

Figure 5. Use case diagram illustrating design principle 3, system externality, in a diabetes mobile app

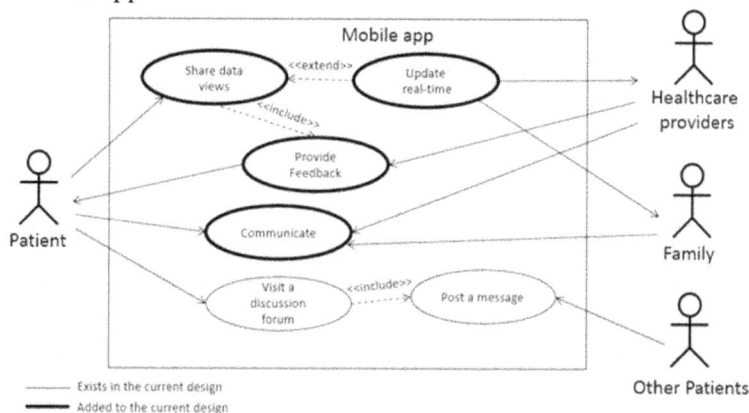

In the GB diabetes app, patients can visit diabetes discussion forums, read, post, and reply to messages but cannot communicate or share data with their healthcare providers or family members. Healthcare providers cannot view and provide feedback on patients' data. Design principle of *system externality* is used when and where a patient-user of a SM system seeks human support struggling with negative feelings caused by the longevity and intensity of the disease conditions. Diabetes mobile apps should have a shared view of the data stored and manipulated in the app accessed by indirect stakeholders, healthcare providers and family members, in real-time. The real-time access to the measurement data stored and manipulated in the diabetes app enables healthcare providers to provide timely feedback to the patients. Unattended patients with negative feelings and frustrations experience negative outcomes in managing their health conditions. Therefore, it is important to immediately attend to the patients' emotional and psychological needs during the conduct of SM.

One of the main advantages of the mobile platforms is their communicative features. Patients will be able to communicate with their healthcare providers and family members via text messages, voice and video calls. Patients with depression and anxiety need more than medical recommendations. Health coaches can communicate with the patients through the communicative capabilities of the mobile platforms at any time and location, to provide supportive guidelines. The need for such support is more critical at the onset of the disease. Patients after diagnosis are most vulnerable to negative emotions and thoughts which can be mitigated by participating in the digital communities, forums, and social media platforms designed and managed for specific diseases to share experiences with other patients with similar conditions. From the GB diabetes app patients can visit discussion forums and boards that are linked to it on the go to read through different topics related to their disease. They can post their questions or respond to other patients' questions and concerns. There are different topics in different categories in the discussion forums for patients with type 1, type 1.5, type 2 diabetes and pre-diabetes.

8. CONCLUSION

SM of chronic diseases is a complex and dynamic process in which patients as human agencies interact with intelligent features and technologies. Technology-based SM plays an important role in achieving SM goals and generating positive health outcomes. Certain characteristics of the digital technologies support specific values of the patients and reduce the complexity of SM process. The design principles proposed in this chapter provide guidelines for designing effective SM systems based on the characteristics of digital technologies, informed by the SM theories, and sensitized to the values of the patients with chronic diseases and conditions. System designers can use these design principles, their descriptions, and illustrative use case diagrams to fully utilize material properties of the digital technologies in their designs. The results of technical investigation in this chapter show how characteristics of digital technologies support specific patients' values and reduce the complexities inherent in designing SM systems, such as data relationships, integration within and between systems, and coordination and communication between indirect stakeholders. Healthcare providers, physicians, and nurses can use such value-sensitive systems in care processes working proactively with the patients and collaboratively managing their chronic conditions and diseases.

REFERENCES

Al-Msie'deen, R., Huchard, M., Seriai, A.-D., Urtado, C., and Vauttier, S. 2014. "Automatic Documentation of [Mined] Feature Implementations from Source Code Elements and Use-Case Diagrams with the REVPLINE Approach.," *International Journal of Software Engineering & Knowledge Engineering* (24:10), pp. 1413–1438.

Bailey, S. C., Belter, L. T., Pandit, A. U., & Carpenter, D. M. (2013). *The Availability*. Functionality, and Quality of Mobile Applications Supporting Medication Selfmanagement.

Baskerville, R., & Pries-Heje, J. 2014. "Design Theory Projectability," in *Information Systems and Global Assemblages. (Re)Configuring Actors, Artefacts, Organizations*, IFIP Advances in Information and Communication Technology, B. Doolin, E. Lamprou, N. Mitev, and L. McLeod (eds.), Springer, Berlin, Heidelberg, pp. 219–232. (https://link.springer.com/chapter/10.1007/978-3-662-45708-5_14)

Bodenheimer, T., Lorig, K., Holman, H., and Grumbach, K. 2002. "Patient Self-Management of Chronic Disease in Primary Care," *JAMA* (288:19), pp. 2469–2475.

Bu, D., Pan, E., Walker, J., Adler-Milstein, J., Kendrick, D., Hook, J. M., Cusack, C. M., Bates, D. W., & Middleton, B. (2007). Benefits of Information Technology–Enabled Diabetes Management. *Diabetes Care*, 30(5), 5. DOI: 10.2337/dc06-2101 PMID: 17322483

Chatterjee, S., Sarker, S., and Fuller, M. A. 2009. "A Deontological Approach to Designing Ethical Collaboration," *Journal of the Association for Information Systems* (10:Special Issue), pp. 138–169.

Conallen, J. 1999. "MODELING WEB APPLICATION ARCHITECTURES with UML.," *Communications of the ACM* (42:10), pp. 63–70.

Cummings, E., & Turner, P. (2009). Patient Self-Management and Chronic Illness: Evaluating Outcomes and Impacts of Information Technology. *Studies in Health Technology and Informatics*, (143), 229–234. PMID: 19380941

Dadgar, M., and Joshi, K. D. 2017. "Value-Sensitive Review and Analysis of Technology-Enabled Self-Management Systems: A Conceptual Investigation," *International Journal of Electronic Healthcare* (9:2/3), p. 157. ().DOI: 10.1504/IJEH.2017.10003175

Dadgar, M., and Joshi, K. D. 2018. "The Role of Information and Communication Technology in Self-Management of Chronic Diseases: An Empirical Investigation through Value Sensitive Design (Forthcoming)," *Journal of the Association for Information Systems (JAIS)* (19:2), pp. 86–112.

Dobing, B., and Parsons, J. 2006. "How UML IS USED.," *Communications of the ACM* (49:5), pp. 109–113.

Friedman, B., Kahn, P. H., & Borning, A. (2008). *Value Sensitive Design and Information Systems, The Handbook of Information and Computer Ethics* (Himma, K. E., & Tavani, H. T., Eds.). John Wiley & Sons, Inc.

Harvey, L. (1990). *Critical Social Research*. Unwin Hyman.

Jacelon, C. S., Gibbs, M. A., & Ridgway, J. V. (2016). Computer Technology for Self-Management: A Scoping Review. *Journal of Clinical Nursing*, 25(9-10), 1179–1192. DOI: 10.1111/jocn.13221 PMID: 26990364

Jacobson, I., Spence, I., and Kerr, B. 2016. "Use-Case 2.0.," *Communications of the ACM* (59:5), pp. 61–69.

Klein, H. K., and Myers, M. D. 1999. "A Set of Principles for Conducting and Evaluating Interpretive Field Studies in Information Systems," *MIS Quarterly* (23:1), pp. 67–93.

Koch, T., Jenkin, P., and Kralik, D. 2004. "Chronic Illness Self-Management: Locating the 'Self,'" *Journal of Advanced Nursing* (48:5), pp. 484–492.

Lamprinos, I., Demski, H., Mantwill, S., Kabak, Y., Hildebrand, C., & Ploessnig, M. (2016). Modular ICT-Based Patient Empowerment Framework for Self-Management of Diabetes: Design Perspectives and Validation Results. *International Journal of Medical Informatics*, 91, 31–43. DOI: 10.1016/j.ijmedinf.2016.04.006 PMID: 27185507

LeRouge, C., Hevner, A. R., and Rosann, W. C. 2007. "It's More than Just Use: An Exploration of Telemedicine Use Quality," *Decision Support Systems* (43:4), pp. 1287–1304.

McDermott, M. S., & While, A. E. (2013). Maximizing the Healthcare Environment: A Systematic Review Exploring the Potential of Computer Technology to Promote Selfmanagement of Chronic Illness in Healthcare Settings. *Patient Education and Counseling*, 92(1), 13–22. DOI: 10.1016/j.pec.2013.02.014 PMID: 23566427

Miles, M. B., & Huberman, A. M. (1994). *Qualitative Data Analysis: An Expanded Sourcebook (Second)*. Sage Publications Inc.

Nijland, N., van Gemert-Pijnen, J., Kelders, S. M., & Seydel, E. R. 2009. "Evaluation of an Internet-Based Application for Supporting Self-Care of Patients with Diabetes Mellitus Type 2," in *eTELEMED*. DOI: 10.1109/eTELEMED.2009.33

Pătraşcu, A. 2014. "Document Management Processes and Use Case Scenarios Elaboration.," *Economic Insights - Trends & Challenges* (66:3), pp. 91–98.

Ryan, P. 2009. "Integrated Theory of Health Behavior Change: Background and Intervention Development," *Clin Nurse Spec* (23:3), pp. 161–172.

Ryan, P., and Sawin, K. J. 2009. "The Individual and Family Self-Management Theory: Background and Perspectives on Context, Process, and Outcomes," *Nursing Outlook* (57:4), pp. 217-225.e6. ().DOI: 10.1016/j.outlook.2008.10.004

Schulman-Green, D., Jaser, S., Martin, F., Alonzo, A., Grey, M., McCorkle, R., Redeker, N. S., Reynolds, N., and Whittemore, R. 2012. "Processes of Self-Management in Chronic Illness," *Journal of Nursing Scholarship* (44:2), pp. 136–144.

Vuong, A. M., Ory, M. G., Begaye, D., & Forjuoh, S. N. (2012). Factors Affecting Acceptability and Usability of Technological Approaches to Diabetes Self-Management: A Case Study. *Diabetes Technology & Therapeutics*, 14(12), 12. DOI: 10.1089/dia.2012.0139 PMID: 23013155

Würfel, D., Lutz, R., & Diehl, S. (2016). Grounded Requirements Engineering: An Approach to Use Case Driven Requirements Engineering. *Journal of Systems and Software*, 117, 645–657. DOI: 10.1016/j.jss.2015.10.024

Yoo, Y., Henfridsson, O., and Lyytinen, K. 2010. "The New Organizing Logic of Digital Innovation: An Agenda for Information Systems Research," *Information Systems Research* (21:4), pp. 724–735.

Chapter 13
Using Social Media Data to Predict Mental Health Issues:
A Tertiary Study

Sumana Haldar
Dakota State University, USA

Omar F. El-Gayar
https://orcid.org/0000-0001-8657-8732
Dakota State University, USA

Sherif El-Gayar
The Valley Health System, USA

ABSTRACT

Addressing the pervasive issue of mental illnesses in the U.S. necessitates innovative approaches. This study explores the potential of social media platforms as valuable sources for detecting mental health issues, leveraging the spontaneous and open expression of users' thoughts and feelings. Previous research has applied machine learning techniques to social media data to predict mental health states, which this study aims to expand by providing a holistic view of the strategies used for identifying mental health concerns through social media analysis. Our research questions focus on the strategies for utilizing social media data, the efficacy of these strategies, the challenges faced, and the broader implications for healthcare delivery. Employing a tertiary investigation approach, we review secondary studies to identify trends and synthesize findings, aiming to offer comprehensive insights and guide future research in mental health service delivery through social media engagement.

DOI: 10.4018/979-8-3693-5237-3.ch013

INTRODUCTION

According to the Center for Disease Control (CDC) 1 in 25 Americans are struggling with conditions such as bipolar disorders, major depression, or schizophrenia (*About Mental Health*, 2024). The widespread prevalence of mental health conditions emphasizes the necessity for creative and groundbreaking methods in identifying and addressing these conditions. Real-time insights into individuals' mental states offer opportunities for effective intervention and support. In that regard, the popularity of various social media platforms, including Twitter, Facebook, WhatsApp, and Instagram, has provided individuals with unprecedented avenues to express their thoughts, feelings, and emotions. Social media platforms have emerged as dynamic spaces where users openly articulate their thoughts and emotions. Social media posts potentially provide a rich source of information that can help in the early detection of mental health conditions.

Accordingly, a broader exploration of the methodologies employed for analyzing social media data to identify mental health issues can be valuable for mental health professionals and researchers. Previous secondary studies have investigated detecting or predicting distinct mental health conditions using specialized machine-learning techniques applied to social media data. For example, Helmy et al. (2023) provided an overview of the methodologies used to detect depression from social media data. Lejeune et al. (2022) explored research utilizing ML with social media data for diagnosing psychotic episodes. This study aims to complement prior research by providing a holistic perspective of the methods and strategies employed for identifying mental health concerns through analyzing social media data, offering insights into implications for delivering mental health services, and guiding future research endeavors. Specifically, we aim to address the following research questions:

1. What strategies are employed to detect mental concerns using social media data?
2. What is the efficacy of the proposed strategies in detecting mental health concerns?
3. What are the challenges, emerging trends, and future directions in the field of mental health analysis using social media data?
4. What practical implications arise from the utilization of social media data, in predicting mental health conditions, and how can these insights be seamlessly incorporated into clinical practice and mental health interventions to enhance healthcare delivery?

To achieve this objective, a tertiary investigation was carried out. According to Kitchenham et al. (2010), a primary study involves conducting empirical research to answer specific research questions, while a secondary study involves examining primary research relevant to specific questions to synthesize findings. A tertiary study examines secondary studies relevant to the same research questions to identify patterns and trends.

The following considerations drive this study; while numerous secondary studies have been conducted to detect or predict mental health conditions from social media data, they typically focus on a single mental health issue. A systematic review is employed in this tertiary study to gain a comprehensive understanding of the strategies, the efficacy of these methods, their implications, and the challenges of using social media data to predict various mental health conditions. This approach ensures that the research is both reproducible and consistent, providing a more holistic view of the field.

This research provides a broader view of how mental health concerns can be identified from social media data, along with challenges, future directions, and implications for the delivery of mental healthcare services. By synthesizing findings across multiple review articles, a comprehensive analysis of the current state-of-the-art in social media-based prediction of early mental health issues is provided. This tertiary study offers valuable implications for researchers and mental health professionals seeking to utilize social media data for proactive mental health monitoring and intervention.

Related work

Prior research has extensively explored the potential of social media data analysis in predicting early signs of different types of mental health issues such as depression, anxiety, suicidal ideation, and Schizophrenia. Several systematic reviews have synthesized findings from these studies, offering insights into the methodologies, challenges, and advancements in this field. Systematic reviews play a crucial role in evaluating the relevance and quality of existing evidence to either support or challenge current practices. Systematic literature reviews (SLR) identify gaps, deficiencies, and trends in the evidence base, informing future research directions (Munn et al., 2018). Scoping reviews serves as invaluable tools for assessing the breadth and depth of literature on a particular topic, providing insights into the volume of available studies and the focus of their inquiries (Munn et al., 2018). In this context, several studies investigated the scope, and limitations of techniques used for predicting mental health from social media data. Wongkoblap et al. (2017) found that despite the progress, challenges remain, particularly concerning the assembly of large, high-quality datasets of social media users with mental disorders. Issues such as biases in data collection methods, consent management, and the selection of appropriate analytics techniques persist, highlighting the need for further research and development in this critical area. Boettcher (2021) provided insights into the scope and nature of studies using Reddit as a primary data source for investigating depression and anxiety. This study suggested a need for deeper conceptual exploration regarding the interpretation of Reddit data within the context of mental health.

While existing reviews have made substantial contributions to understanding the potential of social media data analysis for early mental health prediction, several gaps and challenges remain which include issues related to data privacy, algorithm bias, and limited dataset. Addressing these challenges will be crucial for future studies in the field use of predictive analytics in mental health care. In this paper, a systematic literature review of existing reviews is conducted. By synthesizing findings across multiple review articles, a comprehensive analysis of the current state-of-the-art in social media-based prediction of early mental health issues is provided. The review study offers valuable implications for researchers and mental health professionals seeking to utilize social media data for proactive mental health monitoring and intervention.

Methods

Liberati et al. (2009) provided valuable guidance and methodology for constructing a PRISMA framework, ensuring comprehensive and transparent reporting of systematic reviews and meta-analyses related to healthcare interventions. The PRISMA process guided the selection of articles. A search was conducted for publications focusing on mental health and social media from PubMed, IEEE, ScienceDirect, and Web of Science from January 2013 to December 2023. The following generic search terms were compiled for each database: (("mental disorder" OR "mental health" OR "Anxiety Disorders" OR "Depression" OR "Bipolar Disorder" OR "PTSD" OR "Schizophrenia" OR "Eating Disorders" OR "Disruptive behavior" OR "Neurodevelopmental disorders") AND (predict* OR monitor* OR detect* OR prevent*) AND (social media OR social network OR Twitter OR Facebook OR Reddit) AND Review). This search included Title and Abstract fields. To be included in the study, articles must be a review, written in the English language, and available in full-text version. Studies relating to the impact of social media use on mental health, the impact of cyberbullying on mental health, or the impact of social media on a specific user group have been excluded.

Once a final list of articles is selected for inclusions, we extract the following characteristics of the selected secondary studies: (i) authors, title, and year of publication; (ii) target mental health disorders; (iii) research objectives; (iv) search query;

(v) total number of primary studies; (vi) inclusion/exclusion criteria; (vii) primary findings and (viii) reported limitation.

Results

The query resulted in a total of 297 articles. After eliminating duplicates, 214 unique articles remained. A rigorous screening process based on title, abstract, and full-text review for eligibility ensued, resulting in 20 articles for synthesis. Among these, 11 were identified as review articles. Figure 1 shows the PRISMA process phases with inclusion and exclusion criteria. Table 1 shows the key characteristics of the selected studies. Several studies have focused on exploring the most effective techniques for predicting mental health from social media data, whereas others have highlighted the challenges associated with evaluating construct validity throughout the research process, replicability issues, and ethical problems.

Figure 1. PRISMA chart

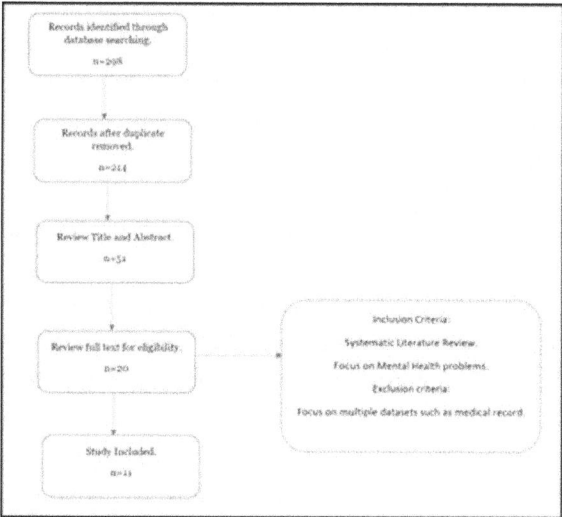

Most of these secondary studies (91%) were published within the last four years (2020–2023). The earliest secondary study included in this research was published in 2017. In the review articles, five studies (45%) focused on depression detection from social media data, one study (9%) focused on depression and anxiety, one study (9%) focused on Schizophrenia/psychotic episodes while others (36%) concentrate on overall mental health and mental wellbeing where various mental health problems such as psychological stress, depression, suicide, postpartum depression, PTSD, Anxiety, OCD, borderline disorder, bipolar disorder, seasonal effective disorder, eating disorder, attention deficit/hyperactivity disorder and sleeping disorder have been investigated.

Studies have generally followed a pattern to predict or identify mental health issues from social media data, which include preprocessing, feature extraction, algorithm used to detect mental health problems, and then finally, validation of the model. Regarding dataset preparation, self-curated datasets are prevalent, as highlighted by Rahman et al. (2020). The Reddit Self-Reported Depression Diagnosis dataset has been used in previous research mentioned by Boettcher (2021). Few approaches have been used for preprocessing, such as Twitter-specific elements like hashtags and a more traditional tokenization method, removing all non-alphanumeric information from the text (Cara et al., 2023). Feature extraction constitutes a critical phase in mental health problem prediction. Numerous feature extraction techniques have been employed, including LIWC and TF-IDF (Rahman et al., 2020). Researchers have extensively explored the utilization of diverse machine learning methodologies, including recent advancements in deep learning, to identify mental health disorders through the analysis of social media data. Additionally, hybrid approaches combining multiple machine-learning techniques have been investigated. Commonly employed algorithms encompass Support Vector Machines, Naïve Bayes, Logistic Regression, Random Forest, Decision Tree, Gaussian Process, K-means, and Artificial Neural Networks (Rahman et al., 2020). N-fold cross-validation is the most common model verification technique.

While there is potential in using social media data for detecting psychotic disorders like schizophrenia, biases may significantly affect the results. These biases arise due to limited access to clinical diagnostic data and small sample sizes (Lejeune et al., 2022). Overfitting, data imbalance issues, and construct validity and replicability problems can be challenging in this field. Including multiple datasets, multiple mental health symptoms, and employing time-based features in the realm of predicting mental health issues through the utilization of social media data needs to be explored further. Boettcher (2021) suggested utilizing insight from Reddit data into clinical application as a practical implication. Chancellor & De Choudhury (2020) and Cara et al. (2023) provided suggestions for enhancing construct validity and replicability to use the mental health prediction application in clinical settings.

Table 1. Analysis of previous studies

Study	Mental health	Research Objectives	Search keywords	Inclusion/ Exclusion criteria	Primary Studies	Primary Findings	Reported Limitation
(A. Helmy et al., 2023)	Depression	Provide an overview and methodologies of depression detection from social media data.	Depression, anxiety, stress, detection, symptoms, social media, machine learning, sentiment analysis, Twitter, Facebook	Exclude non-research publications and those completed before 2016	335	Employing SVM classifier with TFIDF, coupled with suitable preprocessing methods increase accuracy levels.	Exclude publications not meeting search criteria and quality rating
(A. M. Putri et al., 2022)	Depression	Investigate how machine learning algorithms classify depressive and non-depressive content in social media.	Detection, Depression, Machine, Learning, Social, and Media	Include study related to ML and depression. Exclude study with no social media data.	330	Classifying depressive and non-depressive content involves data pre-processing, features addition, classification, and evaluation process.	
(Boettcher, 2021)	Depression and Anxiety	Assess the extent and characteristics of research utilizing Reddit as a primary data source for investigating depression and anxiety.	Reddit, depression, or anxiety.	Excluded for not using Reddit data, depression, and anxiety, and not peer review.	554	There is a greater emphasis on depression compared to anxiety in research. Practical implications often recommended proactive monitoring and outreach initiatives for Reddit users.	Excluding studies without a focus on depression and anxiety like suicidality and eating disorders.
(Cara et al., 2023)	Mental health disorders	Analyze the current landscape of predicting mental health outcomes from Twitter data along with construct validity and replicability, focusing on ML methodologies.	Mental health disorders and well-being, machine learning, and Twitter.	Include study used twitter and focus on mental health disorders excluding specific groups.	1164	Lack of clarity and hindering replicability along with insufficient details regarding data sets, model preprocessing and high-quality ground truth data.	Possibility of missing relevant studies in the search process, exclusion of non-English studies, and lack of detailed analysis on study outcomes.

continued on following page

Table 1. Continued

Study	Mental health	Research Objectives	Search keywords	Inclusion/ Exclusion criteria	Primary Studies	Primary Findings	Reported Limitation
(Chancellor & De Choudhury, 2020)	Mental Health Status	Review methods for predicting mental health status (MHS) on social media.	Mental health, social media	Include peer reviewed studies and exclude meta and literature review.	775	There are challenges in assessing construct validity leading to replicability issue for identifying and predicting MHS throughout the research process.	
(Hasib et al., 2023)	Depression	Gain insights into the application of ML and DL algorithms in developing health analytics solutions for depression.			1108	Diagnosing depression using social network (SN) data poses challenges due to the inherent ambiguity of the disease.	
(Lejeune et al., 2022)	Schizophrenia/ psychotic episode	Explored research utilizing ML with social media data for diagnosing psychotic episodes.	Schizophrenia, AI, and social networks	Include clinical trials and observational studies.	77	There is a lack of access to clinical diagnostic data for model training leading biased in detecting schizophrenia on social media.	Limited number of relevant studies available at the time of review
(Liu et al., 2022)	Depression	Explore machine learning for measuring depressive symptoms via text mining techniques on social media data.	ML, depression detection, social media, and text	Exclude study without focusing ML and textual data from social media.	117	Text analysis strategies like LIWC and word-embedding models to extract features from online text posted by users on social media used for depression prediction.	
(Rahman et al., 2020)	Mental health problems	Explore the effectiveness, challenges, and limitations of detecting mental health problems using OSNs data.	Various social media and various mental health disorders.	Included studies focus on OSN and mental health problems.	222	OSNs cannot fully replace traditional methods like face-to-face interviews or questionnaires.	Restriction to English-language articles and focus on mental health issues.

continued on following page

Table 1. Continued

Study	Mental health	Research Objectives	Search keywords	Inclusion/ Exclusion criteria	Primary Studies	Primary Findings	Reported Limitation
(Salas-Zárate et al., 2022)	Depression	Explored available evidence on the detection of signs of depression on social media.	Depression, mental health, and social media	Exclude studies not focusing depression on social media	334	The research in this area is based on widely used tools worldwide, and the datasets analyzed vary from a few tweets to millions of posts.	
(Wongkoblap et al., 2017)	Mental Health Disorders	Examine the advancement of predictive analytics methods in mental health.	Common mental health disorders, social media, and ML/DL	Exclude studies related to internet addiction, cyberbullying.	448	The results indicate the adaptability of analyzing methods across languages.	

DISCUSSION

Strategies for Detecting Mental Concerns Using Social Media Data

Researchers categorized mental health outcomes as binary or categorical like depressed content vs non-depressed content (A. M. Putri et al., 2022) or differentiate between high and low stress (Chancellor & De Choudhury, 2020) or identify user with certain mental health problem like schizophrenia (Lejeune et al., 2022) or if a user shows or does not show depression (Salas-Zárate et al., 2022). According to the literature, social media mining for detecting mental health condition includes three phases – 1) data preprocessing for feature extraction where data is cleaned for use in the next step, 2) classifying the content using a variety of machine learning algorithms, and 3) evaluating the classification performance of the resulting models.

Text documents are inherently stored as strings, posing a challenge for machine learning algorithms that typically require numerical feature vectors to perform tasks. Therefore, preprocessing raw text is essential to convert it into a format that machine learning algorithms can understand and analyze. The preprocessing phase of text data involves several essential steps, including text cleaning, normalization, tokenization, stop word removal, lemmatization, and word stemming. In the context of model training, annotation involves assigning specific outcomes to each data point used for training (Cara et al., 2023). Ground truth for positive annotation in mental health research can be established through human assessments by domain experts, community or network affiliations indicating mental health issues, self-disclosure of conditions or behaviors, administering screening questionnaires, keyword analysis in social media posts, from previous research, news reports of suicide victims, and medical diagnostic codes from health records while on the other hand the negative dataset can be validated using screening cutoffs or expert validation, random selection of control users from social media or historical datasets (Chancellor & De Choudhury, 2020).

Feature extraction is the process of transforming raw input data into a set of features that are meaningful and useful for machine learning tasks. It involves extracting relevant information from the original data to create a more manageable and descriptive representation (Dara & Tumma, 2018) Feature selection plays a pivotal role in isolating a pertinent subset of features capable of predicting symptoms of mental disorders or accurately labeling participants, while mitigating the risk of overfitting. A systematic approach is necessary to outline all preprocessing steps across different contexts, guiding researchers to achieve optimal results tailored to their specific datasets and language types (A. Helmy et al., 2023). Various machine learning and deep learning algorithms are used to detect mental health issues from social media data. Support vector machines (SVM) is the most common. The most prevalent validation technique was n-fold cross-validation, where the dataset is split into n subsets, each used for validation once while the rest are for training. These strategies can be applied to analyze posts in various languages to identify mental health issues.

Wongkoblap et al. (2017) found that the same analysis method could be used in different languages while, based on Rahman et al. (2020), multilingual text could be challenging to analyze mental health conditions from social media data. Cara et al. (2023) highlighted that datasets constructed in languages other than English often needed to develop their own preprocessing and feature selection tools due to a lack of existing software and readily available tools in those languages.

Efficacy of the Proposed Strategies in Detecting Mental Health Concerns

Construct validity ensures that the labels used for training represent the same construct intended for future predictions, thus ensuring the effectiveness of machine learning algorithms. Previous research has raised concerns regarding the quality of data used to train models and not incorporating established theories from clinical science or psychology for mental health inference. Problems with construct validity in generating data labels may impede the reproducibility and application of this research in practical and clinical settings. (Cara et al., 2023) and (Chancellor & De Choudhury, 2020).

Researchers usually consider mental health outcome as a binary result which may overlook nuances in symptom severity and the potential for comorbidity, particularly prevalent in disorders like anxiety and depression. This approach restricts the model's ability to capture the full complexity of mental health constructs (Cara et al., 2023). Deep learning models which are trained in a specific demographic may struggle to perform well on data from users with different writing styles or cultural backgrounds (Rahman et al., 2020). Lejeune et al. (2022) identified potential bias in detecting early sign of psychotic disorders from social media data due to the limited access to clinical diagnostic data for model training. Consequently, drawing a conclusion regarding the effectiveness of artificial intelligence (AI) in detecting schizophrenia patients on social media remains inconclusive. The question remains: how effective are these methods when an individual with mental health problems does not communicate with others?

Despite the challenges, research has shown that machine learning algorithms trained on social media data can accurately predict mental health problems. The accuracy of machine learning algorithms can vary depending on the dataset and training methods. SVM has proven to be a successful method for text classification and regression tasks, displaying efficacy in categorizing mental health issues due to its capacity to model various data sources, achieve high accuracy, and handle high-dimensional data effectively (A. Helmy et al., 2023)

Challenges and Future Directions

The primary challenges in mental health prediction involve imbalanced datasets, dataset biases, insufficient data, and unstructured textual data. Overfitting problems can happen with insufficient data or an overly complex model with too many parameters. To prevent this issue cross-validation techniques can be used (Salas-Zárate et al., 2022) . Detecting mental health problems on online social networks presents a unique challenge due to the short length of posts. Therefore, developing effective machine learning models for mental health problem detection requires addressing the challenge of understanding mental health issues within the constraints of limited post length (Rahman et al., 2020). Sometimes it can be challenging to understand the targeted audience of the mental health issue, particularly when analyzing data from social media whether the focus is on individuals themselves or on individual tweets or posts remains unclear (Cara et al., 2023). The lack of sociodemographic details and psychological factors complicates accurate detection of mental health from social media (Liu et al., 2022).

Detecting mental health problems over time presents a unique and challenging task due to the varying nature of mental health conditions. Unlike static text classification tasks, mental health conditions can evolve significantly over time (Rahman et al., 2020). Demographic disparities in social media usage, such as higher activity among youth and middle-aged individuals compared to young children and older adults, as well as disparities based on income levels and geographical location, contribute to inherent population biases in studies relying on social media data (Liu et al., 2022).

Sometimes, social networking services implement privacy policies for extracting data, which poses challenges for the researchers during the data preparation phase while gathering public user data (Rahman et al., 2020). The ethical considerations surrounding using social media data for research remain ambiguous, especially when dealing with publicly available information without explicit consent (Wongkoblap et al., 2017). Additionally, questions persist regarding the ethical implications of implementing these systems in real-world practice, including the potential impact of misclassification on patients (Cara et al., 2023). The authors highlighted that although it holds that numerous studies employing social media data might not require ethics approval from institutional boards, as there is no direct involvement of "human participants," the ethical considerations within this field are still complex. More attention is needed to ethical issues in social media research. Further study should consider mechanisms such as informed consent, anonymization, and considering participants' perspectives on data use for health monitoring.

To solve the dataset imbalanced issue, Liu et al. (2022) recommended using the Synthetic Minority Oversampling Technique (SMOTE), which aims to balance the dataset by generating synthetic samples from the minority class. Incorporating additional data types such as images, audio recordings, videos, and user interaction graphs alongside textual content can enhance the prediction of mental health conditions through social media analysis (Wongkoblap et al., 2017). Making a publicly available dataset for establishing benchmark standards to evaluate algorithm performance across different studies while maintaining user privacy could be a problem to address in the future. The researchers can consider adopting symptom-based approaches to capture the complexity of comorbid mental illnesses better, allowing for more accurate detection and diagnosis (Cara et al., 2023). Chronic stress can potentially lead to depression and other disorders over time. Detecting and addressing it early on may be crucial in preventing further mental health complications (Wongkoblap et al., 2017).

Besides traditional machine learning and deep learning algorithms, Internet of Medical Things (IoMT) technology may be used to detect stress based on various physiological changes, such as palm temperature reduction, increased physical activity, and higher sweat rates. Leveraging IoMT technology in building a stress detection system that monitors cortisol (the primary stress hormone) levels, temperature, movement, and sweat rates in real-time is worth further exploration. However, the rapid pace of technological advancement in IoMT necessitates frequent device updates, posing challenges (Hasib et al., 2023).

Using time-based features in social media data presents a promising avenue for further research in mental health monitoring. By treating social media data as a time series, researchers could explore tasks such as identifying optimal intervention points and monitoring well-being trends over time. Given clinicians' interest in using social media for tracking symptom changes between time points, further investigation into this area is essential to realize the practical utility of social media data in mental health monitoring (Cara et al., 2023). To implement the detection of mental health issues from real social networks and provide personalized recommendations, it is crucial to develop a methodology integrating data science with digital interventions. This involves promoting access to health services, offering real-time interventions, sharing health information links, and delivering cognitive behavioral therapy through social media platforms (Wongkoblap et al., 2017). Boettcher (2021) recommended incorporating insights derived from Reddit data into professional mental health practice suggesting applications such as clinical tools or diagnostic aids along with proposing implementing professional oversight and proactive outreach for Reddit users.

Implications for Practice

Chancellor & De Choudhury (2020) suggest adopting methodologies that enhance the validity of measures in this area of research by drawing on literature from clinical psychiatry and psychology and collaborating with domain experts which will facilitate the practical application into clinical practice. Authors also suggested to enhance replicability, the details of positive and negative signs of mental health symptoms, addressing data bias and sampling strategies, and detailing feature selection methods can be added in the reporting. Cara et al. (2023) highlighted that the absence of validated ground truth results in a deficiency of demographic information such as age, gender, or cultural background potentially inclining to performance bias. Researchers interested in exploring this field should prioritize addressing the ethical concerns surrounding research involving human subjects and data privacy on social media platforms. These concerns are still not fully comprehended by ethics boards and the public (Wongkoblap et al., 2017).

Cara et al. (2023) provided two sets of recommendations in mental health inferences from social media data one aiming to enhance the quality, replicability, and transparency and the other one aiming to enable positive outcomes in this research. The authors suggestions include clearly defining prediction tasks, specifying mental health outcomes, detailing preprocessing steps, conducting error analysis, providing code and data availability statements, and including an ethics statement in the research study. Another suggestion emphasizes the importance of aligning research with the needs of the public and patients, promoting secure and ethical sharing of high-quality data and models among research groups, and leveraging the unique benefits of social media data while maintaining the role of mental health professionals. According to Wongkoblap et al. (2017) collaboration with mental health professionals to access authentic social network data from real patients shows promise for enhancing the accuracy and reliability of data used in building predictive models for mental health disorders.

Limitation and Future Research

While this study aimed to encompass all pertinent papers, there is a chance that some were overlooked during the systematic search. This study only includes systematic literature reviews and scoping review studies written in English, focusing on predicting mental health problems from social media data. Future research could broaden the scope by including other data sources, such as medical records or smartphone messaging data, to enhance predictive capabilities in understanding mental health issues.

CONCLUSION

This tertiary study conducted on detecting mental health conditions from social media data highlights several key findings and directions for future research. The study primarily focused on the analysis of several secondary studies related to various mental health disorders, highlighting the utilization of various social media platforms such as Twitter, Facebook, and Reddit for research purposes aimed at exploring strategies, their effectiveness, and implication of predicting mental health from social media data. While significant progress has been made in this field, numerous avenues remain for exploration and improvement. Addressing methodological challenges, construct validity and replicability issue, reliability issues, embracing interdisciplinary collaborations, and prioritizing ethical considerations are essential for advancing the field and developing effective technology-based interventions for mental health care which can be adaptable in clinical settings and personalized mental health treatment approaches will be very useful for the society.

REFERENCES

About Mental Health. (2024, May 20). https://www.cdc.gov/mentalhealth/learn/index.htm

Boettcher, N. (2021). Studies of Depression and Anxiety Using Reddit as a Data Source: Scoping Review. *JMIR Mental Health*, 8(11), e29487. DOI: 10.2196/29487 PMID: 34842560

Cara, N. H. D., Maggio, V., Davis, O. S. P., & Haworth, C. M. A. (2023). Methodologies for Monitoring Mental Health on Twitter: Systematic Review. *Journal of Medical Internet Research*, 25(1), e42734. DOI: 10.2196/42734 PMID: 37155236

Chancellor, S., & De Choudhury, M. (2020). Methods in predictive techniques for mental health status on social media: A critical review. *NPJ Digital Medicine*, 3(1), 1. Advance online publication. DOI: 10.1038/s41746-020-0233-7 PMID: 32219184

Dara, S., & Tumma, P. (2018). Feature Extraction By Using Deep Learning: A Survey. *2018 Second International Conference on Electronics, Communication and Aerospace Technology (ICECA)*, 1795–1801. DOI: 10.1109/ICECA.2018.8474912

Hasib, K. M., Islam, M. R., Sakib, S., Akbar, M., Razzak, I., & Alam, M. S. (2023). Depression Detection From Social Networks Data Based on Machine Learning and Deep Learning Techniques: An Interrogative Survey. *IEEE Transactions on Computational Social Systems*, 10(4), 1568–1586. DOI: 10.1109/TCSS.2023.3263128

Helmy, A., Nassar, R., & Ramadan, N. (2023). Depression Detection from Social Media Platforms: A Systematic Literature Review. 2023 Intelligent Methods, Systems, and Applications (IMSA), 387-393.

Lejeune, A., Robaglia, B.-M., Walter, M., Berrouiguet, S., & Lemey, C. (2022). Use of Social Media Data to Diagnose and Monitor Psychotic Disorders: Systematic Review. *Journal of Medical Internet Research*, 24(9), e36986. DOI: 10.2196/36986 PMID: 36066938

Liberati, A., Altman, D. G., Tetzlaff, J., Mulrow, C., Gøtzsche, P. C., Ioannidis, J. P. A., Clarke, M., Devereaux, P. J., Kleijnen, J., & Moher, D. (2009). The PRISMA statement for reporting systematic reviews and meta-analyses of studies that evaluate health care interventions: Explanation and elaboration. *PLoS Medicine*, 6(7), e1000100. DOI: 10.1371/journal.pmed.1000100 PMID: 19621070

Liu, D., Feng, X. L., Ahmed, F., Shahid, M., & Guo, J. (2022). Detecting and Measuring Depression on Social Media Using a Machine Learning Approach: Systematic Review. *JMIR Mental Health*, 9(3), e27244. DOI: 10.2196/27244 PMID: 35230252

Munn, Z., Peters, M. D. J., Stern, C., Tufanaru, C., McArthur, A., & Aromataris, E. (2018). Systematic review or scoping review? Guidance for authors when choosing between a systematic or scoping review approach. *BMC Medical Research Methodology*, 18(1), 143. DOI: 10.1186/s12874-018-0611-x PMID: 30453902

Putri, A. M., Wijaya, K., Salomo, O. A., & Santoso Gunawan, A. A., & Anderies. (2022). A Review Paper: Accuracy of Machine Learning for Depression Detection in Social Media. *2022 IEEE International Conference on Communication, Networks and Satellite (COMNETSAT)*, 39–45. DOI: 10.1109/COMNETSAT56033.2022.9994553

Rahman, R. A., Omar, K., Mohd Noah, S. A., Danuri, M. S. N. M., & Al-Garadi, M. A. (2020). Application of Machine Learning Methods in Mental Health Detection: A Systematic Review. *IEEE Access : Practical Innovations, Open Solutions*, 8, 183952–183964. DOI: 10.1109/ACCESS.2020.3029154

Salas-Zárate, R., Alor-Hernández, G., Salas-Zárate, M. del P., Paredes-Valverde, M. A., Bustos-López, M., & Sánchez-Cervantes, J. L. (2022). Detecting Depression Signs on Social Media: A Systematic Literature Review. *Health Care*, 10(2), 2. Advance online publication. DOI: 10.3390/healthcare10020291 PMID: 35206905

Wongkoblap, A., Vadillo, M. A., & Curcin, V. (2017). Researching Mental Health Disorders in the Era of Social Media: Systematic Review. *Journal of Medical Internet Research*, 19(6), e7215. DOI: 10.2196/jmir.7215 PMID: 28663166

Chapter 14
Digital Health Technologies for Preventive Cardiology

Shaveta Mala
https://orcid.org/0000-0002-4670-9336
Government Multi Specialty Hospital - Sector 16, Chandigarh, India

Upasna Deep
https://orcid.org/0009-0000-7709-3549
Christian Medical College and Hospital - CMC, Ludhiana, India

Ekta Mala
https://orcid.org/0009-0008-6185-1761
Alchemist Multi-Speciality Hospital, Panchkula, India

Shalom Akhai
https://orcid.org/0000-0002-7533-457X
Maharishi Markandeshwar University (Deemed), India

ABSTRACT

This chapter explores the potential of digital health technologies in preventive cardiology, including telemedicine, wearables, sensors, artificial intelligence, and mobile health platforms. These technologies have shown effectiveness in reducing cardiovascular risk factors and improving patient outcomes. However, barriers to widespread adoption include digital literacy gaps, limited internet access, data privacy concerns, and technical complexities. To overcome these, this chapter proposes strategies like national e-Health guidelines, stakeholder engagement, improved regulatory standards, human-centered design principles, integration with existing healthcare systems, technology infrastructure investments, and fair pricing models.

DOI: 10.4018/979-8-3693-5237-3.ch014

Addressing data security, accessibility, and ethical considerations is crucial for a future of personalized, proactive, and accessible cardiovascular care. The chapter concludes by highlighting the challenges of digital health technologies in preventive cardiology.

1 INTRODUCTION

Cardiovascular diseases (CVDs) are a leading cause of morbidity and mortality worldwide, with risk factors such as hypertension, high cholesterol, diabetes, obesity, smoking, and physical inactivity, emphasizing the need for effective preventive measures. Preventive cardiology, a subspecialty of cardiology, focuses on reducing the risk of developing CVDs by managing risk factors such as hypertension, high cholesterol, diabetes, obesity, smoking, and physical inactivity (Krist et al., 2020; Ciumărnean et al., 2021; Bays et al., 2021). Traditional preventive strategies have been essential, but recent advancements in digital health technologies offer promising new tools to enhance these efforts. While traditional approaches have been effective, the field of preventive cardiology is now undergoing a significant transformation with the integration of digital health technologies. Digital health technologies encompass a wide range of tools, including wearables, sensors, artificial intelligence, telemedicine, and electronic and mobile health platforms (Leclercq et al., 2022; Bhavnani, 2020). These technologies have the potential to revolutionize preventive cardiology by providing innovative ways to monitor, manage, and improve cardiovascular health outcomes. Wearable gadgets, mobile apps, telemedicine platforms, remote monitoring systems, and predictive analytics have become integral in offering personalized and preventative treatment options.

In recent years, digital health interventions have demonstrated significant impact in reducing CVD outcomes through correlated reductions in weight and body mass index (Gold, 2021). Non-invasive mobile digital technologies, such as teleconsultations, smartphone applications, wearables, remote monitoring, and predictive analytics, are now accessible and aid in the optimal care of heart failure patients. These technologies influence patient behaviors and are crucial in the primary and secondary prevention of coronary artery disease (Gray et al., 2022; Mishra et al., 2023; Rashidy et al., 2021).

The integration of digital health technology in preventive cardiology has shown success in lowering risk factors and improving patient outcomes. However, challenges remain, including ensuring equal access and usability for all patients, integrating these technologies into existing healthcare systems, addressing the costs of technology, and managing healthcare consumption (Bayoumy et al., 2021; Burke et al., 2015; Gastounioti et al., 2015; Sharma et al., 2018). Furthermore, the adoption of these technologies raises concerns about privacy and technology acceptance among patients (Pegoraro et al., 2023).

As digital health technologies continue to evolve, new pathways for research and clinical practice emerge, underscoring the need to develop ad hoc management models tailored to specific patient needs and conditions.

2 BACKGROUND AND EPIDEMIOLOGY OF CARDIOVASCULAR DISEASES

Cardiovascular diseases (CVDs) are the leading cause of death globally, accounting for an estimated million deaths each year, representing 31% of all global deaths (Soares et al., 2023). These diseases include coronary artery disease, heart failure, stroke, and hypertension. An estimated 17.9 million people died from CVDs in 2019, representing 32% of all global deaths. Of these deaths, 85% were due to heart attacks and strokes (Henein et al., 2022). Diabetes accounts for 20% of cardiovascular deaths, while hypertension affects 1.28 billion adults aged 30-79. Despite being a major cause of premature death, only 42% of hypertension patients are diagnosed and treated, with 21% having it under control.

The 2030 projected CVD prevalence rate is estimated to increase to 5.26%, with stroke and ischemic heart disease being major contributors. The prevalence of CVDs has reached epidemic proportions due to factors such as aging populations, unhealthy lifestyles, and the global rise in obesity and diabetes. The global prevalence of cardiovascular disease (CVD) is predicted to rise to 5.26% by 2030, with stroke and ischemic heart disease being major contributors. In Europe, diabetes, cardiovascular disease, stroke, and cancers are expected to reach an average of 3990, 4672, and 2046 cases per 100,000. China aims to reduce active smoking in men to 20% prevalence in 2020 and 10% in 2030 to prevent cardiovascular events and 2.9 to 5.7 million deaths over two decades. By 2030, 40.5% of the US population is expected to have CVD (Heidenreich et al., 2011; Moran et al., 2010; Webber et al., 2014; Banerjee and Huth 2020).

Preventive cardiology, a subspecialty of cardiology, focuses on reducing the risk of developing CVDs by managing risk factors such as hypertension, high cholesterol, diabetes, obesity, smoking, and physical inactivity. Digital health technologies like wearables, sensors, artificial intelligence, telemedicine, and mobile health platforms are revolutionizing preventive cardiology by improving cardiovascular health outcomes. These technologies offer personalized treatment options and significantly reduce CVD outcomes through weight and BMI reductions. Non-invasive mobile digital technologies are now accessible for optimal heart failure patient care (Addissouky et al., 2024).

However, challenges remain, such as ensuring equal access, integrating these technologies into existing healthcare systems, addressing technology costs, and managing healthcare consumption. As digital health technologies evolve, new research and clinical practice pathways emerge, necessitating the development of ad hoc management models tailored to specific patient needs.

3 ADVANCEMENTS AND EFFECTIVENESS

Digital health technologies have significantly advanced preventive cardiology, offering innovative solutions to address cardiovascular risk factors. These advancements span various domains, including wearables for arrhythmia detection, interventions targeting risk factors like diabetes and smoking cessation, and multi-risk factor modification through cardiac rehabilitation programs.

- **Wearables for Arrhythmia Detection:** Wearable devices equipped with advanced sensors and algorithms can detect irregular heart rhythms, such as atrial fibrillation, in real-time. These devices continuously monitor the heart's electrical activity, providing valuable data for early detection and intervention. By alerting individuals to potential cardiac abnormalities, wearables empower users to seek timely medical attention, thus reducing the risk of adverse cardiovascular events (Cheung, Krahn & Andrade 2018).
- **Risk Factor Modification in Diabetes and Smoking Cessation:** Digital health interventions targeting modifiable risk factors like diabetes and smoking cessation have shown promising results. Mobile applications and telemedicine platforms offer personalized support and resources to individuals seeking to manage their diabetes or quit smoking. These tools provide education, behavior change strategies, tracking mechanisms, and remote monitoring capabilities, enhancing adherence and improving health outcomes (Rehman et al., 2017; Akinosun et al., 2021).
- **Multi-Risk Factor Modification through Cardiac Rehabilitation:** Cardiac rehabilitation programs leverage digital health technologies to provide comprehensive support for individuals recovering from cardiovascular events or undergoing cardiac procedures (Mala 2021). These programs integrate exercise training, dietary counseling, medication management, and psychosocial support, tailored to each patient's needs. Digital platforms facilitate remote participation, monitoring, and feedback, overcoming barriers to access and adherence associated with traditional in-person programs (Kozik, Isakadze & Martin 2021; Huerne & Eisenberg 2024).

Despite the advancements in digital health technologies, several challenges remain. Validation studies are needed to ensure the accuracy and reliability of these tools across diverse populations. Additionally, scalability issues must be addressed to ensure widespread adoption and accessibility. Furthermore, continuous innovation is essential to keep pace with evolving technological advancements and healthcare needs. Few common digital health technologies being under consideration are shown in **Figure 1**.

Figure 1. Digital health technologies

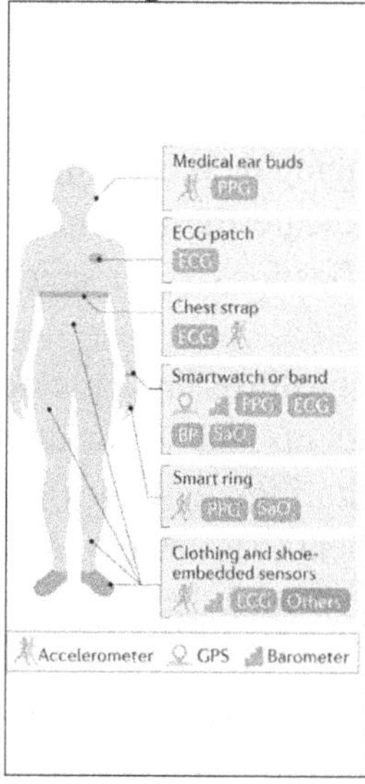

Sensors	Measurements	Clinical applications
Activity		
Accelerometer	Step count, impact force, speed, sedentary time, exercise	• Risk assessment in healthy individuals and those with established CVD • Physical activity behavioural interventions in primary and secondary prevention • Cardiac telerehabilitation • Heart failure management
Barometer	Stair count	
GPS	Distance traveled	
	Calories burned estimated from multiple measurements	
Biometric		
PPG	HR, HRR, HRV, cuff-less BP, SaO_2, cardiac output, stroke volume, pulse-based rhythm detection, sleep and its stages	• Risk prediction in healthy individuals and those with established CVD • Hypertension screening and management • Cardiac telerehabilitation • Arrhythmia screening and diagnosis • Acute coronary syndrome diagnosis • Diagnosis of electrolyte abnormalities such as hyperkalaemia • Long QTc diagnosis • Heart failure management • Medication titration such as β-blockers
ECG	Single-lead and multi-lead ECG, continuous or as-needed ECG monitoring, interval measurements such as QTc, arrhythmia detection and electrolyte abnormality changes	
Oscillometry	Wrist cuff BP	
Other		
Biochemical sensors	Invasive for continuous blood glucose and electrolyte monitoring Non-invasive for sweat and saliva electrolytes and hydration status	• Identifying electrolyte abnormalities • Continuous blood glucose monitoring • Heart failure management
Biomechanical sensors such as ballistocardiograms, seismocardiograms and dielectric sensors	Cardiac output, stroke volume, lung fluid volume, body vibrations, weight	

In conclusion, digital health technologies offer promising solutions for preventive cardiology by enabling early detection, personalized interventions, and comprehensive support for risk factor modification. Through continuous research, validation, and innovation, these technologies have the potential to revolutionize cardiovascular care, improving outcomes and enhancing the quality of life for individuals at risk of CVD.

4 BENEFITS OF DIGITAL HEALTH TECHNOLOGIES IN PREVENTIVE CARDIOLOGY

The integration of digital health technologies into preventive cardiology brings forth a multitude of benefits that significantly enhance the quality of care and patient outcomes. Optimizing processes and strategies consistently leads to enhanced outcomes and improved results (Kumar et al., 2024, Akhai 2023). These benefits extend to various stakeholders, including patients, healthcare providers, and health systems.

1. **Improved Medical Monitoring**: Digital health technologies enable continuous monitoring of key health metrics, such as blood pressure, heart rate, blood glucose levels, and physical activity. Wearable devices and remote monitoring systems provide real-time data, allowing healthcare providers to track patients' progress more effectively. This proactive approach facilitates early detection of abnormalities and timely intervention, leading to better health outcomes.

2. **Adherence to Guidelines**: Digital health tools can help patients adhere to medical guidelines and treatment plans more effectively. Mobile applications and telemedicine platforms offer personalized reminders, educational resources, and tracking mechanisms to support patients in managing their conditions. By empowering patients to take an active role in their healthcare, these technologies promote adherence to recommended lifestyle modifications and medication regimens.

3. **Enhanced Patient-Physician Relationships**: Digital health technologies foster closer collaboration and communication between patients and healthcare providers. Telemedicine consultations and remote monitoring allow for frequent interactions without the need for in-person visits. Patients can easily share data and updates with their providers, leading to more informed decision-making and personalized care plans. This enhanced connectivity strengthens the patient-physician relationship and fosters trust and engagement in the healthcare process.

4. **Remote Monitoring Options**: Digital health technologies enable remote monitoring of patients' health status, particularly beneficial for individuals with chronic conditions or those recovering from cardiovascular events. Remote monitoring systems can detect early warning signs of complications, allowing for timely intervention and prevention of adverse outcomes. This proactive approach reduces the need for frequent hospital visits and empowers patients to manage their health from the comfort of their homes.

5. **Support for Prevention and Management**: Digital health tools offer comprehensive support for both preventive measures and disease management. Mobile applications and online platforms provide educational resources, behavioral interventions, and self-management tools to help individuals adopt healthier lifestyles and manage chronic conditions effectively. By empowering patients with knowledge and resources, digital health technologies play a crucial role in preventing cardiovascular diseases and optimizing outcomes for those already diagnosed.

6. **Cost Savings and Improved Efficiency**: The integration of digital health technologies into preventive cardiology can lead to significant cost savings for health systems. Remote monitoring and telemedicine reduce the need for hospital visits and unnecessary interventions, resulting in lower healthcare expenditures. Moreover, digital tools streamline administrative processes, enhance workflow efficiency, and optimize resource allocation, contributing to overall cost-effectiveness and sustainability.

In conclusion, the integration of digital health technologies into preventive cardiology offers a wide range of benefits that encompass improved monitoring, enhanced adherence, strengthened patient-provider relationships, remote monitoring capabilities, and comprehensive support for prevention and management. By harnessing the power of these technologies, health systems can achieve better outcomes, greater efficiency, and improved patient satisfaction, ultimately advancing the field of preventive cardiology (Sharma et al., 2018; Maddula et al., 2022).

5 POTENTIAL BARRIERS TO WIDESPREAD ADOPTION OF DIGITAL HEALTH TECHNOLOGIES IN PREVENTIVE CARDIOLOGY

The integration of digital health technologies into preventive cardiology faces several barriers that hinder their widespread adoption. These barriers encompass various aspects, including technological, socio-economic, regulatory, and cultural factors. For example, electronic devices when discaded produce e-waste (Aggarwal et el., 2022). Addressing these following barriers is essential to ensure equitable access and maximize the potential benefits of digital health technologies in cardiovascular care (Pegoraro et al., 2023; Smith et al., 2019; Hernandez & Rodriguez 2023; Frederix et al., 2019).

1. **Digital Illiteracy**: Limited digital literacy among both patients and healthcare providers poses a significant barrier to the adoption of digital health technologies. Many individuals may lack the necessary skills to navigate digital platforms effectively, hindering their ability to utilize these tools for preventive cardiology purposes.

2. **Limited Internet Access and Affordability**: Disparities in Internet access and affordability exacerbate existing inequalities in access to digital health technologies. Individuals in underserved communities or low-income households may face challenges accessing reliable internet connectivity and affording the necessary devices to engage with digital health platforms.

3. **Privacy and Security Concerns**: Concerns about data privacy and security represent another barrier to the adoption of digital health technologies. Patients and healthcare providers may be hesitant to use these technologies due to fears of potential data breaches or unauthorized access to sensitive health information.

4. **Low Motivation or Interest in Digital Health**: Some individuals may exhibit low motivation or interest in engaging with digital health technologies, which can impede their adoption. Factors such as skepticism about the effectiveness of digital interventions or a preference for traditional healthcare delivery models may contribute to this barrier.

5. **Limited Technology or Internet Access**: Even in regions where internet access is available, certain populations may still face barriers due to limited access to technology or devices capable of supporting digital health applications. The absence of adequate infrastructure further complicates efforts to promote widespread adoption.

6. **Governance and Legislative Challenges**: Governance and legislative obstacles can also hinder the adoption of digital health technologies in preventive cardiology. Regulatory frameworks may lag behind technological advancements, creating uncertainty and barriers to implementation.

7. **Patient and Staff Acceptance**: Successful implementation of digital health technologies relies on the acceptance and engagement of both patients and healthcare providers. Resistance to change, lack of familiarity with technology, concerns about privacy and security, and skepticism about the effectiveness of digital interventions can impede adoption. Education, training, and stakeholder engagement initiatives are needed to foster acceptance and promote a culture of digital health literacy.

8. **Technical Concerns**: Technical challenges, such as interoperability issues, data integration complexities, and compatibility with existing systems, pose significant barriers to implementation. Digital health solutions must seamlessly integrate with electronic health records (EHRs), clinical workflows, and other healthcare technologies to ensure smooth operation and efficient data exchange. Standardization efforts and collaboration among stakeholders are essential to address technical challenges and promote interoperability.

To overcome these barriers and promote the uptake of digital health technologies in preventive cardiology, targeted strategies are needed. These strategies should include:

- **Establishment of national e-Health guidelines** to provide a framework for the development and implementation of digital health technologies.

- **Engagement of key stakeholders**, including patients, healthcare providers, policymakers, and technology developers, to ensure that digital solutions are aligned with the needs and preferences of end-users.
- **Education initiatives targeting both the health workforce and patients** to improve digital literacy and raise awareness of the potential benefits of digital health technologies.
- **Improvement of regulatory standards** to address privacy and security concerns, ensuring compliance with data governance and privacy regulations.
- **Adoption of human-centered design principles** to develop user-friendly digital health solutions that prioritize usability and accessibility.
- **Integration of digital health technologies with existing healthcare systems and electronic medical records** to facilitate seamless coordination of care.
- **Investment in technology infrastructure** to improve internet/broadband access in underserved areas and increase affordability of digital devices.
- **Pricing digital health technologies fairly and exploring reimbursement options through insurance plans** to enhance affordability and accessibility for all patients.

AI explainability faces challenges due to technological, socio-economic, and regulatory factors. Transparent, interpretable AI models are needed for trust and equitable access to digital health solutions (Akhai 2023; Akhai 2024; Akhai & Kumar 2024). By addressing these barriers and implementing targeted interventions, stakeholders can work towards overcoming the challenges associated with the adoption of digital health technologies in preventive cardiology, ultimately improving cardiovascular outcomes and reducing health disparities.

6 EXAMPLES OF TECHNOLOGIES BEING USED IN PREVENTIVE CARDIOLOGY

Wearable life-detecting devices, such as PPG and ECG sensors, enable real-time data processing, early identification of abnormal heart rhythms, and ongoing monitoring of cardiovascular health. These tools improve patient outcomes by enabling prompt intervention and customized treatment. However, challenges such as accessibility, data security, and regulatory issues must be addressed. Common wearables in preventive cardiology include smart wearables for CVD detection, physical heart monitoring, and wearables that combine machine learning with novel monitoring technologies (Verma et al., 2024). Digital health advances like wearables, sensors, eHealth, mHealth, telemedicine, and artificial intelligence can improve patients' and caregivers' quality of life, reduce healthcare costs, and empower patients and providers. Wearable ECG devices are particularly helpful in preventive cardiology, providing reliable diagnostic data for early identification and treatment of atrial fibrillation and other cardiovascular diseases. Following are few specific technologies being considered (Ullah et al., 2023; Leclercq et al., 2022; Gray et al., 2022; Liang et al., 2023).:

- **Teleconsultations**: Teleconsultations enable remote consultations between patients and healthcare providers, allowing for convenient access to medical advice and monitoring without the need for in-person visits. This technology has proven effective in improving patient engagement and access to preventive cardiology services.
- **Smartphone Applications**: Smartphone applications offer a user-friendly platform for individuals to track their cardiovascular health, monitor vital signs, receive educational resources, and engage in behavior change interventions. These apps play a vital role in promoting healthy behaviors and adherence to treatment plans.
- **Wearables**: Wearable devices, such as smartwatches and fitness trackers, provide continuous monitoring of vital signs, physical activity levels, and even detect irregular heart rhythms. These wearables empower individuals to take control of their cardiovascular health by offering real-time data and alerts for early intervention.
- **Remote Monitoring**: Remote monitoring technologies allow healthcare providers to track patients' health status outside of clinical settings. This approach enables proactive management of cardiovascular conditions, early detection of abnormalities, and timely intervention to prevent adverse events.
- **Predictive Analytics**: Predictive analytics tools leverage data to forecast potential cardiovascular risks, identify patterns, and personalize interventions for individuals at risk. By analyzing large datasets, these technologies enhance risk prediction and support tailored preventive strategies.

These successful digital health technologies in preventive cardiology have revolutionized cardiovascular care by improving patient engagement, promoting healthy behaviors, enhancing monitoring capabilities, and facilitating personalized interventions for better outcomes. **Figure 2** displays examples of technologies used in preventive cardiology. Apart from these there are some secondary digital electronic technologies like automatic climate sensing air conditioners which affect human health (Khang & Akhai 2024). A good climate, including air-conditioned ones, can help prevent heart attacks. Extreme temperatures stress the cardiovascular system, increasing the risk of heart attacks, especially in those with heart disease. Strategies to protect the heart include staying indoors, using air conditioning when needed, dressing appropriately, and staying hydrated. Reducing heat exposure and following basic cooling strategies are also crucial for individuals with existing heart conditions (Akhai et al., 2016; Akhai et al., 2020Akhai et al., 2021; Akhai & Khang 2024).

Figure 2. Examples of technologies used in preventive cardiology.

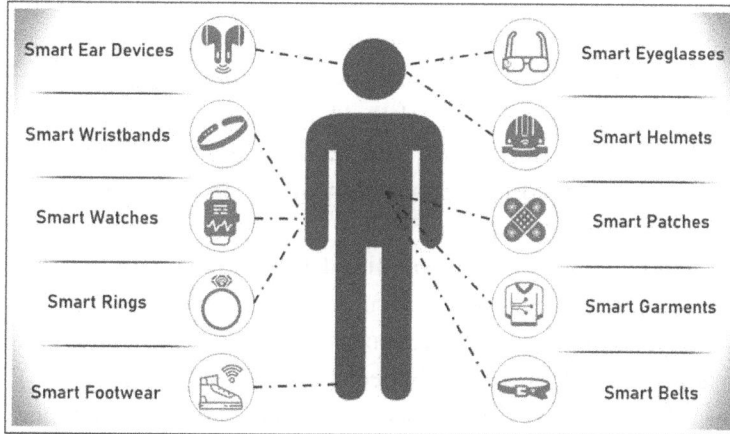

7 DISCUSSION

- Cardiovascular diseases (CVDs) are a significant global health concern, accounting for 31% of all deaths. The projected increase in CVD prevalence by 2030, particularly in stroke and ischemic heart disease, calls for urgent and innovative interventions. This escalating prevalence is driven by aging populations, sedentary lifestyles, poor dietary habits, and the rising incidence of diabetes and hypertension. Regional disparities in CVD prevalence, such as high rates in Europe and ambitious targets set by China to reduce smoking prevalence, highlight the need for tailored interventions.
- Digital health technologies have shown considerable promise in transforming preventive cardiology. Wearables, smartphone applications, telemedicine, and predictive analytics offer multifaceted benefits, including continuous monitoring and real-time data on heart rhythms, risk factor modification, and cardiac rehabilitation. These technologies empower patients with real-time health data, fostering proactive health management.
- However, the effectiveness of these technologies' hinges on rigorous validation studies to ensure their accuracy and reliability across diverse popula-

tions. Scalability and widespread adoption also pose significant challenges, necessitating continuous innovation and integration into existing healthcare systems. Benefits of digital health technologies include improved monitoring and adherence, enhanced patient-physician relationships, cost savings and efficiency, and streamlined administrative processes and efficient resource allocation.

- Barriers to adoption include digital illiteracy and limited access, privacy and security concerns, technical and interoperability issues, and ethical considerations. Addressing these barriers requires targeted strategies, including national e-Health guidelines, stakeholder engagement, education initiatives, improved regulatory standards, and investment in infrastructure. Ensuring fair pricing and exploring reimbursement options through insurance plans can also enhance accessibility.

- Future developments in wearable life detection technologies hold immense potential for enhancing cardiovascular care. Machine learning-based interpretation of biosensor data, novel portable sensors, and personalized care approaches can revolutionize early detection and intervention. However, challenges related to data security, accuracy, and ethical considerations must be addressed to fully realize these benefits.

Overall, digital health technologies offer transformative potential for preventive cardiology, providing innovative solutions to mitigate cardiovascular risk factors and improve patient outcomes. By addressing existing barriers and embracing future innovations, stakeholders can collaborate to usher in a new era of personalized, proactive, and accessible cardiovascular care.

8 CONCLUSIONS

In conclusion:

- Digital health technologies have emerged as powerful tools in the realm of preventive cardiology, offering innovative solutions to mitigate cardiovascular risk factors and improve patient outcomes. From wearable devices for arrhythmia detection to interventions targeting modifiable risk factors like diabetes and smoking cessation, these technologies have demonstrated significant potential in revolutionizing cardiovascular care. Moreover, advancements in remote monitoring systems and predictive analytics have paved the way for personalized and proactive management of cardiovascular conditions.

- Despite the evident benefits, several challenges persist in the widespread adoption of digital health technologies in preventive cardiology. Issues such as digital illiteracy, limited internet access, privacy concerns, and technical complexities pose barriers to equitable access and effective utilization of these technologies. Addressing these barriers requires concerted efforts from stakeholders across the healthcare ecosystem, including policymakers, healthcare providers, technology developers, and patients.
- Moving forward, targeted strategies are needed to overcome these challenges and maximize the potential of digital health technologies in preventive cardiology. Establishing national e-Health guidelines, enhancing digital literacy, improving regulatory standards, and fostering stakeholder engagement are essential steps in promoting the uptake of these technologies. Moreover, investment in technology infrastructure, pricing fairness, and reimbursement mechanisms can further facilitate access and adoption.
- Looking ahead, future developments in wearable life detection technologies hold promise for advancing cardiovascular care. Machine learning-based interpretation of biosensor data, novel portable sensors, and personalized care approaches are poised to revolutionize early detection, evaluation, and intervention in cardiovascular diseases. However, addressing challenges related to data security, accuracy, and ethical considerations remains imperative to realize the full potential of these advancements.

In conclusion, digital health technologies offer a transformative opportunity to enhance preventive cardiology practices, improve patient outcomes, and ultimately reduce the burden of cardiovascular diseases. By addressing existing barriers and embracing future innovations, stakeholders can collaborate to usher in a new era of personalized, proactive, and accessible cardiovascular care.

9 FUTURE DEVELOPMENTS SCOPE

Future advancements in wearable life detection technologies for cardiovascular monitoring may involve machine learning-based interpretation of biosensor data, novel portable sensors, and personalized care approaches. These advancements have the potential to revolutionize cardiovascular care by enabling earlier detection, rapid evaluation, and personalized interventions. Machine learning can facilitate rapid evaluation of hemodynamic consequences of heart failure or arrhythmias, but it is limited by noise and training data. Data security, accessibility, and ownership are challenges associated with data derived from cardiovascular monitoring devices. Novel portable sensors can detect biosignals like cardiac output, blood-pressure levels, and heart rhythm, but they raise concerns about accuracy and actionability within clinical guidelines, medical, legal, and ethical issues. Personalized care approaches can provide more effective interventions for individuals with cardiovascular disease, but they also raise concerns about data security, accessibility, and ownership. Addressing these challenges is crucial to fully realize the potential of these technologies in cardiovascular care.

REFERENCES

Addissouky, T. A., El Sayed, I. E. T., Ali, M. M., Wang, Y., El Baz, A., Elarabany, N., & Khalil, A. A. (2024). Shaping the future of cardiac wellness: Exploring revolutionary approaches in disease management and prevention. *Journal of Clinical Cardiology*, 5(1), 6–29. DOI: 10.33696/cardiology.5.048

Aggarwal, P., Rana, M., & Akhai, S. (2022). Briefings on e-waste hazard until COVID era in India. *Materials Today: Proceedings*, 71(2), 389–393. DOI: 10.1016/j.matpr.2022.09.507

Akhai, S. (2023). Healthcare record management for healthcare 4.0 via blockchain: a review of current applications, opportunities, challenges, and future potential. *Blockchain for Healthcare 4.0, 1*, 211-223.

Akhai, S. (2023). Navigating the potential applications and challenges of intelligent and sustainable manufacturing for a greener future. *Evergreen*, 10(4), 2237–2243. DOI: 10.5109/7160899

Akhai, S. (2024). Towards Trustworthy and Reliable AI The Next Frontier. *Explainable Artificial Intelligence (XAI) in Healthcare, 1*, 119-129.

Akhai, S. (2024). A Review on Optimizations in μ-EDM Machining of the Biomedical Material Ti6Al4V Using the Taguchi Method: Recent Advances Since 2020. *Latest Trends in Engineering and Technology*, 395-402.

Akhai, S., & Khang, A. (2024). Efficient Hospital Waste Treatment and Management Through IoT and Bioelectronics. In *Revolutionizing Automated Waste Treatment Systems: IoT and Bioelectronics* (pp. 126-140). IGI Global. DOI: 10.4018/979-8-3693-6016-3.ch009

Akhai, S., & Khang, A. (2024). Energy Efficiency and Human Comfort: AI and IoT Integration in Hospital HVAC Systems. *Medical Robotics and AI-Assisted Diagnostics for a High-Tech Healthcare Industry*, 93-108.

Akhai, S., & Kumar, V. (2024). Quantum Resilience and Distributed Trust: The Promise of Blockchain and Quantum Computing in Defense. *Sustainable Security Practices Using Blockchain, Quantum and Post-Quantum Technologies for Real Time Applications*, 125-153.

Akhai, S., Mala, S., & Jerin, A. A. (2020). Apprehending air conditioning systems in context to COVID-19 and human health: a brief communication. *International Journal of Healthcare Education & Medical Informatics (ISSN: 2455-9199)*, 7(1&2), 28-30.

Akhai, S., Mala, S., & Jerin, A. A. (2021). Understanding whether air filtration from air conditioners reduces the probability of virus transmission in the environment. *Journal of Advanced Research in Medical Science & Technology (ISSN: 2394-6539), 8*(1), 36-41.

Akhai, S., Singh, V. P., & John, S. (2016). Human performance in industrial design centers with small unit air conditioning systems. *Journal of Advanced Research in Production Industrial Engineering*, 3(2), 5–11.

Akhai, S., Singh, V. P., & John, S. (2016). Investigating Indoor Air Quality for the Split-Type Air Conditioners in an Office Environment and Its Effect on Human Performance. *Journal of Mechanical Civil Engineering*, 13(6), 113–118.

Akinosun, A. S., Polson, R., Diaz-Skeete, Y., De Kock, J. H., Carragher, L., Leslie, S., Grindle, M., & Gorely, T. (2021). Digital technology interventions for risk factor modification in patients with cardiovascular disease: Systematic review and meta-analysis. *JMIR mHealth and uHealth*, 9(3), e21061. DOI: 10.2196/21061 PMID: 33656444

Banerjee, S., & Huth, J. K. (2020). Time-series study of cardiovascular rates in India: A systematic analysis between 1990 and 2017. *Indian Heart Journal*, 72(3), 194–196. DOI: 10.1016/j.ihj.2020.05.014 PMID: 32768021

Bayoumy, K., Gaber, M., Elshafeey, A., Mhaimeed, O., Dineen, E. H., Marvel, F. A., Martin, S. S., Muse, E. D., Turakhia, M. P., Tarakji, K. G., & Elshazly, M. B. (2021). Smart wearable devices in cardiovascular care: Where we are and how to move forward. *Nature Reviews. Cardiology*, 18(8), 581–599. DOI: 10.1038/s41569-021-00522-7 PMID: 33664502

Bays, H. E., Taub, P. R., Epstein, E., Michos, E. D., Ferraro, R. A., Bailey, A. L., Kelli, H. M., Ferdinand, K. C., Echols, M. R., Weintraub, H., Bostrom, J., Johnson, H. M., Hoppe, K. K., Shapiro, M. D., German, C. A., Virani, S. S., Hussain, A., Ballantyne, C. M., Agha, A. M., & Toth, P. P. (2021). Ten things to know about ten cardiovascular disease risk factors. *American Journal of Preventive Cardiology*, 5, 100149. DOI: 10.1016/j.ajpc.2021.100149 PMID: 34327491

Bhavnani, S. P. (2020). Digital health: Opportunities and challenges to develop the next-generation technology-enabled models of cardiovascular care. *Methodist DeBakey Cardiovascular Journal*, 16(4), 296. DOI: 10.14797/mdcj-16-4-296 PMID: 33500758

Burke, L. E., Ma, J., Azar, K. M., Bennett, G. G., Peterson, E. D., Zheng, Y., Riley, W., Stephens, J., Shah, S. H., Suffoletto, B., Turan, T. N., Spring, B., Steinberger, J., & Quinn, C. C. (2015). Current science on consumer use of mobile health for cardiovascular disease prevention: A scientific statement from the American Heart Association. *Circulation*, 132(12), 1157–1213. DOI: 10.1161/CIR.0000000000000232 PMID: 26271892

Cheung, C. C., Krahn, A. D., & Andrade, J. G. (2018). The emerging role of wearable technologies in detection of arrhythmia. *The Canadian Journal of Cardiology*, 34(8), 1083–1087. DOI: 10.1016/j.cjca.2018.05.003 PMID: 30049358

Ciumărnean, L., Milaciu, M. V., Negrean, V., Orășan, O. H., Vesa, S. C., Sălăgean, O., Iluț, S., & Vlaicu, S. I. (2021). Cardiovascular risk factors and physical activity for the prevention of cardiovascular diseases in the elderly. *International Journal of Environmental Research and Public Health*, 19(1), 207. DOI: 10.3390/ijerph19010207 PMID: 35010467

El-Rashidy, N., El-Sappagh, S., Islam, S. R. M., El-Bakry, H., & Abdelrazek, S. (2021). Mobile health in remote patient monitoring for chronic diseases: Principles, trends, and challenges. *Diagnostics (Basel)*, 11(4), 607. DOI: 10.3390/diagnostics11040607 PMID: 33805471

Frederix, I., Caiani, E. G., Dendale, P., Anker, S., Bax, J., Böhm, A., Cowie, M., Crawford, J., de Groot, N., Dilaveris, P., Hansen, T., Koehler, F., Krstačić, G., Lambrinou, E., Lancellotti, P., Meier, P., Neubeck, L., Parati, G., Piotrowicz, E., & van der Velde, E. (2019). ESC e-Cardiology Working Group Position Paper: Overcoming challenges in digital health implementation in cardiovascular medicine. *European Journal of Preventive Cardiology*, 26(11), 1166–1177. DOI: 10.1177/2047487319832394 PMID: 30917695

Gastounioti, A., Golemati, S., Andreadis, I., Kolias, V., & Nikita, K. S. (2015). Cardiovascular disease management via electronic health. In *Telehealth and Mobile Health* (pp. 187–202). CRC Press.

Gold, N., Yau, A., Rigby, B., Dyke, C., Remfry, E. A., & Chadborn, T. (2021). Effectiveness of digital interventions for reducing behavioral risks of cardiovascular disease in nonclinical adult populations: Systematic review of reviews. *Journal of Medical Internet Research*, 23(5), e19688. DOI: 10.2196/19688 PMID: 33988126

Gray, R., Indraratna, P., Lovell, N., & Ooi, S. Y. (2022). Digital health technology in the prevention of heart failure and coronary artery disease. *Cardiovascular Digital Health Journal*, 3(6), S9–S16. DOI: 10.1016/j.cvdhj.2022.09.002 PMID: 36589760

Heidenreich, P. A., Trogdon, J. G., Khavjou, O. A., Butler, J., Dracup, K., Ezekowitz, M. D., Finkelstein, E. A., Hong, Y., Johnston, S. C., Khera, A., Lloyd-Jones, D. M., Nelson, S. A., Nichol, G., Orenstein, D., Wilson, P. W. F., & Woo, Y. J. (2011). Forecasting the future of cardiovascular disease in the United States: A policy statement from the American Heart Association. *Circulation*, 123(8), 933–944. DOI: 10.1161/CIR.0b013e31820a55f5 PMID: 21262990

Henein, M. Y., Cameli, M., Pastore, M. C., & Mandoli, G. E. (2022). COVID-19 severity and cardiovascular disease: An inseparable link. *Journal of Clinical Medicine*, 11(3), 479. DOI: 10.3390/jcm11030479 PMID: 35159931

Hernandez, M. F., & Rodriguez, F. (2023). Health techequity: Opportunities for digital health innovations to improve equity and diversity in cardiovascular care. *Current Cardiovascular Risk Reports*, 17(1), 1–20. DOI: 10.1007/s12170-022-00711-0 PMID: 36465151

Huerne, K., & Eisenberg, M. J. (2024). Advancing Telemedicine in Cardiology: A Comprehensive Review of Evolving Practices and Outcomes in a Post-Pandemic Context. *Cardiovascular Digital Health Journal*, 5(2), 96–110. DOI: 10.1016/j.cvdhj.2024.02.001 PMID: 38765624

Javaid, A., Zghyer, F., Kim, C., Spaulding, E. M., Isakadze, N., Ding, J., Kargillis, D., Gao, Y., Rahman, F., Brown, D. E., Saria, S., Martin, S. S., Kramer, C. M., Blumenthal, R. S., & Marvel, F. A. (2022). Medicine 2032: The future of cardiovascular disease prevention with machine learning and digital health technology. *American Journal of Preventive Cardiology*, 12, 100379. DOI: 10.1016/j.ajpc.2022.100379 PMID: 36090536

Khang, A., & Akhai, S. (2024). Green Intelligent and Sustainable Manufacturing: Key Advancements, Benefits, Challenges, and Applications for Transforming Industry. *Machine Vision and Industrial Robotics in Manufacturing*, 405-417.

Kozik, M., Isakadze, N., & Martin, S. S. (2021). Mobile health in preventive cardiology: Current status and future perspective. *Current Opinion in Cardiology*, 36(5), 580–588. DOI: 10.1097/HCO.0000000000000891 PMID: 34224437

Krist, A. H., Davidson, K. W., Mangione, C. M., Barry, M. J., Cabana, M., Caughey, A. B., Donahue, K., Doubeni, C. A., Epling, J. W.Jr, Kubik, M., Landefeld, S., Ogedegbe, G., Pbert, L., Silverstein, M., Simon, M. A., Tseng, C.-W., & Wong, J. B. (2020). Behavioral counseling interventions to promote a healthy diet and physical activity for cardiovascular disease prevention in adults with cardiovascular risk factors: US Preventive Services Task Force recommendation statement. *Journal of the American Medical Association*, 324(20), 2069–2075. DOI: 10.1001/jama.2020.21749 PMID: 33231670

Kumar, H., Wadhwa, A. S., Akhai, S., & Kaushik, A. (2024). Parametric analysis, modeling and optimization of the process parameters in electric discharge machining of aluminium metal matrix composite. *Engineering Research Express*, 6(2), 025542. DOI: 10.1088/2631-8695/ad4ba9

Kumar, H., Wadhwa, A. S., Akhai, S., & Kaushik, A. (2024). Parametric optimization of the machining performance of Al-SiCp composite using combination of response surface methodology and desirability function. *Engineering Research Express*, 6(2), 025505. DOI: 10.1088/2631-8695/ad38ff

Leclercq, C., Witt, H., Hindricks, G., Katra, R. P., Albert, D., Belliger, A., Cowie, M. R., Deneke, T., Friedman, P., Haschemi, M., Lobban, T., Lordereau, I., McConnell, M. V., Rapallini, L., Samset, E., Turakhia, M. P., Singh, J. P., Svennberg, E., Wadhwa, M., & Weidinger, F. (2022). Wearables, telemedicine, and artificial intelligence in arrhythmias and heart failure: Proceedings of the European Society of Cardiology Cardiovascular Round Table. *Europace*, 24(9), 1372–1383. DOI: 10.1093/europace/euac052 PMID: 35640917

Leclercq, C., Witt, H., Hindricks, G., Katra, R. P., Albert, D., Belliger, A., Cowie, M. R., Deneke, T., Friedman, P., Haschemi, M., Lobban, T., Lordereau, I., McConnell, M. V., Rapallini, L., Samset, E., Turakhia, M. P., Singh, J. P., Svennberg, E., Wadhwa, M., & Weidinger, F. (2022). Wearables, telemedicine, and artificial intelligence in arrhythmias and heart failure: Proceedings of the European Society of Cardiology Cardiovascular Round Table. *Europace*, 24(9), 1372–1383. DOI: 10.1093/europace/euac052 PMID: 35640917

Liang, F., Yang, X., Peng, W., Zhen, S., Cao, W., Li, Q., & Gu, D. (2023). Applications of digital health approaches for cardiometabolic diseases prevention and management in the Western Pacific region. *The Lancet Regional Health. Western Pacific*. PMID: 38456090

Maddula, R., MacLeod, J., McLeish, T., Painter, S., Steward, A., Berman, G., Hamid, A., Abdelrahim, M., Whittle, J., & Brown, S. A. (2022). The role of digital health in the cardiovascular learning healthcare system. *Frontiers in Cardiovascular Medicine*, 9, 1008575. DOI: 10.3389/fcvm.2022.1008575 PMID: 36407438

Mala, S. (2021). Myocardial Injury after Non-Cardiac Surgery and Its Correlation with Mortality-A Brief Review on Its Scenario till 2020. *International Journal of Preventive Cardiology*, 1(1), 29–31.

Mishra, A., Mishra, J., Tiwari, M., Hugo, V., Neto, A. V. L., & Menezes, J. W. M. (2023, March). Digital Health Technology in the Prevention of Heart Failure Coronary Artery Disease. In *Doctoral Symposium on Computational Intelligence* (pp. 593-604). Singapore: Springer Nature Singapore. DOI: 10.1007/978-981-99-3716-5_48

Moran, A., Gu, D., Zhao, D., Coxson, P., Wang, Y. C., Chen, C. S., Liu, J., Cheng, J., Bibbins-Domingo, K., Shen, Y.-M., He, J., & Goldman, L. (2010). Future cardiovascular disease in China: Markov model and risk factor scenario projections from the coronary heart disease policy model–China. *Circulation: Cardiovascular Quality and Outcomes*, 3(3), 243–252. DOI: 10.1161/CIRCOUTCOMES.109.910711 PMID: 20442213

Pegoraro, V., Bidoli, C., Dal Mas, F., Bert, F., Cobianchi, L., Zantedeschi, M., Campostrini, S., Migliore, F., & Boriani, G. (2023). Cardiology in a digital age: opportunities and challenges for e-health: a literature review. *Journal of Clinical Medicine*, 12(13), 4278. DOI: 10.3390/jcm12134278 PMID: 37445312

Rehman, H., Kamal, A. K., Sayani, S., Morris, P. B., Merchant, A. T., & Virani, S. S. (2017). Using mobile health (mHealth) technology in the management of diabetes mellitus, physical inactivity, and smoking. *Current Atherosclerosis Reports*, 19(4), 1–11. DOI: 10.1007/s11883-017-0650-5 PMID: 28243807

Senbekov, M., Saliev, T., Bukeyeva, Z., Almabayeva, A., Zhanaliyeva, M., Aitenova, N., Toishibekov, Y., & Fakhradiyev, I. (2020). The recent progress and applications of digital technologies in healthcare: A review. *International Journal of Telemedicine and Applications*, 2020, 2020. DOI: 10.1155/2020/8830200 PMID: 33343657

Sharma, A., Harrington, R. A., McClellan, M. B., Turakhia, M. P., Eapen, Z. J., Steinhubl, S., Mault, J. R., Majmudar, M. D., Roessig, L., Chandross, K. J., Green, E. M., Patel, B., Hamer, A., Olgin, J., Rumsfeld, J. S., Roe, M. T., & Peterson, E. D. (2018). Using digital health technology to better generate evidence and deliver evidence-based care. *Journal of the American College of Cardiology*, 71(23), 2680–2690. DOI: 10.1016/j.jacc.2018.03.523 PMID: 29880129

Sharma, A., Harrington, R. A., McClellan, M. B., Turakhia, M. P., Eapen, Z. J., Steinhubl, S., Mault, J. R., Majmudar, M. D., Roessig, L., Chandross, K. J., Green, E. M., Patel, B., Hamer, A., Olgin, J., Rumsfeld, J. S., Roe, M. T., & Peterson, E. D. (2018). Using digital health technology to better generate evidence and deliver evidence-based care. *Journal of the American College of Cardiology*, 71(23), 2680–2690. DOI: 10.1016/j.jacc.2018.03.523 PMID: 29880129

Smith, B., & Magnani, J. W. (2019). New technologies, new disparities: The intersection of electronic health and digital health literacy. *International Journal of Cardiology*, 292, 280–282. DOI: 10.1016/j.ijcard.2019.05.066 PMID: 31171391

Soares, L., Leal, T., Faria, A. L., Aguiar, A., & Carvalho, C. (2023). Cardiovascular disease: A review. *Biomedical Journal of Scientific & Technical Research, 51*(3).

Tariq, M. U. (2024). Advanced wearable medical devices and their role in transformative remote health monitoring. In *Transformative Approaches to Patient Literacy and Healthcare Innovation* (pp. 308–326). IGI Global. DOI: 10.4018/979-8-3693-3661-8.ch015

Ullah, M., Hamayun, S., Wahab, A., Khan, S. U., Rehman, M. U., Haq, Z. U., Rehman, K. U., Ullah, A., Mehreen, A., Awan, U. A., Qayum, M., & Naeem, M. (2023). Smart technologies used as smart tools in the management of cardiovascular disease and their future perspective. *Current Problems in Cardiology*, 48(11), 101922. DOI: 10.1016/j.cpcardiol.2023.101922 PMID: 37437703

Verma, R., Akhai, S., & Wadhwa, A. S. (2024). Use of Smart Materials in Physiotherapy. In *Revolutionizing Healthcare Treatment With Sensor Technology* (pp. 300–319). IGI Global. DOI: 10.4018/979-8-3693-2762-3.ch019

Webber, L., Divajeva, D., Marsh, T., McPherson, K., Brown, M., Galea, G., & Breda, J. (2014). The future burden of obesity-related diseases in the 53 WHO European-Region countries and the impact of effective interventions: A modelling study. *BMJ Open*, 4(7), e004787. DOI: 10.1136/bmjopen-2014-004787 PMID: 25063459

Chapter 15
Designing Wearables for Improved Healthcare:
A Survey of Current Trends and Future Directions

Abdullah Wahbeh
https://orcid.org/0000-0002-6894-0192
Slippery Rock University, USA

Mohammad Al-Ramahi
https://orcid.org/0000-0002-8170-8312
Texas A&M University, San Antonio, USA

Omar El-Gayar
https://orcid.org/0000-0001-8657-8732
Dakota State University, USA

Ahmed Elnoshokaty
California State University, San Bernardino, USA

Tareq Nasralah
Northeastern University, USA

ABSTRACT

Recent advancements in healthcare technologies, particularly wearable devices, have significantly enhanced the delivery and efficiency of healthcare. Wearable devices integration with mobile apps provides many functionalities to users including but not limited to vital sign monitoring and physical activity tracking. This chapter is a survey of current trends in wearable design with a particular focus on the impact on improved healthcare delivery. The chapter provides a foundation for the design

DOI: 10.4018/979-8-3693-5237-3.ch015

features of wearable devices, focusing on users' experience, acceptance, adoption, and continuous use of such devices.

INTRODUCTION

Recent advancements in healthcare technologies have significantly enhanced healthcare delivery and improved the healthcare system's efficiency (Kumari & Chander, 2024). These advancements include many tools and technologies, such as electronic medical record systems, telemedicine, mobile health, artificial intelligence, and machine learning (Hope & McPeake, 2022; Rathore & Sharma, 2022). Furthermore, such technologies extend the healthcare delivery after patients receive the necessary care which could result in reduced rehospitalization, reduced mortality rates, and improved quality of life (Hope & McPeake, 2022; Singh et al., 2023).

One such promising technology is wearables. Wearable devices are advanced gadgets that are designed to be worn on the body, mainly as a wristband or smartwatch (Patel et al., 2022). Wearable devices have been used in healthcare for the last few years. Such devices are meant to help enhance patient care through continuous health monitoring (Mettler & Wulf, 2019). Such devices usually offer different features including communication, health monitoring, *and* personalized functionalities. Wearable devices such as smartwatches can be used with smartphone devices to capture different types of data, such as health data, and provide users with access to notifications and messages, even helping them make phone calls (El-Masri et al., 2022). More specialized and advanced wearable devices are equipped with sensors to monitor physiological parameters, such as heart rates and blood pressure, in different settings (El-Masri et al., 2022; Patel et al., 2022).

Furthermore, the increased use of wearable devices resulted in their growing importance in encouraging individuals to manage their own health by providing useful health insights (P. Yang et al., 2021). Wearable devices also provide users with personalization features, recommendations related to self-heath, and features that promote healthier lifestyles (Makeham, 2019; Zhou et al., 2023). Moreover, wearable technology's advanced technological features played a crucial role in managing health crises, such as the COVID-19 pandemic, by enabling the early detection and monitoring of diseases among the population through data collection and analysis techniques (Channa et al., 2021). Overall, wearable devices represent a convergence of technology, healthcare, and personal lifestyle, offering different approaches to health management and maintaining healthy lifestyle.

Wearable devices coupled with mobile apps have enhanced the delivery of healthcare through continuous monitoring of vital signs and physical activities (Lewy, 2015). offer users different health-related functionalities such as tracking activities, vital signs, and sleep tracking (El-Gayar et al., 2021). They also aid in early disease diagnosis and detection by transferring data to healthcare providers (Ibrahim & Ali, 2023). Wearables could also be integrated into clinical practices, and they have the potential to provide healthcare through patient support to make lifestyle changes as well as provide personalized care (Bayoumy et al., 2021).

Designing these devices requires taking into consideration several factors such as user experience, input/output modalities, small form factor, and battery life (Q. Yang et al., 2022). Analysis of social media data, as well as online user reviews, can shed light on the users' perspective on wearable devices, aiding in the improvement of the device design for sustained user engagement (El-Gayar et al., 2019; Erdmier et al., 2016). Such design should focus on functional design features, such as sleep tracking, activity tracking, and steps counter, as well as nonfunctional design features, such as aesthetics, ease of use, and battery lifetime, to enhance user experience and adoption (El-Gayar et al., 2019). Studying such user feedback to address and improve the design features of wearable devices is a crucial step in the design process of wearable devices for enhancing their usability, appeal, continued use, and improved health outcomes.

Wearable design features are critical when it comes to user adoption and satisfaction (Cheung et al., 2019; Karahanoglu & Erbug, 2011). Studying the design features of wearable devices is important since it significantly impacts user experience, adoption, and continued use (El-Gayar et al., 2019, 2021; Esen & Eroğlu, 2018; Hasan & Stannard, 2022). Design features related to the wearable devices' functionality, effectiveness, ergonomics, and aesthetics play a significant role in shaping the user experience with wearable devices (Pustiek et al., 2015). In addition, the acceptance of such devices by end users is related to the usefulness of the device, its compatibility, and accuracy, which in turn can influence user experience and promote the intention to use wearable devices (Lukowicz et al., 2004).

The design of wearable devices for improved healthcare delivery requires the integration of innovative solutions to improve healthcare conditions, improve quality of life, enhance early disease detection, support more effective health conditions monitoring and management, and offer more useful personalized insights to users (Mehta & Sharma, 2023; Sakthi et al., 2022). The use of wearable devices to improve healthcare delivery requires overcoming challenges related to user acceptance, adoption, security, and privacy (Iqbal et al., 2021; Perego et al., 2021). The design process itself plays a major role in addressing these issues while focusing on a user-oriented approach that could help integrate such devices into patients' daily lives (Smuck et al., 2021). Such a design process is critical for innovative, continuous, real-time health monitoring (Jakhar et al., 2022). Overall, wearables design that aims to improve the delivery of care requires a multidisciplinary approach to handle technical challenges, improve user experience, and leverage recent advances such as artificial intelligence, large language models, and the Internet of Things (IoT).

With advances in wearable devices and the rise of generative artificial intelligence (AI) and large language models (LLMs), there remains a need to address the design features of wearable devices. First, considering various perspectives of different users in the design of wearable devices can lead to better adherence and wider audience reach, as well as better addressing the existing challenges in different design paradigms (Romero-Perales et al., 2023). In addition, the successful adoption and use of wearable devices in a clinical setting require several features, such as personalized experiences and integration into healthcare systems, emphasizing the importance of addressing design aspects for effective implementation (Smuck et al., 2021). Furthermore, improving some medical conditions and preventative care using wearable devices requires the need to address design challenges for sustainable self-managed use on a daily basis (Hamari, 2021). Lastly, the evolving nature of wearable technologies demands precise fit testing and iterative human subject involvement throughout the design process, especially for innovative products lacking precedents (Islam et al., 2018).

This chapter is a survey of current trends in wearable design with a particular focus on the impact on improved healthcare delivery. The chapter provides a foundation for the design features of wearable devices, focusing on users' experience, acceptance, adoption, and continuous use of such devices. It emphasizes the role of wearable devices and their effective design in improving healthcare delivery. The outline of the chapter is as follows. First, we provide a survey of application domains application areas of wearable technology and supporting infrastructure within the healthcare domain. Next, we illustrate the critical role of software in wearable devices and provide an overview of software design elements and their impact on user experience. We discuss user interface (UI) design including the key principles for designing intuitive and engaging interfaces. We, then explore factors related to user experience (UX) design, including interaction design, personalization and customization, user education, and accessibility. An important aspect of wearable design is mainly related to software integration and ecosystem connectivity. We discuss smartphone integration and the health and fitness ecosystem in this context. Next, we discuss the role of privacy and security in wearable design, including data privacy and security features. We conclude with a discussion of implications for practice and research focusing on how the integration of wearables in the healthcare system could improve the healthcare delivery process.

REFERENCES

Bayoumy, K., Gaber, M., Elshafeey, A., Mhaimeed, O., Dineen, E. H., Marvel, F. A., Martin, S. S., Muse, E. D., Turakhia, M. P., Tarakji, K. G., & Elshazly, M. B. (2021). Smart wearable devices in cardiovascular care: Where we are and how to move forward. *Nature Reviews. Cardiology*, 18(8), 581–599. DOI: 10.1038/s41569-021-00522-7

Channa, A., Popescu, N., Skibinska, J., & Burget, R. (2021). The Rise of Wearable Devices during the COVID-19 Pandemic: A Systematic Review. *Sensors (Basel)*, 21(17), 17. Advance online publication. DOI: 10.3390/s21175787

Cheung, M. L., Chau, K. Y., Lam, M. H. S., Tse, G., Ho, K. Y., Flint, S. W., Broom, D. R., Tso, E. K. H., & Lee, K. Y. (2019). Examining Consumers' Adoption of Wearable Healthcare Technology: The Role of Health Attributes. *International Journal of Environmental Research and Public Health*, 16(13), 13. Advance online publication. DOI: 10.3390/ijerph16132257

El-Gayar, O., Elnoshokaty, A., & Behrens, A. (2021). Understanding Design Features for Continued Use of Wearables Devices. *Twenty-Seventh Americas Conference on Information Systems*. Americas Conference on Information Systems, Montreal.

El-Gayar, O., Nasralah, T., & Noshokaty, A. E. (2019). Wearable devices for health and wellbeing: Design Insights from Twitter. *Proceedings of the 52nd Hawaii International Conference on System Sciences*, 10. DOI: 10.24251/HICSS.2019.467

El-Masri, M., Al-Yafi, K., & Kamal, M. M. (2022). A Task-Technology-Identity Fit Model of Smartwatch Utilisation and User Satisfaction: A Hybrid SEM-Neural Network Approach. *Information Systems Frontiers*. Advance online publication. DOI: 10.1007/s10796-022-10256-7

Erdmier, C., Hatcher, J., & Lee, M. (2016). Wearable device implications in the healthcare industry. *Journal of Medical Engineering & Technology*, 40(4), 4. Advance online publication. DOI: 10.3109/03091902.2016.1153738

Esen, Ö. C., & Eroğlu, I. (2018). The Effect of Product Technology to Product Acceptance in The User Interaction of Wearable Products – An Assessment of Activity Tracker Product Designed Within The Scope of Health Benefits. *DS 91: Proceedings of NordDesign 2018, Linköping, Sweden, 14th - 17th August 2018*. NordDesign 2018.

Hamari, J. (2021). *Towards the Next Generation of Extended Reality Wearables*. 1–7.

Hasan, M. N.-U., & Stannard, C. R. (2022). Exploring online consumer reviews of wearable technology: The Owlet Smart Sock. *Research Journal of Textile and Apparel, ahead-of-print*(ahead-of-print), Article ahead-of-print. DOI: 10.1108/RJTA-08-2021-0103

Hope, A. A., & McPeake, J. (2022). Healthcare delivery and recovery after critical illness. *Current Opinion in Critical Care*, 28(5), 566–571. DOI: 10.1097/MCC.0000000000000984

Ibrahim, T., & Ali, H. (2023). The Impact of Wearable IoT Devices on Early Disease Detection and Prevention. *International Journal of Applied Health Care Analytics*, 8(8), 8.

Iqbal, S. M. A., Mahgoub, I., Du, E., Leavitt, M. A., & Asghar, W. (2021). Advances in healthcare wearable devices. *NPJ Flexible Electronics*, 5(1), 1–14. DOI: 10.1038/s41528-021-00107-x

Islam, R., Holland, S., Price, B., Georgiou, T., & Mulholland, P. (2018). *Wearables for Long Term Gait Rehabilitation of Neurological Conditions.*

Jakhar, P., Rajagopalan, P., Shukla, M., & Singh, V. (2022). Wearable Devices for Real-time Disease Monitoring in Healthcare. In *Nanosensors for Futuristic Smart and Intelligent Healthcare Systems*. CRC Press. DOI: 10.1201/9781003093534-5

Karahanoglu, A., & Erbug, Ç. (2011). *Perceived qualities of smart wearables: Determinants of user acceptance.* DPPI., DOI: 10.1145/2347504.2347533

Kumari, R., & Chander, S. (2024). Improving healthcare quality by unifying the American electronic medical report system: Time for change. *The Egyptian Heart Journal*, 76(1), 32. DOI: 10.1186/s43044-024-00463-9

Lewy, H. (2015). Wearable technologies – future challenges for implementation in healthcare services. *Healthcare Technology Letters*, 2(1), 1. Advance online publication. DOI: 10.1049/htl.2014.0104

Lukowicz, P., Kirstein, T., & Tröster, G. (2004). Wearable systems for health care applications. *Methods of Information in Medicine*, 43(3), 232–238. DOI: 10.1055/s-0038-1633863

Makeham, M. (2019). My Health Record: Connecting Australians with their own health information. *The HIM Journal*, 48(3), 113–115. DOI: 10.1177/1833358319841511

Mehta, S., & Sharma, D. (2023). Wearable technology in healthcare engineering. In *Emerging Nanotechnologies for Medical Applications* (pp. 227–248). Elsevier. DOI: 10.1016/B978-0-323-91182-5.00005-X

Mettler, T., & Wulf, J. (2019). Physiolytics at the workplace: Affordances and constraints of wearables use from an employee's perspective. *Information Systems Journal*, 29(1), 245–273. DOI: 10.1111/isj.12205

Patel, V., Moosa, S., Sundaram, S., Langer, L., MacMillan, T. E., Cavalcanti, R., Cram, P., Gunaratne, K., Bayley, M., & Wu, R. (2022). Perceptions of patients and nurses regarding the use of wearables in inpatient settings: A mixed methods study. *Informatics for Health & Social Care*, 47(4), 444–452. DOI: 10.1080/17538157.2022.2042304

Perego, P., Scagnoli, M., & Sironi, R. (2021). *Co-design the acceptability of wearables in the healthcare field.* 21–32.

Pustiek, M., Beristain, A., & Kos, A. (2015). Challenges in Wearable Devices Based Pervasive Wellbeing Monitoring. *2015 International Conference on Identification, Information, and Knowledge in the Internet of Things (IIKI)*, 236–243. DOI: 10.1109/IIKI.2015.58

Rathore, P. S., & Sharma, B. K. (2022). Improving Healthcare Delivery System using Business Intelligence. *Journal of IoT in Social, Mobile, Analytics, and Cloud*, 4(1), 11–23. DOI: 10.36548/jismac.2022.1.002

Romero-Perales, E., Sainz-de-Baranda Andujar, C., & López-Ongil, C. (2023). Electronic Design for Wearables Devices Addressed from a Gender Perspective: Cross-Influences and a Methodological Proposal. *Sensors (Basel)*, 23(12), 5483. DOI: 10.3390/s23125483

Sakthi, A. S., Inbamani, A., Elango, R., Niveda, S., Preethi, M., Rajalakshmi, R., & Veerasamy, V. (2022). Healthcare Solutions Using Wearable Devices. In *Smart and Secure Internet of Healthcare Things* (pp. 1–16). CRC Press. DOI: 10.1201/9781003239895-1

Singh, S., Chowdhary, S. K., Rawat, S., & Acharya, B. M. (2023). 5G Revolution Transforming the Delivery in Healthcare. In Swarnkar, T., Patnaik, S., Mitra, P., Misra, S., & Mishra, M. (Eds.), *Ambient Intelligence in Health Care* (pp. 179–188). Springer Nature., DOI: 10.1007/978-981-19-6068-0_17

Smuck, M., Odonkor, C. A., Wilt, J. K., Schmidt, N., & Swiernik, M. A. (2021). The emerging clinical role of wearables: Factors for successful implementation in healthcare. *NPJ Digital Medicine*, 4(1), 1–8. DOI: 10.1038/s41746-021-00418-3

Yang, P., Bi, G., Qi, J., Wang, X., Yang, Y., & Xu, L. (2021). Multimodal wearable intelligence for dementia care in healthcare 4.0: A survey. *Information Systems Frontiers*, ●●●, 1–18. DOI: 10.1007/s10796-021-10163-3

Yang, Q., Mamun, A. A., Hayat, N., Jingzu, G., Hoque, M. E., & Salameh, A. A. (2022). Modeling the Intention and Adoption of Wearable Fitness Devices: A Study Using SEM-PLS Analysis. *Frontiers in Public Health*, 10, 918989. Advance online publication. DOI: 10.3389/fpubh.2022.918989

Zhou, T., Wang, Y., Yan, L., & Tan, Y. (2023). Spoiled for choice? Personalized recommendation for healthcare decisions: A multiarmed bandit approach. *Information Systems Research*, 34(4), 1493–1512. DOI: 10.1287/isre.2022.1191

Chapter 16
Bridging the Gap Between Augmentation and Cognition:
A Comparative Analysis of Wearable and Spatial Augmented Reality for People With aMCI

Martin Böhmer
Martin Luther University Halle-Wittenberg, Germany

Stephan Kuehnel
https://orcid.org/0000-0002-6959-9555
Martin Luther University Halle-Wittenberg, Germany

Johannes Damarowsky
https://orcid.org/0000-0001-8966-5524
Martin Luther University Halle-Wittenberg, Germany

ABSTRACT

This study examines the effectiveness of conventional and spatial augmented reality in assisting individuals with amnestic mild cognitive impairment, which is characterized by memory loss and cognitive challenges. As neurodegenerative diseases become more prevalent in the aging population, AR solutions can improve daily functioning and independence. This study compares the usability and user perceptions of wearable AR and projection-based SAR in augmented living spaces. Results show that SAR significantly reduces cognitive load and anxiety compared to traditional wearable systems. Its intuitive interface and seamless environmental integration lead to improved user satisfaction and higher adoption rates. Participants consis-

DOI: 10.4018/979-8-3693-5237-3.ch016

tently rated spatial augmented reality higher on all usability metrics, suggesting its suitability as a digital health intervention for individuals with aMCI. Adding to the theoretical discourse on the cognitive adoption of innovative digital health solutions, these findings highlight the need for user-centered AR technologies that improve health outcomes.

1. INTRODUCTION

Global demographic shifts have created significant economic and healthcare challenges, particularly a rapidly aging population and an increase in neurodegenerative diseases such as dementia and other cognitive impairments. These conditions, characterized by memory loss, disorientation, and anxiety, have a significant impact on daily life and healthcare systems (Bloom and Canning, 2008; Flicker et al., 1991). Cognitive impairment involves a decline in mental abilities, affecting perception, recognition, memory, thinking, and judgment (von Arnim et al., 2019). While not synonymous with dementia, cognitive impairment is often considered a precursor to such conditions (Gauthier et al., 2006). As posited by cognitive adoption theory, the interaction with technology by individuals with mild cognitive impairment (MCI), which includes but is not limited to the elderly, differs significantly from that of the general population (Böhmer et al., 2024). This requires tailored approaches and intuitive interfaces, as cognitive factors such as task difficulty, cognitive load, and social environment influence technology adoption (Ienca et al., 2021). The study presented here focuses on individuals with amnestic mild cognitive impairment (aMCI), a form of MCI that primarily affects memory but allows for independent living (Petersen, 2016; Petersen et al., 2018; Yu et al., 2017). In particular, multi-domain aMCI, in which memory decline coexists with impairments in other cognitive domains such as executive function, presents additional challenges in daily activities such as understanding complex instructions, using digital tools, or remembering to turn off household appliances (e.g., the stove).

Information technology solutions, especially in the form of Ambient Assisted Living (AAL) systems, offer numerous opportunities to support the lives of elderly and aMCI individuals. These solutions range from technology-enabled transformation of post-acute care (Singh et al., 2011) to fall detection with wearable sensors (Yu et al., 2022) and home activity monitoring (Zhu et al., 2020). Augmented reality (AR) is being explored to assist the elderly and people with aMCI in performing daily tasks. Traditional AR approaches use head-mounted displays (HMDs) that integrate virtual and physical environments (Azuma et al., 2001). However, wearable AR with HMDs has limitations such as limited battery capacity, complex menus, reduced field of view, attention issues, and ergonomic challenges (Biocca et al.,

2007; Steffen et al., 2019). An alternative to wearable AR is spatial AR (SAR), which uses projectors and loudspeakers (Raskar et al., 1998; Vertucci et al., 2023). SAR can reduce cognitive load and increase usability compared to HMD-based AR (Baumeister et al., 2017). Despite its potential, the application of SAR in healthcare and AAL settings is underexplored. Most research has focused on SAR in industrial contexts (Rupprecht et al., 2020; Cardoso et al., 2020; Tavares et al., 2019). In the context of aMCI, isolated SAR applications include projection robots for reminders (Yang et al., 2018) and smart home notifications (Wegerich et al., 2010).

Highly specific services such as telemedicine may not fully address the healthcare needs of aMCI individuals who struggle with dynamic, complex assistance tasks (e.g., recognizing hazards from kitchen appliances or providing therapeutic interventions). SAR, integrated with context reasoning, can enhance context awareness and assistance, facilitating real-time interaction in daily living scenarios. However, there is a notable gap in research comparing wearable AR with projection-based SAR to investigate the potential benefits of SAR for people with aMCI – especially in digital health. Addressing this research gap, our study aims to answer the following research question:

RQ: *How do users with aMCI perceive the performance expectancy, effort expectancy, and anxiety of wearable AR compared to spatial AR in the context of augmented living spaces?*

As such, this study builds on the call for more research on AR by Baker et al. (2023), who emphasize the need for early identification and mitigation of unintended negative consequences of AR. It also incorporates the perspective of Mohammadhossein et al. (2024), who view AR as an emerging technology with barriers to usability and accessibility, to deepen understanding of the impact of AR on this vulnerable population. Through a comparative analysis and subsequent think-aloud session with qualitative analysis of wearable and projection-based AR, this research seeks to provide preliminary data to inform future digital health strategies and interventions tailored to support aging populations and those with cognitive impairments. Thus, our study found that projection-based SAR, in the context of augmented living spaces, achieved higher scores in terms of expected performance and effort as well as reduced scores in anxiety compared to wearable AR among individuals with aMCI. The SAR system was perceived as easier to use, more intuitive, and less anxiety-provoking, potentially promoting higher adoption rates and better health outcomes, confirming the assumptions of our kernel theory of cognitive adoption (Böhmer et al., 2024). Thus, this research contributes to theoretical advances in the cognitive adoption of digital health technologies and provides practical implications for designing more accessible and user-friendly AR systems for vulnerable populations.

In the next sections, we focus on the theoretical foundations of AR in healthcare, spatial augmented reality, and our study context of augmented living spaces. We then present our research design and applied methodologies before presenting our results and delving into the comparative analysis and think-aloud session. Finally, we will discuss the findings and implications of this study and provide interesting areas for future research.

2. THEORETICAL FOUNDATIONS

AR has the potential to improve healthcare by providing digital information overlays that enhance surgery, rehabilitation, and medical education, improving accuracy and patient outcomes. In particular, SAR, an innovative form of AR that integrates real-world surfaces with digital content, offers interactive applications without head-mounted displays, potentially benefiting the elderly and cognitively impaired in augmented environments. Despite their potential, both technologies face challenges in adoption, accessibility, and understanding of their long-term implications, requiring tailored approaches to maximize their benefits and mitigate negative consequences (Baker White et al., 2023). Hence, our study adopts the *analyze with lens*-mechanism proposed by Möller et al. (2022), which includes the use of kernel theories for in-depth analysis of a specific phenomenon to guide the analysis based on concepts in the theory. Therefore, we decided to use *Cognitive Adoption Theory* (Böhmer et al., 2024) as our theoretical lens because it integrates both social-cognitive and cognitive load factors and posits that the adoption of digital health technologies with subsequent health behavior change among people with cognitive impairment, which may or may not (but often does) include the elderly, differs from that of the general population. It not only guides our research design in terms of measures taken, but also as a framework to explore which aspects of cognitive load or self-efficacy influence the usability, accessibility, and learning effort of a digital health technology (i.e., an augmented living space in our case) in terms of its adoption.

2.1. Augmented Reality in Healthcare

The ability to still act in the real world despite being provided with digital information makes AR not only highly interesting but also challenging, with potential applications in surgery, rehabilitation, healthcare training, care, or cognitive neurology (Hoque et al., 2022). While headset-based wearable AR (e.g., Microsoft HoloLens or Apple Vision Pro) is the most widely used form of AR, these technologies have demonstrated significant potential to transform various aspects of healthcare, from surgical precision to medical education. To address the former, AR is used not only in neurosurgery (Masutani et al., 1998) but also in soft tissue surgery (Beller et al., 2007) or catheter-based interventional procedures (Antz et al., 2006; Richmond et al., 2008). Studies such as Guerroudji et al. (2024) and Cotin and Haouchine (2023) have shown that AR can improve the accuracy of complex surgical procedures by superimposing critical anatomical information on the surgical field, thereby reducing errors and improving patient outcomes. In the field of rehabilitation, Ong et al. (2023) presented the ARTHE system, which stages exercises to enhance motor skill recovery, demonstrating superior efficacy compared to traditional methods. The role of AR in medical education is further emphasized in research by Dhar et al. (2021), which highlights its ability to create immersive and interactive learning environments that enhance knowledge retention and practical skills among students. Kriegel et al. (2023) explored the potential of AR to enhance various aspects of children's lives, including education and social interactions, particularly during the COVID-19 pandemic, although they also noted challenges such as accessibility and potential negative health effects. Despite high initial costs, the economic benefits of AR in healthcare have been highlighted by Gómez Bergin and Craven (2023), who advocate for comprehensive economic analyses to understand the long-term financial implications of AR adoption. In addition, AR technologies have been crucial in critical care, as noted by Bruno et al. (2022), where they enhance training and real-time patient monitoring, improving decision-making processes. In addition, as shown by Kanschik et al. (2023), AR tools help visualize complex data and integrate it with real-time patient information to help healthcare providers make informed decisions quickly. Their study suggests that AR, by focusing on its ability to enhance patient monitoring, can significantly improve the efficiency and effectiveness of intensive care units, as well as the accuracy of critical care procedures. In the context of cognitive rehabilitation, Makhataeva et al. (2023) found AR to be effective in improving memory, attention, and problem-solving skills in patients with cognitive impairments. Finally, Tene et al. (2024) provided a comprehensive review that synthesized findings on the use of VR and AR in healthcare education and training, concluding that these immersive technologies significantly improve learning outcomes, engagement, and knowledge retention among healthcare professionals. In addition, AR is also being used to capture brain signals to understand what is happening in the brain as a result of neurodegenerative diseases (Cardin et al., 2016).

Collectively, this body of work underscores the transformative impact of AR in healthcare and presents both opportunities and challenges that warrant further exploration to fully realize their potential in improving medical outcomes, health applications, and education. However, while AR has been around for quite some time now, it is still seen as an emergent technology, and obstacles to using AR are still prevalent (Mohammadhossein et al., 2024), especially among vulnerable populations such as the aging society and individuals with cognitive impairments. Because we need to identify early on any unintended negative consequences of using such technology and develop solutions to mitigate those consequences (White Baker et al., 2023), a tailored approach that carefully navigates the challenges of adoption and optimizes the benefits is essential - as could be done in this context with Spatial Augmented Reality.

2.2. Spatial Augmented Reality

Although the first concept of SAR dates back to the late 1990s (Raskar et al., 1998), its application and use have not gained the same traction as wearable-based approaches. SAR integrates real-world surfaces with projected or audible digital content, enabling interaction without the need for head-mounted displays. These concepts are based on the work of Raskar et al. (1998) on SAR, which introduced the idea of surface shape extraction, rendering methods, and capture artifacts, and have been further developed by subsequent research in the field. Grundhöfer and Iwai (2018) provide a comprehensive overview of the current state-of-the-art algorithms, hardware, and applications of projection mapping in SAR. In particular, current research streams are more focused on technical implementation and cover ontologies and techniques of SAR. Key insights include, among others, error-free compensation methods for projection (Huang et al., 2021), projection manipulation (Miyamoto et al., 2018; Lindlbauer et al., 2017), ideal projection surfaces (Ro et al., 2019), and successful practical applications of SAR in various domains such as cooking assistance for cognitively impaired people (Kosch et al., 2019). These studies highlight the progress and practical benefits of SAR technologies, even though SAR is mainly applied in the manufacturing and maintenance sectors (Uva et al., 2018; Vorraber et al., 2020; Zhou et al., 2012). In terms of feasibility, Di Donato et al. (2015) have done significant work in exploring different surface projections to determine the most appropriate surfaces for SAR. In addition, the exploration of interaction techniques and user interfaces for SAR has expanded, as described in studies by Benko et al. (2012), who explored direct interaction with projected content, and Wilson and Benko (2010), who explored depth-sensing techniques to enhance SAR interactivity. More recently, the use of artificial intelligence to enable projection onto moving objects has also been explored in recent studies (e.g., Gomes et al., 2021; Kobayashi & Hashimoto, 2014; Lee et al., 2019). AI-driven SAR systems can dynamically adjust projections in real time, increasing the versatility and applicability of SAR in dynamic environments. In addition, SAR has found applications in education and training, as demonstrated by Cordeil et al. (2017), who used SAR for collaborative data visualization, highlighting the potential of SAR to transform various domains by providing intuitive and interactive visualization tools.

In summary, the evolution of SAR from its conceptual roots to modern applications underscores its growing importance. However, while the potential of SAR in various domains is clear, its applications and uses remain underexplored, especially in the context of digital health, where only rare isolated applications exist (e.g., Kosch et al., 2019; Yang et al., 2018). The integration of advanced projection techniques, AI, and user interaction methods further expands the capabilities of SAR, paving the way for innovative applications in various fields, especially in digital health, where innovative solutions can be developed based on it.

2.3. Augmented Living Spaces

The concept of Augmented Living Spaces, first introduced by Böhmer et al. (2022) and followed by a detailed technical implementation (Böhmer et al., 2023), uses SAR to immerse users in their environment by projecting relevant information directly into their living space. This innovative approach eliminates the need for potentially cumbersome wearables such as tablets and headsets, making it particularly beneficial for the elderly or those with cognitive impairments. Tailored to individual needs, impairments, and preferences, these augmented living spaces provide comprehensive support for perception, mobility, organization, and medication management, thereby promoting prolonged autonomy without dependence on wearable technology. The implementation involves augmenting specific household objects (e.g., stove, calendar, medication box) with projected widgets consisting of both functional and offering components. These enhancements target areas where aging adults, particularly those with cognitive impairments, often experience declines in cognitive performance (Gauthier et al., 2006; Jongsiriyanyong & Limpawattana, 2018; Petersen et al., 2016; Petersen, 2018). For example, a stove widget may display the operating status and temperature of the stove plates (functional component) along with recipe suggestions (offering component).

Figure 1 shows an example of a SAR-based augmented living space with different widgets. The widgets and their variety are designed to maintain and promote independence for aging people or those with MCI more abstractly while mitigating potential dangers. These SAR-driven environments function as digital health information systems that provide low-threshold, unobtrusive, yet effective and individualized services, addressing the challenges commonly associated with wearable AR for this population (White Baker et al., 2023). To facilitate accessible human-computer interactions, these augmented living spaces use an AI-driven information system to monitor specific zones within the environment.

Figure 1. Exemplary SAR-based augmented living space for individuals with aMCI

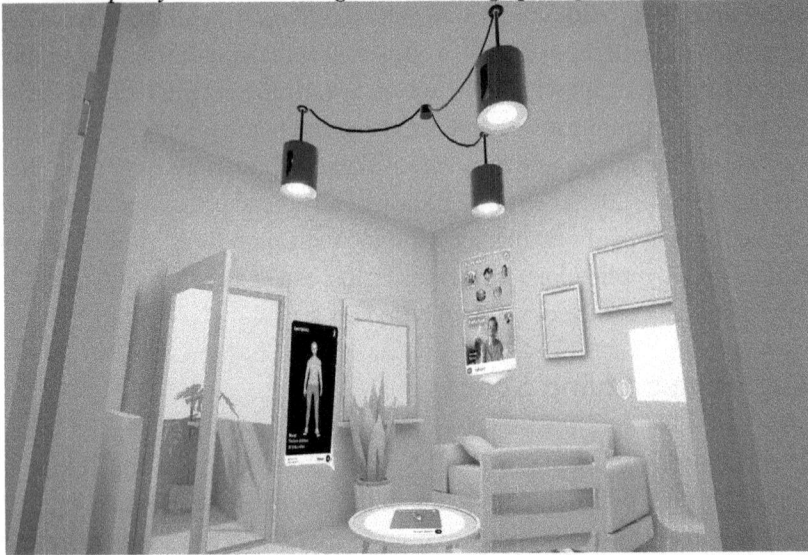

The AI uses a deep learning model trained on synthetic image data to recognize and understand the environment and people, detect objects and people, determine their locations, and infer their contexts. When a person enters a designated zone, the system projects relevant and contextual information directly into their living space at their current location. For example, the system can expand a widget from a minimized icon when a person enters the zone and minimize it again when the person leaves. This mechanism allows the system to highlight potential hazards in the user's immediate environment or guide them through daily tasks without the need for wearable devices. The augmented living spaces are designed to be intuitive and easy to use, responding naturally to the user's location and actions with minimal direct interaction, eliminating the need for explicit commands or complex interfaces.

While pilot studies and preliminary evaluations have shown promising results in terms of perceived usefulness, usability, and adoption, there is still a need to explore whether there is a significant difference between using the same digital health IS (i.e., an augmented living space) in wearable or spatial AR. This is particularly relevant in the context of an aging population, as wearable headsets may not be worn without exception due to attention issues (Biocca et al., 2007) and ergonomic challenges (Steffen et al., 2019). In addition, there is still considerable research to be done on the underlying aspects of their technology adoption that would lead them to prefer one approach over the other.

3. RESEARCH DESIGN

To explore the aforementioned research gap and answer the proposed research question, we will ground our methodology on *experimental research* and *comparative analysis*. Guided by the principles of positivism, experimental research allows for the rigorous testing of research questions and hypotheses by manipulating independent variables and observing their effects on dependent variables, making it suitable for assessing the effectiveness and perceived utility of different AR approaches in controlled settings (Robey, 1996; Straub et al., 2004). This approach allows for causal inference, providing a solid foundation for evaluating wearable-based AR with projection-based SAR. Complementarily, a comparative analysis grounded in the interpretivist paradigm facilitates our intended investigation of the conceptual differences and similarities concerning the usability between the two AR approaches. This methodological approach, which emphasizes qualitative contrasts and contextual interpretation, allows for a nuanced understanding of the applicability and implications of AR in different IS contexts (Kaplan & Duchon, 1988; Stowell & Mingers, 1997). In general, we conducted a mixed methods study (Venkatesh et al., 2013) that included an initial questionnaire-based comparative analysis followed by a qualitatively analyzed think-aloud session to address the shortcomings of the methods considered individually (i.e., to enrich the results of the comparative analysis with in-depth qualitative insights). Such an approach is highly valuable in digital health research, as it combines quantitative rigor with qualitative depth (Creswell & Plano Clark, 2017). Given the qualitative nature of the follow-up think-aloud a smaller sample size for our pilot study is more manageable and allows for in-depth, meaningful analysis (Guest et al., 2006).

Figure 2. Comparative analysis and think-aloud approach

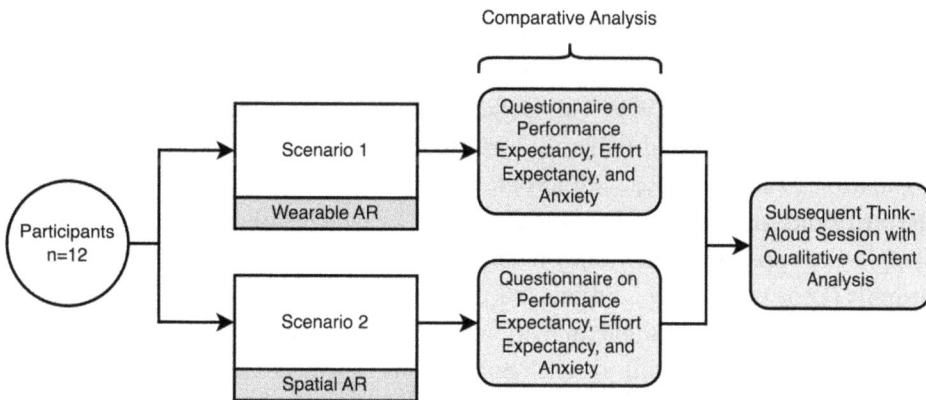

417

As shown in Figure 2, we developed two similar scenarios of augmented living spaces with the same 5 assistive widgets (comparable to the mockup shown in Figure 1), one approached by a wearable AR headset (Scenario 1), the other by SAR (Scenario 2). To reduce bias, participants were randomly assigned to start with either the wearable AR or SAR scenario. After a short introduction, participants were asked to freely use the augmented living space, interact with widgets, and complete small guidance tasks, followed by the questionnaire. After completing both scenarios and questionnaires, all participants gathered in the augmented living space and were asked to express and verbalize their thoughts, feelings, and impressions, and were able to show and discuss them based on the technology of both scenarios.

We based our Likert scale (1=strong disagreement; 7=strong agreement) questionnaire on the constructs of *Performance Expectancy* (PE), *Effort Expectancy* (EE), and *Anxiety* (ANX) from the UTAUT model (Venkatesh et al., 2003) because of their meaningfulness and informative value in our context. In a nutshell, PE assesses the perceived usefulness of the system in terms of helping and achieving performance, EE describes the degree of ease associated with using the system, and ANX describes the intimidation or apprehension associated with using the system. It should be noted that while the UTAUT model treats anxiety as an indirect determinant of behavioral intention, it also posits that anxiety affects how users perceive the ease of using the technology, which in turn affects their intention to use it. For our questionnaire, we inverted the Likert scale for the ANX items, as higher anxiety about using a system typically harms use (which is the opposite for PE and EE).

For the comparative analysis of the questionnaire, we used the non-parametric Wilcoxon Signed Rank test, meaning it does not assume a normal distribution of differences between paired observations (wearable AR and SAR scenario). This characteristic makes it suitable for small sample sizes because it is less sensitive to the underlying distribution of the data than parametric tests such as the paired t-test (Hollander et al., 2013; McCrum-Gardner, 2008). While there is no universally agreed upon minimum sample size for the Wilcoxon Signed Rank Test, statistical guidelines suggest that a sample size of 10-15 pairs can provide adequate power and validity (Conover, 1999; Van Belle, 2008), so our sample size of 12 pairs is within this recommended range. In our specific case, research involving specific populations, such as those with aMCI, often faces recruitment challenges due to the rarity and specific criteria of the condition. In such healthcare contexts, smaller sample sizes are sometimes unavoidable and necessary but can still yield valuable insights (Leon et al., 2011). Julious (2005) suggests that sample sizes as small as 12 can be justified for pilot studies and initial investigations, particularly when working with rare conditions or hard-to-reach populations. Therefore, following Hwang and Salvendy's (2010) 10±2 rule for think-aloud sessions, we argue that the difficulty of recruiting larger samples in rare conditions in empirical settings justifies the use of smaller sample sizes followed by qualitative analysis without compromising the overall goals of the study. Here, the qualitative analysis will provide context and insight into the quantitative results, which is particularly valuable when sample sizes are small (Creswell & Plano Clark, 2017). The qualitative component with the same 12 subjects will help to understand the reasons behind their responses, adding depth to the analysis that compensates for the smaller quantitative sample size.

Table 1. Factor loadings for constructs of both questionnaires

Performance Expectancy (PE1-PE4)	AR	SAR	Effort Expectancy (EE1-EE4)	AR	SAR	Anxiety (ANX1-ANX4)	AR	SAR
Loadings			*Loadings*			*Loadings*		
Usefulness	.785	.699	Clarity	.839	.571	Apprehension	.725	.914
Quickness	.629	.754	Easy to Master	.934	.740	Loss of Information	.689	.582
Productivity	.543	.866	Easy to Use	.779	.998	Hesitation	.463	.845
Chance of Raise*	.856	.792	Easy to Learn	.752	.784	Intimidation	.866	.572
AVE	.510	.609	**AVE**	.687	.621	**AVE**	.491	.554
CCR	.802	.861	**CCR**	.892	.863	**CCR**	.787	.826

To validate the quality of the PE, EE, and ANX constructs, we examined item reliability (loadings), composite construct reliability, and average variance extracted (Hulland, 1999). We assessed item reliability by examining the loadings of the measured items on their respective constructs. As shown in Table 1, confirmatory factor analysis in R indicated that all item loadings exceeded the threshold required to avoid bias (Nunnally, 1978; Hulland, 1999). The average variance extracted (AVE) for all items and artifacts is greater than 0.5, indicating that the variance captured by the construct exceeds measurement error (Fornell & Larcker, 1981). The composite construct reliability (CCR) exceeds the threshold of 0.7 for all items and artifacts (Hulland, 1999; Nunnally, 1978). Based on these criteria, our measurement models with four items each for the constructs PE, EE, and ANX are suitable for evaluation. Our evaluation focused on inferential validity (the relationship between treatment and outcome) and construct validity (accurate measurement) using established measures from previous research (Wohlin et al., 2012; Venkatesh et al., 2003). For the subsequent think-aloud session, we followed the retrospective think-aloud method (van den Haak et al., 2003) to minimize the interference with task performance that can occur with concurrent think-aloud methods. As described in more detail in Section 4.2., the results of this think-aloud session were then content analyzed following Gioia et al.'s (2013) theory-building method, developing first-order informant concepts for induction, as well as second-order themes and aggregate dimensions for abduction and systematic combination of data and theory.

4. RESULTS

While AR in general has the potential to not only transform the healthcare sector, but also provide digital health to vulnerable populations (Hoque et al., 2022), there are still challenges and barriers to adoption, use, and subsequent health behavior change (Mohammadhossein et al., 2024). As shown in Figure 3, our comparative analysis reveals differences in perceived performance expectancy, effort expectancy, and anxiety of wearable AR and SAR approaches among users with aMCI. The box plot in Figure 3 illustrates the distribution and direction of scores of our post-hoc analysis for these constructs across the two AR approaches, where higher scores on the 7-point Likert scale are associated with greater agreement with the item statements and thus imply a positive perception.

Figure 3. Boxplots for the comparative analysis on construct-level

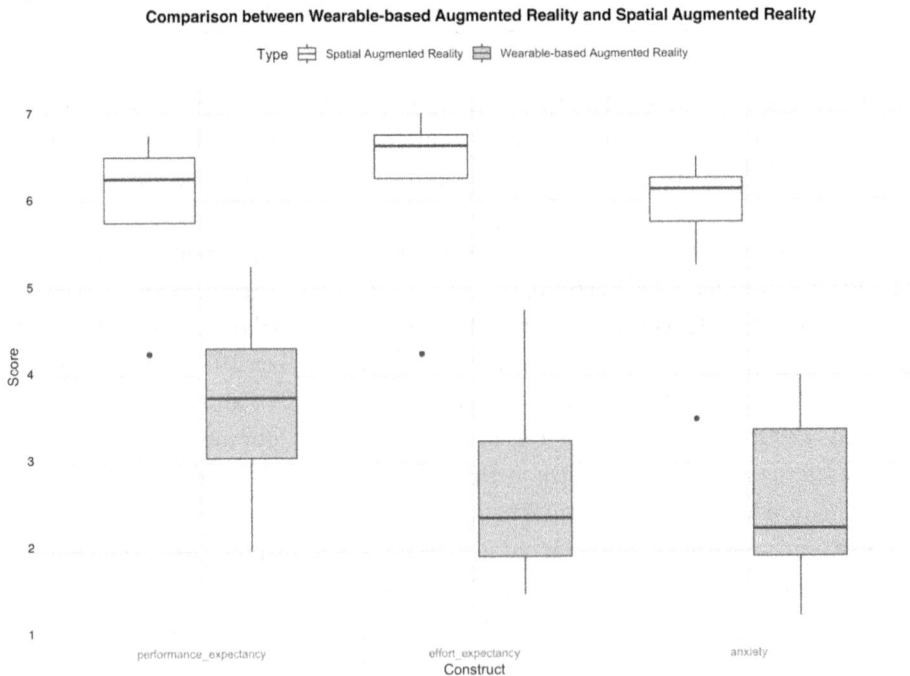

Comparison between Wearable-based Augmented Reality and Spatial Augmented Reality

Regarding PE, users consistently rated the projection-based SAR system higher, with most scores clustering around 6 to 7 (median=6.25), showing high agreement on performance expectancy. The scores for the wearable AR system were lower (median=3.75), with a wider interquartile range, meaning that users may find the goal of the system (i.e., daily support and assistance) reasonable, but not its implementation. In the context of EE, users reported a low expectation of effort, with scores predominantly between 6 and 7 (median=6.60), consistent with the intuitive and indirect nature of SAR. The wearable AR system received lower scores (median=2.40), indicating a higher perceived effort due to the more complex headset and a wider range of user responses. Finally, users reported low levels of anxiety, with scores clustered between 6 and 7 (median=6.15), indicating less perceived intimidation, hesitation, and intimidation. The ANX scores for the wearable AR system were much higher (i.e., they scored lower) with several outliers (median=2.25), indicating strong anxiety about using the system.

4.1. Comparative Analysis of Performance and Effort Expectancy

Table 2 shows the results of the Wilcoxon Signed Rank test both on item- and construct-level for PE, EE, and ANX. On the construct level, PE evaluates the degree to which users believe that the respective AR systems will assist them in achieving improvements in daily task performance (e.g., reminders, warnings, rehabilitation guidance). In our study context of augmented living spaces, especially among people with aMCI, this construct measures the perceived usefulness and effectiveness of the AR approaches in supporting cognitive and functional tasks. The test results for PE at the construct level indicate a highly significant difference (p=0.001***), with users rating significantly higher performance expectancy in terms of perceived usefulness and effectiveness for the projection-based SAR system compared to the wearable AR system. At the item level, users rated the projection-based SAR system as significantly more useful (p=0.007**), likely due to its immediate and indirect presentation of information, which increases its perceived usefulness (PE1). In addition, the SAR system was perceived to be significantly faster in providing information (p=0.003**), an important factor for users who may be experiencing cognitive or functional delays in performing their daily tasks (PE2). In terms of productivity (PE3), users felt that the projection-based SAR system significantly improved their productivity in performing daily tasks such as taking medication, cooking, or reminder/warning (p=0.001***), as it seamlessly integrates helpful information into their environment, reducing the cognitive switching that occurs with wearable AR. Since PE4 (chance of getting a raise) from the original UTAUT model would have no explanatory power in our context, we slightly changed it to "chance of getting health benefits" that users perceive they would get from using the system (which retains the original intention and measure of the item). As expected, there was no significant difference in perceived health benefits between the two AR approaches (p=0.058), indicating that both systems are viewed similarly in terms of providing health information and potential health benefits (e.g., free therapies or programs, massages, treatments). In general, the significant preference suggests that the projection-based SAR system is more effective in assisting users with aMCI to perform daily tasks, likely due to its intuitive and clear presentation of information directly in their environment. This ease of integration reduces cognitive load and increases the perceived usefulness and efficiency of the system, although the outliers and general distribution of the wearable AR approach show that the overall goal of the system (i.e., to assist with daily tasks) is not necessarily perceived negatively.

Table 2. Wilcoxon signed-rank test statistics and p-values on item- and construct-level

Performance Expectancy	p-Value	Effort Expectancy	p-Value	Anxiety	p-Value
Usefulness *(PE1)*	.007**	Clarity *(EE1)*	.005**	Apprehension *(ANX1)*	.009**
Quickness *(PE2)*	.003**	Easy to Master *(EE2)*	.001***	Loss of Information *(ANX2)*	.003**
Productivity *(PE3)*	.001***	Easy to Use *(EE3)*	.001***	Hesitation *(ANX3)*	.001***
Chance of Raise *(PE4)*	.058	Easy to Learn *(EE4)*	.001***	Intimidation *(ANX4)*	.001***
Construct-Level	.001***	*Construct-Level*	.001***	*Construct-Level*	.001***

(*) = p ≤ 0.05; (**) = p ≤ 0.01; (***) = p ≤ 0.001

Next, EE measures the ease and effort required to interact with the augmented environments or AR approaches. This construct is particularly critical for users with aMCI, as increased effort and complexity of interaction may lead to frustration and hinder consistent use/adoption. The test results for EE also showed a highly significant difference (p=0.001***), indicating that the projection-based SAR system was perceived as significantly easier to use than the wearable AR system. At the item level, the projection-based SAR system was significantly clearer (EE1) to understand (p=0.005**), which is critical for users with aMCI facing complex interfaces (e.g., nested menus, complex navigation, interaction design, overlays) that occur with wearable AR. In addition, users found the SAR system significantly easier to use (p=0.001***), likely due to its intuitive and indirect integration into the living environment without the need for additional wearables or prior knowledge/experience (EE2). Regarding EE3, the projection-based SAR system was perceived as significantly easier to use (p=0.001***), ensuring regular engagement and minimizing frustration that would occur with user input, system navigation, equipment, or complexity in wearable AR. Finally, the SAR system was significantly easier to learn (p=0.001***), reflecting its ability to reduce the learning curve for users affected by aMCI due to its intuitive nature (EE4). In general, these findings highlight the importance of minimizing cognitive and physical effort when designing AR systems for people with cognitive impairments. The reduced effort required by the projection-based system likely contributes to higher user satisfaction, adoption, and sustained engagement. The wearable AR approach may be perceived as too complex and cumbersome, especially given the lower technology affinity and competence of older generations.

Lastly, ANX assesses the level of apprehension or discomfort users feel when using the AR systems. High levels of anxiety can severely impact the adoption and effective use of such assisting AR technologies. Here, the test results also showed a highly significant difference (p=0.001***), indicating that users felt significantly lower anxiety, intimidation, or apprehension when using the projection-based SAR system compared to the wearable AR system. At the item level, the projection-based SAR system significantly reduced users' anxiety (ANX1) compared to the wearable AR system (p=0.009**), suggesting that projections elicit less anxious feelings in the context of technology adoption than wearable overlays. Users were also significantly less worried about losing information (ANX2) with the SAR system (p=0.003**), suggesting that wearable AR approaches frighten users into thinking that they could lose a lot of information using the system by pressing the wrong button or losing the assistive overlays. In addition, the projection-based SAR system significantly reduced hesitation (ANX3) in using the augmented living space (0.001***), indicating that the wearable AR system makes users more afraid of making mistakes they cannot correct, which hinders adoption and effective use. Finally, users felt significantly less intimidated (ANX4) by the projection-based SAR system (p=0.001***), indicating that users may feel intimidated by the additional and somewhat bulky headset and the cognitive switch between real-world objects and digital overlays that are more seamless in SAR. In general, this reduced anxiety in the SAR-based approach is crucial for promoting user acceptance and consistent usage, especially among individuals with aMCI who may already experience heightened levels of stress and disorientation.

In conclusion, our pilot comparative analysis between wearable AR and projection-based SAR systems reveals clear differences in user perception and experience, particularly for individuals with aMCI in the context of augmented living spaces. The results underscore the superior performance expectancy, lower effort expectancy, and reduced anxiety associated with the SAR system. Users consistently rated the projection-based SAR system higher in terms of usefulness, ease of use, and comfort, which are critical factors in the adoption and sustained use of AR technologies to assist with daily tasks (Böhmer et al., 2024). These findings highlight the importance of designing AR systems that minimize cognitive and physical effort, thereby increasing user satisfaction and engagement. While the comparative analysis revealed significant differences in the perception of the two AR approaches, the next section, with the subsequent think-aloud session, will delve deeper into the analysis to provide a more detailed understanding of the reasons behind these results.

4.2. Think Aloud Session and Qualitative Analysis

Following the questionnaire and item/construct-based analysis, we conducted a retrospective think-aloud session (van den Haak et al., 2003) with the same participants to gather deeper qualitative insights and their feelings, thoughts, and perceptions of both AR approaches. As shown in Table 3, and following the qualitative theory-building method of Gioia et al. (2013), we first transcribed the participants' expressions and developed inductive first-order concepts (due to space limitations, we decided to omit less relevant passages in the quotes), which were subsequently categorized into second-order themes and aggregate dimensions. Table 3 presents representative quotations from the think-aloud session, organized into first-order concepts. These quotations illustrate the diverse range of user experiences and perceptions regarding wearable-based AR and projection-based SAR systems. The first-order concepts derived from the think-aloud session reveal several key user insights. For example, many participants highlighted the ease of understanding and the intuitiveness of the projection-based SAR system compared to the wearable AR system, which was often described as complex, confusing, and frustrating. In their feedback, participants consistently highlighted the advantages of the projection-based system over the wearable AR system. Many found the projection system easier to understand and use, emphasizing that it provided clear and easily accessible information without requiring much cognitive effort. In contrast, the wearable AR system was often described as confusing, complicated, and anxiety-provoking. Users frequently mentioned that the wearable AR made them anxious and afraid of pressing the wrong buttons and that navigating through it was very challenging.

Table 3. Verbalized thoughts from the think-aloud session and corresponding first-order concepts

Representative think-aloud quotations from participants	1st Order Concepts
"The projection-based system was much easier for me to understand and use because the information was clear and always right where I needed it. [...] The wearable AR was too confusing, and I often didn't know where to look, which was frustrating. It was really hard to get used to the wearable as well, it felt awkward on my head. [...] The projection system just worked without me having to think about it, which made things so much simpler for me."	Projection-based system easier to understand; Wearable AR was confusing and frustrating; Projection system required less cognitive effort; Wearable AR felt awkward
"Using the wearable AR made me very anxious because I was scared of pressing the wrong button. It was also very complicated to navigate. I didn't feel confident using it at all. [...] The projection-based system, however, was more intuitive and really helped ease my stress and anxiety. I could see myself using the projection system every day because it was so much easier and felt more intuitive in general."	Anxiety with wearable AR; Wearable AR was complicated to navigate; Projection system was intuitive; Projection system eased stress
"The projection system was quick to give me information, which made me feel in control and less stressed. But the wearable AR was intimidating and hard to use. There was information everywhere and I felt a bit sick when I used it. This made me more anxious. [...] I liked the healthcare information being projected into the room because it felt like a natural part of my environment and wasn't complicated."	Quick information delivery with projection approach; Wearable AR was intimidating; Wearable AR caused nausea
"The wearable AR was a real struggle for me; I had to keep adjusting the headset, which was annoying and disrupted my focus. Also, I struggled somewhat to walk around the room with the headset as my perspective was not normal. [...] I don't know how to express this, but I didn't feel good wearing the headset. [...] The projection system, on the other hand, was straightforward and took less effort to learn, which made me feel more confident and less anxious."	Struggle with wearable AR adjustments; Wearable AR disrupted focus; Projection system required less effort to learn and was straightforward
"The projection-based system had clear information that was easy to understand and use. [...] I felt overwhelmed with the wearable AR because it needed a lot of adjustments and had a more complex navigation, which made me feel disengaged. I mean, the information was there within the headset but at the same time it was very hard to grasp for me. [...] The projection system would fit well into my daily routine and made me feel more engaged because it wasn't distracting and I wouldn't have to fully focus on it."	Clear information with projection system; Wearable AR was overwhelming and complex; Projection system fit well into daily routine; Disengagement in wearable AR
"I felt much more confident using the projection-based system because it was intuitive and user-friendly. [...] The wearable AR caused a lot of hesitation and anxiety for me because it was complex and I was afraid of making mistakes. [...] I also felt like I couldn't do anything else than using the headset, like for example read something or go to the toilet. The headset always felt restrictive, I didn't like it. The projection system responded quickly to my needs, making it feel more useful and efficient without having to wear something. I could read something and the information was still there where I would need it, and it wouldn't disturb my reading."	Confidence with projection system; Hesitation and stress with wearable AR; Wearable AR felt restrictive; Projection system allowed multitasking

continued on following page

Table 3. Continued

Representative think-aloud quotations from participants	1st Order Concepts
"The wearable AR was hard for me to use and often left me feeling frustrated because I couldn't get it to work right. Things always seemed a little bit blurry and it was hard for me to grasp the information within the headset; I don't know it was just hard for me to have that connection to the real world. [...] The projection system was much easier to use and understand, which helped me stay focused and less frustrated. The health information was always in my line of sight with the projection system, without me having to wear anything. I really liked that approach."	Frustration with wearable AR; Wearable AR had blurry visuals; Projection system was easy to use; Projection system kept health information in line of sight
"I was always worried about making mistakes with the wearable AR or not using it correctly at all, which made me anxious and skeptical about using it. [...] The projection-based system really helped reduce my anxiety and felt like a natural part of my environment, making it easier to use. It required less effort to learn, which boosted my confidence."	Worry about making mistakes with wearable AR; Wearable AR caused stress; Projection system felt natural/intuitive
"The projection system provided information quickly and clearly, which made me feel in control and less stressed. It was really intuitive and somewhat indirect. [...] I could walk around the room and information was displayed directly into my gaze or at certain locations. I don't know but it felt a little bit like magic. [...] The wearable AR took too much effort to use effectively, which made me feel less engaged. It felt more natural and I was indirectly in control with the projection-based system because it was really accessible in my opinion."	Quick and clear information with projection system; Wearable AR required too much effort; Projection system felt natural/intuitive; Projection system allowed for indirect control
"The wearable AR was intimidating and not user-friendly, which made me very skeptical. I couldn't imagine wearing such a thing the whole day; it would make me sick and stressed. [...] It felt weird to wear the headset. [...] The projection system was simple and I didn't have to do anything to get the information, which made me feel more confident. I appreciated that the health information was always in the right place and easy to access with the projection system."	Wearable AR was intimidating; Wearable AR would cause stress if worn all day; Projection system was simple and kept health information accessible
"Using the wearable AR felt like a chore because I had to adjust it constantly, which was very frustrating. It just didn't fit correctly. If I thought about using and adjusting it every day, that would be a big problem. [...] The projection system was easy to use and didn't make me anxious, which made the experience more pleasant. It was more engaging because it required less effort."	Wearable AR felt like a chore; Wearable AR didn't fit correctly; Projection system was easy to use
"The wearable AR often left me feeling confused and stressed because I wasn't sure how to use it properly. It felt so cumbersome. [...] And although there was information in the headset, it was hard to get into the right position, probably because I changed my position; I don't know. [...] The projection-based system was straightforward and boosted my confidence because it was easy to understand and the information was always in the same place for some objects. I felt more engaged with it because it required less effort to use. It felt very accessible."	Wearable AR caused confusion and stress; Wearable AR felt cumbersome; Projection system boosted confidence; Projection system was accessible and easy to use

The projection system was appreciated for its intuitive nature and ability to reduce stress. It fits well into daily routine scenarios, allows for multitasking (i.e., performing daily tasks where headsets are more of an inconvenience), and requires minimal learning due to its intuitive nature. Participants felt that the projection system was more intuitive and significantly helped to reduce their (techno) stress and anxiety. On the other hand, the wearable AR system was criticized for being awkward and requiring frequent adjustments, which distracted from concentration/focus and caused frustration. Users expressed that they had to constantly adjust the wearable AR headset, which they found annoying and distracting. Following this, physical discomfort was a common issue with the wearable AR system, with reports of nausea, blurred vision, and a cumbersome/heavy feel. Users felt overwhelmed with information (i.e., the cognitive switch between real objects and digital overlays) and experienced physical discomfort such as nausea when using wearable AR. In contrast, the projection system was perceived as seamlessly and naturally integrated into the environment, providing quick and clear information that made users feel more in control and less stressed. Overall, the projection-based SAR system's simplicity, intuitive design, and ability to reduce the burden of adoption were consistently mentioned as major benefits, while the wearable AR system was often associated with confusion, complexity, and physical discomfort. The projection-based approach made users feel more confident and engaged because it worked without requiring significant effort, experience, or concentration, simplifying their overall experience.

Based on the corresponding first-order concepts, we developed the second-order themes of *ease of system use*; *effort invested in using the system*; *intuitiveness of the approach*; *emotional response to system use*; *emotional comfort while using the system*; *physical comfort while using the system*; *confidence in using the system*; *engagement evoked by the system*; and *effort to learn how to use the system*. As shown in Figure 4, the participants' feedback on the projection-based system and the wearable AR system reveals clear connections between first-order concepts and several second-order themes. First, ease of use was primarily associated with the projection-based system, which participants described as straightforward and user-friendly. This contrasts sharply with the wearable AR system, which was often perceived as confusing and frustrating. The cognitive effort required to use each system highlights this difference; the projection system required significantly less effort, making it more accessible and less intimidating to use. The intuitiveness of the approach also emerged as a key theme, with the SAR system fitting naturally into users' environments and daily routine scenarios. Participants found it intuitive and easy to integrate, whereas the wearable AR system felt unnatural and required more effort to navigate and understand. Emotional comfort with the system was significantly higher with the projection-based approach. Participants reported feeling more comfortable and less stressed, attributing this to the system's clear and accessible information display. In contrast, the wearable AR system caused discomfort and anxiety, affecting both emotional and physical comfort. Physical comfort was particularly compromised with the wearable AR, leading to issues such as nausea and the need for constant adjustments, while the SAR system allowed users to remain focused without physical strain.

Figure 4. Content analysis and theory building

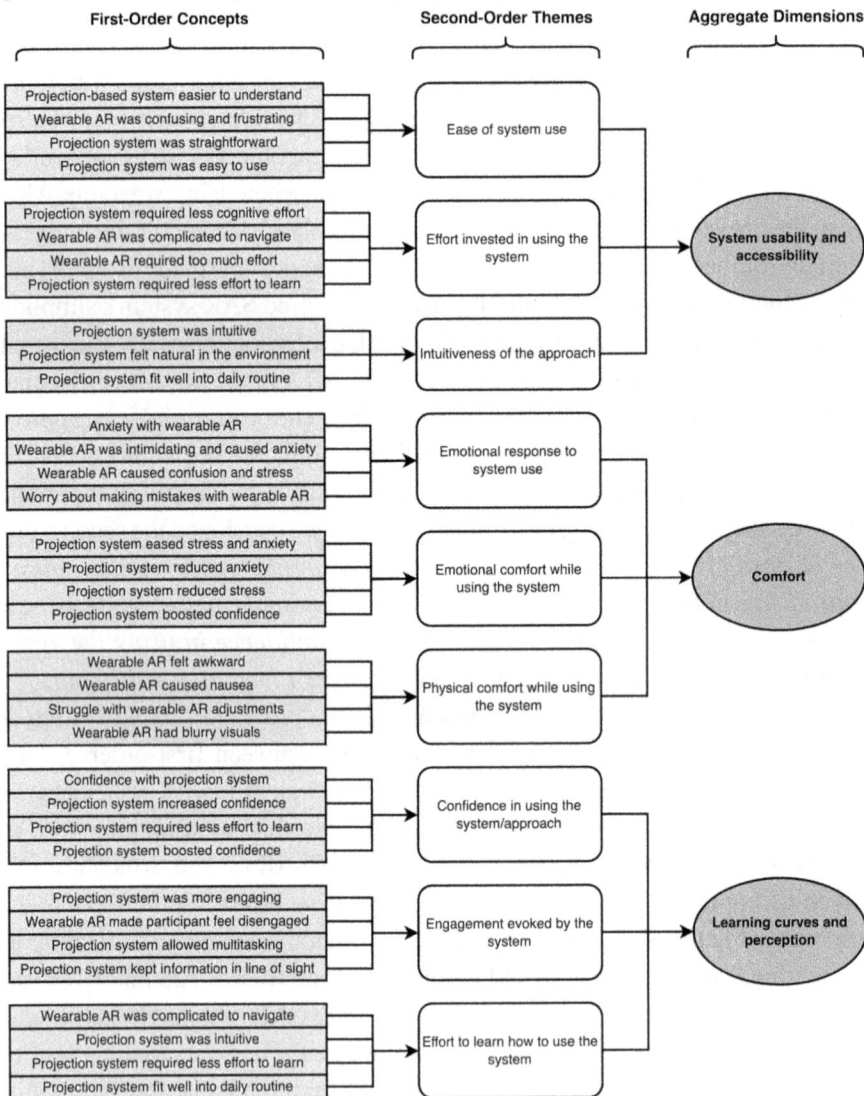

(Gioia et al., 2013)

Furthermore, confidence in the use of the system was another critical factor; the projection system's simplicity and ease of learning increased users' confidence. Participants felt more in control and less intimidated, which improved their overall experience. The engagement generated by the system also favored the projection approach, allowing for multitasking and keeping essential information in view without requiring excessive effort, in stark contrast to wearable AR, which led to disengagement due to its complexity and need for constant adjustment. Finally, the projection system required significantly less effort to learn how to use. Its intuitive design and ease of integration into daily routines made it far more user-friendly compared to the steep learning curve associated with the wearable AR system. Overall, the superior usability and accessibility of the projection-based system, combined with its ability to reduce cognitive and physical effort, seemingly provided a more comfortable, confident, and engaging user experience, underscoring its preference among the participants.

The development of the second-order themes has then resulted in the abductively theory-centered aggregate dimensions of *system usability and accessibility*; *comfort*; and *learning curves and perception* (Figure 4). System usability and accessibility are derived from participants' emphasis on the ease of system use, the minimal effort required to operate the system, and the intuitive nature of the projection-based approach. Comfort then encompasses both emotional and physical comfort, reflecting the participants' experiences of reduced stress and anxiety, as well as the physical ease of using the projection system compared to wearable AR. Finally, learning curves and perception are shaped by the users' confidence in using the system, the level of engagement it evokes, and the effort required to learn and integrate the system into daily routines. Together, these dimensions provide a comprehensive understanding of user experience and preferences, serving as overarching theoretical aspects in terms of technology adoption, use, and integration.

5. DISCUSSION

Since the development and introduction of innovative healthcare solutions is an ever-emerging challenge, IS researchers as well as healthcare and management authorities should be equipped with the relevant knowledge to provide user-centered and needs-oriented services/products. Therefore, we would like to start our discussion by addressing a thought that was probably inevitable in the course of reading this article, especially after the presentation of the results. Our results should be treated with care and in the right context. Thus, it should be noted that the results of our comparative and qualitative analysis so far apply only in our very specific healthcare context, with several implications that arise from what we will elaborate on in this section. It may seem like we are dismissing wearable AR as "bad" or inapplicable, but that is definitely not what we want to prove with our study. Rather, we want to show that other (often neglected) forms of AR may be more appropriate in one context or another - especially for vulnerable populations and innovative digital health solutions. Hence, the findings of our study have the potential to significantly contribute to the theoretical and practical application of innovative digital health solutions, particularly AR technologies, for individuals with cognitive impairment in general, which may or may not include the aging society. By employing the Cognitive Adoption Theory (Böhmer et al., 2024), this research addresses critical gaps in the literature and theoretical discourse concerning the adoption and usability of digital health technologies among vulnerable populations. Moreover, we have identified several practical implications that may lead to more tailored, accessible, and inclusive digital health solutions in the future.

To further showcase the abductively and systematic combining of our theory-centered analysis, the observations and insights from both the questionnaire and think-aloud session revealed some underlying patterns. By beginning the analysis with the participants' raw data (first-order concepts) and moving to higher levels of abstraction (second-order themes and aggregate dimensions), our inductive process ensures that these theoretical concepts are grounded in the data. From our think-aloud observations, the aggregate dimension of system usability and accessibility is central to our model, affecting and being affected by the other dimensions, which is consistent with the digital health adoption construct of cognitive adoption theory (Böhmer et al., 2024). For example, usability directly impacts and is impacted by comfort and engagement, while effort impacts learning curves and perception as well as physical comfort. In addition, intuitiveness interacts with comfort and confidence, while accessibility plays a role in emotional comfort and engagement. At a higher level of abstraction, comfort generally encompasses both emotional and physical comfort and acts as a mediator between system usability and learning curves. In other words, emotional comfort reduces anxiety and increases engagement and confidence, while physical comfort reduces physical strain and increases ease of learning and sustained use - that is, the cognitive adoption of digital health technology. From this perspective, learning curves and perception determine how quickly and effectively users adapt to the system, with confidence affecting and being affected by both system usability and engagement. Learning effort represents the cognitive and physical effort required to master the system. Finally, engagement indicates how actively users interact with the system, which is influenced by comfort, usability, and confidence, and reflects the users' ability to use and adopt the system while performing primary (i.e., some focused activity such as cooking or taking medicine) or secondary (i.e., some activity that is done on the side, such as cleaning up a few things on the way through the living environment) daily life tasks.

5.1. Theoretical Implications

Building on our kernel theory of cognitive adoption in individuals with MCI (Böhmer et al., 2024), which takes into account both cognitive load and social-cognitive factors, we delved deeper into understanding the unique adoption behaviors of this population (Ienca et al., 2021), particularly in the context of health technologies that are largely inaccessible to this vulnerable population (i.e., wearables or HMDs). Here, our study empirically and qualitatively validates some of the constructs of Cognitive Adoption Theory, specifically highlighting the interplay between cognitive load and self-efficacy in the context of digital health technologies. The higher performance expectancy and lower effort expectancy ratings for SAR systems suggest that reducing extraneous cognitive load and increasing relevant cognitive load can significantly improve technology adoption and user satisfaction (Böhmer et al., 2024; Sweller et al., 1998; Paas et al., 2003). Moreover, the lower anxiety levels associated with SAR systems underscore the role of self-efficacy and reciprocal determinism in mitigating negative emotional responses to technology use (Bandura, 2001; Compeau et al., 1999). Thus, by reducing cognitive load and anxiety, SAR systems may, in certain contexts, increase users' confidence in their ability to use the technology effectively, which in turn may lead to greater adoption and sustained use. From a more effect-oriented perspective, these results imply that SAR systems could facilitate health behavior change more effectively than wearable AR by providing more contextually relevant, more accessible, and less intrusive support. The ability of SAR systems to integrate seamlessly into the user's environment and provide real-time assistance without requiring wearable devices addresses the unique needs of individuals with cognitive impairments, aligning with the health behavior change aspects of Cognitive Adoption Theory (Böhmer et al., 2024). Thus, our study's finding that SAR systems reduce cognitive effort and anxiety compared to wearable AR highlights the importance of designing technologies that are not only functional but also cognitively accessible (Sweller, 1988; Sweller et al., 1998) – especially among those with cognitive impairments. Finally, the application of Gioia et al.'s (2013) qualitative content analysis methodology in our study provided a robust framework for theory building, particularly in understanding the differential impact of wearable and projection-based AR systems on individuals with aMCI. By systematically developing a data structure that captured both first-order informant-centered codes and second-order theory-centered themes, we were able to build a grounded theoretical model that elucidated the nuances of technology adoption and usability in this specific context (Magnani & Gioia, 2023) and connected to our kernel theory. This inductive approach ensured that the voices of the participants were at the forefront of our analysis, authentically capturing their experiences and perceptions. Subsequently, the systematic combination of data and theory facilitated abductive reasoning, allowing us to generate plausible explanations for the observed phenomena. In addition, our narrative approach not only made our findings more compelling but also demonstrated clear connections between data and theory, addressing potential criticisms of qualitative research as too impressionistic (Leidner & Gregory, 2024).

Furthermore, our study contributes to the theoretical discourse by comparing the effects of wearable AR and projection-based SAR on these constructs. The results are expected to contribute to empirical and theoretical advances by determining which type of AR minimizes cognitive load and enhances usability in everyday tasks, an area where current literature is sparse, especially in healthcare settings. Previous studies have highlighted the transformative potential of AR in healthcare, emphasizing its applications in surgery, rehabilitation, and education (Guerroudji et al., 2024; Cotin & Haouchine, 2023; Ong et al., 2023). However, these studies primarily focus on wearable AR, with limited exploration of SAR applications, particularly in the context of cognitive impairments. By demonstrating that SAR systems, at least within the scope of this study, significantly reduce cognitive load and anxiety while improving usability and performance expectancy, our findings extend the applicability of AR technologies to more vulnerable populations, consistent with the work of Hoque et al. (2022) and Makhataeva et al. (2023) on AR in cognitive rehabilitation. As a result, our study responds to the need for early identification of unintended negative consequences of wearable AR use and the development of solutions (i.e., a SAR-based system) to mitigate these consequences (White Baker et al., 2023) with a tailored approach that carefully navigates the challenges of adoption and optimizes the benefits.

In addition, our results validate and extend the theoretical propositions of Grundhöfer and Iwai (2018) and Kosch et al. (2019) regarding the practical benefits of SAR. The significantly higher performance and effort expectancy ratings for SAR systems suggest that integrating digital content into real-world surfaces can create more intuitive and accessible user experiences, potentially reducing the technostress creators of techno-complexity, techno-overload, and techno-uncertainty (Nastjuk et al., 2024). This supports the notion that SAR can mitigate the cognitive challenges associated with traditional AR systems, as demonstrated by previous research on error-free compensation methods and projection manipulation (Huang et al., 2021; Miyamoto et al., 2018; Lindlbauer et al., 2017). By addressing this gap, our study generated preliminary data that can inform future digital health strategies and interventions specifically tailored to support the aging population and those with cognitive impairments, a population significantly impacted (and often left out of the equation) by technological advances (Petersen et al., 2018; Yu et al., 2017).

5.2. Practical Implications

From a more practical perspective, the insights from this study may have significant implications for the design and implementation of AR technologies in innovative healthcare settings. The superior performance of SAR systems in terms of usability and user satisfaction, at least in our specific context, suggests that healthcare providers and technology developers should prioritize projection-based AR solutions over wearable devices for aMCI populations. The reduced cognitive load and anxiety associated with SAR systems can lead to higher adoption rates and better health outcomes, as users are more likely to engage consistently with technologies that they find easy to use, accessible, and non-threatening (Ienca et al., 2021; White Baker et al., 2023). In terms of expected performance, our results showed that projection-based SAR is perceived as more effective in improving performance (i.e., assisting with daily tasks). This may be due to better integration into the user's environment, reduced cognitive load, and more seamless interactions. This could also mean that improving the performance-related aspects of wearable-based AR by improving the accuracy, speed, and relevance of the information presented could help close this perception gap. In terms of expected effort, users found projection-based AR significantly easier to use. This may be because it naturally integrates information into the environment without requiring additional user actions, suggesting that simplifying the interface and interaction methods for wearable-based AR and providing more intuitive controls and feedback could help reduce perceived effort. In addition, lower anxiety levels with projection-based AR suggest that users feel more at ease and in control. This may be due to the passive nature of the interaction and the reduction of technical barriers. Therefore, addressing the factors that contribute to anxiety in wearable-based AR, such as improving the user interface to prevent errors and providing more supportive and informative feedback, may help make such systems more user-friendly. In conclusion, as projection-based AR is perceived more favorably across all constructs in our context, our findings suggest that it is better suited for healthcare settings where ease of use, reduced cognitive effort, and reduced anxiety are critical, such as for elderly and cognitively impaired users. Wearable-based AR, on the other hand, needs to improve usability and reduce anxiety-inducing factors to increase user acceptance and satisfaction in this vulnerable population.

Furthermore, the results of our study support a user-centered design approach that takes into account the specific cognitive and emotional needs of people with aMCI. This includes not only simplifying interfaces and minimizing cognitive load but also improving system responsiveness and contextual relevance. By integrating real-time contextual sensors and adaptive AI systems, SAR technologies can provide more personalized and effective support, thereby promoting autonomy and improving the quality of life for users with cognitive impairments (Böhmer et al., 2022). Thus, healthcare managers and decision-makers can use our findings to address strategic management challenges in caring for the elderly and people with neurodegenerative diseases. Our research provides a bird's-eye view of the potential of SAR and context-aware IS, ensuring that technological solutions address the pressing needs of this ever-growing population. The phenomenon of aMCI and older people experiencing barriers to the use of new technologies is widespread, although such technologies are largely beneficial to their use (Tacken et al., 2005). In conclusion, our study highlights the critical role of cognitive and social factors in the adoption of digital health technologies among people with cognitive impairment. The empirical and qualitative validation of the cognitive adoption aspect and the demonstrated benefits of SAR systems provide a solid foundation for future research and development in this area. By addressing both theoretical and practical dimensions, this research provides valuable insights for improving the design and implementation of AR technologies, ultimately contributing to more inclusive and effective digital health solutions.

5.3. Limitations and Future Research

Despite the promising findings of this study, several limitations must be acknowledged. A primary limitation is the relatively small sample size of 12 participants. While this sample size is consistent with statistical guidelines for pilot studies in digital health and preliminary investigations, particularly in the context of specific populations such as individuals with aMCI (Julious, 2005; Leon et al., 2011), it may limit the generalizability of the findings. While our comparative analysis in terms of the Wilcoxon Signed Rank Test is thus limited in statistical power, our study should be treated with sufficient care and rather be seen as a starting point for future research in (S)AR-based digital health. Due to the small sample size, the test may have limited the power to detect small effects, which we tried to overcome by validating our constructs and delving deeper into the reasons behind the test results with our subsequent qualitative think-aloud session. This allowed us to maintain a practical and reasonable sample size for both of our chosen methods. Thus, we encourage more research on the application of AR technologies in digital health, confirming, challenging, or utilizing our findings. Future research should thus aim to include larger and more diverse samples to validate these findings and enhance the robustness of the conclusions (Venkatesh et al., 2013). In this context, our study primarily used a mixed-methods approach, combining quantitative questionnaires with qualitative think-aloud sessions. While this approach provides a rich and nuanced understanding of user experiences (Creswell & Plano Clark, 2017), future research could benefit from incorporating longitudinal studies to assess the long-term effects of AR technology use. This would help identify any lasting benefits or potential drawbacks over time, allowing for a more thorough evaluation of these technologies (Robey, 1996; Straub et al., 2004). An interesting thought that arose before and accompanying this study was the general willingness and openness of individuals to use and adopt (new) technologies in the first place. In our context, the majority of participants were open and somewhat enthusiastic about using both AR technologies, but we also had individuals who were more skeptical and reserved. This led to the thought that even if one approach is perceived as easier to use or more accessible if an individual is generally closed to using new technologies, this will have negative implications for use and adoption. So that would be a very intriguing and interesting avenue for further research.

Subsequently, another limitation relates to the specific demographic and cognitive profiles of the participants. The study focused on individuals with aMCI, and while this provides valuable insights into the usability and acceptance of AR technologies in this group, it may not fully capture the experiences of other populations, such as those with different types of cognitive impairments or different levels of technological proficiency (Ienca et al., 2021; Petersen et al., 2018). Furthermore, the severity or characteristics of aMCI may vary between affected individuals (Petersen, 2016; Petersen et al., 2018; Yu et al., 2017), which may lead to different perceptions even under the same circumstances. Therefore, it would be interesting to see how the severity of aMCI characteristics further affects not only perceptions but also technology adoption. Expanding the research to include such diverse groups could provide a more comprehensive understanding of the effectiveness of AR technologies across different user demographics. Moreover, our research was conducted in a controlled environment, which may not fully reflect the complexities and variabilities of real-world settings. Future studies should explore the implementation of SAR and wearable AR in more naturalistic and varied environments to better understand their adoption, practical applications, and potential challenges in everyday use (Böhmer et al., 2024; White Baker et al., 2023).

6. CONCLUSION

As we witness a demographic shift towards an increasingly elderly society with more prevalent neurodegenerative diseases and a rapid increase in digital health solutions due to technological advances, we need to ensure not only the usefulness and applicability of such solutions but also their adoption to truly trigger the desired health behavior changes. We need to talk to users and vulnerable populations, who are often neglected and overlooked when they would presumably benefit most from these technologies in their daily lives. We need to explore, overcome barriers to use, and tailor information systems to the specific needs and impairments that users may experience. As such, our study is one of many examples where traditional approaches (e.g., in AR/VR or AI) may not work as well as they do in other domains or with different populations. We have shown that SAR can be a promising alternative to wearable AR in digital health for people with cognitive impairments, by delving deeper into the usability, accessibility, and perception aspects of IS technology. Therefore, we encourage more research on usability and adoption mechanisms among vulnerable populations to ensure that these individuals can benefit from digital health solutions as much as the majority of people.

REFERENCES

Antz, M., Chun, K. J., Ouyang, F., & Kuck, K. H. (2006). Ablation of atrial fibrillation in humans using a balloon-based ablation system: Identification of the site of phrenic nerve damage using pacing maneuvers and CARTO. *Journal of Cardiovascular Electrophysiology*, 17(11), 1242–1245. DOI: 10.1111/j.1540-8167.2006.00589.x

Azuma, R., Baillot, Y., Behringer, R., Feiner, S., Julier, S., and MacIntyre, B. (2001). Recent Advances in Augmented Reality. *IEEE Computer Graphics and Applications* (21:6), pp. 34-47.

Bandura, A. (2001). Social cognitive theory: An agentic perspective. *Annual Review of Psychology*, 52(1), 1–26. DOI: 10.1146/annurev.psych.52.1.1

Baumeister, J., Ssin, S.Y., El Sayed, N.A.M., Dorrian, J., Webb, D.P., Walsh, J.A., Simon, T.M., Irlitti, A., Smith, R.T., Kohler, M., and Thomas B.H. 2017. Cognitive Cost of Using Augmented Reality Displays, *IEEE Transactions on Visualization and Computer Graphics* (23:11), pp. 2378-2388.

Beller, S., Hünerbein, M., Lange, T., Eulenstein, S., Gebauer, B., & Schlag, P. M. (2007). Image-guided surgery of liver metastases by three-dimensional ultrasound-based optoelectronic navigation. *British Journal of Surgery*, 94(7), 866–875. DOI: 10.1002/bjs.5712

Benko, H., Jota, R., & Wilson, A. D. (2012). Miragetable: Freehand interaction on a projected augmented reality tabletop. *SIGCHI Conference on Human Factors in Computing Systems*. DOI: 10.1145/2207676.2207704

Biocca, F., Owen, C., Tang, A., & Bohil, C. (2007). Attention issues in spatial information systems: Directing mobile users' visual attention using augmented reality. *Journal of Management Information Systems*, 23(4), 163–184. DOI: 10.2753/MIS0742-1222230408

Bloom, D. E., & Canning, D. (2008). Global demographic change: Dimensions and economic significance. *Population and Development Review*, ●●●, 34.

Böhmer, M., Damarowsky, J., & Kuehnel, S. (2023). Implementing ALiS: Towards a Reference Architecture for Augmented Living Spaces. *Hawaiian Conference on System Sciences* (HICSS).

Böhmer, M., Damarowsky, J., Kühnel, S., Parschat, S., & Mahn, V. A. (2022). Preserve Autonomy–Developing and Implementing a Design Theory for Augmented Living Spaces. *Pacific Asia Conference on Information Systems* (PACIS).

Böhmer, M., Kendziorra, J., & Kuehnel, S. (2024). A Proposal for Theorizing the Cognitive Adoption of Digital Health Technologies for People with Cognitive Impairments, *32nd European Conference on Information Systems (ECIS 2024)*, Paphos (Cyprus).

Bruno, R. R., Wolff, G., Wernly, B., Masyuk, M., Piayda, K., Leaver, S., Erkens, R., Oehler, D., Afzal, S., Heidari, H., Kelm, M., & Jung, C. (2022). Virtual and augmented reality in critical care medicine: The patient's, clinician's, and researcher's perspective. *Critical Care (London, England)*, 26(1), 326. DOI: 10.1186/s13054-022-04202-x

Cardin, S., Ogden, H., Perez-Marcos, D., Williams, J., Ohno, T., & Tadi, T. (2016). Neurogoggles for multimodal augmented reality. *Proceedings of the 7th Augmented Human International Conference 2016*. DOI: 10.1145/2875194.2875242

Cardoso, L.F., Mariano, F.C., and Zorzal, E.R. 2020. A survey of industrial augmented reality, *Computers & Industrial Engineering* (139:1), pp. 1-12.

Compeau, D. R., & Higgins, C. A. (1995). Computer self-efficacy: Development of a measure and initial test. *Management Information Systems Quarterly*, 19(2), 189–211. DOI: 10.2307/249688

Conover, W. J. (1999). *Practical nonparametric statistics*. John Wiley & Sons.

Cordeil, M., Dwyer, T., Klein, K., Laha, B., Marriott, K., & Thomas, B. H. (2017). Immersive collaborative analysis of network connectivity: CAVE-style or head-mounted display? *IEEE Transactions on Visualization and Computer Graphics*, 23(1), 441–450. DOI: 10.1109/TVCG.2016.2599107

Cotin, S., & Haouchine, N. (2023). Augmented Reality for Computer-Guided Interventions. In Springer Handbook of Augmented Reality, 689-707. DOI: 10.1007/978-3-030-67822-7_28

Creswell, J. W., & Clark, V. L. P. (2017). *Designing and conducting mixed methods research*. Sage publications.

Dhar, P., Rocks, T., Samarasinghe, R. M., Stephenson, G., & Smith, C. (2021). Augmented reality in medical education: Students' experiences and learning outcomes. *Medical Education Online*, 26(1), 1953953. DOI: 10.1080/10872981.2021.1953953

Flicker, C., Ferris, S. H., & Reisberg, B. (1991). Mild cognitive impairment in the elderly: Predictors of dementia. *Neurology*, 41(7), 1006–1006. DOI: 10.1212/WNL.41.7.1006

Fornell, C., & Larcker, D. F. (1981). Evaluating Structural Equation Models with Unobservable Variables and Measurement Error. *JMR*, 18(1), 39–50.

Gauthier, S., Reisberg, B., Zaudig, M. et al. 2006. Mild cognitive impairment," *The Lancet* (367:9518), pp. 1262-1270.

Gioia, D. A., Corley, K. G., & Hamilton, A. L. (2013). Seeking qualitative rigor in inductive research: Notes on the Gioia methodology. *Organizational Research Methods*, 16(1), 15–31. DOI: 10.1177/1094428112452151

Gómez Bergin, A. D., & Craven, M. P. (2023). Virtual, augmented, mixed, and extended reality interventions in healthcare: A systematic review of health economic evaluations and cost-effectiveness. *BMC Digital Health*, 1(1), 53. DOI: 10.1186/s44247-023-00054-9

Grundhöfer, A., & Iwai, D. (2018, May). Recent advances in projection mapping algorithms, hardware and applications. *Computer Graphics Forum*, 37(2), 653–675. DOI: 10.1111/cgf.13387

Guerroudji, M. A., Amara, K., & Zenati, N. (2024). Augmented reality aid in diagnostic assistance for breast cancer detection. *Multimedia Tools and Applications*, ●●●, 1–14. DOI: 10.1007/s11042-024-18979-2

Guest, G., Bunce, A., & Johnson, L. (2006). How many interviews are enough? An experiment with data saturation and variability. *Field Methods*, 18(1), 59–82. DOI: 10.1177/1525822X05279903

Hollander, M., Wolfe, D. A., & Chicken, E. (2013). *Nonparametric statistical methods*. John Wiley & Sons.

Hoque, M., Farhad, S., Dewanjee, S., Alom, Z., & Azim, M. (2022). Augmented Reality in Health Care: A Review. In *International Conference on Advanced Computing and Intelligent Engineering*, 305-323.

Huang, B., Sun, T., & Ling, H. (2021). End-to-end full projector compensation. *IEEE Transactions on Pattern Analysis and Machine Intelligence*, 44(6), 2953–2967. DOI: 10.1109/TPAMI.2021.3050124

Hulland, J. (1999). Use of partial least squares (PLS) in strategic management research: A review of four recent studies. *Strategic Management Journal*, 20(2), 195–204. DOI: 10.1002/(SICI)1097-0266(199902)20:2<195::AID-SMJ13>3.0.CO;2-7

Hwang, W., & Salvendy, G. (2010). Number of people required for usability evaluation: The 10±2 rule. *Communications of the ACM*, 53(5), 130–133. DOI: 10.1145/1735223.1735255

Ienca, M., Ferretti, A., Hurst, S., Puhan, M., Lovis, C., & Vayena, E. (2018). Considerations for ethics review of big data health research: A scoping review. *PLoS One*, 13(10), e0204937. DOI: 10.1371/journal.pone.0204937

Jongsiriyanyong, S., & Limpawattana, P. (2018). Mild cognitive impairment in clinical practice: A review article. *American Journal of Alzheimer's Disease and Other Dementias*, 33(8), 500–507. DOI: 10.1177/1533317518791401

Julious, S. A. (2005). Sample size of 12 per group rule of thumb for a pilot study. *Pharmaceutical Statistics*, 4(4), 287–291. DOI: 10.1002/pst.185

Kanschik, D., Bruno, R. R., Wolff, G., Kelm, M., & Jung, C. (2023). Virtual and augmented reality in intensive care medicine: A systematic review. *Annals of Intensive Care*, 13(1), 81. DOI: 10.1186/s13613-023-01176-z

Kaplan, B., & Duchon, D. (1988). Combining qualitative and quantitative methods in information systems research: A case study. *Management Information Systems Quarterly*, 12(4), 571–586. DOI: 10.2307/249133

Kobayashi, D., Hashimoto, N., ... (2014). Spatial augmented reality by using depth-based object tracking, Proceedings of ACM SIGGRAPH '14. ACM, Kosch, T., Wennrich, K., Topp, D., Muntzinger, M., and Schmidt, A. (2019). The digital cooking coach: using visual and auditory in-situ instructions to assist cognitively impaired during cooking, Proceedings of PETRA '19. ACM, New York, USA, 156–163. DOI: 10.1145/2614217.2614226

Kriegel, E. R., Lazarevic, B., Feifer, D. S., ... (2023). Youth and Augmented Reality. In Springer Handbook of Augmented Reality, 709-741. DOI: 10.1007/978-3-030-67822-7_29

Lee, Y. Y., Lee, J. H., Ahmed, B., Son, M. G., & Lee, K. H. (2019). A New Projection-based Exhibition System for a Museum. *Journal on Computing and Cultural Heritage*, 12(2), 1–17. DOI: 10.1145/3275522

Leidner, D. E., & Gregory, R. W. (2024). About Theory and Theorizing. *Journal of the Association for Information Systems*, 25(3), 501–521. DOI: 10.17705/1jais.00886

Leon, A. C., Davis, L. L., & Kraemer, H. C. (2011). The role and interpretation of pilot studies in clinical research. *Journal of Psychiatric Research*, 45(5), 626–629. DOI: 10.1016/j.jpsychires.2010.10.008

Magnani, G., & Gioia, D. (2023). Using the Gioia Methodology in international business and entrepreneurship research. *International Business Review*, 32(2), 102097. DOI: 10.1016/j.ibusrev.2022.102097

Makhataeva, Z., Akhmetov, T., & Varol, H. A. (2023). Augmented Reality for Cognitive Impairments. In Springer Handbook of Augmented Reality, 765-793. DOI: 10.1007/978-3-030-67822-7_31

Masutani, Y., Dohi, T., Yamane, F., Iseki, H., & Takakura, K. (1998). Augmented reality visualization system for intravascular neurosurgery. Computer Aided Surgery [ISCAS]. *Computer Aided Surgery*, 3(5), 239–247. DOI: 10.3109/10929089809149845

McCrum-Gardner, E. (2008). Which is the correct statistical test to use? *British Journal of Oral & Maxillofacial Surgery*, 46(1), 38–41. DOI: 10.1016/j.bjoms.2007.09.002

Miyamoto, J., Koike, H., & Amano, T. (2018). Gaze navigation in the real world by changing visual appearance of objects using projector-camera system. *Proceedings of VRST*, 2018, 1–5. DOI: 10.1145/3281505.3281537

Mohammadhossein, N., Richter, A., & Richter, S. (2024). "What's the matter with Augmented Reality"–Obstacles to using AR and strategies to address them. PACIS 2024 Proceedings.

Möller, F., Schoormann, T., Strobel, G., & Hansen, M. R. P. (2022). Unveiling the Cloak: Kernel Theory Use in Design Science Research. *Proceedings of the International Conference on Information Systems*.

Nastjuk, I., Trang, S., Grummeck-Braamt, J. V., Adam, M. T., & Tarafdar, M. (2024). Integrating and synthesising technostress research: A meta-analysis on technostress creators, outcomes, and IS usage contexts. *European Journal of Information Systems*, 33(3), 361–382. DOI: 10.1080/0960085X.2022.2154712

Nunnally, J. C. (1978). *Psychometric Theory* (2nd ed.). McGraw-Hill.

Ong, S. K., Zhao, M. Y., & Nee, A. Y. C. (2023). Augmented Reality-Assisted Healthcare Exercising Systems. In Springer Handbook of Augmented Reality, pp. 743-763. DOI: 10.1007/978-3-030-67822-7_30

Paas, F., Renkl, A., & Sweller, J. (2003). Cognitive Load Theory and instructional design: Recent developments. *Educational Psychologist*, 38(1), 1–4. DOI: 10.1207/S15326985EP3801_1

Petersen, R.C. (2016). Mild cognitive impairment. *CONTINUUM: Lifelong Learning in Neurology*, 22(2 Dementia), 404-418.

Petersen, R. C., Lopez, O., & Armstrong, M. J.. (2018). Practice guideline update summary: Mild cognitive impairment: Report of the Guideline Development, Dissemination, and Implementation Subcommittee of the American Academy of Neurology. *Neurology*, 90(3), 126–135. DOI: 10.1212/WNL.0000000000004826

Raskar, R., Welch, G., & Fuchs, H. (1998). Spatially Augmented Reality, *First International Workshop on Augmented Reality*, San Francisco.

Richmond, L., Rajappan, K., Voth, E., Rangavajhala, V., Earley, M. J., Thomas, G., Harris, S., Sporton, S. C., & Schilling, R. J. (2008). Validation of computed tomography image integration into the EnSite NavX mapping system to perform catheter ablation of atrial fibrillation. *Journal of Cardiovascular Electrophysiology*, 19(8), 821–827. DOI: 10.1111/j.1540-8167.2008.01127.x

Ro, H., Park, Y. J., Byun, J. H., & Han, T. D. (2019). Display methods of projection augmented reality based on deep learning pose estimation, *Proceedings of ACM SIGGRAPH 2019*, ACM. DOI: 10.1145/3306214.3338608

Robey, D. (1996). Research commentary: diversity in information systems research: threat, promise, and responsibility. *Information Systems Research*, (7:4), 400-408.

Rupprecht, P., Kueffner-Mccauley, and H., Schlund, S. (2020). Information provision utilizing a dynamic projection system in industrial site assembly, *Procedia CIRP* (93:1), pp. 1182-1187.

Singh, R., Mathiassen, L., Stachura, M. E., & Astapova, E. V. (2011). Dynamic capabilities in home health: IT-enabled transformation of post-acute care. *Journal of the Association for Information Systems*, 12(2), 2. DOI: 10.17705/1jais.00257

Steffen, J. H., Gaskin, J. E., Meservy, T. O., Jenkins, J. L., & Wolman, I. (2019). Framework of affordances for virtual reality and augmented reality. *Journal of Management Information Systems*, 36(3), 683–729. DOI: 10.1080/07421222.2019.1628877

Stowell, F., & Mingers, J. (1997). *Information Systems: An Emerging Discipline?* McGraw-Hill Education.

Straub, D., Boudreau, M. C., & Gefen, D. (2004). Validation guidelines for IS positivist research. *Communications of the Association for Information systems*, (13:1), 24.

Sweller, J. (1988). Cognitive load during problem solving: Effects on learning. *Cognitive Science*, 12(2), 257–285. DOI: 10.1207/s15516709cog1202_4

Sweller, J., Van Merriënboer, J. J., & Paas, F. G. (1998). Cognitive architecture and instructional design. *Educational Psychology Review*, 10(3), 251–296. DOI: 10.1023/A:1022193728205

Tacken, M., Marcellini, F., Mollenkopf, H., Ruoppila, I., & Szeman, Z. (2005). Use and acceptance of new technology by older people. Findings of the international MOBILATE survey: 'Enhancing mobility in later life'. *Gerontechnology (Valkenswaard)*, 3(3), 126–137. DOI: 10.4017/gt.2005.03.03.002.00

Tavares, P., Costa, C.M., Rocha, L., Malaca, P., Costa, P., Moreira, A.P., Sousa, A., and Veiga, G. 2019. Collaborative Welding System using BIM for Robotic Reprogramming and Spatial Augmented Reality, *Automation in Construction* (106:1), pp. 1-12.

Tene, T., Vique López, D. F., Valverde Aguirre, P. E., Orna Puente, L. M., & Vacacela Gomez, C. (2024). Virtual reality and augmented reality in medical education: An umbrella review. *Frontiers in Digital Health*, 6, 1365345. DOI: 10.3389/fdgth.2024.1365345

Uva, A. E., Gattullo, M., Manghisi, V. M., Spagnulo, D., Cascella, G. L., & Fiorentino, M. (2018). Evaluating the effectiveness of spatial augmented reality in smart manufacturing: A solution for manual working stations. *International Journal of Advanced Manufacturing Technology*, 94(1-4), 509–521. DOI: 10.1007/s00170-017-0846-4

Van Belle, G. (2011). *Statistical Rules of Thumb*. John Wiley & Sons.

Van Den Haak, M., De Jong, M., & Jan Schellens, P. (2003). Retrospective vs. concurrent think-aloud protocols: Testing the usability of an online library catalogue. *Behaviour & Information Technology*, 22(5), 339–351. DOI: 10.1080/0044929031000

Venkatesh, V., Brown, S. A., & Bala, H. (2013). Bridging the qualitative-quantitative divide: Guidelines for conducting mixed methods research in information systems. *Management Information Systems Quarterly*, 37(1), 21–54. DOI: 10.25300/MISQ/2013/37.1.02

Venkatesh, V., Morris, M. G., Davis, G. B., & Davis, F. D. (2003). User acceptance of information technology: Toward a unified view. *Management Information Systems Quarterly*, 27(3), 425–478. DOI: 10.2307/30036540

Vertucci, R., D'Onofrio, S., Ricciardi, S., & De Nino, M. (2023). History of Augmented Reality, In: Nee, A.Y.C., Ong, S.K. (eds) *Springer Handbook of Augmented Reality*. Springer Handbooks. Springer, Cham. DOI: 10.1007/978-3-030-67822-7_2

Von Arnim, C. A. F., Bartsch, T., Jacobs, A. H., Holbrook, J., Bergmann, P., Zieschang, T., Polidori, M. C., & Dodel, R. (2019). Diagnosis and treatment of cognitive impairment. *Zeitschrift für Gerontologie und Geriatrie*, 52(4), 309–315. DOI: 10.1007/s00391-019-01560-0

Vorraber, W., Gasser, J., Webb, H., Neubacher, D., & Url, P. (2020). Assessing augmented reality in production: Remote-assisted maintenance with HoloLens. *Procedia CIRP*, 88, 139–144. DOI: 10.1016/j.procir.2020.05.025

Wegerich, A., Dzaack, J., & Rötting, M. (2010). Optimizing Virtual Superimpositions: User–centered Design for a UAR Supported Smart Home System. IFAC Proceedings Volumes, 43(13), 71-76.

White Baker, E., Eden, R., & Xue, Y. (2023). Health Information Systems Research: Opportunities to Further Advance the Field. *Communications of the Association for Information Systems*, 53(1), 984–1002. DOI: 10.17705/1CAIS.05342

Wilson, A. D., & Benko, H. (2010, October). Combining multiple depth cameras and projectors for interactions on, above and between surfaces. In *Proceedings of the 23nd annual ACM symposium on User interface software and technology*, 273-282. DOI: 10.1145/1866029.1866073

Wohlin, C., Runeson, P., Höst, M., Ohlsson, M. C., Regnell, B., & Wesslén, A. (2012). *Experimentation in software engineering* (Vol. 236). Springer. DOI: 10.1007/978-3-642-29044-2

Yang, Y., Park, Y. J., Ro, H., Chae, S., & Han, T. D. (2018). *CARe-bot: Portable Projection-based AR Robot for Elderly, Companion of HRI 2018*. ACM. DOI: 10.1145/3173386.3177528

Yu, J., Lam, C. L., & Lee, T. M. (2017). White matter microstructural abnormalities in amnestic mild cognitive impairment: A meta-analysis of whole-brain and ROI-based studies. *Neuroscience and Biobehavioral Reviews*, 83, 405–416. DOI: 10.1016/j.neubiorev.2017.10.026

Yu, S., Chai, Y., Chen, H., Brown, R. A., Sherman, S. J., & Nunamaker, J. F.Jr. (2021). Fall detection with wearable sensors: A hierarchical attention-based convolutional neural network approach. *Journal of Management Information Systems*, 38(4), 1095–1121. DOI: 10.1080/07421222.2021.1990617

Zhou, J., Lee, I., Thomas, B., Menassa, R., Farrant, A., & Sansome, A. (2012). In-situ support for automotive manufacturing using spatial augmented reality. *The International Journal of Virtual Reality: a Multimedia Publication for Professionals*, 11(1), 33–41. DOI: 10.20870/IJVR.2012.11.1.2835

Zhu, H., Samtani, S., Chen, H., & Nunamaker, J. F.Jr. (2020). Human identification for activities of daily living: A deep transfer learning approach. *Journal of Management Information Systems*, 37(2), 457–483. DOI: 10.1080/07421222.2020.1759961

Chapter 17
Enhancing the Fight of Breast Cancer in Namibia Through Awareness and Online Social Network Support

Valerianus Hashiyana
University of Namibia, Namibia

Fosia Shavuka
University of Namibia, Namibia

Willbard Kamati
https://orcid.org/0009-0007-1834-0491
University of Namibia, Namibia

ABSTRACT

Breast cancer is a leading cause of cancer-related deaths globally, particularly affecting developing countries. In Namibia, it is the most prevalent cancer type, highlighting the need for enhanced awareness and early detection strategies, especially in rural areas. This study evaluated the knowledge and awareness of breast cancer among Namibian women, identifying gaps and exploring the development of an online support group. The research collected qualitative data from randomly selected participants in the Khomas region through questionnaires, as well as secondary data from online archives, which included a comprehensive literature review and observation of the existing structures and systems in place. The study employed interpretive phenomenological analysis and qualitative content analysis to

DOI: 10.4018/979-8-3693-5237-3.ch017

interpret the collected data. It emphasized the importance of psychosocial support for patients and caregivers, suggesting the establishment of an online support group platform to facilitate emotional and moral support, ultimately enhancing the fight against breast cancer in Namibia.

INTRODUCTION

Breast cancer is a group of diseases during which cells in breast tissue change and subdivide uncontrolled, typically leading to a lump or mass. Carcinoma can begin in several parts of the breast nevertheless; 50 -75 percent begin within the lobules (milk glands) or within the ducts that connect the lobules to the nipple. Breast cancer can spread when the cancer cells get into the blood or lymph system and are carried to other parts of the body (El-Sharkawy, 2014). Consistent with Joseph, Mkandawire, and Luginah (2016), in resource-poor settings, carcinoma is usually diagnosed in late stages, and even when diagnosed, treatment could also be inadequate or expensive. As a result, morbidity, mortality, and economic costs associated with breast cancer are increasing in developing nations.

The Cancer Association of Namibia

The Cancer Association of Namibia (CAN) is a non-governmental organization that's mandated to teach the overall public about the prevention, early detection, and dangers of cancer, and supply support as best as possible in Namibia. In 2017 it published the Namibian National Cancer Registry (NNCR) for Cancer Incidences in Namibia 2010-2014. The report indicated that the incidence of cancer was sub-stantially higher in 2014 than in previous years. A complete of 11 248 cases were recorded, 45.6% males and 54.7% females. Breast and prostate cancer have the highest prevalence in each gender respectively. CAN's ex-Chief Executive Officer Reinette Koegelenberg said " fear, complacency, and ignorance are very dangerous, and people should recover from being frightened of going for screening, as early detection greatly increases the probabilities for successful treatment and increased survival rate" (2014). Additionally, she articulated that an outsized number of girls do not have the required information thus breast cancer is usually diagnosed too late. CAN has been campaigning for several years and lots of people are aware, but they still don't choose to screen, which is why the organization is putting more effort into education. A nurse at the cancer care center, Selma Elishi has approached the Ministry of Education about adding cancer awareness education into the varsity curriculum to broader cancer awareness in Namibia. Consistent to a piece of writing published in The Namibian Newspaper "Fighting Cancer in Namibia", on average about 3,000 Namibians are diagnosed with cancer annually; and with a small population of just over two million, it's alarming (2016). The article gave instructions on necessary lifestyle changes that will reduce one's chance of developing cancer. Nghitanwa, Haitembu, and Hatupopi (2019) recommend strengthening breast cancer awareness programs within the Ministry of Health and Social Services to disseminate information regarding breast cancer.

Cancer Treatment

The screening of breast cancer normally happens at private and public facilities in the country in Namibia. Although it is normally affordable at public hospitals, most public hospitals in Namibia are currently overcrowded and ill-equipped in terms of equipment and medications. Similarly, private hospitals and oncologists are extremely expensive that an average Namibian may not be able to afford. Furthermore, preventing breast cancer involves adopting lifestyle choices and medical interventions that can reduce risk factors. The one method that is mostly enforced in Namibia includes living a healthy lifestyle, and self-examination which involves one checking for lumps on their own breasts and going for regular check-ups at health facilities.

Jamal et al. (2012) researched the Cancer Burden in Africa. The research proved that although the cancer burden keeps growing, cancer continues to receive low public priority health in Africa. Jamal et al also stated that this might partially be due to the overall lack of awareness among policymakers, the overall public, and therefore the international private and public health sector concerning the magnitude of cancer burden. The World Health Organization (WHO) (2010) explained that prevention is the foremost feasible and cost-effective mechanism to regulate cancer. It is often achieved by educating people about the danger and risk factors. Nakwafila (2017), WHO, CAN, and Jamal all have reassured that the majority of cancer patients come to medical attention late in the course of the disease. Consistent with Jamal et al., increasing public awareness of early signs and symptoms should increase the detection of cancer at earlier stages when there are simpler options for treatment, resulting in a far better prognosis.

Public campaigns and mass awareness campaigns can play a crucial role in the prevention of breast cancer by educating people about risk factors, early detection, and lifestyle changes. Mass awareness efforts often build community support for breast cancer survivors and those at risk, creating networks where people feel supported in their journey toward prevention and treatment. Hence this encourages the community and more women to be proactive about their health.

One of the objectives of cancer treatment is the enhancement of patients' quality of life through cancer programs, which should establish standards for improving the patient's well-being (Usta, 2012). When giving nurture to persons with life-threatening illnesses like cancer, caregivers are confronted with physical and emotional challenges and it has been found that the impact of a cancer diagnosis is bigger on relations than it is on patients (LeSeure & Chongkham-ang, 2015). Social support may be a critical, yet underutilized resource when undergoing cancer care. Underutilization occurs when patients fail to hunt out information, material assistance, and emotional support from family and friends or when family and friends fail to satisfy the individualized needs and preferences of patients (Skeels, Unruh, Powell & Pratt, 2020). Psychosocial groups are developed to assist cancer patients and caregivers with comprehensive, social, and academic support. Consistent with Loibl and Ledere (2014), it's been shown that failure to deal with supportive care during cancer treatment can cause reduced compliance to therapy and, as a consequence, worse outcomes.

Caregivers play a vital role in supporting breast cancer patients and their families by providing emotional, physical, medical and transportation assistance. They help manage treatment schedules, offer comfort during medical procedures, and assist with daily activities. Supporters, including family members or designated caregivers, ensure adherence to treatment plans by encouraging patients to follow prescribed treatments and attend appointments.

Similarly, healthcare workers can also enhance treatment adherence through clear communication, individualized care plans, building trust, and ongoing monitoring of progress. Involving patients in decision-making, providing education about the importance of compliance, and addressing challenges to care are crucial items to consider. Counselling and psychological support for breast cancer patients often involve psychotherapy and peer support groups, aimed at helping patients cope with emotional challenges, fear, and anxiety. These methods focus on improving mental well-being, resilience, and overall quality of life during treatment.

CAN staff give moral support and physical assistance to thousands of cancer patients through their support groups. They pursue to scale back the death rate and combat the social stigma related to breast cancer. 2018 Mayo Clinic staff stated that "online support groups offer more frequent or flexible participation, opportunities for people that might not have local face-to-face support groups and a degree of privacy or anonymity. Group members tend to feel easier discussing their emotions, and experiences, venting their frustrations, and discussing their daily struggles, including discussing treatment options, side effects, and symptom management with others who have been through the experience as against a physician, family, and friends who might not be ready to understand them well (Turner,2017).

Cancer Treatment vs. Technology

Technological innovations significantly enhance the detection, treatment, prevention, and care of breast cancer patients. Artificial intelligence (AI) is increasingly utilized to analyse medical data, predict outcomes, and assist in breast cancer diagnosis, contributing to earlier detection, more accurate treatments, and improved patient outcomes.

Online support groups are relatively safe places to ask questions and therefore the participants don't get to worry about being judged or being seen to be ignorant about their condition. These support groups put forth convenience as patients who are homebound can participate without having to go away from their homes. Plus, the groups are available anytime and therefore the patient doesn't get to plan for any meeting or commute to a gathering. Group members may prefer to not disclose their identity, which makes it easier for them to vent their frustrations or opinions without the fear of being recognized.

Motivation

This research was sparked by the concerning breast cancer statistics in Namibia, revealing a troubling gap in awareness, education, and support services, particularly for women in remote areas who are disproportionately affected by late-stage detection and lack of psychosocial support. The aim is to address this disparity by promoting widespread screening to detect breast cancer early, emphasizing the importance of self-examination for high-risk women, and ensuring that cancer facilities are easily accessible throughout Namibia. It's essential to dispel fears about the screening process, highlighting its simplicity, effectiveness, and safety. Mass screening remains the most effective method for reducing breast cancer mortality until primary prevention strategies are developed. Therefore, efforts must be intensified to make screening programs more efficient, cost-effective, and appealing to women.

The development of the ICare application was prompted by the scarcity of support groups for cancer patients and their families, particularly outside major urban centers like Oshakati and Windhoek. Through online support groups, ICare aims to bridge this gap, providing accessible psychosocial support to breast cancer patients and their caregivers regardless of their geographical location. This holistic approach considers the emotional and mental well-being of patients and their support networks, recognizing the importance of comprehensive care throughout the treatment journey.

Research Objectives

This project is dedicated to fostering awareness of Breast and Prostate Cancer while simultaneously combating the associated stigma and fear. It is committed to empowering individuals by equipping them with knowledge to recognize early signs and symptoms, thereby facilitating prompt medical intervention. Moreover, the initiative seeks to educate the public about the primary risk factors contributing to these cancers. Beyond mere awareness, the project endeavours to establish a robust social support network catering to both patients and caregivers. By facilitating connections between individuals traversing similar journeys, it aims to cultivate a sense of solidarity and understanding within the community. The overarching objective is to provide a comprehensive platform where individuals can access guidance on various aspects of their lives affected by cancer, including communication strategies with family members, navigating professional challenges, managing financial and insurance matters, or simply finding solace in sharing their experiences with others. Through innovative approaches tailored to the context of Namibia, this endeavour aspires to instil hope and foster a sense of empowerment among cancer patients and caregivers alike.

LITERATURE REVIEW

Access to cancer treatment and adherence is often influenced by a number of factors including affordability, and support (Pazvakawambwa & Embela, 2017). Similarly, studies have shown that breast cancer survival is equally influenced by age, region and ethnicity, marital status, menopausal stage (for women) and education (Pazvakawambwa & Embela, 2017).

Research in this scope is increasing rapidly across the world (Wortman, n.d). There is stigma or moral opprobrium associated with prevalent chronic illness not only with being ill but also for "giving in" to a major chronic illness. Social support is one of the effective strategies set for assisting cancer patients with managing and enhancing their quality of life even in low-resource settings because not all cancer treatments are curative (Usta, 2012). Social support is believed to have positive effects on a wide variety of outcomes, including physical health, mental well-being, and social functioning (Wortman, n.d). The study has evaluated three distinct Online Cancer Support Groups platforms.

The Association of Cancer of South Africa (CANSA) has put forward several awareness and online Cancer Support programs. They have implemented a website that provides awareness and related information on cancer. It has three different Facebook groups; CANSA Survivors Champions of Hope which has about 3800 members. This group is for cancer survivors and peers who are facing similar challenges may chat online. CANSA Caring is a group for caregivers, while CANSA TLC is a childhood cancer group for children and parents/guardians affected by cancer. Group members receive encouragement from fellow members and share stories. On top of that, CANSA has two additional programs. The Survivor Program, a free online weekly email course written to help survivors cope better, and the CANSA CancerCare Coping Kit (CD) Audio Program. The kit gives information to empower and support people dealing with a cancer diagnosis, treatment, possible complications, and changes in body image, emotions, and social issues. Links to subscribe to the weekly emails, as well as to download the Coping Kit are on the CANSA website. Lastly, online queries may be posted on their Facebook, Twitter, and Instagram Pages or via the website, email, and WhatsApp groups which are multilingual for English, Afrikaans, Xhosa, Zulu, Sotho, and SiSwati.

Adopting Facebook groups for communication building may offer basic benefits such as a large number of active users, easy setup, and familiar features but it comes with risks too. Policy changes may have a substantial impact on your group and there is nothing you can do about it. These groups are extremely limited and you can't expand or build new features. The group further needs to confirm Facebook's terms of service or its shutdown (Finn, 2017), it's more advantageous to take time and build your community on your property/ platform.

Cancer.Net Mobile is a mobile application that provides the latest oncology-approved cancer information by the American Society of Clinical Oncology ASCO. It presents information, logs medications, tracks symptoms, and links questions. Users can enter appointment details, view upcoming appointments, and appointment history, and sync with their device calendar. There is a section to furnish information about their health workers. Know Cancer is a similar Cancer Social Network and Resource Hub that offers similar functionalities as the above–mentioned application. It is dedicated to connecting, educating, and empowering all people affected by many forms of Cancer. It offers additional resources such as cancer clinical trials, cancer camps, and cancer treatment centres. Foremost, it's not user-friendly. Users experience trouble logging back into their profiles. There are no predefined groups according to the data provided by the user or features allowing them to create or add friends. Both these platforms focused on a large subset of cancer patients, thus overloading its users with information. They lacked the needed components that will be delivered by this project.

ICare application offers information, emotional, and social interaction support options. The requirements of cancer survivors and patients are well addressed through online social networking interfaces to impact real-world relationships by facilitating employment, volunteering, and advocacy opportunities. It doesn't replace the social and awareness structure currently in situ, but it reinforces it. The above-mentioned support groups target forging new relationships. In contrast, thereto, this study further targeted strengthening existing relationships (friends and family). To assist them dispel myths and improve communication by giving appropriate information regarding cancer. However, it only didn't focus on coping skills, awareness, and social support but it includes support for several projects held by CAN for financial assistance and other Outreach Cancer Community programs.

The creation of Facebook, Twitter, and Instagram Pages for this project will allow the user to follow and obtain information from the appliance through their social networking sites. Discussion boards are utilized to coordinate efforts to vary or amend the present system in situ, local policies, and obstacles faced by cancer patients in Namibia. The groups are peer-led by someone with cancer experience either patient, family, or friends. It makes it easier for group members to speak freely because they share a standard experience or concern. Additionally, it offers basic features like Reminders for medication, appointments, and other special occasions, password protection, and self-created public groups. Alongside interesting information, facts, and recommendations on Breast cancer. A journal will allow the user to record notes from conversations with the healthcare team or support network. Importantly it aimed to suit the five basic core values set for support groups by the Cancer Council Victoria which are Respect, Empowerment, Compassion/ Empathy, Integrity, and Confidentiality.

The project targeted breast cancer, targeting a particular population is an important characteristic of effective awareness (Masculine, n.d). Attention is diverted to prevention, early signs and symptoms, and screening. Information about where, how, and when to request screening in Namibia is going to be added. Awareness concentrates on what is often gained by changing behavior regarding cancer and what would be lost if they don't undergo screening like surgery if the disease is caught at a complicated stage. The research focus is set on the goals of Breast Cancer in Namibia, the present situation, and therefore the gap that needs to be closed. A Study by Maskor et al (2018) suggests that participants are going to be convinced by hearing it from the "horse mouth", hence it'll work on including testimonies from breast survivors.

Socioeconomic factors like lower income, level of education, cultural beliefs, and screening practices appear to affect the treatment as well as the survival of breast cancer (Ali, Aziz-Ali, Suhail & Ali, 2018). Social-cultural factors for this cancer type are going to be investigated to understand community needs. Literature has uncovered that, as stated by Asobayire and Barley (2014) breast cancer social-culture factors included gender inequality and therefore the prevailing influence of traditional health practitioners. The knowledge, awareness, and attitude of girls towards breast cancer could also be improved by the involvement of their partners/ spouses. Women during a study by Elewonibi and BeLue (2017) indicated that their families served as a source of encouragement and motivation to remain getting into breast cancer screening to stay healthy. This study aimed to develop and implement culturally relevant cancer prevention interventions, strategies, and proposals to beat screening barriers in an attempt to extend breast cancer participation and awareness among Namibian women.

METHODOLOGY

This section outlines the actions taken to investigate the research problem and therefore, the rationale for the application of specific procedures or techniques used to identify, select the sample, the methods of data collection, process, and analyse information applied to understand the matter, thereby, allowing the reader to critically evaluate a study's overall validity and reliability.

Methodological Approach

"A research design is a plan, structure, and strategy of investigation so conceived as to obtain answers to research questions or problems" Ranjit Kumar (2011). The sole aim of a research design is to make sure that the evidence obtained from the study will enable the researcher to answer the initial questions as unambiguously as possible. The sort of research problem determines the sort of research design to be implemented. Research methods are specific procedures or techniques that the researcher utilizes to gather and analyze data. These methods depend upon the sort of knowledge needed to answer research questions (MacDonald & Headlam, 2009).

The descriptive research design approach was accustomed to accurately describing the connection between the concepts and answering the research questions. The qualitative research methodology was used to better understand the correlation between awareness and early diagnosis, online support groups, accessibility, and psychosocial treatment. There are different ways in which it is often used to capture, contextualize, interpret, and understand qualitative research data.

Methods of Data Collection

Surveys were administered to get general breast and prostate cancer knowledge from randomly selected participants from a population of 100 people in Khomas region. Different questionnaires directly collected original data relating to support groups from randomly sampled cancer patients and caregivers. Secondary data from online archival were explored. It constituted what was learned from the literature reviewed and observation of the current system. The secondary data collection method assisted with acquiring data that spanned over longer timescales and broader geographical locations.

Surveys were distributed on the Internet. Qualitative data collected was evaluated by interpreting patterns and describing participant's perceptions and experiences. The data outcome was implemented into a well-fitted solution that better answered the study's research questions.

Methods of Analysis

This study has used interpretive phenomenological and qualitative content analysis approaches to analyse and interpret data collected. Interpretive phenomenology was used to understand the background of the patients and caretakers about their experiences with breast cancer.

Content analysis was used to evaluate patterns within the content of the data obtained against the literature reviewed. This was done by identifying the frequency with which an idea appeared and by identifying patterns of deeper underlying interpretation of some data. This was easily done, against the questions asked in the surveys. Data was exported into Excel files, which made it easier in groups with different charts.

RESEARCH ETHICS

As stated by Akaranga and Makau (2016), research ethics is important in our daily life research endeavours and requires that researchers should protect the dignity of their subjects and publish well the information that is researched.

The study has applied a few policies to ensure authenticity, and integrity and protect social norms and morals. This study has been carried out according to the study designs stipulated in the proposal. It is appropriate and proportionate to the research objectives. It aimed to answer the research questions and not only collect data. Every participant who took part in the data collection process has undertaken consent, which explicitly states that their participation was voluntary and that they may choose to not continue taking part without any implications. Benefits and risks were clearly stated and confidentiality was highly upheld.

The data collected was handled appropriately and can fully be disclosed. No results were fabricated, falsified, or intentionally omitted to constitute misconduct. All biases or limitations have been discussed in the Limitations Section. No conflict of interest has influenced the methodological part of this research. Every party that took part in this study fitted the appropriate sample of the study. No personal opinions have been employed in the outcome of this research. Work that has been taken from others has been well-referenced and acknowledged to avoid plagiarism and copyright fraud. Any omissions were unintentional. No part of this paper has been done/contributed by another party that wasn't acknowledged.

DESIGN AND IMPLEMENTATION

This section explicitly describes the design, the type of tools used to build this system and the general layout of the ICare Application, how the different segments and activities are interlinked.

Software Development Process Model

The iterative model was employed to materialize the proposed project. The iterative model, shown in Figure 1, focuses on initial, simplified, implementation which then progressively gains more complexity and a broader feature set until the final system is complete (Summerville, 2011). At each iteration, design modifications are made, and new functional capabilities are added.

Figure 1. Iterative process model

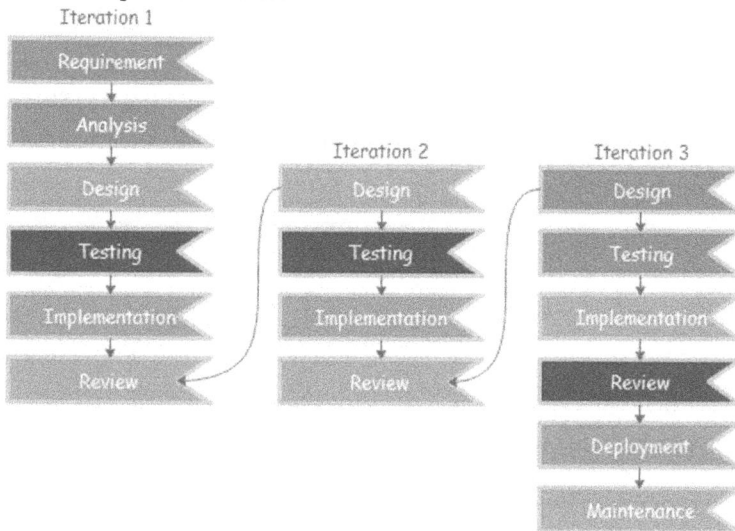

SYSTEM DESIGN

The design of the system will be accomplished by outlining a well-detailed flow graph of the system, and entity relationship diagrams explicitly showing different components are related to each other. The components will be developed module by module iteratively. Each activity will be interlinked and interconnected through the Firebase real-time database. The system will be designed according to the requirements specified. Figure 2 shows the system architecture.

Figure 2. ICare system architecture

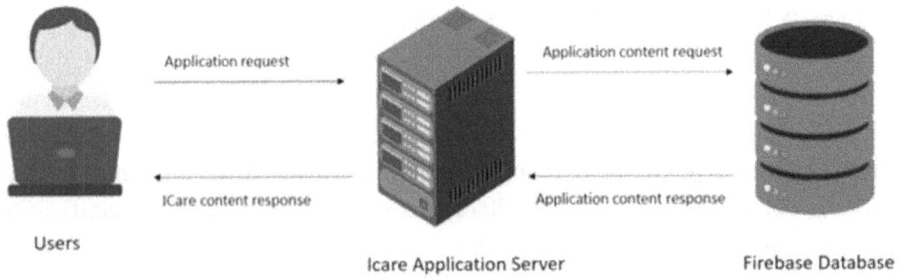

Figure 3 illustrates the system workflow which details how the system presents the user with an option to login if they have not logged in already. Thereafter, the user is presented with options including awareness, support treatment etc.

Figure 3. ICare system workflow

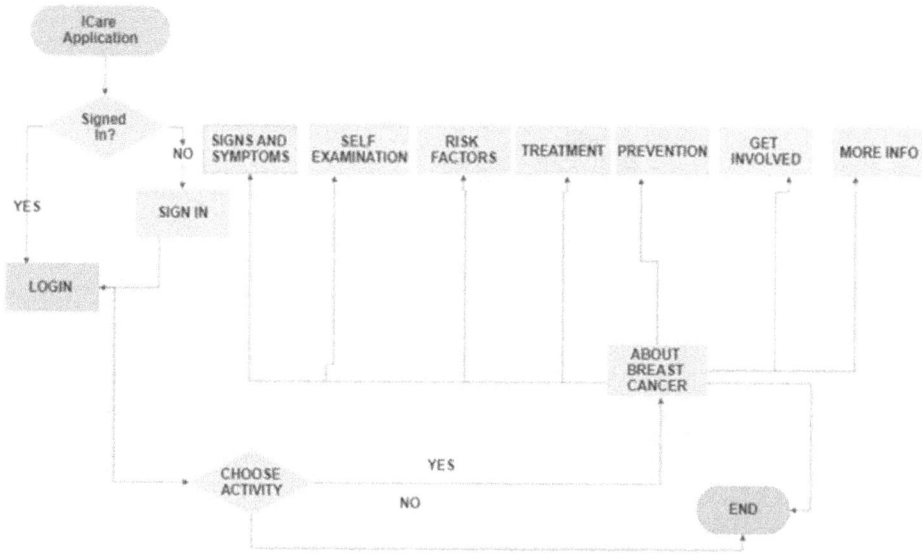

SYSTEM TESTING

Software developed at each iteration went through all the different testing, Unit testing, Component testing, and Integration testing phases. After the software development was completed, System Testing was done to test the system as a whole. It was tested against different test cases, inputting different inputs to see if the system behaves as was intended to, and to ensure that it meets the prescribed requirements.

RESULTS

Participants Age

As illustrated in the following diagrams, data collected from both surveys show that more young people in the age range of 20-39 years took part in both studies compared to other age groups. This shown in Figure 4 and 5 below.

Age of the Participants that took part in the Surveys

Figure 4. General knowledge participants age

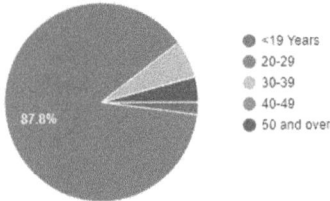

Figure 5. Patients and caregivers' participants' age

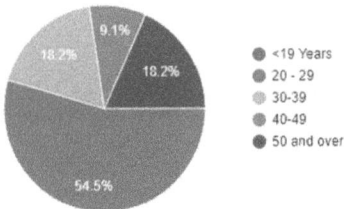

Participants Gender, Self-examination, Signs and Symptoms

Results show that more Females took part in the study as shown in Figure 6. Although, more than half of them do not perform self-examination, about 57.1% of those that perform self-examination know what to look for as demonstrated in Figure 7 and 8. As shown in Figure 9, a new lump or thickening in the breast prevails is one of the well-known breast cancer signs, deducing that little is known about the other easily noticeable breast cancer signs and symptoms.

Gender of the Participant Do you regularly observe/feel your breast

Figure 6. Participants gender

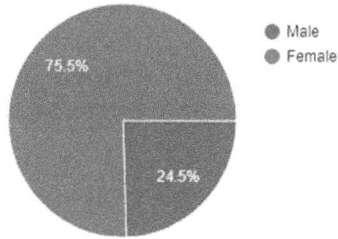

Figure 7. Regularly observe

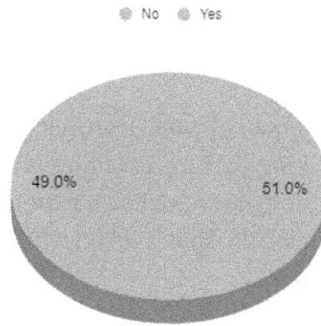

Figure 8. Know what to check for

Do you feel confident that you know what to look for when feeling/observing /checking your breast?

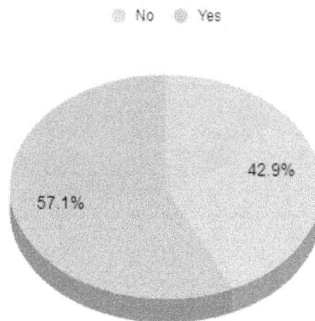

Figure 9. Signs and symptoms

Which of the following do you think are the highest risk factors contributing to Breast Cancer?

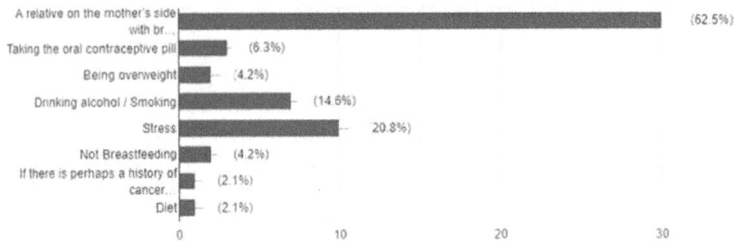

Breast Medical Check-ups

It's observed that a high number of women are generally not invested in performing self-examination, nor taking part in screening activities. Results have shown that less than 15% of the participants have had a mammogram in the last two years as indicated in Figure 10. Figure 11 shows a variety of reasons why women rarely go for medical breast check-ups.

Figure 10. Mammogram in the past two years

Have you had a mammogram / breast check in the last two years?

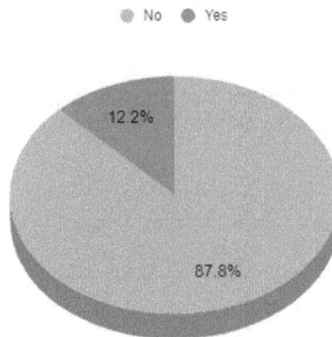

Figure 11. Why women don't go in for check-ups

Why do you think woman don't go in for Breast Cancer check ups regularly?

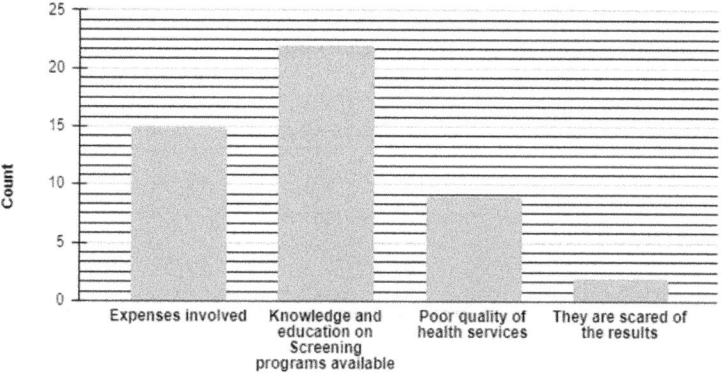

Early Detection

It's alarming to notice that there were participants who still think that early detection of breast cancer has no advantage at all. Regardless, the good outweighs the bad since more than 70% of the participants know the ultimate advantage of early breast cancer detection. Figure 12 illustrates that.

Figure 12. What to do if you notice changes in your breast

What advantages do you think comes with Early Breast Cancer detection?

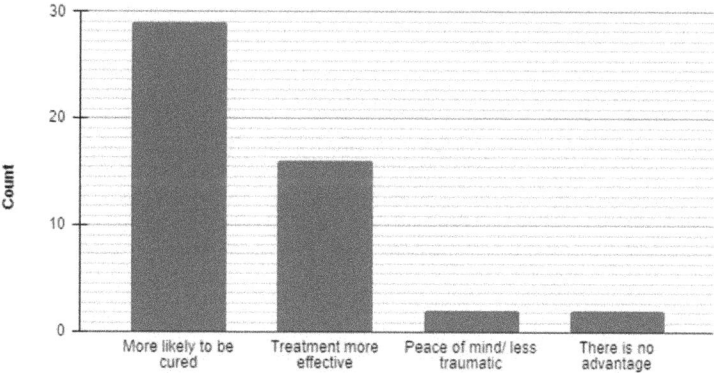

Risk Factors and Source of Information

More than 60% of the participants do not know that breast cancer may be caused by other factors other than having a breast cancer history in the family. Factors such as consumption of alcohol and drugs may too influence your chances of developing breast cancer. Figures shown in Figure 13.

Figure 13. Risk factors

Which of the following do you think are the highest risk factors contributing to Breast Cancer?

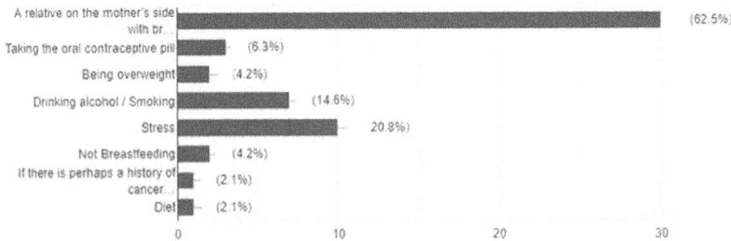

Figure 14 shows the platforms where participants were most likely to get breast cancer. Participants were asked to choose their preferred and convenient way to receive breast cancer-related information. In the technological era, it's not surprising that most participants prefer the Internet as the main medium to get breast cancer-related information. Results are shown in Figure 15.

Figure 14. Where information is obtained

Where do you obtain information related to breast health, cancer and problems?

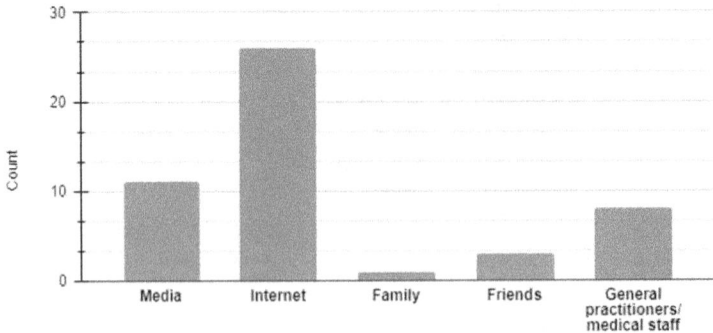

Figure 15. Preferred ways to obtain information

What is your preferred way(s) of receiving breast cancer information?

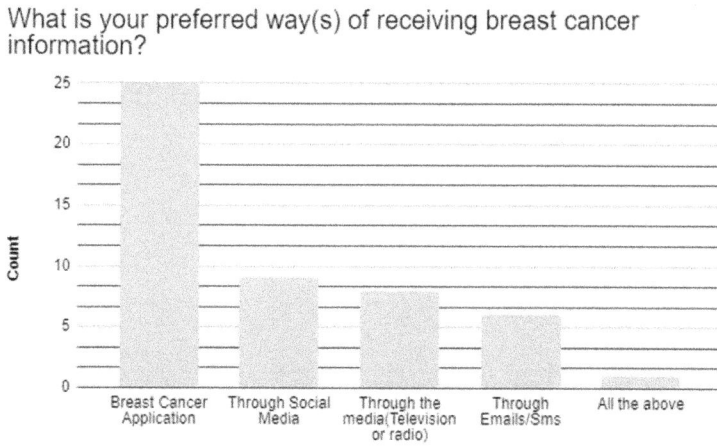

AWARENESS IN NAMIBIA

General Breast Cancer Knowledge Survey

Data collected indicates that the Breast Cancer in Namibia is insufficient as about 29.8% of the participants disagree that the Awareness campaigns currently in place are doing enough justice to evenly distribute breast cancer knowledge in Namibia. This is shown in Figure 16.

Figure 16. Breast cancer awareness in Namibia

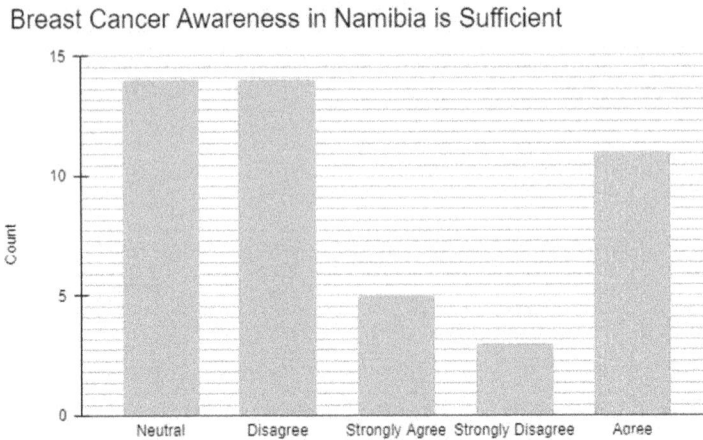

Breast Cancer Awareness in Namibia is Sufficient

The last question in this survey asked for input from participants on what contributions they think might enhance the fight against Breast Cancer in Namibia. Different opinions and suggestions were aired but more than 60% agreed that awareness needs to be diversified across the country, some stating that there should be health practitioners checking up on our women in villages and giving them the necessary information, they need, especially during baby's injection days because that's when a lot of women come together, "Increase awareness by providing and educating the nation about breast cancer. Because honestly, only 1/ 10 people in the northern region of the country know about it. And most people die from it because it's detected too late. So, more emphasis must be put on educating school kids and parents at community meetings about breast cancer."

Participants are convinced that the youth and the education sector might be the best tool to channel breast cancer-related information, "Breast cancer screening should be compulsory to all women aged 14 to above like Tetanus toxoid. Having breast cancer associations at school or having a health practitioner assigned at every organization may add more attention to the disease." Two more wrote "Women should be educated about breast cancer at a younger age and they need to make Breast cancer an open discussion". "The youth should actively get involved, educate them on breast cancer (host seminars) because I feel the youth gets the information across faster."

Results demonstrate that awareness may reach a greater audience if multiple platforms are used to spread the word across, with some contemplating that breast cancer-related advertisements on national television should be free, and that additional forms of spreading awareness would truly be helpful, such as the use of more media and the internet. Some aforesaid that "sending regular short messages to all cell phone numbers like they do games would make a big difference." with some suggesting that they need the stigma around cancer removed and more avail access to Breast cancer facilities countrywide.

Lastly, many emphasized factors that may increase breast cancer and what to do once diagnosed with breast cancer. Some gave advice such as "stop smoking and drinking alcohol", "in case you see some change on your breast visit a doctor" and to always go for check-ups and eat healthy. All in all, most responses point to better ways to complement and enhance the fight against breast cancer in Namibia.

Breast Cancer Patients and Caregivers Survey

According to the results, only 10% of the breast cancer diagnoses were done through a routine breast cancer screening procedure, and a significant number have indicated that the awareness campaigns currently in place have assisted them in some way in their cancer journey. These figures are summarized in Figure 17 and Figure 18.

Figure 17. How breast cancer was diagnosed

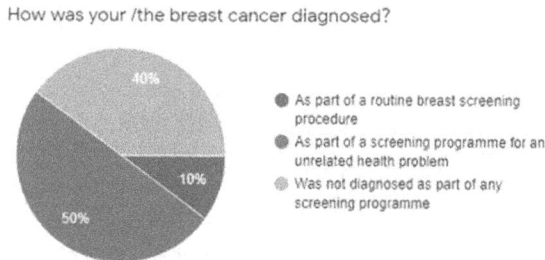

How was your /the breast cancer diagnosed?

- As part of a routine breast screening procedure
- As part of a screening programme for an unrelated health problem
- Was not diagnosed as part of any screening programme

Figure 18. Has awareness assisted in any way

Have you always been given enough information about your / the cancer care and treatment, in a way that you could understand?

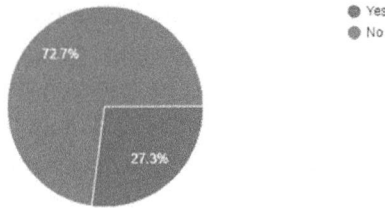

Diagnosis

A cancer diagnosis may bring a set of different emotions and thoughts. Most patients feared the unknown, pain, and suffering to be endured after the diagnosis. These fears and mixed emotions are highlighted in Figure 19.

Figure 19. Worst fear after the diagnosis

What was your worst fear(s) after the diagnosis?

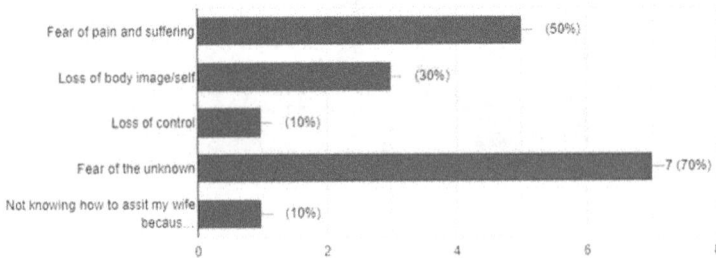

Information Presented During Treatment

The study aimed to analyse how the patients and their caregivers were involved in the whole cancer journey, how they have been treated, and recommendations on what they wished was done for them. Figure 20 indicates that most cancer patients received all the information regarding their treatment all at once, which may be overwhelming and frightening to some patients, and only 18.2% received information at each stage of their treatment.

Figure 20. How information was presented

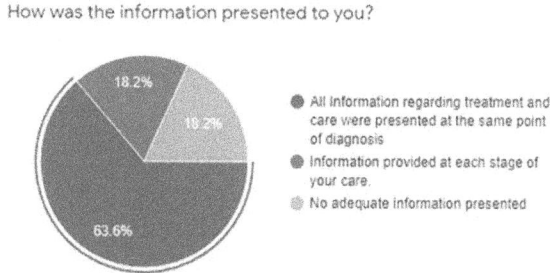

How was the information presented to you?

18.2%

18.2%

63.6%

● All information regarding treatment and care were presented at the same point of diagnosis

● Information provided at each stage of your care.

● No adequate information presented

Figure 21 shows that, although 63.6% of the participants have received all information regarding their treatment and care at once, only 27.3% of that data was adequate and well understood by the patient or caregiver.

Figure 21. Was information enough

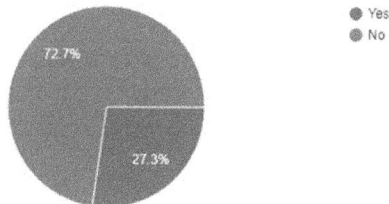

Have you always been given enough information about your / the cancer care and treatment, in a way that you could understand?

72.7%

27.3%

● Yes
● No

There was a tire regarding the involvement of patients and their caregivers in choosing the treatment options that were presented to them. Results are shown in figure 22 below.

Figure 22. Involved in choosing treatment options

Were you involved as much as you wanted to be in deciding which treatment options were best for you / for your family member(for Caregivers)?

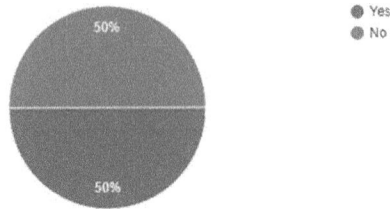

Psychosocial Care and Support Groups

Results in this subsection give analyses of information presented about the psychosocial treatment of both the patients and caregivers. Overall, the results show that the emotional aspect of the breast cancer treatment was neglected for both the patients and their caregivers.

Figure 23 and Figure 24 indicate that merely, over 50% of the patients/ caregivers were not given any information about support groups or referred to any.

Figure 23. Support groups information given

Were you given information about available patient/ caregivers groups or peer support supports?

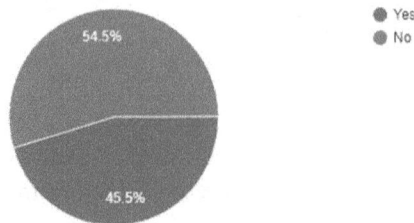

Figure 24. Psychological support given

What Psychological support was made available for your immediate family and friends?

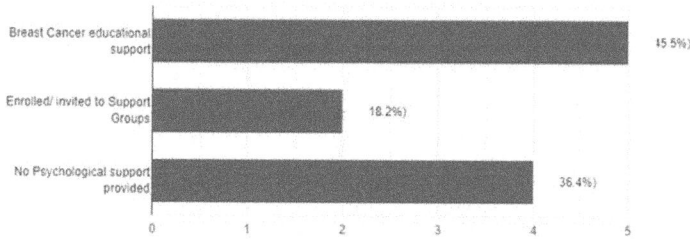

With all these alarming figures, over 90% of the participants agreed that the mental well-being of breast cancer patients contributes greatly to their treatment and well-being as shown in Figure 25. With the minimum access to support groups, question 15 of the survey, asked for which way the participants wished to participate in support groups. The majority voted for an online platform, shown in Figure 26.

Figure 25. Emotional and mental well-being of patients

Do you think the mental and emotional well being of a cancer patients contributes to the overall Treatment of the disease?

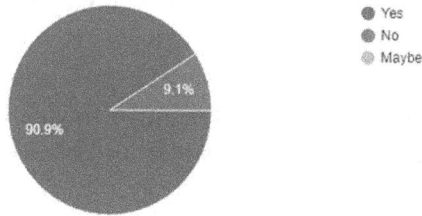

Figure 26. Preferred platform

Joining support groups is proven to offer Psychological support . How would you prefer to part take in these groups?

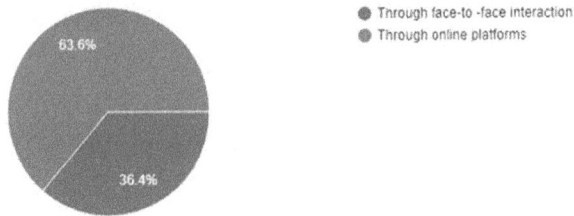

● Through face-to -face interaction
● Through online platforms

63.6%

36.4%

Breast Cancer Patients / Caregivers' Cancer Journey

The last three questions in the Breast Cancer Patients and Caregivers were open-ended, which required the respondents to elaborate on their points, to help see things from their perspective.

Question 16 asked for advice that respondents would give to someone that just been diagnosed with breast cancer. Respondents gave encouraging and motivating guidance. Having a good support system, educating yourself on the disease, and having a positive mindset are some of the prevalent advice given. "Educate yourself more on the treatment choices and how you may make your loved one more comfortable. "Enrol in support groups so you engage with people with the same experience" "Educate yourself on the available information on breast cancer. The doctors, especially the public sector, won't give enough information." Always be hopeful, strong, calm, and positive. Lastly, it is treatable with a good prognosis. Those were some of the responses given.

Question 17 inquired about what better ways participants believed could help improve the lives of cancer patients and their caregivers. The responses varied greatly, but emphasis was placed on providing more financial resources to breast cancer programs, especially in the public health sector. The government in this context was pointed out to improve service delivery in this regard by investing resources in educating its nation on breast cancer to avoid late prognosis and for the patients and caregivers to be well informed on what to expect and how to go about it. "They need financial assistance and to be given the best treatment. The government should invest in better treatment options for their patients because their service isn't ideal." "Caregivers and families need to be educated so they understand cancer better, to be able to provide the best care to their loved ones."

Respondents focused on emotional support too, some suggested that "It's very important to have people that have the same experience as you." and that it is good to encourage and give them good moral support". Hence, it comes down to how everyone has a role to play in making the cancer journey for both the patient and their loved ones easier and bearable. All the result correlates to the findings in the literature reviews that early detection of breast cancer is by far the most efficient way to lower mortality rates, as there are more treatment options and a better chance for survival.

In conclusion, question 18 solicits one thing the respondents wished that they had known at the beginning of their breast cancer journey. Around 40% of them wished they knew that there were different treatment options available and that breast cancer was indeed easily curable, some stated "There are a lot of treatment choices. I wish the government could educate the kids in schools about cancers because the cases of cancers in Namibia keep rising rapidly and less is done to educate the nation." "Breast cancer is not a death sentence"

One respondent pointed out that feeling any lump in the breast is worth asking a qualified healthcare professional about so that it's diagnosed and treated early for better survival and shorter chemotherapy sessions. Lastly, one particular participant wished they knew or had someone to talk to who was going through the same thing.

Feedback from I Care

This section reports the evaluation results of the I Care Application. A total of 13 participants took part in the survey. Figure 27 shows the type of feedback given by the participants.

Figure 27. Feedback type

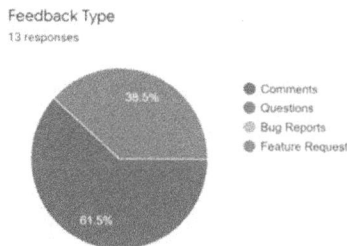

The following diagram shows the summarized data from the survey. Results in Figure 28 prove that participants were satisfied with the overall use of the application. Figure 29 shows that more than 60% of the participants are content that they can collaborate with other users on these applications. Additionally, Figure 30 shows that all the respondents are likely to recommend the software to family and friends.

Figure 28. System ease of use

How Satisfied are you with this System Ease of Use?
13 responses

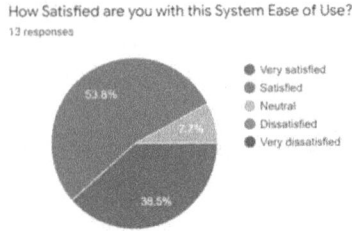

- Very satisfied
- Satisfied
- Neutral
- Dissatisfied
- Very dissatisfied

Figure 29. Ability to collaborate with other users

How Satisfied are you with the ability to collaborate with other users on this software
13 responses

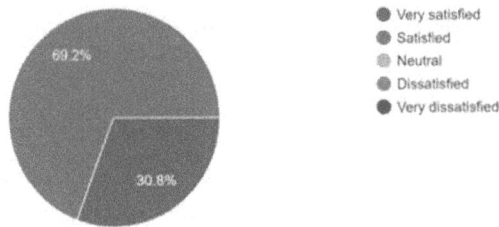

- Very satisfied
- Satisfied
- Neutral
- Dissatisfied
- Very dissatisfied

Figure 30. Recommending the application

Considering your complete experience with our software, how likely would you be to recommend its use to a friend or colleague?
13 responses

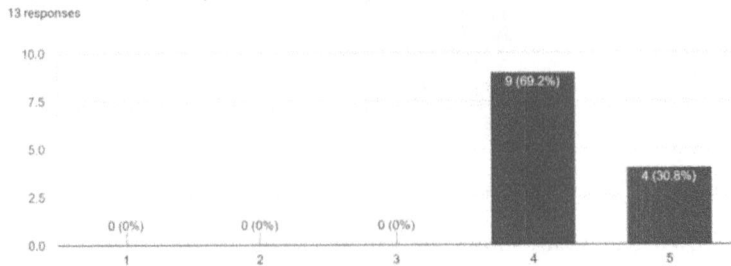

Participants gave a few suggestions and comments on the system. Suggestions included adding privacy settings to the groups. One respondent stated, "It would be amazing if the app could have video features too, where people can meet and discuss via video sessions." Some recommended adding additional features and easily understandable information. Overall, the application proved to be warmly designed and easy to use.

DISCUSSION

This section establishes the relationship between the results in the Results Section. It elaborates on the importance, meaning, and relevance of the results obtained. The main driver of this research is the high mortality rates of breast cancer in Namibia and the lack of online support groups for Breast Cancer Patients and Caregivers. The objectives of the study are to enhance the fight against breast cancer by finding different ways to efficiently increase awareness of Breast Cancer. Hence promoting early breast cancer detection, which increases the success rate of treatment. It proposed to create a system to increase access to support groups for both patients and caregivers in a way that is more beneficial to them to complement the practices currently in place. This section is subdivided into three sections.

Breast Cancer Knowledge and Awareness in Namibia

The young female community made up the highest number of participants in the study. It can be deduced that more young females are more open and willing to learn and discuss about Breast Cancer. This correlates with the study done by Elewonibi and BeLue (2017), which states that families can serve as a source of encouragement and motivation for women to go in for breast cancer screening to stay healthy. Hence a need to involve families, friends, and partners to improve the knowledge, awareness, and attitude of women toward breast cancer.

The results indicate that a lot still has to be done to increase the knowledge base of breast cancer to a wider population in Namibia. It demonstrates that women in rural areas are left out or little attention is given to them. The data suggests that the ultimate way to successfully cure and treat breast cancer is by having an early prognosis. All this may be achieved by investing more time and resources in educating about breast cancer through ways and platforms that are widely used / accessible by the targeted population. This analysis supports the theory made by CAN and WHO about the main causes of late breast cancer diagnosis in Namibia, and worldwide.

Psychosocial care through Support Groups

The results agree with the study by Usta (2012) that social support is one of the effective strategies set for assisting cancer patients with managing and enhancing their quality of life even in low-resource settings because not all cancer treatments are curative. Analysis shows that having someone to talk to and share feelings with proves to be beneficial to patients and caregivers. Although it's neglected, there are conducive approaches to provide psychosocial support. This study adds to existing knowledge a platform that allows patients and caregivers to interact with fellow patients/caregivers effortlessly and conveniently.

ICare System Review

Evaluation done on the system shows that the overall application is easy to use as the application is warmly designed and the themes present tranquillity. The implementation of such a system offers great help as it saves time and offers conveniences for patients and caregivers to engage with each other. It provides ad quant breast cancer information and other important features such as a journal for note taking, task and reminder management through the schedule, etc.

CONCLUSION

This research was set to answer three questions. Foremost, from the qualitative analysis of the data, it can be concluded that teaching a larger women population about breast cancer, will intensify their awareness and familiarity, which will make it easier for them to notice and detect breast cancer signs and symptoms earlier. The results indicate having an online platform to provide emotional and moral support is more suitable for patients and their caretakers.

The fight against breast cancer may be strengthened by investing and evenly distributing resources for breast cancer awareness and treatment. The public, health, and sectors should invest more time in implementing breast cancer education in the Education sector, to reach young people and avail more breast cancer facilities country-wide.

This research intends to emphasize channelling the same attention, coverage, and resources through awareness as well as education for breast cancer as it is done for other diseases in Namibia. it aims to change the views of policymakers, the general public, and the international private and public health sector, by highlighting the unaccounted factors in the current Breast Cancer Initiatives and Campaigns. It aspires to expand the coverage of Breast Cancer awareness and education to the people who need it. It will concentrate on aiding cancer organizations to utilize on-hand resources in curbing the disease rather than employing them in costs that might be encountered in the administrative work of the organization. The goal is to involve everyone, from the education, public, and private sectors to the general public. These sectors are compelled to incorporate Breast Cancer awareness and educative activities in their policies. Women make up to 50% of these sectors, it's only fair to cater for their wellbeing too.

RECOMMENDATIONS

Due to the limited time and expertise, I would recommend the implementation of extra features on the Application. Audio and video may be incorporated to facilitate live group sessions, which are even more exacting and more like the traditional group sessions, only this time is done through the application. The groups should be led by a facilitator who will be responsible for managing the group. Group discussion features should be integrated in such a way that the facilitator has the role of choosing the topic to be discussed and other aspects of the discussions.

This study further, recommends the implementation of machine learning in the system to cater to smart search and personalized

The study couldn't reach a greater women population, I would highly suggest that more resources should be devoted to trying to reach people out of reach, especially in rural areas.

Due to the findings discovered, this study recommends that all sectors should be involved in the fight against breast cancer in Namibia. It shouldn't only be left on the shoulders of CAN and the health sector to raise awareness. Cancer knowledge should be implemented in the education curriculum. Organizations should implement policies and laws that cater to the well-being of their employees by hosting activities, workshops, or seminars that educate about diseases and other pressing matters.

Research may branch too, into finding factors that are hindering the country's capacity and capabilities in combating cancer, with such a small population.

ACKNOWLEDGMENTS

The authors would like to express their unlimited gratitude and appreciation to the Department of Computing, Mathematical and Statistical Science that made this research study possible.

REFERENCES

Ahmedin Jemal, F. B. (2012). Cancer Burden in Africa and Opportunities for Prevention. *American Cancer Society*, 1-24.

Alice Asobayire, R. B. (2015). Women's Cultural Perceptions and Attitudes Towards Breast Cancer: Northern Ghana. *Health Promotion International*, 30(3), 647–657. DOI: 10.1093/heapro/dat087 PMID: 24474424

Bilikisu Elewonibi, R. B. (2016). *The influence of socio-cultural factors on breast cancer screening behaviors in Lagos*.

Brain Oldenburg, C. T. (2015). Using New Technologies to Improve the Prevention and Management of Chronic Conditions in Populations. *Annual Review of Public Health*, 36(1), 483–505. DOI: 10.1146/annurev-publhealth-031914-122848 PMID: 25581147

Finn, G. (2017). *Why You Shouldn't Use Facebook Groups To Build a Community*. Retrieved from Cypress North: www.google.com/amp/s/cypressnorth.com/social -media/shouldnt-build-community-using-Facebook-groups/amp

FreeQDA. (n.d.). Retrieved from SourceForge: https://sourceforge.net/projects/freeqda

Gulshan Bano Ali, S. A. (2008). Socio-Cultural Factors Affecting the Treatment of Breast Cancer Among Pakistani Women and Potential Strategies to Prevent Breast Cancer- A Narrative Review. *Open Access Journal Of Reproductive System And Sexual Disorders*, 146-151.

Headlam, S. M. (2009). Research Methods Handbook Introductory guide to research methods for social research.

Herron, L.-M. (2005). *Building Effective Cancer Support Groups*. The Cancer Council Australia.

Individual, Group & Online Support. (n.d.). Retrieved from CANSA website: https://www.cansa.org.za/cansas-care-support/cancer-counselling/

Jacob, B., & Weiss, E. S. (2013). Recommendation for the Design, Implementation, and Evaluation of Social Support in Online Communities, Networks, and Groups. *Journal of Biomedical Informatics*, ●●●, 970–976.

JavaTpoint. (2018). *Iterative Model*. Retrieved from JavaTPoint website: https://www.javatpoint.com/software-engineering-iterative-model

Joseph Kangmennaang, P. M. (2017). Breast cancer screening among women in Namibia: explaining the effect of health insurance coverage and access to information on screening behaviors.

Masiuliene, L. (2015). *The key features of successful awareness-raising campaigns*. European Lifelong Learning Program.

Maskor, N.A., M. A. (2018). Strategy for Effective Cancer Awareness Program. *Journal of Global Oncology*, ●●●, 1–20.

Mavis Machirori, C. P. (2018). Study on the relationship between Black man, culture, and prostate cancer beliefs. *Cogent Medicine*, ●●●, 1–13.

McKenziel F, Z. A. (2018). Breast Cancer Awareness in Sub-Saharan Africa. *ABC -DO cohort: African Breast Cancer- Disparities in Outcomes study*, 721-730.

Meredith M. Skeels, K. T. (2010). Catalyzing Social Support for Breast Cancer Patients.

Muhammad Akram, M. I. (2017). Awareness and current knowledge of breast cancer.

Nakwafila, O. (2017). *Knowledge and attitudes towards prostate cancer screening amongst men in Oshana Region*.

Namibia, C. A. (2019). *Company Profile and Fact Sheet*. Cancer Association of Namibia.

Namibia, C. A. (n.d.). *Cancer Registry*. Retrieved from Cancer Association of Namibia (W030): www.can.org.na/?page_id=493

Newspaper, T. N. (2016). *Fighting cancer in Namibia*.

Nghitanwa Emma Maano*, H. T. (2019). Awareness and perception of women of reproductive age (15-49) regarding breast cancer at Okuryangava clinic, Namibia.

Observatory, G. (2011). *mHealth: New horizons for health through mobile technologies*. Switzerland: World Health Organization.

Oncology, A. S. (n.d.). *Cancer.Net Mobile*. Retrieved from Cancer.Net: https://www.cancer.net/navigating-cancer-care/managing-your-care/cancernet-mobile

Organization, W. H. (2010, January). *Cancer Fact Sheet.* Retrieved from World Health Organization: www.who.int/cancer/fact-sheet/

Organization, W. H. (2014). *Namibia Cancer Profile.* World Health Organization.

Pazvakawambwa, L., & Embela, S. P. (2017). Prevalence, trends and risk factors of Breast Cancer Mortality in Namibia: 200-2015. Retrieved from https://repository .unam.edu.na/server/api/core/bitstreams/fcc5998a-c36f-454f-ba31-285d6d79513a/ content

Peeranuch LeSeure, S. C. (2015). The Experience of Caregivers Living with Cancer Patients: A Systematic Review and Meta-Synthesis. *Journal of Personalized Medicine*, 5(4), 406–439. DOI: 10.3390/jpm5040406 PMID: 26610573

Prev., A. P. (2011). RESEARCH METHODOLOGY a step-by-step guide for beginners. 1751–1763.

Rakibul, M., & Islam, B. B. (n.d.). Barriers to Cervical Cancer and Breast Cancer Screening Uptake in Low-Income and Middle-Income Countries. *Systematic Reviews.*

Rebecca, L., & Siegel, K. D. (2020). Cancer Statistics 2020. *American Cancer Society*, 7-30.

Sam Wambugu, C. V. (2014). mHealth for Health Information Systems in Low-and-Middle-Income Countries: Challenges and Opportunities in Data Quality, Privacy and Security. *MEASURE Evaluation*, 1-20.

Sommerville, I. (2011). *Software Engineering* (9th ed.). Pearson Education Inc.

Staff, M. C. (2018, June 26). *Stress management.* Retrieved from Mayo Clinic: www.mayoclinic.org/healthy-lifestyle/stress-management/in-depth/support-groups/ art-20044655

Sun, T. N. (2014). Breast cancer: Knowing is best. Windhoek.

Susan, S., & Hendrick, E. C. (2010). Practical Model for Psychosocial Care. *Journal of Oncology Practice / American Society of Clinical Oncology*, ●●●, 34–36. PMID: 20539730

Sylla, B. S. C. W. (2012). Cancer burden in Africa in 2030. *International Agency for Research on Cancer*, 1-2.

Taylor, K. (2015). How digital technology is transforming health and social care. *Deloitte Center for Health Solutions*, 2-37.

Usta, Y. Y. (2012). Importance of Social Support in Cancer Patients. *Asian Pacific Journal of Cancer Prevention*, 13(8), 3569–3572. DOI: 10.7314/APJCP.2012.13.8.3569 PMID: 23098436

Welcome to Know Cancer. (n.d.). Retrieved from Know Cancer: https://www.knowcancer.com/

Wortman, C. B. (1984, May). Social Support and the Cancer Patient: Conceptual and Methodologic Issues. *Cancer*, 53(S10), 2339–2360. DOI: 10.1002/cncr.1984.53.s10.2339 PMID: 6367944

KEY TERMS AND THEIR DEFINITIONS

Awareness: knowledge and understanding that something is happening or exists.

Breast Cancer: is a disease in which abnormal breast cells grow out of control and form tumours.

Cancer Association: A non-governmental organization that's mandated to teach the overall public about the prevention, early detection, and dangers of cancer, and supply support as best as possible.

Caregivers: People who gives care to people who need help taking care of themselves.

ICare: A model developed through collaboration between the Office of Patient Experience and an interdisciplinary focus group, including representatives in different roles across the hospital, patients, and steering committees.

Patients: A person receiving or registered in health care providing institution to receive medical treatment.

Prevention strategies: Activities targeted to a specific population or the larger community that are designed to be implemented before the onset of problems as a means to prevent substance abuse or its detrimental effects from occurring.

Psychosocial Support: *Actions that address both psychological and social needs of individuals, families and* communities.

Support Groups: Gathering of people facing common issues to share what's troubling them.

Chapter 18
The Impact and Significance of Diabetes Mellitus as a Global Health Challenge

Ayesha Thanthrige

https://orcid.org/0009-0001-0518-2849

La Trobe University, Australia

Nilmini Wickramasinghe

La Trobe University, Australia

ABSTRACT

Diabetes mellitus is a critical global health problem affecting millions of individuals and imposing a significant economic burden worldwide. A RLR across multiple selected databases was conducted to provide a detailed analysis regarding the significance of diabetes as a disease, with a particular focus on the evolving role of digital health interventions in diabetes management. Key areas discussed include global prevalence and projections, economic costs, complications and comorbidities, psychological factors, and history of diabetes understanding. The review includes studies conducted both before and after the COVID-19 pandemic to provide a comprehensive understanding of how digital health technologies, such as mobile health applications, telemedicine have evolved and been adapted in response to the pandemic's challenges. The paper also discusses the advancement and features of self-management methods. By examining this evolution, the study provides new insights into the effectiveness, challenges, and future potential of these technologies in enhancing diabetes care.

DOI: 10.4018/979-8-3693-5237-3.ch018

1. INTRODUCTION

Diabetes mellitus is a chronic metabolic condition categorised by high blood glucose levels which has emerged as one of the most significant global health problems of the 21st century. Referring to the International Diabetes Federation, 2021 approximately 537 million adults globally were living with diabetes in 2021. This alarming situation is observed not limited to high-income developed countries but also in low and middle-income developing countries, where healthcare systems are often less utilised to manage the disease effectively (World Health Organization, 2024). The burden of diabetes extends beyond individual health condition, also significantly impacting healthcare systems and economies. In 2021, global healthcare spending on diabetes was estimated at USD 966 billion (International Diabetes Federation, 2021). Therefore, this fact further highlighting the need for effective management and prevention strategies for diabetes (Nadeau et al., 2016; Nguyen et al., 2016).

Diabetes is categorized into three forms namely Type 1, Type 2, and Gestational diabetes. Type 1 diabetes is a state where the immune system affect insulin producing beta cells in the pancreas. It often begins in childhood or teenage years and requires lifelong insulin therapy (Morone, 2019; Wojahn et al., 2014). Type 2 diabetes, the most common type which is related to insulin resistance and typically develops in adults, although it is commonly can be seen in younger people due to increasing obesity rates (Bertsimas et al., 2017; Tomlin & Asimakopoulou, 2014). Gestational diabetes appears during pregnancy and increases the risk of developing type 2 diabetes later in life for both the child and mother (Alqudah et al., 2019; Fareed et al., 2023).

Over time, diabetes can cause severe damage on blood vessels throughout the body. Diabetes primarily affecting the heart, eyes, kidneys, and nerves. This vascular damage significantly increases the risk of serious health complications for individuals with diabetes, including heart attack, stroke, and kidney failure. Additionally, diabetes can lead to permanent vision loss by damaging the blood vessels in the eyes (World Health Organization, 2023). Cardiovascular problems are the foremost cause of death among people with diabetes. The progression to kidney failure requires costly treatments such as dialysis or kidney transplantation (Blonde et al., 2022). Neuropathy or nerve damage can lead to severe outcomes like foot ulcers and amputations (Chun & Hong, 2015). Diabetic retinopathy is the prominent cause of blindness among elders and can be commonly seen with Type 1 diabetes patients (Hall et al., 2016).

Self-management is the foundation of effective diabetes care, involving routine activities such as monitoring blood glucose levels, engaging in physical activities, adhering to dietary advices, and taking medicines as prescribed by the healthcare provider (Goyal et al., 2016). The evolution of healthcare technology, particularly during and after the COVID-19 pandemic, has significantly transformed diabetes management. Advanced digital health tools such as Continuous glucose monitoring (CGM) systems, mobile health (mHealth) applications, and telemedicine platforms have facilitated patients by providing real-time data, personalized feedback, and remote support (Brørs et al., 2020; Pekmezaris et al., 2020). The pandemic has accelerated the adoption and integration of these digital health solutions, revealing both their potential benefits and the challenges associated with widespread implementation. Further, integration with 5th Generation (5G) technology in healthcare contributes for further improving diabetes management. 5G's high-speed connectivity and low latency enable continuous communication between devices, ensuring more effective use of CGM systems, insulin pumps, and telehealth services (Beck & Greenwood, 2017; Duran Souza et al., 2017). These technologies support personalized self-management, which is essential for improving health outcomes and reducing the burden on healthcare systems (Desveaux et al., 2016).

Despite these advancements, significant gaps remain in current diabetes care. Many individuals lack access to the support systems and required resources to manage their condition effectively. Majority of diabetic patients living in low-and middle-income countries, and every year 1.5 million deaths are related with diabetes (World Health Organization, 2024). There is also a need for more comprehensive and integrated management strategies that incorporate medical, psychological, and social aspects for diabetes management (Mendenhall et al., 2016). Given the rapid technological advancements and the shift in healthcare dynamics post COVID-19, there is a critical need to assess how these changes have impacted diabetes care and identify areas where further innovation is required. This paper attempt to provide an overview of the significance of diabetes as a disease, examining its prevalence, complications, economic impacts, and psychological challenges. By highlighting these aspects, the study emphasises the urgent need for integrated management strategies that leverage advanced healthcare technologies and provide continuous support to individuals with diabetes. Furthermore, it explores the evolution of self-management practices and the transformative potential of 5G technology and other digital solutions to enhance diabetes care in the post pandemic era, offering insights into future research directions to improve outcomes and quality of life for people living with diabetes.

2. METHODOLOGY

2.1 Study Design

The methodology of this literature review is designed to systematically examine the significance of diabetes mellitus, focusing on its prevalence, economic impacts, complications, psychological challenges, and management strategies. Additionally, this study focuses on the evolving role of digital health interventions in diabetes management, particularly in the context of the post COVID-19 era, to understand how technological advancements have been adapted and integrated in response to recent healthcare challenges. This study utilized a rapid literature review (RLR) approach, adhering to the PRISMA guidelines, to ensure comprehensive reporting of the review process (Page et al., 2021).

2.2 Research Question

How have digital health interventions evolved and impacted diabetes management, particularly in the post COVID-19 period?

2.3 Search Strategy

To explore the role of digital health interventions and the significance of diabetes management practices as a disease, a literature search was conducted across multiple academic databases. The databases included MEDLINE, Scopus, CINAHL, and IEEE Xplore. The search strategy was developed to capture a wide range of studies that provide a rapid review of the current state of knowledge regarding the prevalence, complications, economic impacts, psychological challenges, digital health interventions, and management strategies related to diabetes. The search strategy included both pre and post COVID-19 studies to provide a comprehensive understanding of the evolution and adaptation of digital health technologies over time. The search results were imported into Endnote and removed duplicates via the tool itself and then uploaded into Covidence software for management.

The specific search terms and Boolean operators used were: ("Diabetes Mellitus" OR "Diabetes Management") AND ("Digital Health" OR "mHealth" OR "Telemedicine" OR "5G" OR "Artificial Intelligence" OR "Remote Monitoring") AND ("COVID-19" OR "Pandemic") AND ("Prevalence" OR "Complications" OR "Economic Impact" OR "Psychological Factors"). The search was limited to articles published from 2014 onwards to ensure the relevance and inclusion of the most recent developments. The search results were imported into Endnote, where duplicates were identified and removed. The remaining articles were then uploaded into Covidence software for further management and screening.

2.4 Inclusion and Exclusion Criteria

To ensure the relevance and quality of the studies considered for the study, specific inclusion and exclusion criteria were considered.

Inclusion Criteria:
- Studies focusing on the global prevalence of diabetes, economic impacts, complications associated with diabetes, psychological impacts, digital health interventions in diabetes management particularly post COVID-19
- Articles published from 2014 onwards to ensure the relevance and latest information.
- Articles written in English to facilitate analysis and interpretation.

Exclusion Criteria:
- Studies not related to digital health interventions in diabetes management or without discussing significance of the disease.
- Non-English articles and publications before 2014.

2.5 Screening and Full-Text Review

The selection process involved a two-step screening approach. Initially, titles and abstracts of the articles recognized through the search were reviewed for relevance against the inclusion and exclusion criteria. Articles that met the inclusion criteria based on their titles and abstracts were then subjected to a full-text review. The screening also prioritized studies that provided insights into the changes in digital health adoption and integration due to the COVID-19 pandemic.

2.6 Data Extraction and Synthesis

A consistent data extraction form was maintained to extract the relevant information from the selected studies systematically. The extracted data included,

- Study characteristics (author, year, country, study design)
- Sample characteristics (sample size, population demographics)
- Key findings related to diabetes prevalence, complications, economic impacts, psychological challenges, and digital health interventions.
- Management strategies and interventions discussed in the studies.

The data were synthesized qualitatively to provide an inclusive overview of the significance of diabetes. A thematic analysis approach was employed to identify and categorize the main themes and sub-themes emerging from the data, with a specific focus on the evolution of digital health technologies in diabetes care before and after the COVID-19 pandemic (see table 1 for overview of the included studies.

3. RESULTS

A total of 6,136 articles were imported for screening from the Medline, CINAHL, IEEE Xplore, and Scopus databases. After an initial screening, 675 duplicates were identified manually, and 312 duplicates were identified by Covidence. Additionally, 941 articles were excluded due to being out of the publication year range, and 3,771 articles were out of scope. This left 437 studies to be screened, of which 185 were found to be irrelevant and 110 full texts were not available. Of the 142 full-text studies assessed for eligibility, 110 were excluded for several reasons, resulting in eighteen studies being included in the final review (Refer Figure 1). The included studies span both pre and post COVID-19 periods to provide a comprehensive analysis of how digital health interventions in diabetes management have evolved over time.

Figure 1. PRISMA flow diagram

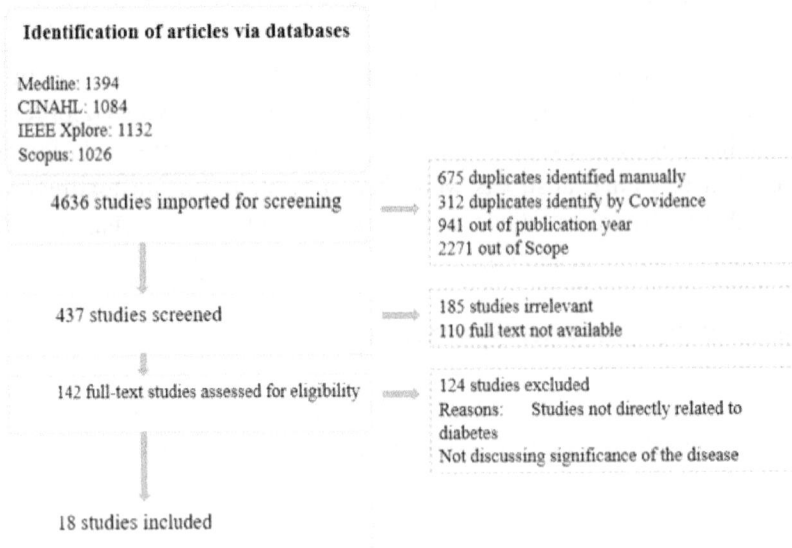

Identification of articles via databases

Medline: 1394
CINAHL: 1084
IEEE Xplore: 1132
Scopus: 1026

| 4636 studies imported for screening | ⟶ | 675 duplicates identified manually
312 duplicates identify by Covidence
941 out of publication year
2271 out of Scope |

| 437 studies screened | ⟶ | 185 studies irrelevant
110 full text not available |

| 142 full-text studies assessed for eligibility | ⟶ | 124 studies excluded
Reasons: Studies not directly related to diabetes
Not discussing significance of the disease |

18 studies included

3.1 Prevalence and Projections

Diabetes is known as a critical global health issue, with an estimated 537 million adults living with the condition in 2021. This number is expected to rise significantly, reaching 783 million by 2045 (International Diabetes Federation, 2021). The increase in diabetes prevalence is observed globally, with both high income and low to middle income countries experiencing rising rates. The prevalence varies widely across different regions and populations. For instance, America has the highest prevalence rates, whereas regions in Africa, although currently lower in prevalence, are experiencing rapid increases (World Health Organization, 2024). The COVID-19 pandemic has worsened diabetes management challenges due to limited healthcare accessibility and restrictions, highlighting the critical need for innovative digital health solutions (Moglia et al., 2022). For example, the UK National Health Authority reported on diabetes patients who died after contracting COVID-19. Between March 1, 2020, and May 11, 2020, there were 23,804 deaths. Among these, 31.4% (7,466) were patients with type 2 diabetes, and 1.5% (365) were patients with type 1 diabetes. The report highlighted that over 30% of the deaths were associated with diabetes patients (Subramanian & Sreekantan Thampy, 2021). Since diabetes has a massive impact on global health and well-being, it is crucial to improve prevention and treatment methods of diabetes (Chen et al., 2018).

Table 1. Summary of the included studies

Characteristics	Number of studies (n = 18)
Year of publication	
2017	2
2018	3
2019	5
2021	4
2022	2
2023	2
Location	
High income countries (HIC)	6
Low-middle income countries (LMIC)	4
Diabetes types	
Type 1 diabetes	0
Type 2 diabetes	1
Mix (Type 1/Type 2/Gestational)	17

3.2 Economic Impact

Diabetes causes a significant economic burden on healthcare systems worldwide. In 2021, global healthcare spending on diabetes was approximately USD 966 billion, a 316% increase over the last 15 years (International Diabetes Federation, 2021). This financial burden occurs from direct costs such as hospital admissions, medications, and medical supplies, as well as indirect costs connected to loss of productivity and long-lasting disability. Low and middle-income countries bear a share of this burden due to limited healthcare resources and higher prevalence rates. For example, a study by Ames et al. (2020) highlighted that healthcare service utilization and costs among youth with diabetes mellitus are higher compared to individuals without chronic conditions. This has increased the healthcare burden for diabetes management consumes a huge portion of healthcare budgets, further worsening economic disparities. The study found that youth with diabetes had higher utilization of healthcare services, which highlight the ongoing need for strong medical care and resources in managing diabetes (Ames et al., 2021). The inclusion of both pre and post pandemic studies allows for understanding how digital health interventions can potentially manage these economic burdens by improving access to care and optimizing resource utilization.

3.3 Complications and Comorbidities

Diabetes is associated with numerous complications that significantly contribute to increased deaths. Major complications include cardiovascular disease, kidney failure, neuropathy, retinopathy, and diabetic foot ulcers. Cardiovascular complications are the leading cause of death among individuals with diabetes. Additionally, stroke and hypertension are prevalent among people with diabetes, further increasing the burden on healthcare systems (Dagliati et al., 2018). Heart disease, diabetes, hypertension, and chronic kidney disease are prevalent among the elderly population in developing countries, posing significant challenges due to limited medical resources. Chronic diseases account for approximately 80% of all deaths in these regions, highlighting the critical need for effective management strategies (Wu et al., 2021). In the study, chronic diseases such as diabetes, heart disease, kidney disease, and hypertension were monitored, with accuracy and specificity exceeding 85%, and sensitivity not lower than 75%. These conditions often require long-term treatment and management, impacting the quality of life for the elderly and leading to substantial medical expenses. Digital health interventions, such as AI-driven decision support systems and telehealth, offer potential solutions for better managing these complications by enabling timely predictions and personalized care strategies (Wu et al., 2021).

3.4 Psychological Factors

Managing diabetes extends beyond physical health to significant psychological challenges. Diabetes distress and depression are common among individuals with diabetes and can adversely affect their ability to manage their condition. A study by Hertroijs et al. (2019) found that among people with type 2 diabetes mellitus, diabetes-related distress was a significant concern, with various demographic factors influencing its prevalence. Depression is also common, with diabetic individuals having doubled the risk of developing depression compared to the general population (Vesselkov et al., 2018). Healthcare systems designed to assist individuals with depression in returning to their normal lives (El-Rashidy et al., 2021). These psychological factors impose the need of continuous education, emotional support, and encouragement to help individuals adhere to their treatment plans and maintain optimal health outcomes (Hertroijs et al., 2019). The integration of digital health platforms, such as mobile apps and telepsychiatry, has shown promise in addressing these psychological needs by providing remote support and personalized mental health interventions.

3.5 Historical Analysis of Self-Management in Diabetes Care

The concept of self-management in diabetes care has evolved significantly over the years. Initially, diabetes management was primarily led by healthcare providers. However, advancements in healthcare technology and a growing understanding of the importance of patient engagement have changed the focus towards personalized and proactive self-management approaches.

Initially, self-management involved manual record-keeping of blood glucose levels and manual injections of insulin. With the advancement of digital solutions, especially with 5G-enabled devices, patients can now benefit from CGM systems and insulin pumps that adjust insulin delivery in real time (Chen et al., 2018; Zhu et al., 2023). Digital health platforms have evolved to integrate data from multiple sources, providing a holistic view of a patient's health. These platforms employ artificial intelligence (AI) to offer personalized insights and recommendations for diabetes management (Mohanta et al., 2019; Taimoor & Rehman, 2022). The review findings emphasise that while these advancements began before COVID-19, the pandemic significantly accelerated their adoption and integration into routine care practices, particularly telemedicine and remote monitoring. The smartphones have led to the development of mHealth applications that provide educational content, medication reminders, dietary tracking, and exercise logging, empowering patients in their self-management routines (El-Rashidy et al., 2021). With advancements in telehealth, patients can have regular follow-ups with their healthcare providers from the comfort of their homes, ensuring that their self-management plans are real time and up-to-date and effective (Andres et al., 2019; Moglia et al., 2022) which is vital when it comes to the situation like Covid-19 pandemic (Moglia et al., 2022). Wearable technology has become more sophisticated and advanced method, allowing for the monitoring of not just glucose levels but also other important signs that can impact diabetes management. These devices can generate alerts to patients and their clinicians if intervention is needed to manage the condition (Chen et al., 2018; Giordanengo et al., 2019). Digital tools have changed certain characteristics of diabetes management from providers to patients compared to initial diabetes management methods and engagement in their health decisions. This shift is supported by the real-time nature and accessibility of digital health data (Twohig et al., 2019; Wu et al., 2021). The application of predictive analytics in diabetes self-management helps anticipate potential complications and provides guidance on preventive measures, improving long-term outcomes for patients (Dagliati et al., 2018). The advancement of self-management in diabetes care through digital solutions has significantly transformed the approach to managing this chronic condition, making it more proactive, personalized, and patient-centered. These findings indicate the need for further exploration into the sustained impact of these digital tools in the evolving healthcare landscape.

Another important advancement in digital health technology is that integration of 5G Technology in Diabetes Care. The initial adoption of 5G technology in healthcare was marked by theoretical development and potential applications. Studies like Latif et al. (2017) discussed the innovative potential of 5G in healthcare, while Bertsimas et al. (2017) emphasized personalized diabetes management using electronic medical records. Also, the integration of 5G with wearable devices for real-time blood glucose monitoring has demonstrated improved patient outcomes. Chen et al. (2018) and showcased how these technologies enable continuous monitoring and timely interventions. During the COVID-19 pandemic, there was a notable increase in 5G-enabled telemedicine systems. Moglia et al. (2022) reviewed the role of 5G in remote patient care, highlighting its importance in maintaining stability and continuous patient care during the pandemic. As 5G technology matured, strategies have been implemented to addressing challenges such as infrastructure needs and data security. Studies by Devi et al. (2023) and Mohanta et al. (2019) highlighted these issues, emphasizing the need for robust cybersecurity measures and scalable infrastructure. Taimoor and Rehman (2022) discussed the potential of these technologies to provide personalized care and improve health outcomes. The findings illustrate that while 5G and similar technologies were being explored before the pandemic, their practical application and value were more clearly demonstrated during the COVID-19 era, which serves as a catalyst for broader adoption and future research.

4. DISCUSSION

Diabetes mellitus has emerged as one of the most significant global health problems, affecting millions of individuals worldwide. The increasing prevalence of diabetes causes a substantial challenge to healthcare systems globally. This alarming trend is driven by several factors, including urbanization, aging populations, and lifestyle changes such as unhealthy diets and physical inactivity. The global burden of diabetes is not limited to high-income countries, but also low and middle-income countries are experiencing growing rates, often without the necessary healthcare resources to manage the disease effectively. The COVID-19 pandemic further worsened these challenges by disrupting access to healthcare services and accelerating the need for innovative, digital solutions in diabetes management.

The economic impact of diabetes is high, and this includes direct medical costs such as hospital admissions, medications, and medical supplies, as well as indirect costs related to loss of productivity and long-term disability. The financial burden is particularly high in low and middle-income countries, where healthcare resources are limited, and the capacity to manage chronic diseases is insufficient. Effective management and prevention strategies are essential to mitigate these economic impacts and improve health outcomes. The integration of digital health interventions, such as telemedicine and mHealth applications, provides potential cost saving solutions by optimizing resource utilization and expanding access to care, particularly in limited resources settings.

Diabetes is associated with a range of serious complications, which significantly contribute to deaths among individuals with the disease. Cardiovascular disease is the leading cause of death in diabetic patients, with the risk of heart disease being two to four times higher in individuals with diabetes compared to those without diabetes. Stroke and hypertension are also common among diabetic individuals, further increasing the burden on healthcare systems. These complications not only affect the health and quality of life of individuals but also cause significant economic burden on healthcare systems. Managing these complications requires comprehensive and continuous care, which can be quite challenging for low and middle-income countries due to lack of access to the resources. Digital health technologies, such as AI-driven predictive analytics and remote monitoring, offer innovative ways to manage these complications by enabling early detection and personalized care strategies that can help reduce both mortality and costs associated with diabetes complications. Managing diabetes extends beyond physical health to include significant psychological challenges. Diabetes distress, characterized by feelings of frustration, worry, and burnout related to managing the disease common among diabetic patients. These psychological factors demand continuous education, emotional support, and encouragement to help patients to adhere to their treatment plans has been identified as some common themes. Therefore, it is important to note that integrated care approaches that address both diabetes and mental health are essential for improving outcomes. The adoption of telehealth platforms and digital mental health tools can play a critical role in providing remote psychological support, which has become particularly relevant in the post COVID-19 period when in-person consultations may be limited.

The evolution of diabetes care has highlighted the importance of personalized self-management. Unlike the traditional diabetes management approach, the advancements in healthcare technology emphasise the importance of patient engagement in proactive self-management approaches. Therefore, the advanced digital health tools such as CGM systems, mHealth applications, and telemedicine have empowered patients to take an active role in managing their condition. Also, telehealth enables regular monitoring with healthcare providers from the comfort of patients' homes, ensuring that their self-management plans are effective. Wearable technology has become more sophisticated, allowing for the monitoring glucose levels but also other signs that can impact diabetes management. Predictive analytics, enabled by advanced technologies such as AI and machine learning (ML), help to predict potential complications and provide guidance on preventive measures, improving long-term outcomes for individuals with diabetics. These advancements were significantly enhanced during the COVID-19 pandemic, which highlighted the need for flexible, remote management options to ensure continuity of care.

The integration of 5G technology in diabetes care offers significant potential to enhance self-management and improve health outcomes. The studies highlighted the benefits of 5G in personalized diabetes management using electronic medical records and wearable devices for real-time blood glucose monitoring. Particularly, during the COVID-19 pandemic, there was a notable increase in 5G-enabled telemedicine applications. Telemedicine allowed for the continuity of care during the pandemic, demonstrating the importance of 5G in remote patient care. The integration of 5G with wearable devices and the Internet of Things (IoT) has improved patient outcomes by enabling continuous monitoring and timely interventions. However, the adoption of 5G technology also faces challenges such as infrastructure needs and data security. Despite these challenges, the pandemic demonstrated the importance of investing in digital infrastructure and cybersecurity to support broader adoption of these technologies, which are essential for enhancing diabetes management in future healthcare landscapes. The findings of this study emphasize the urgent need for comprehensive management strategies that incorporate advanced healthcare technologies and continuous support for individuals with diabetes. Healthcare systems must address both the physical and psychological matters can be caused by diabetes.

Prevention of diabetes is a critical component of reducing its global impact. Lifestyle interventions, including healthy eating, regular physical activity, and weight management, have been shown to significantly reduce the risk of developing type 2 diabetes. Public health campaigns and community programs play a vital role in raising awareness about these preventive measures so that it can prevent the progression from pre-diabetes to diabetes. Digital health tools, such as mobile apps that promote healthy behaviours and provide real time feedback, have proven to be effective in supporting lifestyle interventions and could be scaled up to reach broader populations in both high- and low-income settings.

5. LIMITATIONS AND FUTURE STUDIES

This study has several limitations that need to be acknowledged. Firstly, the literature search was confined to articles published in English and from the year 2014 onwards. This may have excluded significant studies published in other languages or prior to 2014, potentially limiting the insights and data available for analysis. However, this timeframe was chosen to focus on more recent developments in digital health interventions and their relevance to contemporary diabetes management practices, especially considering the impact of the COVID-19 pandemic. Another limitation is the limited number of included studies, only 18 papers met the inclusion criteria for this review. This relatively small number of studies reflects a potential gap in the current literature on the specific focus of this study the impact and evolution of digital health interventions in diabetes management, particularly in the context of the post COVID-19 period. The limited number of studies could be attributed to the emerging nature of this research area and the lack of comprehensive studies that evaluate the integration and effectiveness of advanced technologies such as 5G, AI, and mHealth in diabetes care. This gap in the literature suggests a need for more focused research to explore and validate these technological solutions and their long-term benefits for diabetes management. Moreover, while this study highlights the benefits of digital health interventions, such as mHealth applications and telemedicine, it does not delve deeply into the specific challenges and barriers to their implementation, particularly in low and middle-income countries. Issues such as digital literacy, access to technology, infrastructure limitations, and data privacy concerns need to be explored in detail in future research to provide a deeper understanding of these interventions' feasibility and effectiveness in diverse settings.

6. CONCLUSIONS

Diabetes mellitus, as a chronic metabolic disorder, remains a significant global health challenge affecting millions of people worldwide. The complexity of diabetes management extends beyond managing blood glucose levels and it involves addressing a range of complications, economic burdens, and psychological challenges that impact both individuals and healthcare systems. The COVID-19 pandemic has further highlighted these challenges, disrupted traditional care models and emphasized the need for innovative, digital solutions in diabetes management. This study provides a comprehensive review of the evolving role of digital health interventions, such as mHealth applications, telemedicine, continuous glucose monitoring (CGM) systems, and 5G-enabled remote monitoring, in enhancing diabetes care. While these technologies have shown significant potential in improving patient engagement, self-management, and care continuity especially during the pandemic there remain substantial gaps in research and implementation. The findings of this study suggest that advanced digital health technologies, when integrated into comprehensive management strategies, can help mitigate the economic and healthcare burden of diabetes by optimizing resource utilization, improving access to care, and supporting personalized treatment plans. However, there are still significant barriers to their widespread adoption, including infrastructure limitations, digital literacy, data privacy concerns, and unequal access to technology, particularly in low and middle-income countries. Investigating these barriers is critical to ensuring that digital health interventions are accessible, equitable, and sustainable. To maximize the benefits of these technological advancements, healthcare systems must invest in digital infrastructure, provide training and support for both healthcare providers and patients, and develop policies that protect data privacy and security. Furthermore, future research should focus on generating real world evidence of the long term impact of digital health tools on health outcomes, cost-effectiveness, and patient satisfaction. By addressing these gaps, stakeholders can better integrate these innovations into standard diabetes care practices and ultimately improve the quality of life for people living with diabetes.

REFERENCES

Alqudah, A., McMullan, P., Todd, A., O'Doherty, C., McVey, A., McConnell, M., O'Donoghue, J., Gallagher, J., Watson, C. J., & McClements, L. (2019). Service evaluation of diabetes management during pregnancy in a regional maternity hospital: Potential scope for increased self-management and remote patient monitoring through mHealth solutions. *BMC Health Services Research*, 19(1), 662. https://doi.org/https://dx.doi.org/10.1186/s12913-019-4471-9. DOI: 10.1186/s12913-019-4471-9 PMID: 31514743

Ames, J. L., Massolo, M. L., Davignon, M. N., Qian, Y., & Croen, L. A. (2021). Healthcare service utilization and cost among transition-age youth with autism spectrum disorder and other special healthcare needs. *Autism*, 25(3), 705–718. DOI: 10.1177/1362361320931268 PMID: 32583679

Andres, E., Meyer, L., Zulfiqar, A.-A., Hajjam, M., Talha, S., Bahougne, T., Erve, S., Hajjam, J., Doucet, J., Jeandidier, N., & Hajjam El Hassani, A. (2019). Telemonitoring in diabetes: Evolution of concepts and technologies, with a focus on results of the more recent studies. *Journal of Medicine and Life*, 12(3), 203–214. https://doi.org/https://dx.doi.org/10.25122/jml-2019-0006. DOI: 10.25122/jml-2019-0006 PMID: 31666818

Beck, J., Greenwood, D. A., Blanton, L., Bollinger, S. T., Butcher, M. K., Condon, J. E., Cypress, M., Faulkner, P., Fischl, A. H., Francis, T., Kolb, L. E., Lavin-Tompkins, J. M., MacLeod, J., Maryniuk, M., Mensing, C., Orzeck, E. A., Pope, D. D., Pulizzi, J. L., Reed, A. A., & Wang, J. (2017). 2017 National Standards for Diabetes Self-Management Education and Support. *Diabetes Spectrum*, 30(4), 301–314. DOI: 10.2337/ds17-0067 PMID: 29151721

Bertsimas, D., Kallus, N., Weinstein, A. M., Ying Daisy, Z., & Zhuo, Y. D. (2017). Personalized Diabetes Management Using Electronic Medical Records. *Diabetes Care*, 40(2), 210–217. DOI: 10.2337/dc16-0826 PMID: 27920019

Blonde, L., Umpierrez, G. E., Reddy, S. S., McGill, J. B., Berga, S. L., Bush, M., Chandrasekaran, S., DeFronzo, R. A., Einhorn, D., Galindo, R. J., Gardner, T. W., Garg, R., Garvey, W. T., Hirsch, I. B., Hurley, D. L., Izuora, K., Kosiborod, M., Olson, D., Patel, S. B., & Weber, S. L. (2022). American Association of Clinical Endocrinology Clinical Practice Guideline: Developing a Diabetes Mellitus Comprehensive Care Plan—2022 Update [Article]. *Endocrine Practice*, 28(10), 923–1049. DOI: 10.1016/j.eprac.2022.08.002 PMID: 35963508

Brørs, G., Norman, C. D., & Norekvål, T. M. (2020). Accelerated importance of eHealth literacy in the COVID-19 outbreak and beyond. *European Journal of Cardiovascular Nursing*, 19(6), 458–461. DOI: 10.1177/1474515120941307 PMID: 32667217

Chen, M., Yang, J., Zhou, J., Hao, Y., Zhang, J., & Youn, C. H. (2018). 5G-Smart Diabetes: Toward Personalized Diabetes Diagnosis with Healthcare Big Data Clouds. *IEEE Communications Magazine*, 56(4), 16–23. DOI: 10.1109/MCOM.2018.1700788

Chun, J., & Hong, J. (2015). Relationships between presynaptic inhibition and static postural sway in subjects with and without diabetic neuropathy [Article]. *Journal of Physical Therapy Science*, 27(9), 2697–2700. DOI: 10.1589/jpts.27.2697 PMID: 26504271

Dagliati, A., Sacchi, L., Tibollo, V., Cogni, G., Teliti, M., Martinez-Millana, A., Traver, V., Segagni, D., Posada, J., Ottaviano, M., Fico, G., Arredondo, M. T., De Cata, P., Chiovato, L., & Bellazzi, R. (2018). A dashboard-based system for supporting diabetes care. *Journal of the American Medical Informatics Association : JAMIA*, 25(5), 538–547. https://doi.org/https://dx.doi.org/10.1093/jamia/ocx159. DOI: 10.1093/jamia/ocx159 PMID: 29409033

Desveaux, L., Agarwal, P., Shaw, J., Hensel, J. M., Mukerji, G., Onabajo, N., Marani, H., Jamieson, T., Bhattacharyya, O., Martin, D., Mamdani, M., Jeffs, L., Wodchis, W. P., Ivers, N. M., & Bhatia, R. S. (2016). A randomized wait-list control trial to evaluate the impact of a mobile application to improve self-management of individuals with type 2 diabetes: A study protocol. *BMC Medical Informatics and Decision Making*, 16(1), 144. https://ovidsp.ovid.com/ovidweb.cgi?T=JS&PAGE=reference&D=med13&NEWS=N&AN=27842539. DOI: 10.1186/s12911-016-0381-5 PMID: 27842539

Devi, D. H., Duraisamy, K., Armghan, A., Alsharari, M., Aliqab, K., Sorathiya, V., Das, S., & Rashid, N. (2023). 5G Technology in Healthcare and Wearable Devices: A Review. *Sensors (Basel)*, 23(5), 2519. DOI: 10.3390/s23052519 PMID: 36904721

El-Rashidy, N., El-Sappagh, S., Riazul Islam, S. M., El-Bakry, H. M., & Abdelrazek, S. (2021). Mobile health in remote patient monitoring for chronic diseases: Principles, trends, and challenges. *Diagnostics (Basel)*, 11(4), 607. DOI: 10.3390/diagnostics11040607 PMID: 33805471

Fareed, N., Swoboda, C., Singh, P., Boettcher, E., Wang, Y., Venkatesh, K., & Strouse, R. (2023). Developing and testing an integrated patient mHealth and provider dashboard application system for type 2 diabetes management among Medicaid-enrolled pregnant individuals based on a user-centered approach: Mixed-methods study [Article]. *Digital Health*, 9, 20552076221144181. Advance online publication. DOI: 10.1177/20552076221144181 PMID: 36644662

Giordanengo, A., Årsand, E., Woldaregay, A. Z., Bradway, M., Grottland, A., Hartvigsen, G., Granja, C., Torsvik, T., & Hansen, A. H. (2019). Design and prestudy assessment of a dashboard for presenting self-collected health data of patients with diabetes to clinicians: Iterative approach and qualitative case study [Article]. *JMIR Diabetes*, 4(3), e14002. Advance online publication. DOI: 10.2196/14002 PMID: 31290396

Goyal, S., Morita, P., Lewis, G. F., Yu, C., Seto, E., & Cafazzo, J. A. (2016). The Systematic Design of a Behavioural Mobile Health Application for the Self-Management of Type 2 Diabetes. *Canadian Journal of Diabetes*, 40(1), 95–104. https://doi.org/https://dx.doi.org/10.1016/j.jcjd.2015.06.007. DOI: 10.1016/j.jcjd.2015.06.007 PMID: 26455762

Hall, C. E., Hall, A. B., Kok, G., Mallya, J., & Courtright, P. (2016). A needs assessment of people living with diabetes and diabetic retinopathy [Article]. *BMC Research Notes*, 9(1), 56. Advance online publication. DOI: 10.1186/s13104-016-1870-4 PMID: 26829927

Hertroijs, D. F. L., Brouwers, M. C. G. J., Elissen, A. M. J., Schaper, N. C., & Ruwaard, D. (2019). Relevant patient characteristics for estimating healthcare needs according to healthcare providers and people with type 2 diabetes: A Delphi survey. *BMC Health Services Research*, 19(1), 575. https://doi.org/https://dx.doi.org/10.1186/s12913-019-4371-z. DOI: 10.1186/s12913-019-4371-z PMID: 31419980

International Diabetes Federation. (2021). IDF Diabetes Atlas (10th ed.). Retrieved from https://diabetesatlas.org/atlas/tenth-edition/

Latif, S., Qadir, J., Farooq, S., & Imran, M. A. (2017). How 5G wireless (and Concomitant Technologies) will revolutionize healthcare? [Article]. *Future Internet*, 9(4), 93. Advance online publication. DOI: 10.3390/fi9040093

Mendenhall, E., McMurry, H. S., Shivashankar, R., Narayan, K. M. V., Tandon, N., & Prabhakaran, D. (2016). Normalizing diabetes in Delhi: A qualitative study of health and health care. *Anthropology & Medicine*, 23(3), 295–310. DOI: 10.1080/13648470.2016.1184010 PMID: 27328175

Moglia, A., Georgiou, K., Marinov, B., Georgiou, E., Berchiolli, R. N., Satava, R. M., & Cuschieri, A. (2022). 5G in Healthcare: From COVID-19 to Future Challenges [Article]. *IEEE Journal of Biomedical and Health Informatics*, 26(8), 4187–4196. DOI: 10.1109/JBHI.2022.3181205 PMID: 35675255

Mohanta, B., Das, P., & Patnaik, S. (2019, May 25-26). 2019). Healthcare 5.0: A Paradigm Shift in Digital Healthcare System Using Artificial Intelligence, IOT and 5G Communication. 2019 International Conference on Applied Machine Learning (ICAML), Morone, J. (2019). Systematic review of sociodemographic representation and cultural responsiveness in psychosocial and behavioral interventions with adolescents with type 1 diabetes. *Journal of Diabetes*, 11(7), 582–592. https://doi.org/https://dx.doi.org/10.1111/1753-0407.12889 PMID: 30565425

Nadeau, K. J., Anderson, B. J., Berg, E. G., Chiang, J. L., Chou, H., Copeland, K. C., Hannon, T. S., Huang, T. T. K., Lynch, J. L., Powell, J., Sellers, E., Tamborlane, W. V., & Zeitler, P. (2016). Youth-Onset Type 2 Diabetes Consensus Report: Current Status, Challenges, and Priorities. *Diabetes Care*, 39(9), 1635–1642. https://doi.org/https://dx.doi.org/10.2337/dc16-1066. DOI: 10.2337/dc16-1066 PMID: 27486237

Nguyen, H. D., Chitturi, S., & Maple-Brown, L. J. (2016). Management of diabetes in Indigenous communities: Lessons from the Australian Aboriginal population. *Internal Medicine Journal*, 46(11), 1252–1259. https://doi.org/https://dx.doi.org/10.1111/imj.13123. DOI: 10.1111/imj.13123 PMID: 27130346

Page, M. J., McKenzie, J. E., Bossuyt, P. M., Boutron, I., Hoffmann, T. C., Mulrow, C. D., Shamseer, L., Tetzlaff, J. M., Akl, E. A., Brennan, S. E., Chou, R., Glanville, J., Grimshaw, J. M., Hróbjartsson, A., Lalu, M. M., Li, T., Loder, E. W., Mayo-Wilson, E., McDonald, S., & Moher, D. (2021). The PRISMA 2020 statement: An updated guideline for reporting systematic reviews. *BMJ (Clinical Research Ed.)*, 372(71), n71. Advance online publication. DOI: 10.1136/bmj.n71 PMID: 33782057

Pekmezaris, R., Williams, M. S., Pascarelli, B., Finuf, K. D., Harris, Y. T., Myers, A. K., Taylor, T., Kline, M., Patel, V. H., Murray, L. M., McFarlane, S. I., Pappas, K., Lesser, M. L., Makaryus, A. N., Martinez, S., Kozikowski, A., Polo, J., Guzman, J., Zeltser, R., & Granville, D. (2020). Adapting a home telemonitoring intervention for underserved Hispanic/Latino patients with type 2 diabetes: An acceptability and feasibility study [Article]. *BMC Medical Informatics and Decision Making*, 20(1), 324. Advance online publication. DOI: 10.1186/s12911-020-01346-0 PMID: 33287815

Souza, D. J., Barbosa Baptista, M. H., dos Santos Gomides, D., & Emilia Pace, A. (2017). Adherence to diabetes mellitus care at three levels of health care. *Anna Nery School Journal of Nursing / Escola Anna Nery Revista de Enfermagem, 21*(4), 1-9. https://doi.org/DOI: 10.1590/2177-9465-EAN-2017-0045

Subramanian, G., & Sreekantan Thampy, A. (2021). Implementation of Blockchain Consortium to Prioritize Diabetes Patients' Healthcare in Pandemic Situations [Article]. *IEEE Access : Practical Innovations, Open Solutions*, 9, 162459–162475. DOI: 10.1109/ACCESS.2021.3132302

Taimoor, N., & Rehman, S. (2022). Reliable and Resilient AI and IoT-Based Personalised Healthcare Services: A Survey [Article]. *IEEE Access : Practical Innovations, Open Solutions*, 10, 535–563. DOI: 10.1109/ACCESS.2021.3137364

Tomlin, A., & Asimakopoulou, K. (2014). Supporting behaviour change in older people with type 2 diabetes. *British Journal of Community Nursing*, 19(1), 22–27. http://ez.library.latrobe.edu.au/login?url=https://search.ebscohost.com/login.aspx?direct=true&db=cul&AN=103994423&login.asp&site=ehost-live&scope=site. DOI: 10.12968/bjcn.2014.19.1.22 PMID: 24800323

Twohig, P. A., Rivington, J. R., Gunzler, D., Daprano, J., & Margolius, D. (2019). Clinician dashboard views and improvement in preventative health outcome measures: A retrospective analysis. *BMC Health Services Research*, 19(1), 475. https://doi.org/https://dx.doi.org/10.1186/s12913-019-4327-3. DOI: 10.1186/s12913-019-4327-3 PMID: 31296211

Vesselkov, A., Hämmäinen, H., & Töyli, J. (2018). Technology and value network evolution in telehealth [Article]. *Technological Forecasting and Social Change*, 134, 207–222. DOI: 10.1016/j.techfore.2018.06.011

Wojahn, R. D., Foeger, N. C., Gelberman, R. H., & Calfee, R. P. (2014). Long-term outcomes following a single corticosteroid injection for trigger finger. [Comment in: J Bone Joint Surg Am. 2014 Nov 19;96(22) [:e191 PMID: 25410519] [. *The Journal of Bone and Joint Surgery. American Volume*, 96(22), 1849–1854. https://www.ncbi.nlm.nih.gov/pubmed/25410519. DOI: 10.2106/JBJS.N.00004 PMID: 25410501

World Health Organization. (2023). Global report on diabetes. Retrieved from https://www.who.int/news-room/fact-sheets/detail/diabetes

World Health Organization. (2024). World health statistics 2024. Retrieved from https://www.who.int/data/gho/publications/world-health-statistics

Wu, J., Chang, L., & Yu, G. (2021). Effective Data Decision-Making and Transmission System Based on Mobile Health for Chronic Disease Management in the Elderly. *IEEE Systems Journal*, 15(4), 5537–5548. DOI: 10.1109/JSYST.2020.3024816

Zhu, T., Kuang, L., Daniels, J., Herrero, P., Li, K., & Georgiou, P. (2023). IoMT-Enabled Real-Time Blood Glucose Prediction With Deep Learning and Edge Computing [Article]. *IEEE Internet of Things Journal*, 10(5), 3706–3719. DOI: 10.1109/JIOT.2022.3143375

Compilation of References

Abawajy, J. H., & Hassan, M. M. (2017). Federated Internet of Things and Cloud Computing Pervasive Patient Health Monitoring System. *IEEE Communications Magazine*, 55(1), 48–53. DOI: 10.1109/MCOM.2017.1600374CM

Abdel-Basset, M., Abduallah Gamal, Gunasekaran Manogaran, Le Hoang Son, & Long, H. V. (. (2019). A novel group decision making model based on neutrosophic sets for heart disease diagnosis. *Multimedia Tools and Applications*, •••, 1–26. DOI: 10.1007/s11042-019-07742-7

Abdi, J., Al-Hindawi, A., Ng, T., & Vizcaychipi, M. P. (2018). Scoping review on the use of socially assistive robot technology in elderly care. *BMJ Open*, 8(2), e018815. DOI: 10.1136/bmjopen-2017-018815 PMID: 29440212

Abdur Rahman, M., Rashid, M. M., Le Kernec, J., Philippe, B., Barnes, S. J., Fioranelli, F., Yang, S., Romain, O., Abbasi, Q. H., Loukas, G., & Imran, M. (2019). A Secure Occupational Therapy Framework for Monitoring Cancer Patients' Quality of Life. *Sensors (Basel)*, 19(23), 5258. Advance online publication. DOI: 10.3390/s19235258 PMID: 31795384

About Mental Health. (2024, May 20). https://www.cdc.gov/mentalhealth/learn/index.htm

Addante, F., Gaetani, F., Patrono, L., Sancarlo, D., Sergi, I., & Vergari, G. (2019). An Innovative AAL System Based on IoT Technologies for Patients with Sarcopenia. *Sensors (Basel)*, 19(22), 4951. Advance online publication. DOI: 10.3390/s19224951 PMID: 31739396

Addissouky, T. A., El Sayed, I. E. T., Ali, M. M., Wang, Y., El Baz, A., Elarabany, N., & Khalil, A. A. (2024). Shaping the future of cardiac wellness: Exploring revolutionary approaches in disease management and prevention. *Journal of Clinical Cardiology*, 5(1), 6–29. DOI: 10.33696/cardiology.5.048

Aggarwal, P., Rana, M., & Akhai, S. (2022). Briefings on e-waste hazard until COVID era in India. *Materials Today: Proceedings*, 71(2), 389–393. DOI: 10.1016/j.matpr.2022.09.507

Ahmadi, H., Arji, G., Shahmoradi, L., Safdari, R., Nilashi, M., & Alizadeh, M. (2018). The application of internet of things in healthcare: A systematic literature review and classification. *Universal Access in the Information Society*. Advance online publication. DOI: 10.1007/s10209-018-0618-4

Ahmedin Jemal, F. B. (2012). Cancer Burden in Africa and Opportunities for Prevention. *American Cancer Society*, 1-24.

Ahmed, S. (2019). BYOD, Personal Area Networks (PANs) and IOT: Threats to Patients Privacy. In Visvizi, A., & Lytras, M. D. (Eds.), *Research & Innovation Forum 2019* (pp. 403–410). Springer International Publishing., DOI: 10.1007/978-3-030-30809-4_36

Akhai, S. (2023). Healthcare record management for healthcare 4.0 via blockchain: a review of current applications, opportunities, challenges, and future potential. *Blockchain for Healthcare 4.0, 1*, 211-223.

Akhai, S. (2024). A Review on Optimizations in μ-EDM Machining of the Biomedical Material Ti6Al4V Using the Taguchi Method: Recent Advances Since 2020. *Latest Trends in Engineering and Technology*, 395-402.

Akhai, S. (2024). Towards Trustworthy and Reliable AI The Next Frontier. *Explainable Artificial Intelligence (XAI) in Healthcare, 1*, 119-129.

Akhai, S., & Khang, A. (2024). Efficient Hospital Waste Treatment and Management Through IoT and Bioelectronics. In *Revolutionizing Automated Waste Treatment Systems: IoT and Bioelectronics* (pp. 126-140). IGI Global. DOI: 10.4018/979-8-3693-6016-3.ch009

Akhai, S., & Khang, A. (2024). Energy Efficiency and Human Comfort: AI and IoT Integration in Hospital HVAC Systems. *Medical Robotics and AI-Assisted Diagnostics for a High-Tech Healthcare Industry*, 93-108.

Akhai, S., & Kumar, V. (2024). Quantum Resilience and Distributed Trust: The Promise of Blockchain and Quantum Computing in Defense. *Sustainable Security Practices Using Blockchain, Quantum and Post-Quantum Technologies for Real Time Applications*, 125-153.

Akhai, S., Mala, S., & Jerin, A. A. (2020). Apprehending air conditioning systems in context to COVID-19 and human health: a brief communication. *International Journal of Healthcare Education & Medical Informatics (ISSN: 2455-9199), 7*(1&2), 28-30.

Akhai, S., Mala, S., & Jerin, A. A. (2021). Understanding whether air filtration from air conditioners reduces the probability of virus transmission in the environment. *Journal of Advanced Research in Medical Science & Technology (ISSN: 2394-6539), 8*(1), 36-41.

Akhai, S. (2023). Navigating the potential applications and challenges of intelligent and sustainable manufacturing for a greener future. *Evergreen*, 10(4), 2237–2243. DOI: 10.5109/7160899

Akhai, S., Singh, V. P., & John, S. (2016). Human performance in industrial design centers with small unit air conditioning systems. *Journal of Advanced Research in Production Industrial Engineering*, 3(2), 5–11.

Akhai, S., Singh, V. P., & John, S. (2016). Investigating Indoor Air Quality for the Split-Type Air Conditioners in an Office Environment and Its Effect on Human Performance. *Journal of Mechanical Civil Engineering*, 13(6), 113–118.

Akhtar, M., Haleem, A., & Javaid, M. (2024). Exploring the advent of Medical 4.0: A bibliometric analysis systematic review and technology adoption insights. Informatics and Health, 16-28. DOI: 10.1016/j.infoh.2023.10.001

Akinosun, A. S., Polson, R., Diaz-Skeete, Y., De Kock, J. H., Carragher, L., Leslie, S., Grindle, M., & Gorely, T. (2021). Digital technology interventions for risk factor modification in patients with cardiovascular disease: Systematic review and meta-analysis. *JMIR mHealth and uHealth*, 9(3), e21061. DOI: 10.2196/21061 PMID: 33656444

Al Mamun, K. A., Alhussein, M., Sailunaz, K., & Islam, M. S. (2017). Cloud based framework for Parkinson's disease diagnosis and monitoring system for remote healthcare applications. *Future Generation Computer Systems*, 66, 36–47. DOI: 10.1016/j.future.2015.11.010

Aleisa, N., & Renaud, K. (2017). Privacy of the Internet of Things: A Systematic Literature Review. *Proceedings of the 50th Hawaii International Conference on System Sciences*, 10. DOI: 10.24251/HICSS.2017.717

Alexandre, R., & Postolache, O. (2018). Wearable and IoT Technologies Application for Physical Rehabilitation. *2018 International Symposium in Sensing and Instrumentation in IoT Era (ISSI)*, 1–6. DOI: 10.1109/ISSI.2018.8538058

Al-Fuqaha, A., Guizani, M., Mohammadi, M., Aledhari, M., & Ayyash, M. (2015). Internet of Things: A Survey on Enabling Technologies, Protocols, and Applications. *IEEE Communications Surveys Tutorials, 17*(4), 2347–2376. *IEEE Communications Surveys and Tutorials.* Advance online publication. DOI: 10.1109/COMST.2015.2444095

Alhussein, M. (2017). Monitoring Parkinson's disease in smart cities. *IEEE Access : Practical Innovations, Open Solutions*, 5, 19835–19841. DOI: 10.1109/ACCESS.2017.2748561

Alice Asobayire, R. B. (2015). Women's Cultural Perceptions and Attitudes Towards Breast Cancer: Northern Ghana. *Health Promotion International*, 30(3), 647–657. DOI: 10.1093/heapro/dat087 PMID: 24474424

Ali, R., Hussain, A., Nazir, S., Khan, S., & Khan, H. (2023). Intelligent Decision Support Systems—An Analysis of Machine Learning and Multicriteria Decision-Making Methods. *Applied Sciences (Basel, Switzerland)*, 13(22), 12426. Advance online publication. DOI: 10.3390/app132212426

Aljahdali, M., Abokhamees, R., Bensenouci, A., Brahimi, T., & Bensenouci, M. (2018). IoT based assistive walker device for frail &visually impaired people. *2018 15th Learning and Technology Conference (L&T)*, 171–177. DOI: 10.1109/LT.2018.8368503

Al-Khafajiy, M., Baker, T., Chalmers, C., Asim, M., Kolivand, H., Fahim, M., & Waraich, A. (2019). Remote health monitoring of elderly through wearable sensors. In *Multimedia Tools and Applications* (Vol. 78, Issue 17, pp. 24681–24706). SPRINGER. DOI: 10.1007/s11042-018-7134-7

Alkhalidy, H., Wang, Y., & Liu, D. (2018). Dietary flavonoids in the prevention of T2D: An overview. *Nutrients*, 10(4), 438. DOI: 10.3390/nu10040438 PMID: 29614722

Almogren, A. (2019). An automated and intelligent parkinson disease monitoring system using wearable computing and cloud technology. *Cluster Computing*, 22(1), 2309–2316. DOI: 10.1007/s10586-017-1591-z

Al-Msie'deen, R., Huchard, M., Seriai, A.-D., Urtado, C., and Vauttier, S. 2014. "Automatic Documentation of [Mined] Feature Implementations from Source Code Elements and Use-Case Diagrams with the REVPLINE Approach.," *International Journal of Software Engineering & Knowledge Engineering* (24:10), pp. 1413–1438.

Alqudah, A., McMullan, P., Todd, A., O'Doherty, C., McVey, A., McConnell, M., O'Donoghue, J., Gallagher, J., Watson, C. J., & McClements, L. (2019). Service evaluation of diabetes management during pregnancy in a regional maternity hospital: Potential scope for increased self-management and remote patient monitoring through mHealth solutions. *BMC Health Services Research*, 19(1), 662. https://doi.org/https://dx.doi.org/10.1186/s12913-019-4471-9. DOI: 10.1186/s12913-019-4471-9 PMID: 31514743

AL-Rousan, N., & AL-Najjar, H.. (2020). Data analysis of coronavirus COVID-19 epidemic in South Korea based on recovered and death cases. *Journal of Medical Virology*, 92(9), 1603–1608. DOI: 10.1002/jmv.25850 PMID: 32270521

Al-Taee, M. A., Al-Nuaimy, W., Muhsin, Z. J., & Al-Ataby, A. (2017). Robot Assistant in Management of Diabetes in Children Based on the Internet of Things. *IEEE Internet of Things Journal*, 4(2), 437–445. DOI: 10.1109/JIOT.2016.2623767

Altulaihan, E. A., Alismail, A., & Frikha, M. (2023). A survey on web application penetration testing. *Electronics (Basel)*, 12(5), 1229. DOI: 10.3390/electronics12051229

Al-Turjman, F., Hasan, M. Z., & Al-Rizzo, H. (2019). Task scheduling in cloud-based survivability applications using swarm optimization in IoT. *Transactions on Emerging Telecommunications Technologies*, 30(8), e3539. DOI: 10.1002/ett.3539

Alzheimer's Society. (2024). Local dementia statistics. URL: https://www.alzheimers.org.uk/about-us/policy-and-influencing/local-dementia-statistics

American Cancer Society. (2023). *Melanoma skin cancer*. Retrieved from https://www.cancer.org/cancer/melanoma-skin-cancer.html

Ames, J. L., Massolo, M. L., Davignon, M. N., Qian, Y., & Croen, L. A. (2021). Healthcare service utilization and cost among transition-age youth with autism spectrum disorder and other special healthcare needs. *Autism*, 25(3), 705–718. DOI: 10.1177/1362361320931268 PMID: 32583679

Andres, E., Meyer, L., Zulfiqar, A.-A., Hajjam, M., Talha, S., Bahougne, T., Erve, S., Hajjam, J., Doucet, J., Jeandidier, N., & Hajjam El Hassani, A. (2019). Telemonitoring in diabetes: Evolution of concepts and technologies, with a focus on results of the more recent studies. *Journal of Medicine and Life*, 12(3), 203–214. https://doi.org/https://dx.doi.org/10.25122/jml-2019-0006. DOI: 10.25122/jml-2019-0006 PMID: 31666818

Antz, M., Chun, K. J., Ouyang, F., & Kuck, K. H. (2006). Ablation of atrial fibrillation in humans using a balloon-based ablation system: Identification of the site of phrenic nerve damage using pacing maneuvers and CARTO. *Journal of Cardiovascular Electrophysiology*, 17(11), 1242–1245. DOI: 10.1111/j.1540-8167.2006.00589.x

Arora, P., Kumar, H., & Panigrahi, B. K. (2020). Prediction and analysis of COVID-19 positive cases using deep learning models: A descriptive case study of India. *Chaos, Solitons, and Fractals*, 139, 110017. Advance online publication. DOI: 10.1016/j.chaos.2020.110017 PMID: 32572310

Arpaia, P., D'Errico, G., De Paolis, L. T., Moccaldi, N., & Nuccetelli, F. (2021). A narrative review of mindfulness-based interventions using virtual reality. *Mindfulness*, 1–16.

ArunKumar, K. E., Kalaga, D. V., Kumar, C. M. S., Chilkoor, G., Kawaji, M., & Brenza, T. M. (2021). Forecasting the dynamics of cumulative COVID-19 cases (confirmed, recovered and deaths) for top-16 countries using statistical machine learning models: Auto-Regressive Integrated Moving Average (ARIMA) and Seasonal Auto-Regressive Integrated Moving Average (SARIMA). *Applied Soft Computing*, 103, 107161.

Asghari, P., Rahmani, A. M., & Javadi, H. H. S. (2019a). A medical monitoring scheme and health-medical service composition model in cloud-based IoT platform. *Transactions on Emerging Telecommunications Technologies*, 30(6), e3637. Advance online publication. DOI: 10.1002/ett.3637

Asghari, P., Rahmani, A. M., & Javadi, H. H. S. (2019b). Internet of Things applications: A systematic review. *Computer Networks*, 148, 241–261. DOI: 10.1016/j.comnet.2018.12.008

Astell, A. J., McGrath, C., & Dove, E. (2020). 'That's for old so and so's!': Does identity influence older adults' technology adoption decisions? *Ageing and Society*, 40(7), 1550–1576. DOI: 10.1017/S0144686X19000230

Atieh, A. (2021). The Next Generation Cloud technologies: A Review On Distributed Cloud, Fog And Edge Computing and Their Opportunities and Challenges. ResearchBerg Review of Science and Technology, 1-15. Retrieved from https://www.researchberg.com/index.php/rrst/article/view/18

Attallah, O., & Sharkas, M. (2021). Intelligent Dermatologist Tool for Classifying Multiple Skin Cancer Subtypes by Incorporating Manifold Radiomics Features Categories. *Contrast Media & Molecular Imaging*, 2021, 1–14. Advance online publication. DOI: 10.1155/2021/7192016 PMID: 34621146

Atzori, L., Iera, A., & Morabito, G. (2010). The Internet of Things: A survey. *Computer Networks*, 54(15), 2787–2805. DOI: 10.1016/j.comnet.2010.05.010

Azimi, I., Anzanpour, A., Rahmani, A. M., Pahikkala, T., Levorato, M., Liljeberg, P., & Dutt, N. (2017). HiCH: Hierarchical Fog-Assisted Computing Architecture for Healthcare IoT. *ACM Transactions on Embedded Computing Systems, 16*(5, SI). DOI: 10.1145/3126501

Azuma, R., Baillot, Y., Behringer, R., Feiner, S., Julier, S., and MacIntyre, B. (2001). Recent Advances in Augmented Reality. *IEEE Computer Graphics and Applications* (21:6), pp. 34-47.

Baandrup, L., & Jennum, P. J. (2021). Effect of a dynamic lighting intervention on circadian rest-activity disturbances in cognitively impaired, older adults living in a nursing home: A proof-of-concept study. *Neurobiology of Sleep and Circadian Rhythms*, 11, 100067. DOI: 10.1016/j.nbscr.2021.100067 PMID: 34095610

Bae, J.-H., & Lee, H.-K. (2018). User Health Information Analysis With a Urine and Feces Separable Smart Toilet System. *IEEE Access : Practical Innovations, Open Solutions*, 6, 78751–78765. DOI: 10.1109/ACCESS.2018.2885234

Baig, M. M., Afifi, S., GholamHosseini, H., & Mirza, F. (2019). A systematic review of wearable sensors and IoT-based monitoring applications for older adults–a focus on ageing population and independent living. *Journal of Medical Systems*, 43(8), 1–11. DOI: 10.1007/s10916-019-1365-7 PMID: 31203472

Bailey, S. C., Belter, L. T., Pandit, A. U., & Carpenter, D. M. (2013). *The Availability*. Functionality, and Quality of Mobile Applications Supporting Medication Selfmanagement.

Baker, S., & Xiang, W. (2023). Artificial Intelligence of Things for Smarter Healthcare: A Survey of Advancements, Challenges, and Opportunities. *IEEE Communications Surveys and Tutorials*, 25(2), 1261–1293. DOI: 10.1109/COMST.2023.3256323

Balandina, E., Balandin, S., Koucheryavy, Y., & Mouromtsev, D. (2015). IoT Use Cases in Healthcare and Tourism. *2015 IEEE 17th Conference on Business Informatics, 2*, 37–44. DOI: 10.1109/CBI.2015.16

Baltagi, B. H., Lagravinese, R., Moscone, F., & Tosetti, E. (2017). Health Care Expenditure and Income: A Global Perspective. *Health Economics*, 26(7), 863–874. DOI: 10.1002/hec.3424 PMID: 27679983

Bandura, A. (1971). *Social learning theory* (Vol. 1). Prentice Hall.

Bandura, A. (2001). Social cognitive theory: An agentic perspective. *Annual Review of Psychology*, 52(1), 1–26. DOI: 10.1146/annurev.psych.52.1.1

Banerjee, S., & Huth, J. K. (2020). Time-series study of cardiovascular rates in India: A systematic analysis between 1990 and 2017. *Indian Heart Journal*, 72(3), 194–196. DOI: 10.1016/j.ihj.2020.05.014 PMID: 32768021

Banki, M., Farsinia, F., & Ghasemi, S. (2023). Artificial intelligence in management and prognosis of melanoma: A literature review. *Open Access Research Journal of Biology and Pharmacy*, 8(2), 023–026. Advance online publication. DOI: 10.53022/oarjbp.2023.8.2.0029

Baños, R. M., Etchemendy, E., Carrillo-Vega, A., & Botella, C. (2021). Positive psychological interventions and information and communication technologies. In *Research Anthology on Rehabilitation Practices and Therapy* (pp. 1648–1668). IGI Global.

Basanta, H., Huang, Y., & Lee, T. (2016). Intuitive IoT-based H2U healthcare system for elderly people. *2016 IEEE 13th International Conference on Networking, Sensing, and Control (ICNSC)*, 1–6. DOI: 10.1109/ICNSC.2016.7479018

Baskerville, R., & Pries-Heje, J. 2014. "Design Theory Projectability," in *Information Systems and Global Assemblages. (Re)Configuring Actors, Artefacts, Organizations*, IFIP Advances in Information and Communication Technology, B. Doolin, E. Lamprou, N. Mitev, and L. McLeod (eds.), Springer, Berlin, Heidelberg, pp. 219–232. (https://link.springer.com/chapter/10.1007/978-3-662-45708-5_14)

Basulo-Ribeiro, J., & Teixeira, L. (2024). The Future of Healthcare with Industry 5.0: Preliminary Interview-Based Qualitative Analysis. *Future Internet*, 16(3), 68. DOI: 10.3390/fi16030068

Basu, S., & Campbell, R. H. (2020). Going by the numbers: Learning and modeling COVID-19 disease dynamics. *Chaos, Solitons, and Fractals*, 138, 110140. DOI: 10.1016/j.chaos.2020.110140 PMID: 32834585

Baumeister, J., Ssin, S.Y., El Sayed, N.A.M., Dorrian, J., Webb, D.P., Walsh, J.A., Simon, T.M., Irlitti, A., Smith, R.T., Kohler, M., and Thomas B.H. 2017. Cognitive Cost of Using Augmented Reality Displays, *IEEE Transactions on Visualization and Computer Graphics* (23:11), pp. 2378-2388.

Bayoumy, K., Gaber, M., Elshafeey, A., Mhaimeed, O., Dineen, E. H., Marvel, F. A., Martin, S. S., Muse, E. D., Turakhia, M. P., Tarakji, K. G., & Elshazly, M. B. (2021). Smart wearable devices in cardiovascular care: Where we are and how to move forward. *Nature Reviews. Cardiology*, 18(8), 581–599. DOI: 10.1038/s41569-021-00522-7 PMID: 33664502

Bays, H. E., Taub, P. R., Epstein, E., Michos, E. D., Ferraro, R. A., Bailey, A. L., Kelli, H. M., Ferdinand, K. C., Echols, M. R., Weintraub, H., Bostrom, J., Johnson, H. M., Hoppe, K. K., Shapiro, M. D., German, C. A., Virani, S. S., Hussain, A., Ballantyne, C. M., Agha, A. M., & Toth, P. P. (2021). Ten things to know about ten cardiovascular disease risk factors. *American Journal of Preventive Cardiology*, 5, 100149. DOI: 10.1016/j.ajpc.2021.100149 PMID: 34327491

Beam, A. L., & Kohane, I. S. (2018). Big data and machine learning in health care. *Journal of the American Medical Association*, 319(13), 1317–1318. DOI: 10.1001/jama.2017.18391 PMID: 29532063

Beck, J., Greenwood, D. A., Blanton, L., Bollinger, S. T., Butcher, M. K., Condon, J. E., Cypress, M., Faulkner, P., Fischl, A. H., Francis, T., Kolb, L. E., Lavin-Tompkins, J. M., MacLeod, J., Maryniuk, M., Mensing, C., Orzeck, E. A., Pope, D. D., Pulizzi, J. L., Reed, A. A., & Wang, J. (2017). 2017 National Standards for Diabetes Self-Management Education and Support. *Diabetes Spectrum*, 30(4), 301–314. DOI: 10.2337/ds17-0067 PMID: 29151721

Bedaf, S., Marti, P., Amirabdollahian, F., & de Witte, L. (2018). A multi-perspective evaluation of a service robot for seniors: The voice of different stakeholders. *Disability and Rehabilitation. Assistive Technology*, 13(6), 592–599. DOI: 10.1080/17483107.2017.1358300 PMID: 28758532

Beeler, P. E., Bates, D. W., & Hug, B. L. (2014). Clinical decision support systems. *Swiss Medical Weekly*, 144(5152), w14073–w14073. PMID: 25668157

Behnood, A., Mohammadi Golafshani, E., & Hosseini, S. M. (2020). Determinants of the infection rate of the COVID-19 in the U.S. using ANFIS and virus optimization algorithm (VOA). *Chaos, Solitons, and Fractals*, 139, 110051. DOI: 10.1016/j.chaos.2020.110051 PMID: 32834605

Behrens, D. A., Rauner, M. S., & Caulkins, J. P. (2008). Modelling the spread of hepatitis c via commercial tattoo parlours: Implications for public health interventions. *OR-Spektrum*, 30(2), 269–288. DOI: 10.1007/s00291-007-0090-7

Behroozi, M., & Sami, A. (2016). A multiple-classifier framework for Parkinson's disease detection based on various vocal tests. *International Journal of Telemedicine and Applications*, 2016, 2016. DOI: 10.1155/2016/6837498 PMID: 27190506

Belard, A., Buchman, T., Forsberg, J., Potter, B. K., Dente, C. J., Kirk, A., & Elster, E. (2017). Precision diagnosis: A view of the clinical decision support systems (CDSS) landscape through the lens of critical care. *Journal of Clinical Monitoring and Computing*, 31(2), 261–271. DOI: 10.1007/s10877-016-9849-1 PMID: 26902081

Beller, S., Hünerbein, M., Lange, T., Eulenstein, S., Gebauer, B., & Schlag, P. M. (2007). Image-guided surgery of liver metastases by three-dimensional ultrasound-based optoelectronic navigation. *British Journal of Surgery*, 94(7), 866–875. DOI: 10.1002/bjs.5712

Benko, H., Jota, R., & Wilson, A. D. (2012). Miragetable: Freehand interaction on a projected augmented reality tabletop. *SIGCHI Conference on Human Factors in Computing Systems*. DOI: 10.1145/2207676.2207704

Bennett, J., Stevens, G., Mathers, C., Bonita, R., Rehm, J., Kruk, M., . . . Ezzati, M. (2018). NCD Countdown 2030: worldwide trends in non-communicable disease mortality and progress towards Sustainable Development Goal target 3.4. The Lancet, 0140-6736. DOI: 10.1016/S0140-6736(18)31992-5

BenYishay, A., & Mobarak, A. M. (2019). Social learning and incentives for experimentation and communication. *The Review of Economic Studies*, 86(3), 976–1009. DOI: 10.1093/restud/rdy039

Berenson, R. A., & Rich, E. C. (2010). US Approaches to Physician Payment: The Deconstruction of Primary Care. *Journal of General Internal Medicine*, 25(6), 613–618. DOI: 10.1007/s11606-010-1295-z PMID: 20467910

Berkes, F. (2009). Evolution of co-management: Role of knowledge generation, bridging organizations and social learning. *Journal of Environmental Management*, 90(5), 1692–1702. DOI: 10.1016/j.jenvman.2008.12.001 PMID: 19110363

Berman, B., & Berman, C. (2016). Current approaches to the diagnosis and management of skin cancer. *The Journal of Clinical and Aesthetic Dermatology*, 9(6), 26–33. https://jcadonline.com/current-approaches-to-the-diagnosis-and-management-of-skin-cancer/

Bertsimas, D., Kallus, N., Weinstein, A. M., Ying Daisy, Z., & Zhuo, Y. D. (2017). Personalized Diabetes Management Using Electronic Medical Records. *Diabetes Care*, 40(2), 210–217. DOI: 10.2337/dc16-0826 PMID: 27920019

Beuscher, L. M., Fan, J., Sarkar, N., Dietrich, M. S., Newhouse, P. A., Miller, K. F., & Mion, L. C. (2017). Socially assistive robots: Measuring older adults' perceptions. *Journal of Gerontological Nursing*, 43(12), 35–43. DOI: 10.3928/00989134-20170707-04 PMID: 28700074

Bhatia, M., Kaur, S., & Sood, S. K. (2020). IoT-Inspired Smart Toilet System for Home-Based Urine Infection Prediction. *ACM Transactions on Computing for Healthcare*, 1(3), 1–25. DOI: 10.1145/3379506

Bhatia, M., & Sood, S. K. (2017). A comprehensive health assessment framework to facilitate IoT-assisted smart workouts: A predictive healthcare perspective. *Computers in Industry*, 92–93, 50–66. DOI: 10.1016/j.compind.2017.06.009

Bhatt, H., Shah, V., Shah, K., Shah, R., & Shah, M. (2023). State-of-the-art machine learning techniques for melanoma skin cancer detection and classification: A comprehensive review. *Intelligent Medicine*, 3(3), 180–190. Advance online publication. DOI: 10.1016/j.imed.2022.08.004

Bhavnani, S. P. (2020). Digital health: Opportunities and challenges to develop the next-generation technology-enabled models of cardiovascular care. *Methodist De-Bakey Cardiovascular Journal*, 16(4), 296. DOI: 10.14797/mdcj-16-4-296 PMID: 33500758

Bian, C., Ye, B., Hoonakker, A., & Mihailidis, A. (2021). Attitudes and perspectives of older adults on technologies for assessing frailty in home settings: A focus group study. *BMC Geriatrics*, 21(1), 298. DOI: 10.1186/s12877-021-02252-4 PMID: 33964887

Bilikisu Elewonibi, R. B. (2016). *The influence of socio-cultural factors on breast cancer screening behaviors in Lagos.*

Biocca, F., Owen, C., Tang, A., & Bohil, C. (2007). Attention issues in spatial information systems: Directing mobile users' visual attention using augmented reality. *Journal of Management Information Systems*, 23(4), 163–184. DOI: 10.2753/MIS0742-1222230408

Biran Achituv, D., & Haiman, L. (2016). Physicians' attitudes toward the use of IoT medical devices as part of their practice. [OJAKM]. *Online Journal of Applied Knowledge Management*, 4(2), 128–145. DOI: 10.36965/OJAKM.2016.4(2)128-145

Bisio, I., Garibotto, C., Lavagetto, F., & Sciarrone, A. (2019). Towards IoT-Based eHealth Services: A Smart Prototype System for Home Rehabilitation. *2019 IEEE Global Communications Conference (GLOBECOM)*, 1–6. DOI: 10.1109/GLOBE-COM38437.2019.9013194

Blonde, L., Umpierrez, G. E., Reddy, S. S., McGill, J. B., Berga, S. L., Bush, M., Chandrasekaran, S., DeFronzo, R. A., Einhorn, D., Galindo, R. J., Gardner, T. W., Garg, R., Garvey, W. T., Hirsch, I. B., Hurley, D. L., Izuora, K., Kosiborod, M., Olson, D., Patel, S. B., & Weber, S. L. (2022). American Association of Clinical Endocrinology Clinical Practice Guideline: Developing a Diabetes Mellitus Comprehensive Care Plan—2022 Update [Article]. *Endocrine Practice*, 28(10), 923–1049. DOI: 10.1016/j.eprac.2022.08.002 PMID: 35963508

Bloom, D. E., & Canning, D. (2008). Global demographic change: Dimensions and economic significance. *Population and Development Review*, ●●●, 34.

Blowers, M., Iribarne, J., Colbert, E., & Kott, A. (2016). The Future Internet of Things and Security of its Control Systems. *arXiv:1610.01953[Cs]*. http://arxiv.org/abs/1610.01953 DOI: 10.1007/978-3-319-32125-7_16

Bodenheimer, T., Lorig, K., Holman, H., and Grumbach, K. 2002. "Patient Self-Management of Chronic Disease in Primary Care," *JAMA* (288:19), pp. 2469–2475.

Bodenreider, O. (2004). The Unified Medical Language System (UMLS): Integrating biomedical terminology. *Nucleic Acids Research*, 32(Database issue), D267–D270. DOI: 10.1093/nar/gkh061 PMID: 14681409

Boettcher, N. (2021). Studies of Depression and Anxiety Using Reddit as a Data Source: Scoping Review. *JMIR Mental Health*, 8(11), e29487. DOI: 10.2196/29487 PMID: 34842560

Böhmer, M., Damarowsky, J., & Kuehnel, S. (2023). Implementing ALiS: Towards a Reference Architecture for Augmented Living Spaces. *Hawaiian Conference on System Sciences* (HICSS).

Böhmer, M., Damarowsky, J., Kühnel, S., Parschat, S., & Mahn, V. A. (2022). Preserve Autonomy–Developing and Implementing a Design Theory for Augmented Living Spaces. *Pacific Asia Conference on Information Systems* (PACIS).

Böhmer, M., Kendziorra, J., & Kuehnel, S. (2024). A Proposal for Theorizing the Cognitive Adoption of Digital Health Technologies for People with Cognitive Impairments, *32nd European Conference on Information Systems (ECIS 2024)*, Paphos (Cyprus).

Bollino, R., Bovenzi, G., Cipolletta, F., Docimo, L., Gravina, M., Marrone, S., . . . Sansone, C. (2022). Synergy-Net: Artificial Intelligence at the Service of Oncological Prevention. In *Intelligent Systems Reference Library* (Vol. 211). Retrieved from https://doi.org/DOI: 10.1007/978-3-030-79161-2_16

Bolognia, J. L., Schaffer, J. V., & Cerroni, L. (2018). *Dermatology*. Elsevier Health Sciences.

Bonoto, B. C., de Araújo, V. E., Godói, I. P., de Lemos, L. L. P., Godman, B., Bennie, M., & Alvares, J. (2017). Efficacy of mobile health applications in improving health outcomes in patients with diabetes: A systematic review and meta-analysis. *BMJ Open*, 7(8), e012194. DOI: 10.1136/bmjopen-2016-012194

Borgohain, T., Kumar, U., & Sanyal, S. (2015). Survey of Security and Privacy Issues of Internet of Things. *arXiv:1501.02211[Cs]*. http://arxiv.org/abs/1501.02211

Brain Oldenburg, C. T. (2015). Using New Technologies to Improve the Prevention and Management of Chronic Conditions in Populations. *Annual Review of Public Health*, 36(1), 483–505. DOI: 10.1146/annurev-publhealth-031914-122848 PMID: 25581147

Broadbent, E., Tamagawa, R., Kerse, N., Knock, B., Patience, A., & MacDonald, B. (2009, September). Retirement home staff and residents' preferences for healthcare robots. In RO-MAN 2009-The 18th IEEE International Symposium on Robot and Human Interactive Communication (pp. 645-650). IEEE.

Brørs, G., Norman, C. D., & Norekvål, T. M. (2020). Accelerated importance of eHealth literacy in the COVID-19 outbreak and beyond. *European Journal of Cardiovascular Nursing*, 19(6), 458–461. DOI: 10.1177/1474515120941307 PMID: 32667217

Brownie, S., & Horstmanshof, L. (2011). The management of loneliness in aged care residents: An important therapeutic target for gerontological nursing. *Geriatric Nursing*, 32(5), 318–325. DOI: 10.1016/j.gerinurse.2011.05.003 PMID: 21831481

Brownsell, S., & Hawley, M. S. (2004). Automatic fall detectors and the fear of falling. *Journal of Telemedicine and Telecare*, 10(5), 262–266. DOI: 10.1258/1357633042026251 PMID: 15494083

Bruno, R. R., Wolff, G., Wernly, B., Masyuk, M., Piayda, K., Leaver, S., Erkens, R., Oehler, D., Afzal, S., Heidari, H., Kelm, M., & Jung, C. (2022). Virtual and augmented reality in critical care medicine: The patient's, clinician's, and researcher's perspective. *Critical Care (London, England)*, 26(1), 326. DOI: 10.1186/s13054-022-04202-x

Bu, D., Pan, E., Walker, J., Adler-Milstein, J., Kendrick, D., Hook, J. M., Cusack, C. M., Bates, D. W., & Middleton, B. (2007). Benefits of Information Technology–Enabled Diabetes Management. *Diabetes Care*, 30(5), 5. DOI: 10.2337/dc06-2101 PMID: 17322483

Burke, L. E., Ma, J., Azar, K. M., Bennett, G. G., Peterson, E. D., Zheng, Y., Riley, W., Stephens, J., Shah, S. H., Suffoletto, B., Turan, T. N., Spring, B., Steinberger, J., & Quinn, C. C. (2015). Current science on consumer use of mobile health for cardiovascular disease prevention: A scientific statement from the American Heart Association. *Circulation*, 132(12), 1157–1213. DOI: 10.1161/CIR.0000000000000232 PMID: 26271892

Buzachis, A., Bernava, G. M., Busa, M., Pioggia, G., & Villari, M. (2018). Towards the Basic Principles of Osmotic Computing: A Closed-Loop Gamified Cognitive Rehabilitation Flow Model. *2018 IEEE 4th International Conference on Collaboration and Internet Computing (CIC)*, 446–452. DOI: 10.1109/CIC.2018.00067

Caddy, B. (2019, September 19). *Wearable tech and regulation: What laws do wearables need to follow?* Wareable. https://www.wareable.com/health-and-wellbeing/wearable-tech-and-regulation-5678

Cai, D., Ardakany, A. R., & Ay, F. (2021). Deep Learning-Aided Diagnosis of Autoimmune Blistering Diseases. medRxiv, 2021-11.

Çakan, S. (2020). Dynamic analysis of a mathematical model with health care capacity for COVID-19 pandemic. *Chaos, Solitons, and Fractals*, 139, 110033. Advance online publication. DOI: 10.1016/j.chaos.2020.110033 PMID: 32834594

Canhoto, A. I., & Arp, S. (2017). Exploring the factors that support adoption and sustained use of health and fitness wearables. *Journal of Marketing Management*, 33(1–2), 32–60. DOI: 10.1080/0267257X.2016.1234505

Cano Porras, D., Siemonsma, P., Inzelberg, R., Zeilig, G., & Plotnik, M. (2018). Advantages of virtual reality in the rehabilitation of balance and gait: Systematic review. *Neurology*, 90(22), 1017–1025. DOI: 10.1212/WNL.0000000000005603 PMID: 29720544

Cara, N. H. D., Maggio, V., Davis, O. S. P., & Haworth, C. M. A. (2023). Methodologies for Monitoring Mental Health on Twitter: Systematic Review. *Journal of Medical Internet Research*, 25(1), e42734. DOI: 10.2196/42734 PMID: 37155236

Cardin, S., Ogden, H., Perez-Marcos, D., Williams, J., Ohno, T., & Tadi, T. (2016). Neurogoggles for multimodal augmented reality. *Proceedings of the 7th Augmented Human International Conference 2016*. DOI: 10.1145/2875194.2875242

Cardoso, L.F., Mariano, F.C., and Zorzal, E.R. 2020. A survey of industrial augmented reality, *Computers & Industrial Engineering* (139:1), pp. 1-12.

Carey, R. M., & Whelton, P. K. (2020). Evidence for the universal blood pressure goal of< 130/80 mm Hg is strong: Controversies in hypertension-pro side of the argument. *Hypertension*, 76(5), 1384–1390. DOI: 10.1161/HYPERTENSIONA-HA.120.14647 PMID: 32951472

Cavallari, R., Martelli, F., Rosini, R., Buratti, C., & Verdone, R. (2014). A Survey on Wireless Body Area Networks: Technologies and Design Challenges. *IEEE Communications Surveys and Tutorials*, 16(3), 1635–1657. DOI: 10.1109/SURV.2014.012214.00007

Cengiz, D., & Korkmaz, F. (2023). Effectiveness of a nurse-led personalized patient engagement program to promote type 2 diabetes self-management: A randomized controlled trial. *Nursing & Health Sciences*, 25(4), 571–584. DOI: 10.1111/nhs.13048 PMID: 37670722

Cennamo, K., & Kalk, D. (2019). *Real world instructional design: An iterative approach to designing learning experiences*. Routledge. DOI: 10.4324/9780203712207

Chancellor, S., & De Choudhury, M. (2020). Methods in predictive techniques for mental health status on social media: A critical review. *NPJ Digital Medicine*, 3(1), 1. Advance online publication. DOI: 10.1038/s41746-020-0233-7 PMID: 32219184

Chang, W.-J., Chen, L.-B., Hsu, C.-H., Chen, J.-H., Yang, T.-C., & Lin, C.-P. (2020). MedGlasses: A Wearable Smart-Glasses-Based Drug Pill Recognition System Using Deep Learning for Visually Impaired Chronic Patients. *IEEE Access : Practical Innovations, Open Solutions*, 8, 17013–17024. DOI: 10.1109/ACCESS.2020.2967400

Channa, A., Popescu, N., Skibinska, J., & Burget, R. (2021). The Rise of Wearable Devices during the COVID-19 Pandemic: A Systematic Review. *Sensors (Basel)*, 21(17), 17. Advance online publication. DOI: 10.3390/s21175787

Chatterjee, S., Sarker, S., and Fuller, M. A. 2009. "A Deontological Approach to Designing Ethical Collaboration," *Journal of the Association for Information Systems* (10:Special Issue), pp. 138–169.

Cheng, V. W. S., Davenport, T., Johnson, D., Vella, K., & Hickie, I. B. (2019). Gamification in apps and technologies for improving mental health and well-being: Systematic review. *JMIR Mental Health*, 6(6), e13717. DOI: 10.2196/13717 PMID: 31244479

Chen, M., Ma, Y., Li, Y., Wu, D., Zhang, Y., & Youn, C.-H. (2017). Wearable 2.0: Enabling Human-Cloud Integration in Next Generation Healthcare Systems. *IEEE Communications Magazine*, 55(1), 54–61. DOI: 10.1109/MCOM.2017.1600410CM

Chen, M., Yang, J., Zhou, J., Hao, Y., Zhang, J., & Youn, C. H. (2018). 5G-Smart Diabetes: Toward Personalized Diabetes Diagnosis with Healthcare Big Data Clouds. *IEEE Communications Magazine*, 56(4), 16–23. DOI: 10.1109/MCOM.2018.1700788

Chen, T. L., Bhattacharjee, T., Beer, J. M., Ting, L. H., Hackney, M. E., Rogers, W. A., & Kemp, C. C. (2017). Older adults' acceptance of a robot for partner dance-based exercise. *PLoS One*, 12(10), e0182736. DOI: 10.1371/journal.pone.0182736 PMID: 29045408

Chen, X., & Ibrahim, Z. (2023). A Comprehensive Study of Emotional Responses in AI-Enhanced Interactive Installation Art. *Sustainability (Basel)*, 15(22), 15830. DOI: 10.3390/su152215830

Cheruvu, S., Kumar, A., Smith, N., & Wheeler, D. M. (2020). Connectivity Technologies for IoT. In Cheruvu, S., Kumar, A., Smith, N., & Wheeler, D. M. (Eds.), *Demystifying Internet of Things Security: Successful IoT Device/Edge and Platform Security Deployment* (pp. 347–411). Apress., DOI: 10.1007/978-1-4842-2896-8_5

Cheung, C. C., Krahn, A. D., & Andrade, J. G. (2018). The emerging role of wearable technologies in detection of arrhythmia. *The Canadian Journal of Cardiology*, 34(8), 1083–1087. DOI: 10.1016/j.cjca.2018.05.003 PMID: 30049358

Cheung, M. L., Chau, K. Y., Lam, M. H. S., Tse, G., Ho, K. Y., Flint, S. W., Broom, D. R., Tso, E. K. H., & Lee, K. Y. (2019). Examining Consumers' Adoption of Wearable Healthcare Technology: The Role of Health Attributes. *International Journal of Environmental Research and Public Health*, 16(13), 13. Advance online publication. DOI: 10.3390/ijerph16132257

Chimmula, V. K. R., & Zhang, L. (2020). Time series forecasting of COVID-19 transmission in Canada using LSTM networks. *Chaos, Solitons, and Fractals*, 135, 109864. Advance online publication. DOI: 10.1016/j.chaos.2020.109864 PMID: 32390691

Chiu, H. Y., & Wang, H. T. (2021). The impact of artificial intelligence on dermatology. *Dermatologic Clinics*, 39(4), 417–423. DOI: 10.1016/j.det.2021.05.002

Choi, A., Noh, S., & Shin, H. (2020). Internet-Based Unobtrusive Tele-Monitoring System for Sleep and Respiration. *IEEE Access : Practical Innovations, Open Solutions*, 8, 76700–76707. DOI: 10.1109/ACCESS.2020.2989336

Choukou, M. A., Zhu, X., Malwade, S., Dhar, E., & Abdul, S. S. (2022). Digital Health Solutions Transforming Long-Term Care and Rehabilitation. In *Healthcare Information Management Systems: Cases, Strategies, and Solutions* (pp. 301–316). Springer International Publishing. DOI: 10.1007/978-3-031-07912-2_19

Chu, L., Chen, H. W., Cheng, P. Y., Ho, P., Weng, I. T., Yang, P. L., Chien, S.-E., Tu, Y.-C., Yang, C.-C., Wang, T.-M., Fung, H. H., & Yeh, S. L. (2019). Identifying features that enhance older adults' acceptance of robots: A mixed methods study. *Gerontology*, 65(4), 441–450. DOI: 10.1159/000494881 PMID: 30844813

Chung, J., Demiris, G., Thompson, H. J., Chen, K. Y., Burr, R., Patel, S., & Fogarty, J. (2017). Feasibility testing of a home-based sensor system to monitor mobility and daily activities in Korean American older adults. *International Journal of Older People Nursing*, 12(1), e12127. DOI: 10.1111/opn.12127 PMID: 27431567

Chun, J., & Hong, J. (2015). Relationships between presynaptic inhibition and static postural sway in subjects with and without diabetic neuropathy [Article]. *Journal of Physical Therapy Science*, 27(9), 2697–2700. DOI: 10.1589/jpts.27.2697 PMID: 26504271

Ciumărnean, L., Milaciu, M. V., Negrean, V., Orăan, O. H., Vesa, S. C., Sălăgean, O., Iluț, S., & Vlaicu, S. I. (2021). Cardiovascular risk factors and physical activity for the prevention of cardiovascular diseases in the elderly. *International Journal of Environmental Research and Public Health*, 19(1), 207. DOI: 10.3390/ijerph19010207 PMID: 35010467

CMS. (2019). *Historical National Health Expenditure Accounts*. Centers for Medicare & Medicaid Services. https://www.cms.gov/Research-Statistics-Data -and-Systems/Statistics-Trends-and-Reports/NationalHealthExpendData/Na tionalHealthAccountsHistorical

Cohen, C., Kampel, T., & Verloo, H. (2016). Acceptability of an intelligent wireless sensor system for the rapid detection of health issues: Findings among home-dwelling older adults and their informal caregivers. *Patient Preference and Adherence*, ●●●, 1687–1695. PMID: 27660417

Cohen, J. (1960). A Coefficient of Agreement for Nominal Scales. *Educational and Psychological Measurement*, 20(1), 37–46. Advance online publication. DOI: 10.1177/001316446002000104

Compeau, D. R., & Higgins, C. A. (1995). Computer self-efficacy: Development of a measure and initial test. *Management Information Systems Quarterly*, 19(2), 189–211. DOI: 10.2307/249688

Conallen, J. 1999. "MODELING WEB APPLICATION ARCHITECTURES with UML.," *Communications of the ACM* (42:10), pp. 63–70.

Conover, W. J. (1999). *Practical nonparametric statistics*. John Wiley & Sons.

Cordeil, M., Dwyer, T., Klein, K., Laha, B., Marriott, K., & Thomas, B. H. (2017). Immersive collaborative analysis of network connectivity: CAVE-style or head-mounted display? *IEEE Transactions on Visualization and Computer Graphics*, 23(1), 441–450. DOI: 10.1109/TVCG.2016.2599107

Corno, F., Russis, L. D., & Roffarello, A. M. (2016). A Healthcare Support System for Assisted Living Facilities: An IoT Solution. *2016 IEEE 40th Annual Computer Software and Applications Conference (COMPSAC)*, *1*, 344–352. DOI: 10.1109/COMPSAC.2016.29

Correa, D. (2019). *Fitness Trackers Market Projected To Display A Robust Growth With a CAGR of 19.6% by 2023*. MarketWatch. https://www.marketwatch.com/press-release/fitness-trackers-market-projected-to-display-a-robust-growth-with-a-cagr-of-196-by-2023-2019-09-18

Correction, S. E. E., & This, F. O. R. (2022). *Evaluation of individual and ensemble probabilistic forecasts of COVID-19 mortality in the United States. 119*(15). https://doi.org/DOI: 10.1073/pnas.2113561119/-/DCSupplemental.Published

Cotin, S., & Haouchine, N. (2023). Augmented Reality for Computer-Guided Interventions. In Springer Handbook of Augmented Reality, 689-707. DOI: 10.1007/978-3-030-67822-7_28

Cotler, J. L. (2016). *The impact of online teaching and learning about emotional intelligence, Myers Briggs personality dimensions and mindfulness on personal and social awareness*. State University of New York at Albany.

Cotler, J. L., DiTursi, D., Goldstein, I., Yates, J., & Del Belso, D. (2017). A mindful approach to teaching. *Information Systems Education Journal*, 15(1), 12.

Creswell, J. W., & Clark, V. L. P. (2017). *Designing and conducting mixed methods research*. Sage publications.

Cui, S., Wang, Y., Wang, D., Sai, Q., Huang, Z., & Cheng, T. C. E. (2021). A two-layer nested heterogeneous ensemble learning predictive method for COVID-19 mortality. *Applied Soft Computing*, 113, 107946. DOI: 10.1016/j.asoc.2021.107946 PMID: 34646110

Cummings, E., & Turner, P. (2009). Patient Self-Management and Chronic Illness: Evaluating Outcomes and Impacts of Information Technology. *Studies in Health Technology and Informatics*, (143), 229–234. PMID: 19380941

D'Errico, G., Barba, M. C., Gatto, C., Nuzzo, B. L., Nuccetelli, F., Luca, V. D., & Paolis, L. T. D. (2023, September). Measuring the Effectiveness of Virtual Reality for Stress Reduction: Psychometric Evaluation of the ERMES Project. In *International Conference on Extended Reality* (pp. 484-499). Cham: Springer Nature Switzerland. DOI: 10.1007/978-3-031-43401-3_32

Dadgar, M., and Joshi, K. D. 2017. "Value-Sensitive Review and Analysis of Technology-Enabled Self-Management Systems: A Conceptual Investigation," *International Journal of Electronic Healthcare* (9:2/3), p. 157. ().DOI: 10.1504/IJEH.2017.10003175

Dadgar, M., and Joshi, K. D. 2018. "The Role of Information and Communication Technology in Self-Management of Chronic Diseases: An Empirical Investigation through Value Sensitive Design (Forthcoming)," *Journal of the Association for Information Systems (JAIS)* (19:2), pp. 86–112.

Dagliati, A., Sacchi, L., Tibollo, V., Cogni, G., Teliti, M., Martinez-Millana, A., Traver, V., Segagni, D., Posada, J., Ottaviano, M., Fico, G., Arredondo, M. T., De Cata, P., Chiovato, L., & Bellazzi, R. (2018). A dashboard-based system for supporting diabetes care. *Journal of the American Medical Informatics Association : JAMIA*, 25(5), 538–547. https://doi.org/https://dx.doi.org/10.1093/jamia/ocx159. DOI: 10.1093/jamia/ocx159 PMID: 29409033

Daniels, N. (2001). Justice, health, and healthcare. *The American Journal of Bioethics*, 1(2), 2–16. DOI: 10.1162/152651601300168834 PMID: 11951872

Dara, S., & Tumma, P. (2018). Feature Extraction By Using Deep Learning: A Survey. *2018 Second International Conference on Electronics, Communication and Aerospace Technology (ICECA)*, 1795–1801. DOI: 10.1109/ICECA.2018.8474912

Dash, S., Shakyawar, S. K., Sharma, M., & Kaushik, S. (2019). Big data in healthcare: Management, analysis and future prospects. *Journal of Big Data*, 6(1), 1–25. DOI: 10.1186/s40537-019-0217-0

Davis, F. (1989). Perceived Usefulness, Perceived Ease of Use, and User Acceptance of Information Technology. *Management Information Systems Quarterly*, 13(3), 319–340. DOI: 10.2307/249008

De Grood, C., Raissi, A., Kwon, Y., & Santana, M. J. (2016). Adoption of e-health technology by physicians: A scoping review. *Journal of Multidisciplinary Healthcare*, 9, 335–344. DOI: 10.2147/JMDH.S103881 PMID: 27536128 de la Iglesia, D. H., Sales Mendes, A., Villarrubia Gonzalez, G., Jimenez-Bravo, D. M., & de Paz Santana, J. F. (2020). Connected Elbow Exoskeleton System for Rehabilitation Training Based on Virtual Reality and Context-Aware. In *Sensors* (Vol. 20, Issue 3). MDPI. DOI: 10.3390/s20030858

De Sousa Barroca, J. D. (2021). Verification and validation of knowledge-based clinical decision support systems-a practical approach: A descriptive case study at Cambio CDS.

Demark-Wahnefried, W., Clipp, E., Lipkus, I., Lobach, D., Snyder, D. C., Sloane, R., Peterson, B., Macri, J. M., Rock, C. L., McBride, C. M., & Kraus, W. E. (2007). Main Outcomes of the FRESH START Trial: A Sequentially Tailored, Diet and Exercise Mailed Print Intervention Among Breast and Prostate Cancer Survivors. *Journal of Clinical Oncology*, 25(19), 2709–2718. DOI: 10.1200/JCO.2007.10.7094 PMID: 17602076

Demiris, G., Oliver, D. P., Giger, J., Skubic, M., & Rantz, M. (2009). Older adults' privacy considerations for vision based recognition methods of eldercare applications. *Technology and Health Care*, 17(1), 41–48. DOI: 10.3233/THC-2009-0530 PMID: 19478404

Deng, S., Zhao, H., Fang, W., Yin, J., Dustdar, S., & Zomaya, A. (2020). Edge Intelligence: The Confluence of Edge Computing and Artificial Intelligence. *IEEE Internet of Things Journal*, 7(8), 2327–4662. DOI: 10.1109/JIOT.2020.2984887

Deodhar, S., Chen, J., Wilson, M., Bisset, K., Barrett, C., & Marathe, M. (2015). EpiCaster: An integrated web application for situation assessment and forecasting of global epidemics. *Proceedings of the 6th ACM Conference on Bioinformatics, Computational Biology and Health Informatics*, 156–165. DOI: 10.1145/2808719.2808735

Dermatology Online Journal. (2016). *Nonmelanoma skin cancer*. Retrieved from https://escholarship.org/uc/item/5k10x6k7

Desveaux, L., Agarwal, P., Shaw, J., Hensel, J. M., Mukerji, G., Onabajo, N., Marani, H., Jamieson, T., Bhattacharyya, O., Martin, D., Mamdani, M., Jeffs, L., Wodchis, W. P., Ivers, N. M., & Bhatia, R. S. (2016). A randomized wait-list control trial to evaluate the impact of a mobile application to improve self-management of individuals with type 2 diabetes: A study protocol. *BMC Medical Informatics and Decision Making*, 16(1), 144. https://ovidsp.ovid.com/ovidweb.cgi?T=JS&PAGE=reference&D=med13&NEWS=N&AN=27842539. DOI: 10.1186/s12911-016-0381-5 PMID: 27842539

Devarajan, M., & Ravi, L. (2018). Intelligent cyber–physical system for an efficient detection of Parkinson disease using fog computing. *Multimedia Tools and Applications*, ●●●, 1–25.

Devi, D. H., Duraisamy, K., Armghan, A., Alsharari, M., Aliqab, K., Sorathiya, V., Das, S., & Rashid, N. (2023). 5G Technology in Healthcare and Wearable Devices: A Review. *Sensors (Basel)*, 23(5), 2519. DOI: 10.3390/s23052519 PMID: 36904721

Dhar, P., Rocks, T., Samarasinghe, R. M., Stephenson, G., & Smith, C. (2021). Augmented reality in medical education: Students' experiences and learning outcomes. *Medical Education Online*, 26(1), 1953953. DOI: 10.1080/10872981.2021.1953953

Di Mascolo, M., & Gouin, A. (2013). A generic simulation model to assess the performance of sterilization services in health establishments. *Health Care Management Science*, 16(1), 45–61. DOI: 10.1007/s10729-012-9210-2 PMID: 22886097

Dickinson, K. M., Clifton, P. M., Burrell, L. M., Barrett, P. H. R., & Keogh, J. B. (2014). Postprandial effects of a high salt meal on serum sodium, arterial stiffness, markers of nitric oxide production and markers of endothelial function. *Atherosclerosis*, 232(1), 211–216. DOI: 10.1016/j.atherosclerosis.2013.10.032 PMID: 24401240

Dimitrov, D. V. (2016). Medical Internet of Things and Big Data in Healthcare. *Healthcare Informatics Research*, 22(3), 156. DOI: 10.4258/hir.2016.22.3.156 PMID: 27525156

Dineen-Griffin, S., Garcia-Cardenas, V., Williams, K., & Benrimoj, S. I. (2019). Helping patients help themselves: A systematic review of self-management support strategies in primary health care practice. *PLoS One*, 14(8), e0220116. DOI: 10.1371/journal.pone.0220116 PMID: 31369582

Din, I., Almogren, A., Guizani, M., & Zuair, M. (2019). A Decade of Internet of Things: Analysis in the Light of Healthcare Applications. *IEEE Access : Practical Innovations, Open Solutions*, 7, 89967–89979. DOI: 10.1109/ACCESS.2019.2927082

Din, I., Guizani, M., Hassan, S., Kim, B., Khan, M. K., Atiquzzaman, M., & Ahmed, S. H. (2019). The Internet of Things: A Review of Enabled Technologies and Future Challenges. *IEEE Access : Practical Innovations, Open Solutions*, 7, 7606–7640. DOI: 10.1109/ACCESS.2018.2886601

Dionyssiotis, Y. (2012). Analyzing the problem of falls among older people. *International Journal of General Medicine*, ●●●, 805–813. DOI: 10.2147/IJGM.S32651 PMID: 23055770

Dobing, B., and Parsons, J. 2006. "How UML IS USED.," *Communications of the ACM* (49:5), pp. 109–113.

Downing, G. J., Boyle, S. N., Brinner, K. M., & Osheroff, J. A. (2009). Information management to enable personalized medicine: Stakeholder roles in building clinical decision support. *BMC Medical Informatics and Decision Making*, 9(1), 1–11. DOI: 10.1186/1472-6947-9-44 PMID: 19814826

Drigas, A., Mitsea, E., & Skianis, C. (2022). Subliminal Training Techniques for Cognitive, Emotional and Behavioral Balance. The Role of Emerging Technologies. *Technium Soc. Sci. J.*, 33, 164.

Drigas, A., Mitsea, E., & Skianis, C. (2022). Virtual reality and metacognition training techniques for learning disabilities. *Sustainability (Basel)*, 14(16), 10170. DOI: 10.3390/su141610170

Du-Harpur, X., Watt, F. M., Luscombe, N. M., & Lynch, M. D. (2020). What is AI? Applications of artificial intelligence to dermatology. *British Journal of Dermatology*, 183(3), 423–430. Advance online publication. DOI: 10.1111/bjd.18880 PMID: 31960407

Durnell, L. A. (2018). *Emotional Reaction of Experiencing Crisis in Virtual Reality (VR)/360* (Doctoral dissertation, Fielding Graduate University).

Ebert, D. D., Harrer, M., Apolinário-Hagen, J., & Baumeister, H. (2019). Digital interventions for mental disorders: key features, efficacy, and potential for artificial intelligence applications. *Frontiers in Psychiatry: Artificial Intelligence, Precision Medicine, and Other Paradigm Shifts*, 583-627.

Edoh, T., & Degila, J. (2019). IoT-enabled health monitoring and assistive systems for in place aging dementia patient and elderly. In Internet of Things (IoT) for Automated and Smart Applications. IntechOpen., 10. 5772/intechopen.86247. DOI: 10.5772/intechopen.86247

Eger, H., Chacko, S., El-Gamal, S., Gerlinger, T., Kaasch, A., Meudec, M., Munshi, S., Naghipour, A., Rhule, E., Sandhya, Y. K., & Uribe, O. L. (2024). Towards a Feminist Global Health Policy: Power, intersectionality, and transformation. *PLOS Global Public Health*, 4(3), e0002959. DOI: 10.1371/journal.pgph.0002959 PMID: 38451969

El Zein, B., Elrashidi, A., Dahlan, M., Al Jarwan, A., & Jabbour, G. (2024). Nano and Society 5.0: Advancing the Human-Centric Revolution.

El-Gayar, O., Elnoshokaty, A., & Behrens, A. (2021). Understanding Design Features for Continued Use of Wearables Devices. *Twenty-Seventh Americas Conference on Information Systems*. Americas Conference on Information Systems, Montreal.

El-Gayar, O., Ambati, L. S., & Nawar, N. (2020). Wearables, Artificial intelligence, and the Future of Healthcare. In *AI and Big Data's Potential for Disruptive Innovation* (pp. 104–129). IGI GLOBAL., DOI: 10.4018/978-1-5225-9687-5.ch005

El-Gayar, O., Nasralah, T., & Elnoshokaty, A. (2019, January 8). Wearable Devices for Health and Wellbeing: Design Insights from Twitter. *HICSS 52. Hawaii International Conference on System Sciences*. DOI: 10.24251/HICSS.2019.467

El-Gayar, O., Timsina, P., Nawar, N., & Eid, W. (2013). Mobile applications for diabetes self-management: Status and potential. *Journal of Diabetes Science and Technology*, 7(1), 247–262. DOI: 10.1177/193229681300700130 PMID: 23439183

El-Masri, M., Al-Yafi, K., & Kamal, M. M. (2022). A Task-Technology-Identity Fit Model of Smartwatch Utilisation and User Satisfaction: A Hybrid SEM-Neural Network Approach. *Information Systems Frontiers*. Advance online publication. DOI: 10.1007/s10796-022-10256-7

Elor, A., & Kurniawan, S. (2020). The ultimate display for physical rehabilitation: A bridging review on immersive virtual reality. *Frontiers in Virtual Reality*, 1, 585993. DOI: 10.3389/frvir.2020.585993

El-Rashidy, N., El-Sappagh, S., Islam, S. R. M., El-Bakry, H., & Abdelrazek, S. (2021). Mobile health in remote patient monitoring for chronic diseases: Principles, trends, and challenges. *Diagnostics (Basel)*, 11(4), 607. DOI: 10.3390/diagnostics11040607 PMID: 33805471

El-Tamer, M. B., & Wang, P. L. (2017). Cost-effectiveness of skin cancer screening and early detection programs. *The Journal of Dermatology*, 44(9), 1149–1155. DOI: 10.1111/1346-8138.13717

Emerson, L. C., & Berge, Z. L. (2018). Microlearning: Knowledge management applications and competency-based training in the workplace. *Knowledge Management & E-Learning*, 10(2), 125–132.

England Transformation Directorate, N. H. S. (2020). Acoustic monitoring integrated with electronic care planning. Available at: https://transform.england.nhs.uk/ai-lab/explore-all-resources/understand-ai/acoustic-monitoring-integrated-electronic-care-planning/

Enshaeifar, S., Barnaghi, P., Skillman, S., Markides, A., Elsaleh, T., Acton, S. T., Nilforooshan, R., & Rostill, H. (2018). The Internet of Things for Dementia Care. *IEEE Internet Computing*, 22(1), 8–17. DOI: 10.1109/MIC.2018.112102418

Erdmier, C., Hatcher, J., & Lee, M. (2016). Wearable device implications in the healthcare industry. *Journal of Medical Engineering & Technology*, 40(4), 4. Advance online publication. DOI: 10.3109/03091902.2016.1153738

Esen, Ö. C., & Eroğlu, I. (2018). The Effect of Product Technology to Product Acceptance in The User Interaction of Wearable Products – An Assessment of Activity Tracker Product Designed Within The Scope of Health Benefits. *DS 91: Proceedings of NordDesign 2018, Linköping, Sweden, 14th - 17th August 2018.* NordDesign 2018.

Esteva, A., Kuprel, B., Novoa, R. A., Ko, J., Swetter, S. M., Blau, H. M., & Thrun, S. (2017). Dermatologist-level classification of skin cancer with deep neural networks. *Nature*, 542(7639), 115–118. DOI: 10.1038/nature21056 PMID: 28117445

Ettaloui, N., Arezki, S., & Gadi, T. (2023, November). An Overview of Blockchain-Based Electronic Health Record and Compliance with GDPR and HIPAA. In *The International Conference on Artificial Intelligence and Smart Environment* (pp. 405-412). Cham: Springer Nature Switzerland. DOI: 10.56294/dm2023166

Ezer, N., Fisk, A. D., & Rogers, W. A. (2009, October). More than a servant: Self-reported willingness of younger and older adults to having a robot perform interactive and critical tasks in the home. []. Sage CA: Los Angeles, CA: SAGE Publications.]. *Proceedings of the Human Factors and Ergonomics Society Annual Meeting*, 53(2), 136–140. DOI: 10.1177/154193120905300206 PMID: 25349553

Faggella, D. (2020, March). *Machine Learning for Medical Diagnostics—4 Current Applications.* Emerj. https://emerj.com/ai-sector-overviews/machine-learning-medical-diagnostics-4-current-applications/

Fareed, N., Swoboda, C., Singh, P., Boettcher, E., Wang, Y., Venkatesh, K., & Strouse, R. (2023). Developing and testing an integrated patient mHealth and provider dashboard application system for type 2 diabetes management among Medicaid-enrolled pregnant individuals based on a user-centered approach: Mixed-methods study [Article]. *Digital Health*, 9, 20552076221144181. Advance online publication. DOI: 10.1177/20552076221144181 PMID: 36644662

Farnikova, K., Krobot, A., & Kanovsky, P. (2012). Musculoskeletal problems as an initial manifestation of Parkinson's disease: A retrospective study. *Journal of the Neurological Sciences*, 319(1–2), 102–104. DOI: 10.1016/j.jns.2012.05.002 PMID: 22656184

Fatima, M., Khan, M. A., Shaheen, S., Almujally, N. A., & Wang, S. H. (2023). B2C3NetF2: Breast cancer classification using an end-to-end deep learning feature fusion and satin bowerbird optimization controlled Newton Raphson feature selection. *CAAI Transactions on Intelligence Technology*, 8(4), 1374–1390. Advance online publication. DOI: 10.1049/cit2.12219

Fatima, S. A. (2020). IoT enabled Smart Monitoring of Coronavirus empowered with Fuzzy Inference System. *International Journal of Advance Research. Ideas and Innovations in Technology*, 6(1), 8.

Fendos, J. (2020, April 29). How surveillance technology powered South Korea's COVID-19 response. *Brookings*. https://www.brookings.edu/techstream/how-surveillance-technology-powered-south-koreas-covid-19-response/

Fenton, R. (2019, November). 5 Common Medical Device Regulatory Compliance Problems Faced in 2019 [Qualio]. *Medical-Device-Regulatory-Compliance*. https://www.qualio.com/blog/medical-device-regulatory-compliance

Fico, G., Hernanzez, L., Cancela, J., Dagliati, A., Sacchi, L., Martinez-Millana, A., Posada, J., Manero, L., Verdú, J., Facchinetti, A., Ottaviano, M., Zarkogianni, K., Nikita, K., Groop, L., Gabriel-Sanchez, R., Chiovato, L., Traver, V., Merino-Torres, J. F., Cobelli, C., & Arredondo, M. T. (2019). What do healthcare professionals need to turn risk models for type 2 diabetes into usable computerized clinical decision support systems? Lessons learned from the MOSAIC project. *BMC Medical Informatics and Decision Making*, 19(1), 1–16. DOI: 10.1186/s12911-019-0887-8 PMID: 31419982

Finn, G. (2017). *Why You Shouldn't Use Facebook Groups To Build a Community*. Retrieved from Cypress North: www.google.com/amp/s/cypressnorth.com/social-media/shouldnt-build-community-using-Facebook-groups/amp

Flicker, C., Ferris, S. H., & Reisberg, B. (1991). Mild cognitive impairment in the elderly: Predictors of dementia. *Neurology*, 41(7), 1006–1006. DOI: 10.1212/WNL.41.7.1006

Fogg, B. J. (2009). A behavior model for persuasive design. *Proceedings of the 4th international conference on persuasive technology*. ACM, 2009. DOI: 10.1145/1541948.1541999

Fogg, B. J., & Fogg, G. E. (2003). *Persuasive Technology: Using Computers to Change What We Think and Do*. Morgan Kaufmann. DOI: 10.1016/B978-155860643-2/50011-1

Folland, S., Goodman, A. C., & Stano, M. (2024). *The economics of health and health care: Pearson new international edition*. Routledge.

Fornell, C., & Larcker, D. F. (1981). Evaluating Structural Equation Models with Unobservable Variables and Measurement Error. *JMR*, 18(1), 39–50.

Fraenkel, L., & Fried, T. R. (2010). Individualized medical decision making: Necessary, achievable, but not yet attainable. *Archives of Internal Medicine*, 170(6), 566–569. DOI: 10.1001/archinternmed.2010.8 PMID: 20308644

Frank, E., Trigg, L., Holmes, G., & Witten, I. H. (2000). Technical note: Naive Bayes for regression. *Machine Learning*, 41(1), 5–25. DOI: 10.1023/A:1007670802811

Franzini, L., Ardigo, D., Valtuena, S., Pellegrini, N., Del Rio, D., Bianchi, M. A., Scazzina, F., Piatti, P. M., Brighenti, F., & Zavaroni, I. (2012). Food selection based on high total antioxidant capacity improves endothelial function in a low cardiovascular risk population. *Nutrition, Metabolism, and Cardiovascular Diseases*, 22(1), 50–57. DOI: 10.1016/j.numecd.2010.04.001 PMID: 20674303

Frederix, I., Caiani, E. G., Dendale, P., Anker, S., Bax, J., Böhm, A., Cowie, M., Crawford, J., de Groot, N., Dilaveris, P., Hansen, T., Koehler, F., Krstačić, G., Lambrinou, E., Lancellotti, P., Meier, P., Neubeck, L., Parati, G., Piotrowicz, E., & van der Velde, E. (2019). ESC e-Cardiology Working Group Position Paper: Overcoming challenges in digital health implementation in cardiovascular medicine. *European Journal of Preventive Cardiology*, 26(11), 1166–1177. DOI: 10.1177/2047487319832394 PMID: 30917695

FreeQDA. (n.d.). Retrieved from SourceForge: https://sourceforge.net/projects/freeqda

Friedman, B., Kahn, P. H., & Borning, A. (2008). *Value Sensitive Design and Information Systems, The Handbook of Information and Computer Ethics* (Himma, K. E., & Tavani, H. T., Eds.). John Wiley & Sons, Inc.

Future Care Lab in Japan. (living lab): a project of caregiving improvement produced by the Sompo Holdings Group. https://futurecarelab.com/en/about/

Gabrielli, S., Kimani, S., & Catarci, T. (2017). The design of microlearning experiences: A research agenda (on microlearning).

Gastounioti, A., Golemati, S., Andreadis, I., Kolias, V., & Nikita, K. S. (2015). Cardiovascular disease management via electronic health. In *Telehealth and Mobile Health* (pp. 187–202). CRC Press.

Gatouillat, A., Badr, Y., Massot, B., & Sejdic, E. (2018). Internet of Medical Things: A Review of Recent Contributions Dealing With Cyber-Physical Systems in Medicine. *IEEE Internet of Things Journal*, 5(5), 3810–3822. DOI: 10.1109/JIOT.2018.2849014

Gauthier, S., Reisberg, B., Zaudig, M. et al. 2006. Mild cognitive impairment," *The Lancet* (367:9518), pp. 1262-1270.

Ghaffar Nia, N., Kaplanoglu, E., & Nasab, A. (2023). Evaluation of artificial intelligence techniques in disease diagnosis and prediction. *Discover Artificial Intelligence*, 3(1), 5. Advance online publication. DOI: 10.1007/s44163-023-00049-5

Ghamari, M., Janko, B., Sherratt, R., Harwin, W., Piechockic, R., & Soltanpur, C. (2016). A Survey on Wireless Body Area Networks for eHealthcare Systems in Residential Environments. *Sensors (Basel)*, 16(6), 831. DOI: 10.3390/s16060831 PMID: 27338377

Ghosal, S., Sengupta, S., Majumder, M., & Sinha, B. (2020). Linear Regression Analysis to predict the number of deaths in India due to SARS-CoV-2 at 6 weeks from day 0 (100 cases - March 14th 2020). *Diabetes & Metabolic Syndrome*, 14(January), 311–315. DOI: 10.1016/j.dsx.2020.03.017 PMID: 32298982

Gioia, D. A., Corley, K. G., & Hamilton, A. L. (2013). Seeking qualitative rigor in inductive research: Notes on the Gioia methodology. *Organizational Research Methods*, 16(1), 15–31. DOI: 10.1177/1094428112452151

Giordanengo, A., Årsand, E., Woldaregay, A. Z., Bradway, M., Grottland, A., Hartvigsen, G., Granja, C., Torsvik, T., & Hansen, A. H. (2019). Design and prestudy assessment of a dashboard for presenting self-collected health data of patients with diabetes to clinicians: Iterative approach and qualitative case study [Article]. *JMIR Diabetes*, 4(3), e14002. Advance online publication. DOI: 10.2196/14002 PMID: 31290396

Giurgiu, L. (2017). Microlearning an evolving elearning trend. *Science Bulletin*, 22(1), 18–23. DOI: 10.1515/bsaft-2017-0003

Gold, N., Yau, A., Rigby, B., Dyke, C., Remfry, E. A., & Chadborn, T. (2021). Effectiveness of digital interventions for reducing behavioral risks of cardiovascular disease in nonclinical adult populations: Systematic review of reviews. *Journal of Medical Internet Research*, 23(5), e19688. DOI: 10.2196/19688 PMID: 33988126

Gómez Bergin, A. D., & Craven, M. P. (2023). Virtual, augmented, mixed, and extended reality interventions in healthcare: A systematic review of health economic evaluations and cost-effectiveness. *BMC Digital Health*, 1(1), 53. DOI: 10.1186/s44247-023-00054-9

Gostin, L. O., Levit, L. A., & Nass, S. J. (Eds.). (2009). *Beyond the HIPAA privacy rule: enhancing privacy, improving health through research*.

Gövercin, M., Költzsch, Y., Meis, M., Wegel, S., Gietzelt, M., Spehr, J., Winkelbach, S., Marschollek, M., & Steinhagen-Thiessen, E. (2010). Defining the user requirements for wearable and optical fall prediction and fall detection devices for home use. *Informatics for Health & Social Care*, 35(3-4), 177–187. DOI: 10.3109/17538157.2010.528648 PMID: 21133771

Gövercin, M., Meyer, S., Schellenbach, M., Steinhagen-Thiessen, E., Weiss, B., & Haesner, M. (2016). SmartSenior@ home: Acceptance of an integrated ambient assisted living system. Results of a clinical field trial in 35 households. *Informatics for Health & Social Care*, 41(4), 430–447. DOI: 10.3109/17538157.2015.1064425 PMID: 26809357

Goyal, S., Morita, P., Lewis, G. F., Yu, C., Seto, E., & Cafazzo, J. A. (2016). The Systematic Design of a Behavioural Mobile Health Application for the Self-Management of Type 2 Diabetes. *Canadian Journal of Diabetes*, 40(1), 95–104. https://doi.org/https://dx.doi.org/10.1016/j.jcjd.2015.06.007. DOI: 10.1016/j.jcjd.2015.06.007 PMID: 26455762

Gray, R., Indraratna, P., Lovell, N., & Ooi, S. Y. (2022). Digital health technology in the prevention of heart failure and coronary artery disease. *Cardiovascular Digital Health Journal*, 3(6), S9–S16. DOI: 10.1016/j.cvdhj.2022.09.002 PMID: 36589760

Greger, M., & Stone, G. (2016). *How not to die: discover the foods scientifically proven to prevent and reverse disease*. Pan Macmillan.

Grundhöfer, A., & Iwai, D. (2018, May). Recent advances in projection mapping algorithms, hardware and applications. *Computer Graphics Forum*, 37(2), 653–675. DOI: 10.1111/cgf.13387

Guerroudji, M. A., Amara, K., & Zenati, N. (2024). Augmented reality aid in diagnostic assistance for breast cancer detection. *Multimedia Tools and Applications*, •••, 1–14. DOI: 10.1007/s11042-024-18979-2

Guest, G., Bunce, A., & Johnson, L. (2006). How many interviews are enough? An experiment with data saturation and variability. *Field Methods*, 18(1), 59–82. DOI: 10.1177/1525822X05279903

Guizzo, E. (2010). *France developing advanced humanoid robot Romeo.* IEEE Spectrum Automaton Blog.

Gulshan Bano Ali, S. A. (2008). Socio-Cultural Factors Affecting the Treatment of Breast Cancer Among Pakistani Women and Potential Strategies to Prevent Breast Cancer- A Narrative Review. *Open Access Journal Of Reproductive System And Sexual Disorders*, 146-151.

Gupta, D., Sundaram, S., Khanna, A., Hassanien, A. E., & De Albuquerque, V. H. C. (2018). Improved diagnosis of Parkinson's disease using an optimized crow search algorithm. *Computers & Electrical Engineering*, 68, 412–424. DOI: 10.1016/j.compeleceng.2018.04.014

Gupta, P., Saini, D., & Verma, R. (2022). *Healthcare Solutions Using Machine Learning and Informatics.* Auerbach Publications., DOI: 10.1201/9781003322597

Gusev, M., Ristov, S., Prodan, R., Dzanko, M., & Bilic, I. (2017). Resilient IoT eHealth solutions in case of disasters. *2017 9th International Workshop on Resilient Networks Design and Modeling (RNDM)*, 1–7. DOI: 10.1109/RNDM.2017.8093024

Gutierrez-Madronal, L., La Blunda, L., Wagner, M. F., & Medina-Bulo, I. (2019). Test Event Generation for a Fall-Detection IoT System. *IEEE Internet of Things Journal*, 6(4), 6642–6651. DOI: 10.1109/JIOT.2019.2909434

Hadi, M. S., Lawey, A. Q., El-Gorashi, T. E. H., & Elmirghani, J. M. H. (2019). Patient-Centric Cellular Networks Optimization Using Big Data Analytics. *IEEE Access : Practical Innovations, Open Solutions*, 7, 49279–49296. DOI: 10.1109/ACCESS.2019.2910224

Haenssle, H. A., Fink, C., & Schneider, B. W. (2018). Man against machine: Diagnostic performance of a deep learning convolutional neural network for dermoscopic melanoma detection in comparison to 58 dermatologists. *Annals of Oncology : Official Journal of the European Society for Medical Oncology*, 29(8), 1836–1842. DOI: 10.1093/annonc/mdy166 PMID: 29846502

Hagège, H., Ourmi, M. E., Shankland, R., Arboix-Calas, F., Leys, C., & Lubart, T. (2023). Ethics and Meditation: A New Educational Combination to Boost Verbal Creativity and Sense of Responsibility. *Journal of Intelligence*, 11(8), 155. DOI: 10.3390/jintelligence11080155 PMID: 37623538

Haghi, M., Neubert, S., Geissler, A., Fleischer, H., Stoll, N., Stoll, R., & Thurow, K. (2020). A Flexible and Pervasive IoT Based Healthcare Platform for Physiological and Environmental Parameters Monitoring. *IEEE Internet of Things Journal*, 7(6), 1–1. DOI: 10.1109/JIOT.2020.2980432

Hall, A., Wilson, C. B., Stanmore, E., & Todd, C. (2017). Implementing monitoring technologies in care homes for people with dementia: A qualitative exploration using normalization process theory. *International Journal of Nursing Studies*, 72, 60–70. DOI: 10.1016/j.ijnurstu.2017.04.008 PMID: 28494333

Hall, C. E., Hall, A. B., Kok, G., Mallya, J., & Courtright, P. (2016). A needs assessment of people living with diabetes and diabetic retinopathy [Article]. *BMC Research Notes*, 9(1), 56. Advance online publication. DOI: 10.1186/s13104-016-1870-4 PMID: 26829927

Hamari, J. (2021). *Towards the Next Generation of Extended Reality Wearables*. 1–7.

Harvey, L. (1990). *Critical Social Research*. Unwin Hyman.

Hasan, M. N.-U., & Stannard, C. R. (2022). Exploring online consumer reviews of wearable technology: The Owlet Smart Sock. *Research Journal of Textile and Apparel, ahead-of-print*(ahead-of-print), Article ahead-of-print. DOI: 10.1108/RJTA-08-2021-0103

Hasib, K. M., Islam, M. R., Sakib, S., Akbar, M., Razzak, I., & Alam, M. S. (2023). Depression Detection From Social Networks Data Based on Machine Learning and Deep Learning Techniques: An Interrogative Survey. *IEEE Transactions on Computational Social Systems*, 10(4), 1568–1586. DOI: 10.1109/TCSS.2023.3263128

Hassan, M. K., El Desouky, A. I., Elghamrawy, S. M., & Sarhan, A. M. (2019). A Hybrid Real-time remote monitoring framework with NB-WOA algorithm for patients with chronic diseases. *Future Generation Computer Systems*, 93, 77–95. DOI: 10.1016/j.future.2018.10.021

Hassan, N. H., Salwana, E., Drus, S., Maarop, N., Samy, G. N., & Ahmad, N. A. (2018). Proposed Conceptual Iot-Based Patient Monitoring Sensor for Predicting and Controlling Dengue. *International Journal of Grid and Distributed Computing*, 11(4), 127–134. DOI: 10.14257/ijgdc.2018.11.4.11

Hayek, A., Telawi, S., Boercsoek, J., Daou, R. A. Z., & Halabi, N. (2020). Smart wearable system for safety-related medical IoT application: Case of epileptic patient working in industrial environment. *Health and Technology, 10*(1, SI), 363–372. DOI: 10.1007/s12553-019-00335-2

HCPO. (2013). *Pharmaceutical Compliance and Adherence Packaging Trade Organizations*. https://www.hcpconline.org/

Headlam, S. M. (2009). Research Methods Handbook Introductory guide to research methods for social research.

Heerink, M., Kröse, B., Evers, V., & Wielinga, B. (2010). Assessing acceptance of assistive social agent technology by older adults: the almere model.

Heerink, M., Kröse, B., Wielinga, B. J., & Evers, V. (2006). Studying the acceptance of a robotic agent by elderly users. *International Journal of Assistive Robotics and Mechatronics*, 7(3), 33–43.

Heerink, M., Kröse, B., Wielinga, B., & Evers, V. (2009, September). Measuring the influence of social abilities on acceptance of an interface robot and a screen agent by elderly users. In *People and Computers XXIII Celebrating People and Technology*. BCS Learning & Development. DOI: 10.14236/ewic/HCI2009.54

Heidenreich, P. A., Trogdon, J. G., Khavjou, O. A., Butler, J., Dracup, K., Ezekowitz, M. D., Finkelstein, E. A., Hong, Y., Johnston, S. C., Khera, A., Lloyd-Jones, D. M., Nelson, S. A., Nichol, G., Orenstein, D., Wilson, P. W. F., & Woo, Y. J. (2011). Forecasting the future of cardiovascular disease in the United States: A policy statement from the American Heart Association. *Circulation*, 123(8), 933–944. DOI: 10.1161/CIR.0b013e31820a55f5 PMID: 21262990

Heijmans, M., Habets, J. G., Herff, C., Aarts, J., Stevens, A., Kuijf, M. L., & Kubben, P. L. (2019). Monitoring Parkinson's disease symptoms during daily life: A feasibility study. *NPJ Parkinson's Disease*, 5(1), 1–6. DOI: 10.1038/s41531-019-0093-5 PMID: 31583270

Helmy, A., Nassar, R., & Ramadan, N. (2023). Depression Detection from Social Media Platforms: A Systematic Literature Review. 2023 Intelligent Methods, Systems, and Applications (IMSA), 387-393.

Henein, M. Y., Cameli, M., Pastore, M. C., & Mandoli, G. E. (2022). COVID-19 severity and cardiovascular disease: An inseparable link. *Journal of Clinical Medicine*, 11(3), 479. DOI: 10.3390/jcm11030479 PMID: 35159931

Hernandez, M. F., & Rodriguez, F. (2023). Health techequity: Opportunities for digital health innovations to improve equity and diversity in cardiovascular care. *Current Cardiovascular Risk Reports*, 17(1), 1–20. DOI: 10.1007/s12170-022-00711-0 PMID: 36465151

Herrmann, E., Call, J., Hernández-Lloreda, M. V., Hare, B., & Tomasello, M. (2007). Humans have evolved specialized skills of social cognition: The cultural intelligence hypothesis. *Science*, 317(5843), 1360–1366. DOI: 10.1126/science.1146282 PMID: 17823346

Herron, L.-M. (2005). *Building Effective Cancer Support Groups*. The Cancer Council Australia.

Hertroijs, D. F. L., Brouwers, M. C. G. J., Elissen, A. M. J., Schaper, N. C., & Ruwaard, D. (2019). Relevant patient characteristics for estimating healthcare needs according to healthcare providers and people with type 2 diabetes: A Delphi survey. *BMC Health Services Research*, 19(1), 575. https://doi.org/https://dx.doi.org/10.1186/s12913-019-4371-z. DOI: 10.1186/s12913-019-4371-z PMID: 31419980

HITInfrastructure. (2017, May 15). *Remote Monitoring, Operations Drive Healthcare IoT Adoption*. HITInfrastructure. https://hitinfrastructure.com/news/remote-monitoring-operations-drive-healthcare-iot-adoption

Hollander, M., Wolfe, D. A., & Chicken, E. (2013). *Nonparametric statistical methods*. John Wiley & Sons.

Holt, S. (2022). Virtual reality, augmented reality and mixed reality: For astronaut mental health; and space tourism, education and outreach. *Acta Astronautica*.

Hope, A. A., & McPeake, J. (2022). Healthcare delivery and recovery after critical illness. *Current Opinion in Critical Care*, 28(5), 566–571. DOI: 10.1097/MCC.0000000000000984

Hoque, M., Farhad, S., Dewanjee, S., Alom, Z., & Azim, M. (2022). Augmented Reality in Health Care: A Review. In *International Conference on Advanced Computing and Intelligent Engineering*, 305-323.

Hoseinpour Dehkordi, A., Alizadeh, M., Derakhshan, P., Babazadeh, P., & Jahandideh, A. (2020). Understanding epidemic data and statistics: A case study of COVID-19. *Journal of Medical Virology*, 92(7), 868–882. DOI: 10.1002/jmv.25885 PMID: 32329522

Hou, C., Carter, B., Hewitt, J., Francisa, T., & Mayor, S. (2016). Do mobile phone applications improve glycemic control (HbA1c) in the self-management of diabetes? A systematic review, meta-analysis, and GRADE of 14 randomized trials. *Diabetes Care*, 39(11), 2089–2095. DOI: 10.2337/dc16-0346 PMID: 27926892

Https://www.kaggle.com/sudalairajkumar/covid19-in-india. (n.d.). *Covid-19 in India*.

Huang, B., Sun, T., & Ling, H. (2021). End-to-end full projector compensation. *IEEE Transactions on Pattern Analysis and Machine Intelligence*, 44(6), 2953–2967. DOI: 10.1109/TPAMI.2021.3050124

Huerne, K., & Eisenberg, M. J. (2024). Advancing Telemedicine in Cardiology: A Comprehensive Review of Evolving Practices and Outcomes in a Post-Pandemic Context. *Cardiovascular Digital Health Journal*, 5(2), 96–110. DOI: 10.1016/j.cvdhj.2024.02.001 PMID: 38765624

Hu, F., Xie, D., & Shen, S. (2013). On the Application of the Internet of Things in the Field of Medical and Health Care. *2013 IEEE International Conference on Green Computing and Communications and IEEE Internet of Things and IEEE Cyber, Physical and Social Computing*, 2053–2058. DOI: 10.1109/GreenCom-iThings-CPSCom.2013.384

Hulland, J. (1999). Use of partial least squares (PLS) in strategic management research: A review of four recent studies. *Strategic Management Journal*, 20(2), 195–204. DOI: 10.1002/(SICI)1097-0266(199902)20:2<195::AID-SMJ13>3.0.CO;2-7

Hung, L., Liu, C., Woldum, E., Au-Yeung, A., Berndt, A., Wallsworth, C., Horne, N., Gregorio, M., Mann, J., & Chaudhury, H. (2019). The benefits of and barriers to using a social robot PARO in care settings: A scoping review. *BMC Geriatrics*, 19(1), 1–10. DOI: 10.1186/s12877-019-1244-6 PMID: 31443636

Hussain, A., Wenbi, R., da Silva, A. L., Nadher, M., & Mudhish, M. (2015). Health and emergency-care platform for the elderly and disabled people in the Smart City. *Journal of Systems and Software*, 110, 253–263. DOI: 10.1016/j.jss.2015.08.041

Hwang, G. J., Chang, C. Y., & Ogata, H. (2022). The effectiveness of the virtual patient-based social learning approach in undergraduate nursing education: A quasi-experimental study. *Nurse Education Today*, 108, 105164. DOI: 10.1016/j.nedt.2021.105164 PMID: 34627030

Hwang, W., & Salvendy, G. (2010). Number of people required for usability evaluation: The 10 ± 2 rule. *Communications of the ACM*, 53(5), 130–133. DOI: 10.1145/1735223.1735255

Ibrahim, T., & Ali, H. (2023). The Impact of Wearable IoT Devices on Early Disease Detection and Prevention. *International Journal of Applied Health Care Analytics*, 8(8), 8.

Ienca, M., Ferretti, A., Hurst, S., Puhan, M., Lovis, C., & Vayena, E. (2018). Considerations for ethics review of big data health research: A scoping review. *PLoS One*, 13(10), e0204937. DOI: 10.1371/journal.pone.0204937

Igwaran, A., & Okoh, A. I. (2019). Human campylobacteriosis: A public health concern of global importance. *Heliyon*, 5(11), e02814. DOI: 10.1016/j.heliyon.2019.e02814 PMID: 31763476

Iio, T., Shiomi, M., Kamei, K., Sharma, C., & Hagita, N. (2016). Social acceptance by senior citizens and caregivers of a fall detection system using range sensors in a nursing home. *Advanced Robotics*, 30(3), 190–205. DOI: 10.1080/01691864.2015.1120241

Ikram, M. A., Alshehri, M. D., & Hussain, F. K. (2015). Architecture of an IoT-based system for football supervision (IoT Football). *2015 IEEE 2nd World Forum on Internet of Things (WF-IoT)*, 69–74. DOI: 10.1109/WF-IoT.2015.7389029

Imam-Fulani, Y. O., Faruk, N., Sowande, O. A., Abdulkarim, A., Alozie, E., Usman, A. D., Adewole, K. S., Oloyede, A. A., Chiroma, H., Garba, S., Imoize, A. L., Baba, B. A., Musa, A., Adediran, Y. A., & Taura, L. S. (2023). 5G frequency standardization, technologies, channel models, and network deployment: Advances, challenges, and future directions. *Sustainability (Basel)*, 15(6), 5173. DOI: 10.3390/su15065173

Inan, O. T., Tenaerts, P., Prindiville, S. A., Reynolds, H. R., Dizon, D. S., Cooper-Arnold, K., Turakhia, M., Pletcher, M. J., Preston, K. L., Krumholz, H. M., Marlin, B. M., Mandl, K. D., Klasnja, P., Spring, B., Iturriaga, E., Campo, R., Desvigne-Nickens, P., Rosenberg, Y., Steinhubl, S. R., & Califf, R. M. (2020). Digitizing clinical trials. *Digital Medicine*, 3(1), 1. Advance online publication. DOI: 10.1038/s41746-020-0302-y PMID: 32821856

Ince Yenilmez, M. (2015). Economic and social consequences of population aging the dilemmas and opportunities in the twenty-first century. *Applied Research in Quality of Life*, 10(4), 735–752. DOI: 10.1007/s11482-014-9334-2

Individual, Group & Online Support. (n.d.). Retrieved from CANSA website: https://www.cansa.org.za/cansas-care-support/cancer-counselling/

International Diabetes Federation. (2021). IDF Diabetes Atlas (10th ed.). Retrieved from https://diabetesatlas.org/atlas/tenth-edition/

Internet Of Things | Definition of Internet Of Things by Merriam-Webster. (n.d.). Retrieved January 29, 2020, from https://www.merriam-webster.com/dictionary/Internet%20of%20Things

Iqbal, S., Mahgoub, I., Du, E., Leavitt, M., & Asghar, W. (2021). Advances in healthcare wearable devices. npj Flexible Electronics, 2397-4621. DOI: 10.1038/s41528-021-00107-x

Islam, R., Holland, S., Price, B., Georgiou, T., & Mulholland, P. (2018). *Wearables for Long Term Gait Rehabilitation of Neurological Conditions*.

ITU. (2012, June 15). *Overview of the Internet of Things*. https://Www.Itu.Int/ITU-T/Recommendations/Rec.Aspx?rec=Y.2060

Jacelon, C. S., Gibbs, M. A., & Ridgway, J. V. (2016). Computer Technology for Self-Management: A Scoping Review. *Journal of Clinical Nursing*, 25(9-10), 1179–1192. DOI: 10.1111/jocn.13221 PMID: 26990364

Jacob, B., & Weiss, E. S. (2013). Recommendation for the Design, Implementation, and Evaluation of Social Support in Online Communities, Networks, and Groups. *Journal of Biomedical Informatics*, ●●●, 970–976.

Jacobson, C., & Karjalainen, P. (2019). *Embracing Internet of Medical Things: A multiple case study of contextual factors' influence on the implementation of IoT healthcare solutions* [Gothenburg University]. https://gupea.ub.gu.se/handle/2077/61406

Jacobson, I., Spence, I., and Kerr, B. 2016. "Use-Case 2.0.," *Communications of the ACM* (59:5), pp. 61–69.

Jadhakhan, F., Blake, H., Hett, D., & Marwaha, S. (2022). Efficacy of digital technologies aimed at enhancing emotion regulation skills: Literature review. *Frontiers in Psychiatry*, 13, 809332. DOI: 10.3389/fpsyt.2022.809332 PMID: 36159937

Jakhar, P., Rajagopalan, P., Shukla, M., & Singh, V. (2022). Wearable Devices for Real-time Disease Monitoring in Healthcare. In *Nanosensors for Futuristic Smart and Intelligent Healthcare Systems*. CRC Press. DOI: 10.1201/9781003093534-5

Jara, A. J., Zamora, M. A., & Skarmeta, A. F. (2012). Knowledge Acquisition and Management Architecture for Mobile and Personal Health Environments Based on the Internet of Things. *2012 IEEE 11th International Conference on Trust, Security and Privacy in Computing and Communications*, 1811–1818. DOI: 10.1109/TrustCom.2012.194

Javaid, A., Zghyer, F., Kim, C., Spaulding, E. M., Isakadze, N., Ding, J., Kargillis, D., Gao, Y., Rahman, F., Brown, D. E., Saria, S., Martin, S. S., Kramer, C. M., Blumenthal, R. S., & Marvel, F. A. (2022). Medicine 2032: The future of cardiovascular disease prevention with machine learning and digital health technology. *American Journal of Preventive Cardiology*, 12, 100379. DOI: 10.1016/j.ajpc.2022.100379 PMID: 36090536

JavaTpoint. (2018). *Iterative Model*. Retrieved from JavaTPoint website: https://www.javatpoint.com/software-engineering-iterative-model

Jeong, S. (2019). Insurers Want to Know How Many Steps You Took Today. *The New York Times*, 3.

Jiang, Y., Qin, Y., Kim, I., & Wang, Y. (2017). Towards an IoT-based upper limb rehabilitation assessment system. *2017 39th Annual International Conference of the IEEE Engineering in Medicine and Biology Society (EMBC)*, 2414–2417. DOI: 10.1109/EMBC.2017.8037343

Jiang, Y. (2020). Combination of wearable sensors and internet of things and its application in sports rehabilitation. In *Computer Communications* (Vol. 150, pp. 167–176). ELSEVIER., DOI: 10.1016/j.comcom.2019.11.021

Ji, X., Chun, S. A., Wei, Z., & Geller, J. (2023). Twitter sentiment classification for measuring public health concerns. *Social Network Analysis and Mining*, 5, 1–25. PMID: 32226558

Johansson-Pajala, R. M., & Gustafsson, C. (2022). Significant challenges when introducing care robots in Swedish elder care. *Disability and Rehabilitation. Assistive Technology*, 17(2), 166–176. DOI: 10.1080/17483107.2020.1773549 PMID: 32538206

Jones, C., Thornton, J., & Wyatt, J. C. (2021). Enhancing trust in clinical decision support systems: A framework for developers. *BMJ Health & Care Informatics*, 28(1), e100247. DOI: 10.1136/bmjhci-2020-100247 PMID: 34088721

Jongsiriyanyong, S., & Limpawattana, P. (2018). Mild cognitive impairment in clinical practice: A review article. *American Journal of Alzheimer's Disease and Other Dementias*, 33(8), 500–507. DOI: 10.1177/1533317518791401

Jonkman, N. H., Schuurmans, M. J., Jaarsma, T., Shortridge-Baggett, L. M., Hoes, A. W., & Trappenburg, J. C. (2016, December). Self-management interventions: Proposal and validation of a new operational definition. *Journal of Clinical Epidemiology*, 80, 34–42. DOI: 10.1016/j.jclinepi.2016.08.001 PMID: 27531245

Jopowicz, A., Wiśniowska, J., & Tarnacka, B. (2022). Cognitive and physical intervention in metals' dysfunction and neurodegeneration. *Brain Sciences*, 12(3), 345. DOI: 10.3390/brainsci12030345 PMID: 35326301

Joseph Kangmennaang, P. M. (2017). Breast cancer screening among women in Namibia: explaining the effect of health insurance coverage and access to information on screening behaviors.

Julious, S. A. (2005). Sample size of 12 per group rule of thumb for a pilot study. *Pharmaceutical Statistics*, 4(4), 287–291. DOI: 10.1002/pst.185

Kadarina, T. M., & Priambodo, R. (2017). Preliminary design of Internet of Things (IoT) application for supporting mother and child health program in Indonesia. *2017 International Conference on Broadband Communication, Wireless Sensors and Powering (BCWSP)*, 1–6. DOI: 10.1109/BCWSP.2017.8272576

Kalaivani, A., & Karpagavalli, S. (2022). Skin Disease Identification and Classification Optimization Study Using Random Forest Boosted Deep Learning Neural Networks. *NeuroQuantology : An Interdisciplinary Journal of Neuroscience and Quantum Physics*, 20(8), 197.

Kamalov, F., Cherukuri, A. K., & Thabtah, F. (2022). Machine learning applications to Covid-19: a state-of-the-art survey. *2022 Advances in Science and Engineering Technology International Conferences, ASET 2022*, 1–6. DOI: 10.1109/ASET53988.2022.9734959

Kamalov, F., Rajab, K., Cherukuri, A. K., Elnagar, A., & Safaraliev, M. (2022). Deep learning for Covid-19 forecasting: State-of-the-art review. *Neurocomputing*, 511, 142–154. DOI: 10.1016/j.neucom.2022.09.005 PMID: 36097509

Kang, J. J., Adibi, S., Larkin, H., & Luan, T. (2015). Predictive data mining for Converged Internet of Things: A Mobile Health perspective. *2015 International Telecommunication Networks and Applications Conference (ITNAC)*, 5–10. DOI: 10.1109/ATNAC.2015.7366781

Kanschik, D., Bruno, R. R., Wolff, G., Kelm, M., & Jung, C. (2023). Virtual and augmented reality in intensive care medicine: A systematic review. *Annals of Intensive Care*, 13(1), 81. DOI: 10.1186/s13613-023-01176-z

Kapil, V., Khambata, R. S., Robertson, A., Caulfield, M. J., & Ahluwalia, A. (2015). Dietary nitrate provides sustained blood pressure lowering in hypertensive patients: A randomized, phase 2, double-blind, placebo-controlled study. *Hypertension*, 65(2), 320–327. DOI: 10.1161/HYPERTENSIONAHA.114.04675 PMID: 25421976

Kaplan, B., & Duchon, D. (1988). Combining qualitative and quantitative methods in information systems research: A case study. *Management Information Systems Quarterly*, 12(4), 571–586. DOI: 10.2307/249133

Karahanoglu, A., & Erbug, Ç. (2011). *Perceived qualities of smart wearables: Determinants of user acceptance*. DPPI., DOI: 10.1145/2347504.2347533

Karayaneva, Y., Baker, S., Tan, B., & Jing, Y. (2018, July). Use of low-resolution infrared pixel array for passive human motion movement and recognition. In Proceedings of the 32nd international BCS human computer interaction conference. BCS Learning & Development. DOI: 10.14236/ewic/HCI2018.143

Karayaneva, Y., Sharifzadeh, S., Jing, Y., & Tan, B. (2023). Human activity recognition for AI-enabled healthcare using low-resolution infrared sensor data. *Sensors (Basel)*, 23(1), 478. DOI: 10.3390/s23010478 PMID: 36617075

Karayaneva, Y., Sharifzadeh, S., Li, W., Jing, Y., & Tan, B. (2021). Unsupervised Doppler radar based activity recognition for e-healthcare. *IEEE Access : Practical Innovations, Open Solutions*, 9, 62984–63001. DOI: 10.1109/ACCESS.2021.3074088

Kario, K., Tomitani, N., Kanegae, H., Yasui, N., Nishizawa, M., Fujiwara, T., Shigezumi, T., Nagai, R., & Harada, H. (2017). Development of a New ICT-Based Multisensor Blood Pressure Monitoring System for Use in Hemodynamic Biomarker-Initiated Anticipation Medicine for Cardiovascular Disease: The National IMPACT Program Project. *Progress in Cardiovascular Diseases*, 60(3), 435–449. DOI: 10.1016/j.pcad.2017.10.002 PMID: 29108929

Kari, T., Koivunen, S., Frank, L., Makkonen, M., & Moilanen, P. (2017). The expected and perceived well-being effects of short-term self-tracking technology use. *International Journal of Networking and Virtual Organisations*, 17(4), 354–370. DOI: 10.1504/IJNVO.2017.088498

Kaushalya, S. A. D. S., Kulawansa, K. A. D. T., & Firdhous, M. F. M. (2019). Internet of Things for Epidemic Detection: A Critical Review. In Bhatia, S. K., Tiwari, S., Mishra, K. K., & Trivedi, M. C. (Eds.), *Advances in Computer Communication and Computational Sciences* (pp. 485–495). Springer., DOI: 10.1007/978-981-13-6861-5_42

Ke, C., Lou, V. W. Q., Tan, K. C. K., Wai, M. Y., & Chan, L. L. (2020). Changes in technology acceptance among older people with dementia: The role of social robot engagement. *International Journal of Medical Informatics*, 141, 104241. DOI: 10.1016/j.ijmedinf.2020.104241 PMID: 32739611

Khan, I., Zeb, K., Mahmood, A., Uddin, W., & Khan, M. A. Saif-ul-Islam, & Kim, H. J. (2019). Healthcare Monitoring System and transforming Monitored data into Real time Clinical Feedback based on IoT using Raspberry Pi. *2019 2nd International Conference on Computing, Mathematics and Engineering Technologies (iCoMET)*, 1–6. DOI: 10.1109/ICOMET.2019.8673393

Khan, S. F. (2017). Health care monitoring system in Internet of Things (IoT) by using RFID. *2017 6th International Conference on Industrial Technology and Management (ICITM)*, 198–204. DOI: 10.1109/ICITM.2017.7917920

Khanam, N., & Kumar, R. (2022). Recent Applications of Artificial Intelligence in Early Cancer Detection. *Current Medicinal Chemistry*, 29(25), 4410–4435. Advance online publication. DOI: 10.2174/0929867329666220222154733 PMID: 35196970

Khang, A., & Akhai, S. (2024). Green Intelligent and Sustainable Manufacturing: Key Advancements, Benefits, Challenges, and Applications for Transforming Industry. *Machine Vision and Industrial Robotics in Manufacturing*, 405-417.

Khan, M. A., Uddin, M. F., & Gupta, N. (2014). Seven V's of Big Data understanding Big Data to extract value. *Proceedings of the 2014 Zone 1 Conference of the American Society for Engineering Education*, 1–5. DOI: 10.1109/ASEEZone1.2014.6820689

Khosla, R., Nguyen, K., & Chu, M. T. (2017). Human robot engagement and acceptability in residential aged care. *International Journal of Human-Computer Interaction*, 33(6), 510–522. DOI: 10.1080/10447318.2016.1275435

Kim, J. T. (2018). Application of machine and deep learning algorithms in intelligent clinical decision support systems in healthcare. *Journal of Health & Medical Informatics*, 9(5), 321. DOI: 10.4172/2157-7420.1000321

Kiran Kumar, M., & Divya Udayan, J. (2019). A survey of machine learning techniques for cancer disease prediction and diagnosis. *Indian Journal of Public Health Research & Development*, 10(4), 157. Advance online publication. DOI: 10.5958/0976-5506.2019.00682.X

Klein, H. K., and Myers, M. D. 1999. "A Set of Principles for Conducting and Evaluating Interpretive Field Studies in Information Systems," *MIS Quarterly* (23:1), pp. 67–93.

Klímová, B., & Kuča, K. (2019). Internet of things in the assessment, diagnostics and treatment of Parkinson's disease. *Health and Technology*, 9(2), 87–91. DOI: 10.1007/s12553-018-0257-z

Kobayashi, D., Hashimoto, N., ... (2014). Spatial augmented reality by using depth-based object tracking, Proceedings of ACM SIGGRAPH '14. ACM, Kosch, T., Wennrich, K., Topp, D., Muntzinger, M., and Schmidt, A. (2019). The digital cooking coach: using visual and auditory in-situ instructions to assist cognitively impaired during cooking, Proceedings of PETRA '19. ACM, New York, USA, 156–163. DOI: 10.1145/2614217.2614226

Koch, T., Jenkin, P., and Kralik, D. 2004. "Chronic Illness Self-Management: Locating the 'Self,'" *Journal of Advanced Nursing* (48:5), pp. 484–492.

Ko, J., Lu, C., Srivastava, M. B., Stankovic, J. A., Terzis, A., & Welsh, M. (2010). Wireless Sensor Networks for Healthcare. *Proceedings of the IEEE*, 98(11), 1947–1960. DOI: 10.1109/JPROC.2010.2065210

Korchut, A., Szklener, S., Abdelnour, C., Tantinya, N., Hernández-Farigola, J., Ribes, J. C., Skrobas, U., Grabowska-Aleksandrowicz, K., Szczęśniak-Stańczyk, D., & Rejdak, K. (2017). Challenges for service robots—Requirements of elderly adults with cognitive impairments. *Frontiers in Neurology*, 8, 228. DOI: 10.3389/fneur.2017.00228 PMID: 28620342

Kozik, M., Isakadze, N., & Martin, S. S. (2021). Mobile health in preventive cardiology: Current status and future perspective. *Current Opinion in Cardiology*, 36(5), 580–588. DOI: 10.1097/HCO.0000000000000891 PMID: 34224437

Kriegel, E. R., Lazarevic, B., Feifer, D. S., ... (2023). Youth and Augmented Reality. In Springer Handbook of Augmented Reality, 709-741. DOI: 10.1007/978-3-030-67822-7_29

Krishnan, B., Babu, S., Shaji, S. P., Tamanampudi, A. S. R., & Sanagapati, S. S. S. (2016). Software based gateway with distributed flow environment for medical IoT in rural areas. *2016 IEEE International Conference on Advanced Networks and Telecommunications Systems (ANTS)*, 1–5. DOI: 10.1109/ANTS.2016.7947858

Krist, A. H., Davidson, K. W., Mangione, C. M., Barry, M. J., Cabana, M., Caughey, A. B., Donahue, K., Doubeni, C. A., Epling, J. W.Jr, Kubik, M., Landefeld, S., Ogedegbe, G., Pbert, L., Silverstein, M., Simon, M. A., Tseng, C.-W., & Wong, J. B. (2020). Behavioral counseling interventions to promote a healthy diet and physical activity for cardiovascular disease prevention in adults with cardiovascular risk factors: US Preventive Services Task Force recommendation statement. *Journal of the American Medical Association*, 324(20), 2069–2075. DOI: 10.1001/jama.2020.21749 PMID: 33231670

Krittanawong, C., & Virk, H. S. (2021). AI education for healthcare professionals: A vital component for future healthcare. *Health Informatics Journal*, 27(2), 133–139. DOI: 10.1177/1460458220986314

Kumar Lilhore, U., Simaiya, S., Sharma, Y. K., Kaswan, K. S., Rao, K. B. V. B., Rao, V. V. R. M., Baliyan, A., Bijalwan, A., & Alroobaea, R. (2024). A precise model for skin cancer diagnosis using hybrid U-Net and improved MobileNet-V3 with hyperparameters optimization. *Scientific Reports*, 14(1), 4299. DOI: 10.1038/s41598-024-54212-8 PMID: 38383520

Kumar, H., Wadhwa, A. S., Akhai, S., & Kaushik, A. (2024). Parametric analysis, modeling and optimization of the process parameters in electric discharge machining of aluminium metal matrix composite. *Engineering Research Express*, 6(2), 025542. DOI: 10.1088/2631-8695/ad4ba9

Kumar, H., Wadhwa, A. S., Akhai, S., & Kaushik, A. (2024). Parametric optimization of the machining performance of Al-SiCp composite using combination of response surface methodology and desirability function. *Engineering Research Express*, 6(2), 025505. DOI: 10.1088/2631-8695/ad38ff

Kumari, R., & Chander, S. (2024). Improving healthcare quality by unifying the American electronic medical report system: Time for change. *The Egyptian Heart Journal*, 76(1), 32. DOI: 10.1186/s43044-024-00463-9

Kumar, S. (2021). Abstract PO-056: Importance of artificial intelligence, machine learning deep learning in the field of medicine on the future role of the physician. *Clinical Cancer Research*, 27(5, Supplement), PO-056. Advance online publication. DOI: 10.1158/1557-3265.ADI21-PO-056

Kushimo, O. O., Salau, A. O., Adeleke, O. J., & Olaoye, D. S. (2023). Deep learning model to improve melanoma detection in people of color. *Arab Journal of Basic and Applied Sciences*, 30(1), 92–102. Advance online publication. DOI: 10.1080/25765299.2023.2170066

La, H. J., Jung, H. T., & Kim, S. D. (2015). Extensible Disease Diagnosis Cloud Platform with Medical Sensors and IoT Devices. *2015 3rd International Conference on Future Internet of Things and Cloud*, 371–378. DOI: 10.1109/FiCloud.2015.65

Laitinen, A., Niemelä, M., & Pirhonen, J. (2019). Recognizing Vulnerability, Agency, and Subjectivity in Robot-based, Robot-assisted, and Teleoperated Elderly Care. *Techné: Research in Philosophy and Technology*.

Laitinen, A., & Pirhonen, J. (2019). Ten forms of recognition and misrecognition in long-term care for older people. *Sats*, 20(1), 53–78. DOI: 10.1515/sats-2016-0017

Laland, K. N. (2004). Social learning strategies. *Animal Learning & Behavior*, 32(1), 4–14. DOI: 10.3758/BF03196002 PMID: 15161136

Lamprinos, I., Demski, H., Mantwill, S., Kabak, Y., Hildebrand, C., & Ploessnig, M. (2016). Modular ICT-Based Patient Empowerment Framework for Self-Management of Diabetes: Design Perspectives and Validation Results. *International Journal of Medical Informatics*, 91, 31–43. DOI: 10.1016/j.ijmedinf.2016.04.006 PMID: 27185507

Landi, H. (2019). *Healthcare data breaches cost an average $6.5M: Report*. Fierce Healthcare. https://www.fiercehealthcare.com/tech/healthcare-data-breach-costs -average-6-45m-60-higher-than-other-industries-report

Landis, J. R., & Koch, G. G. (1977). The Measurement of Observer Agreement for Categorical Data. *Biometrics*, 33(1), 159–174. DOI: 10.2307/2529310 PMID: 843571

Latif, G., Shankar, A., Alghazo, J. M., Kalyanasundaram, V., Boopathi, C. S., & Jaffar, M. A. (2020). I-CARES: advancing health diagnosis and medication through IoT. In *Wireless Networks* (Vol. 26, Issues 4, SI, pp. 2375–2389). Springer. DOI: 10.1007/s11276-019-02165-6

Latif, S., Qadir, J., Farooq, S., & Imran, M. A. (2017). How 5G wireless (and Concomitant Technologies) will revolutionize healthcare? [Article]. *Future Internet*, 9(4), 93. Advance online publication. DOI: 10.3390/fi9040093

Latkin, C. A., & Knowlton, A. R. (2015). Social network assessments and interventions for health behavior change: A critical review. *Behavioral Medicine (Washington, D.C.)*, 41(3), 90–97. DOI: 10.1080/08964289.2015.1034645 PMID: 26332926

Lau, W. L., Reizes, J., Timchenko, V., Kara, S., & Kornfeld, B. (2015). Heat and mass transfer model to predict the operational performance of a steam sterilisation autoclave including products. *International Journal of Heat and Mass Transfer*, 90, 800–811. DOI: 10.1016/j.ijheatmasstransfer.2015.06.089

Law, A. M., & Kelton, W. D. (2000). *Simulation modeling and analysis* (Vol. 3). McGraw-Hill New York.

Lazaro, M. J. S., Lim, J., Kim, S. H., & Yun, M. H. (2020). Wearable Technologies: Acceptance Model for Smartwatch Adoption Among Older Adults. In Gao, Q., & Zhou, J. (Eds.), Lecture Notes in Computer Science: Vol. 12207. *Human Aspects of IT for the Aged Population. Technologies, Design and User Experience. HCII 2020*. Springer. DOI: 10.1007/978-3-030-50252-2_23

Leclercq, C., Witt, H., Hindricks, G., Katra, R. P., Albert, D., Belliger, A., Cowie, M. R., Deneke, T., Friedman, P., Haschemi, M., Lobban, T., Lordereau, I., McConnell, M. V., Rapallini, L., Samset, E., Turakhia, M. P., Singh, J. P., Svennberg, E., Wadhwa, M., & Weidinger, F. (2022). Wearables, telemedicine, and artificial intelligence in arrhythmias and heart failure: Proceedings of the European Society of Cardiology Cardiovascular Round Table. *Europace*, 24(9), 1372–1383. DOI: 10.1093/europace/euac052 PMID: 35640917

Lee, L. Y., Lim, W. M., Teh, P. L., Malik, O. A. S., & Nurzaman, S. (2020). Understanding the interaction between older adults and soft service robots: Insights from robotics and the technology acceptance model. *AIS Transactions on Human-Computer Interaction*, 12(3), 125–145. DOI: 10.17705/1thci.00132

Leen, J. L., & Juurlink, D. N. (2019). Carfentanil: A narrative review of its pharmacology and public health concerns. *Canadian Journal of Anaesthesia*, 66(4), 414–421. DOI: 10.1007/s12630-019-01294-y PMID: 30666589

Lee, Y. Y., Lee, J. H., Ahmed, B., Son, M. G., & Lee, K. H. (2019). A New Projection-based Exhibition System for a Museum. *Journal on Computing and Cultural Heritage*, 12(2), 1–17. DOI: 10.1145/3275522

Lehto, T., Oinas-Kukkonen, H., Pätiälä, T., & Saarelma, O. (2013). Virtual health coaching for consumers: a persuasive systems design perspective. *International Journal of Networking and Virtual Organisations 4, 13*(1), 24-41.

Leidner, D. E., & Gregory, R. W. (2024). About Theory and Theorizing. *Journal of the Association for Information Systems*, 25(3), 501–521. DOI: 10.17705/1jais.00886

Lejeune, A., Robaglia, B.-M., Walter, M., Berrouiguet, S., & Lemey, C. (2022). Use of Social Media Data to Diagnose and Monitor Psychotic Disorders: Systematic Review. *Journal of Medical Internet Research*, 24(9), e36986. DOI: 10.2196/36986 PMID: 36066938

Lemmer, K., Mielke, M., Pauli, G., & Beekes, M. (2004). Decontamination of surgical instruments from prion proteins: In vitro studies on the detachment, destabilization and degradation of prpsc bound to steel surfaces. *The Journal of General Virology*, 85(12), 3805–3816. DOI: 10.1099/vir.0.80346-0 PMID: 15557254

Leon, A. C., Davis, L. L., & Kraemer, H. C. (2011). The role and interpretation of pilot studies in clinical research. *Journal of Psychiatric Research*, 45(5), 626–629. DOI: 10.1016/j.jpsychires.2010.10.008

LeRouge, C., Hevner, A. R., and Rosann, W. C. 2007. "It's More than Just Use: An Exploration of Telemedicine Use Quality," *Decision Support Systems* (43:4), pp. 1287–1304.

Lethbridge, T. C., Sim, S. E., & Singer, J. (2005). Studying software engineers: Data collection techniques for software field studies. *Empirical Software Engineering*, 10(3), 311–341. DOI: 10.1007/s10664-005-1290-x

Lewy, H. (2015). Wearable technologies – future challenges for implementation in healthcare services. *Healthcare Technology Letters*, 2(1), 1. Advance online publication. DOI: 10.1049/htl.2014.0104

Li, W., Xu, Y., Tan, B., & Piechocki, R. J. (2017, June). Passive wireless sensing for unsupervised human activity recognition in healthcare. In 2017 13th International Wireless Communications and Mobile Computing Conference (IWCMC) (pp. 1528-1533). IEEE. DOI: 10.1109/IWCMC.2017.7986511

Liang, F., Yang, X., Peng, W., Zhen, S., Cao, W., Li, Q., & Gu, D. (2023). Applications of digital health approaches for cardiometabolic diseases prevention and management in the Western Pacific region. *The Lancet Regional Health. Western Pacific*. PMID: 38456090

Liao, D., Shu, L., Liang, G., Li, Y., Zhang, Y., Zhang, W., & Xu, X. (2019). Design and evaluation of affective virtual reality system based on multimodal physiological signals and self-assessment manikin. *IEEE Journal of Electromagnetics, RF and Microwaves in Medicine and Biology*, 4(3), 216–224. DOI: 10.1109/JERM.2019.2948767

Liao, H., He, Y., Wu, X., Wu, Z., & Bausys, R. (2023). Reimagining multi-criterion decision making by data-driven methods based on machine learning: A literature review. *Information Fusion*, 12, 101970. Advance online publication. DOI: 10.1016/j.inffus.2023.101970

Li, B., Dong, Q., Downen, R. S., Tran, N., Jackson, J. H., Pillai, D., Zaghloul, M., & Li, Z. (2019). A wearable IoT aldehyde sensor for pediatric asthma research and management. *Sensors and Actuators. B, Chemical*, 287, 584–594. DOI: 10.1016/j.snb.2019.02.077 PMID: 31938011

Liberati, A., Altman, D. G., Tetzlaff, J., Mulrow, C., Gøtzsche, P. C., Ioannidis, J. P. A., Clarke, M., Devereaux, P. J., Kleijnen, J., & Moher, D. (2009). The PRISMA statement for reporting systematic reviews and meta-analyses of studies that evaluate health care interventions: Explanation and elaboration. *PLoS Medicine*, 6(7), e1000100. DOI: 10.1371/journal.pmed.1000100 PMID: 19621070

Lie, M. L., Lindsay, S., & Brittain, K. (2016). Technology and trust: Older people's perspectives of a home monitoring system. *Ageing and Society*, 36(7), 1501–1525. DOI: 10.1017/S0144686X15000501

Li, J., Ma, Q., Chan, A. H., & Man, S. (2019). Health monitoring through wearable technologies for older adults: Smart wearables acceptance model. *Applied Ergonomics*, 75, 162–169. DOI: 10.1016/j.apergo.2018.10.006 PMID: 30509522

Lim, S. S., Vos, T., Flaxman, A. D., Danaei, G., Shibuya, K., Adair-Rohani, H., & Pelizzari, P. M. (2012). A comparative risk assessment of burden of disease and injury attributable to 67 risk factors and risk factor clusters in 21 regions, 1990–2010: A systematic analysis for the Global Burden of Disease Study 2010. *Lancet*, 380(9859), 2224–2260. DOI: 10.1016/S0140-6736(12)61766-8 PMID: 23245609

Lin, W.-Y., Chou, W.-C., Tsai, T.-H., Lin, C.-C., & Lee, M.-Y. (2016). Development of a Wearable Instrumented Vest for Posture Monitoring and System Usability Verification Based on the Technology Acceptance Model. *Sensors (Basel)*, 16(12), 2172. DOI: 10.3390/s16122172 PMID: 27999324

Li, S., Xu, L. D., & Zhao, S. (2015). The internet of things: A survey. *Information Systems Frontiers*, 17(2), 243–259. DOI: 10.1007/s10796-014-9492-7

Liu, D., Feng, X. L., Ahmed, F., Shahid, M., & Guo, J. (2022). Detecting and Measuring Depression on Social Media Using a Machine Learning Approach: Systematic Review. *JMIR Mental Health*, 9(3), e27244. DOI: 10.2196/27244 PMID: 35230252

Liu, K., Madrigal, E., Chung, J. S., Parekh, M., Kalahar, C. S., Nguyen, D., & Harris, O. A. (2023). Preliminary Study of Virtual-reality-guided Meditation for Veterans with Stress and Chronic Pain. *Alternative Therapies in Health and Medicine*, 29(6). PMID: 34559692

Liu, Y., Niu, J., Yang, L., & Shu, L. (2014). eBPlatform: An IoT-based system for NCD patients homecare in China. *2014 IEEE Global Communications Conference*, 2448–2453. DOI: 10.1109/GLOCOM.2014.7037175

Li, W., Tan, B., & Piechocki, R. (2018). Passive radar for opportunistic monitoring in e-health applications. *IEEE Journal of Translational Engineering in Health and Medicine*, 6, 1–10. DOI: 10.1109/JTEHM.2018.2791609 PMID: 29456898

Li, W., Tan, B., Xu, Y., & Piechocki, R. J. (2018). Log-likelihood clustering-enabled passive RF sensing for residential activity recognition. *IEEE Sensors Journal*, 18(13), 5413–5421. DOI: 10.1109/JSEN.2018.2834739

Li, X., Gunal, M., & Shiau, J. Y. 2009, March. Computational modeling for improving usability design workflow. In *2009 International Conference on Networking, Sensing and Control* (pp. 679-684). IEEE.

Lopez, G., Shuzo, M., & Yamada, I. (2011). New healthcare society supported by wearable sensors and information mapping-based services. *International Journal of Networking and Virtual Organisations*, 9(3), 233–247. DOI: 10.1504/IJN-VO.2011.042481

Louie, W. Y. G., McColl, D., & Nejat, G. (2014). Acceptance and attitudes toward a human-like socially assistive robot by older adults. *Assistive Technology*, 26(3), 140–150. DOI: 10.1080/10400435.2013.869703 PMID: 26131794

Lou, Z., Wang, L., Jiang, K., Wei, Z., & Shen, G. (2020). Reviews of wearable healthcare systems: Materials, devices and system integration. *Materials Science and Engineering R Reports*, 24, 100523. Advance online publication. DOI: 10.1016/j.mser.2019.100523

Lowell, V. L., & Yang, M. (2023). Authentic learning experiences to improve online instructor's performance and self-efficacy: The design of an online mentoring program. *TechTrends*, 67(1), 112–123. DOI: 10.1007/s11528-022-00770-5

Lozano, R., Naghavi, M., Foreman, K., Lim, S., Shibuya, K., Aboyans, V., & Remuzzi, G. (2012). Global and regional mortality from 235 causes of death for 20 age groups in 1990 and 2010: A systematic analysis for the Global Burden of Disease Study 2010. *Lancet*, 380(9859), 2095–2128. DOI: 10.1016/S0140-6736(12)61728-0 PMID: 23245604

Lukowicz, P., Kirstein, T., & Tröster, G. (2004). Wearable systems for health care applications. *Methods of Information in Medicine*, 43(3), 232–238. DOI: 10.1055/s-0038-1633863

Luo, G., & Gao, S. J. (2020). Global health concerns stirred by emerging viral infections. *Journal of Medical Virology*, 92(4), 399–400. DOI: 10.1002/jmv.25683 PMID: 31967329

Luo, X., Liu, T., Liu, J., Guo, X., & Wang, G. (2012). Design and implementation of a distributed fall detection system based on wireless sensor networks. *EUR-ASIP Journal on Wireless Communications and Networking*, 2012(1), 1–13. DOI: 10.1186/1687-1499-2012-118

Ma, B., Li, C., Wu, Z., Huang, Y., van der Zijp-Tan, A. C., Tan, S., Li, D., Fong, A., Basetty, C., Borchert, G. M., Benton, R., Wu, B., & Huang, J. (2019). Muscle fatigue detection and treatment system driven by internet of things. In *BMC Medical Informatics and Decision Making* (Vol. 19, Issues 7, SI). BMC. DOI: 10.1186/s12911-019-0982-x

Maçorano, R. D. N. A. (2020). *Exploratory Psychometric Validation and Efficacy Assessment Study of Social Phobia Treatment based on Augmented and Virtual Reality Serious Games and Biofeedback* (Doctoral dissertation, Universidade de Lisboa (Portugal)).

Maddula, R., MacLeod, J., McLeish, T., Painter, S., Steward, A., Berman, G., Hamid, A., Abdelrahim, M., Whittle, J., & Brown, S. A. (2022). The role of digital health in the cardiovascular learning healthcare system. *Frontiers in Cardiovascular Medicine*, 9, 1008575. DOI: 10.3389/fcvm.2022.1008575 PMID: 36407438

Magnani, G., & Gioia, D. (2023). Using the Gioia Methodology in international business and entrepreneurship research. *International Business Review*, 32(2), 102097. DOI: 10.1016/j.ibusrev.2022.102097

Magsi, H., Sodhro, A. H., Chachar, F. A., Abro, S. A. K., Sodhro, G. H., & Pirbhulal, S. (2018). Evolution of 5G in Internet of medical things. *2018 International Conference on Computing, Mathematics and Engineering Technologies (iCoMET)*, 1–7. DOI: 10.1109/ICOMET.2018.8346428

Maiti, A., Chatterjee, B., Ashour, A. S., & Dey, N. (2019). Computer-aided Diagnosis of Melanoma: A Review of Existing Knowledge and Strategies. *Current Medical Imaging*, 16(7), 835–854. Advance online publication. DOI: 10.2174/1573405615 666191210104141 PMID: 33059554

Makeham, M. (2019). My Health Record: Connecting Australians with their own health information. *The HIM Journal*, 48(3), 113–115. DOI: 10.1177/1833358319841511

Makhataeva, Z., Akhmetov, T., & Varol, H. A. (2023). Augmented Reality for Cognitive Impairments. In Springer Handbook of Augmented Reality, 765-793. DOI: 10.1007/978-3-030-67822-7_31

Maksimović, D., Vujovic, V., & Perisic, B. (2016). Do It Yourself solution of Internet of Things Healthcare System: Measuring body parameters and environmental parameters affecting health. *Journal of Information Systems Engineering & Management*, 1(1), ●●●. DOI: 10.20897/lectito.201607

Mala, S. (2021). Myocardial Injury after Non-Cardiac Surgery and Its Correlation with Mortality-A Brief Review on Its Scenario till 2020. *International Journal of Preventive Cardiology*, 1(1), 29–31.

Malki, Z., Atlam, E. S., Hassanien, A. E., Dagnew, G., Elhosseini, M. A., & Gad, I. (2020). Association between weather data and COVID-19 pandemic predicting mortality rate: Machine learning approaches. *Chaos, Solitons, and Fractals*, 138, 110137. DOI: 10.1016/j.chaos.2020.110137 PMID: 32834583

Manatarinat, W., Poomrittigul, S., & Tantatsanawong, P. (2019). Narrowband-Internet of Things (NB-IoT) System for Elderly Healthcare Services. *2019 5th International Conference on Engineering, Applied Sciences and Technology (ICEAST)*, 1–4. DOI: 10.1109/ICEAST.2019.8802604

Market Research Future. (2018, April). *Telemedicine Market Size, Trends, Growth, Share, Industry Forecast Till 2023*. https://www.marketresearchfuture.com/reports/telemedicine-market-2216

Marossi, C., Mariani, V., Arenas, A., Brondino, M., de Carvalho, C. V., Costa, P., . . . Pasini, M. (2023, July). Mindfulness Lessons in a Virtual Natural Environment to Cope with Work-Related Stress. In *International Conference in Methodologies and intelligent Systems for Techhnology Enhanced Learning* (pp. 227-238). Cham: Springer Nature Switzerland. DOI: 10.1007/978-3-031-41226-4_24

Marvaso, G., Pepa, M., Volpe, S., Mastroleo, F., Zaffaroni, M., Vincini, M. G., & Jereczek-Fossa, B. A. (2022). Virtual and Augmented Reality as a Novel Opportunity to Unleash the Power of Radiotherapy in the Digital Era: A Scoping Review. *Applied Sciences (Basel, Switzerland)*, 12(22), 11308. DOI: 10.3390/app122211308

Mashiyama, S., Hong, J., & Ohtsuki, T. (2015, June). Activity recognition using low resolution infrared array sensor. In *2015 IEEE International Conference on Communications (ICC)* (pp. 495-500). IEEE. DOI: 10.1109/ICC.2015.7248370

Masiuliene, L. (2015). *The key features of successful awareness-raising campaigns.* European Lifelong Learning Program.

Maskor, N.A., M. A. (2018). Strategy for Effective Cancer Awareness Program. *Journal of Global Oncology*, ●●●, 1–20.

Masutani, Y., Dohi, T., Yamane, F., Iseki, H., & Takakura, K. (1998). Augmented reality visualization system for intravascular neurosurgery. Computer Aided Surgery [IS-CAS]. *Computer Aided Surgery*, 3(5), 239–247. DOI: 10.3109/10929089809149845

Matthews, K., & Industry Voice. (2020, April 3). *How AI and IoT Are Changing Daily Operations in Hospitals.* Healthcare Innovation. https://www.hcinnovationgroup.com/analytics-ai/article/21132663/how-ai-and-iot-are-changing-daily-operations-in-hospitals

Mavis Machirori, C. P. (2018). Study on the relationship between Black man, culture, and prostate cancer beliefs. *Cogent Medicine*, ●●●, 1–13.

Ma, W. T., Yan, W. X., Fu, Z., & Zhao, Y. Z. (2011). A Chinese cooking robot for elderly and disabled people. *Robotica*, 29(6), 843–852. DOI: 10.1017/S0263574711000051

Ma, X., Gao, H., Xu, H., & Bian, M. (2019). An IoT-based task scheduling optimization scheme considering the deadline and cost-aware scientific workflow for cloud computing. *EURASIP Journal on Wireless Communications and Networking*, 2019(1), 249. DOI: 10.1186/s13638-019-1557-3

Ma, Y., Zhang, P., Tang, Y., Pan, C., Li, G., Liu, N., Hu, Y., & Tang, Z. (2020). Artificial intelligence: The dawn of a new era for cutting-edge technology based diagnosis and treatment for stroke. *Brain Hemorrhages*, 1(1), 1–5. Advance online publication. DOI: 10.1016/j.hest.2020.01.006

McCann, M., Donnelly, M., & O'Reilly, D. (2012). Gender differences in care home admission risk: Partner's age explains the higher risk for women. *Age and Ageing*, 41(3), 416–419. DOI: 10.1093/ageing/afs022 PMID: 22510517

McCreadie, C., & Tinker, A. (2005). The acceptability of assistive technology to older people. *Ageing and Society*, 25(1), 91–110. DOI: 10.1017/S0144686X0400248X

McCrum-Gardner, E. (2008). Which is the correct statistical test to use? *British Journal of Oral & Maxillofacial Surgery*, 46(1), 38–41. DOI: 10.1016/j.bjoms.2007.09.002

McDermott, M. S., & While, A. E. (2013). Maximizing the Healthcare Environment: A Systematic Review Exploring the Potential of Computer Technology to Promote Selfmanagement of Chronic Illness in Healthcare Settings. *Patient Education and Counseling*, 92(1), 13–22. DOI: 10.1016/j.pec.2013.02.014 PMID: 23566427

McGlynn, S. A., Kemple, S. C., Mitzner, T. L., King, C. H., & Rogers, W. A. (2014, September). Understanding older adults' perceptions of usefulness for the paro robot. [). Sage CA: Los Angeles, CA: SAGE Publications.]. *Proceedings of the Human Factors and Ergonomics Society Annual Meeting*, 58(1), 1914–1918. DOI: 10.1177/1541931214581400 PMID: 31320791

McGushin, A., de Barros, E. F., Floss, M., Mohammad, Y., Ndikum, A. E., Ngenda-hayo, C., Oduor, P. A., Sultana, S., Wong, R., & Abelsohn, A. (2023). The World Organization of Family Doctors Air Health Train the Trainer Program: Lessons learned and implications for planetary health education. *The Lancet. Planetary Health*, 7(1), e55–e63. DOI: 10.1016/S2542-5196(22)00218-2 PMID: 36608949

McKenziel F, Z. A. (2018). Breast Cancer Awareness in Sub-Saharan Africa. *ABC -DO cohort: African Breast Cancer- Disparities in Outcomes study*, 721-730.

McKinsey Global Institute. (2015, June). *The Internet of Things: Mapping the Value Beyond the Hype*. McKinsey & Company. https://www.mckinsey.com/~/media/McKinsey/Industries/Technology%20Media%20and%20Telecommunications/High%20Tech/Our%20Insights/The%20Internet%20of%20Things%20The%20value%20of%20digitizing%20the%20physical%20world/The-Internet-of-things-Mapping-the-value-beyond-the-hype.ashx

Mehta, S., & Sharma, D. (2023). Wearable technology in healthcare engineering. In *Emerging Nanotechnologies for Medical Applications* (pp. 227–248). Elsevier. DOI: 10.1016/B978-0-323-91182-5.00005-X

Melarkode, N., Srinivasan, K., Qaisar, S. M., & Plawiak, P. (2023). AI-Powered Diagnosis of Skin Cancer: A Contemporary Review, Open Challenges and Future Research Directions. *Cancers (Basel)*, 15(4), 1183. Advance online publication. DOI: 10.3390/cancers15041183 PMID: 36831525

Mendenhall, E., McMurry, H. S., Shivashankar, R., Narayan, K. M. V., Tandon, N., & Prabhakaran, D. (2016). Normalizing diabetes in Delhi: A qualitative study of health and health care. *Anthropology & Medicine*, 23(3), 295–310. DOI: 10.1080/13648470.2016.1184010 PMID: 27328175

Meola, A. (2020). *IoT Healthcare in 2020: Companies, devices, use cases and market stats*. Business Insider. https://www.businessinsider.com/iot-healthcare

Mer, A., & Virdi, A. S. (2023). Navigating the paradigm shift in HRM practices through the lens of artificial intelligence: A post-pandemic perspective. *The Adoption and Effect of Artificial Intelligence on Human Resources Management, Part A*, 123-154.

Meredith M. Skeels, K. T. (2010). Catalyzing Social Support for Breast Cancer Patients.

Mettler, T., & Wulf, J. (2019). Physiolytics at the workplace: Affordances and constraints of wearables use from an employee's perspective. *Information Systems Journal*, 29(1), 245–273. DOI: 10.1111/isj.12205

Midha, S., & Singh, K. (2023). Happiness-Enhancing Strategies Among Indians. In *Religious and Spiritual Practices in India: A Positive Psychological Perspective* (pp. 341–368). Springer Nature Singapore. DOI: 10.1007/978-981-99-2397-7_15

Mieronkoski, R., Azimi, I., Rahmani, A. M., Aantaa, R., Terävä, V., Liljeberg, P., & Salanterä, S. (2017). The Internet of Things for basic nursing care-A scoping review. *International Journal of Nursing Studies*, 69, 78–90. DOI: 10.1016/j.ijnurstu.2017.01.009 PMID: 28189116

Mihailidis, A., Cockburn, A., Longley, C., & Boger, J. (2008). The acceptability of home monitoring technology among community-dwelling older adults and baby boomers. *Assistive Technology*, 20(1), 1–12. DOI: 10.1080/10400435.2008.10131927 PMID: 18751575

Miles, M. B., & Huberman, A. M. (1994). *Qualitative Data Analysis: An Expanded Sourcebook (Second)*. Sage Publications Inc.

Mills, J.-A., Marks, E., Reynolds, T., & Cieza, A. (2017). Rehabilitation: Essential along the Continuum of Care. In Jamison, D. T., Gelband, H., Horton, S., Jha, P., Laxminarayan, R., Mock, C. N., & Nugent, R. (Eds.), *Disease Control Priorities: Improving Health and Reducing Poverty* (3rd ed.). The International Bank for Reconstruction and Development / The World Bank., https://www.ncbi.nlm.nih.gov/books/NBK525298/ DOI: 10.1596/978-1-4648-0527-1_ch15

Mincolelli, G., Imbesi, S., Marchi, M., & Giacobone, G. A. (2019). New Domestic Healthcare. Co-designing Assistive Technologies for Autonomous Ageing at Home. *The Design Journal*, 22(1), 503–516. DOI: 10.1080/14606925.2019.1595435

Miner, N. (2022). *Stairway to Heaven: Breathing Mindfulness into Virtual Reality* (Doctoral dissertation, Northeastern University).

Minerva, R., Biru, A., & Rotondi, D. (2015). Towards a definition of the Internet of Things (IoT). *IEEE Internet Initiative*, 1, 1–86.

Miraz, M. H., Excell, P. S., & Ali, M. (2016). User interface (UI) design issues for multilingual users: A case study. *Universal Access in the Information Society*, 15(3), 431–444. DOI: 10.1007/s10209-014-0397-5

Mishra, A., Mishra, J., Tiwari, M., Hugo, V., Neto, A. V. L., & Menezes, J. W. M. (2023, March). Digital Health Technology in the Prevention of Heart Failure Coronary Artery Disease. In *Doctoral Symposium on Computational Intelligence* (pp. 593-604). Singapore: Springer Nature Singapore. DOI: 10.1007/978-981-99-3716-5_48

Mitzner, T. L., Smarr, C. A., Beer, J. M., Chen, T. L., Springman, J. M., Prakash, A., & Rogers, W. A. (2011). *Older adults' acceptance of assistive robots for the home*. Georgia Institute of Technology.

Miyamoto, J., Koike, H., & Amano, T. (2018). Gaze navigation in the real world by changing visual appearance of objects using projector-camera system. *Proceedings of VRST*, 2018, 1–5. DOI: 10.1145/3281505.3281537

Moglia, A., Georgiou, K., Marinov, B., Georgiou, E., Berchiolli, R. N., Satava, R. M., & Cuschieri, A. (2022). 5G in Healthcare: From COVID-19 to Future Challenges [Article]. *IEEE Journal of Biomedical and Health Informatics*, 26(8), 4187–4196. DOI: 10.1109/JBHI.2022.3181205 PMID: 35675255

Mohammadhossein, N., Richter, A., & Richter, S. (2024). "What's the matter with Augmented Reality"–Obstacles to using AR and strategies to address them. PACIS 2024 Proceedings.

Mohammed, M. N., Hazairin, N. A., Al-Zubaidi, S., Mustapha, S., & Yusuf, E. (2020). Toward a Novel Design for Coronavirus Detection and Diagnosis System Using IoT Based Drone Technology. *International Journal of Psychosocial Rehabilitation*, 24(7), 10.

Mohammed, Z. K., Mohammed, M. A., Abdulkareem, K. H., Zebari, D. A., Lakhan, A., Marhoon, H. A., Nedoma, J., & Martinek, R. (2024). A metaverse framework for IoT-based remote patient monitoring and virtual consultations using AES-256 encryption. *Applied Soft Computing*, 158, 111588. DOI: 10.1016/j.asoc.2024.111588

Mohanta, B., Das, P., & Patnaik, S. (2019, May 25-26). 2019). Healthcare 5.0: A Paradigm Shift in Digital Healthcare System Using Artificial Intelligence, IOT and 5G Communication. 2019 International Conference on Applied Machine Learning (ICAML), Morone, J. (2019). Systematic review of sociodemographic representation and cultural responsiveness in psychosocial and behavioral interventions with adolescents with type 1 diabetes. *Journal of Diabetes*, 11(7), 582–592. https://doi.org/https://dx.doi.org/10.1111/1753-0407.12889 PMID: 30565425

Moher, D., Liberati, A., Tetzlaff, J., Altman, D. G., & Group, T. P. (2009). Preferred Reporting Items for Systematic Reviews and Meta-Analyses: The PRISMA Statement. *PLoS Medicine*, 6(7), e1000097. DOI: 10.1371/journal.pmed.1000097 PMID: 19621072

Molka-Danielsen, J., Carter, B. W., & Creelman, A. (2009). Empathy in virtual learning environments. *International journal of Networking and Virtual Organisations, 6*(2), 123-139.

Möller, F., Schoormann, T., Strobel, G., & Hansen, M. R. P. (2022). Unveiling the Cloak: Kernel Theory Use in Design Science Research. *Proceedings of the International Conference on Information Systems*.

Mora, H., Gil, D., Terol, R. M., Azorin, J., & Szymanski, J. (2017). An IoT-Based Computational Framework for Healthcare Monitoring in Mobile Environments. *Sensors (Basel)*, 17(10), 2302. Advance online publication. DOI: 10.3390/s17102302 PMID: 28994743

Moran, A., Gu, D., Zhao, D., Coxson, P., Wang, Y. C., Chen, C. S., Liu, J., Cheng, J., Bibbins-Domingo, K., Shen, Y.-M., He, J., & Goldman, L. (2010). Future cardiovascular disease in China: Markov model and risk factor scenario projections from the coronary heart disease policy model–China. *Circulation: Cardiovascular Quality and Outcomes*, 3(3), 243–252. DOI: 10.1161/CIRCOUTCOMES.109.910711 PMID: 20442213

Mori, M. (1970). The uncanny valley. *Energy*, 7(4), 33–35.

Moyle, W., Bramble, M., Jones, C., & Murfield, J. (2016). Care staff perceptions of a social robot called Paro and a look-alike Plush Toy: A descriptive qualitative approach. *Aging & Mental Health*, 22(3), 330–335. DOI: 10.1080/13607863.2016.1262820 PMID: 27967207

Muhammad Akram, M. I. (2017). Awareness and current knowledge of breast cancer.

Muhammad, G., Rahman, S. M. M., Alelaiwi, A., & Alamri, A. (2017). Smart Health Solution Integrating IoT and Cloud: A Case Study of Voice Pathology Monitoring. *IEEE Communications Magazine*, 55(1), 69–73. DOI: 10.1109/MCOM.2017.1600425CM

Mumtaj, S. Y., & Umamakeswari, A. (2017). Neuro fuzzy based healthcare system using IoT. *2017 International Conference on Energy, Communication, Data Analytics and Soft Computing (ICECDS)*, 2299–2303. DOI: 10.1109/ICECDS.2017.8389863

Munn, Z., Peters, M. D. J., Stern, C., Tufanaru, C., McArthur, A., & Aromataris, E. (2018). Systematic review or scoping review? Guidance for authors when choosing between a systematic or scoping review approach. *BMC Medical Research Methodology*, 18(1), 143. DOI: 10.1186/s12874-018-0611-x PMID: 30453902

Myint, S. H. (1994). Human coronaviruses: A brief review. *Reviews in Medical Virology*, 4(1), 35–46. DOI: 10.1002/rmv.1980040108

Nabi, K. N. (2020). Forecasting COVID-19 pandemic: A data-driven analysis. *Chaos, Solitons, and Fractals*, 139, 110046. DOI: 10.1016/j.chaos.2020.110046 PMID: 32834601

Nadeau, K. J., Anderson, B. J., Berg, E. G., Chiang, J. L., Chou, H., Copeland, K. C., Hannon, T. S., Huang, T. T. K., Lynch, J. L., Powell, J., Sellers, E., Tamborlane, W. V., & Zeitler, P. (2016). Youth-Onset Type 2 Diabetes Consensus Report: Current Status, Challenges, and Priorities. *Diabetes Care*, 39(9), 1635–1642. https://doi.org/https://dx.doi.org/10.2337/dc16-1066. DOI: 10.2337/dc16-1066 PMID: 27486237

Nakwafila, O. (2017). *Knowledge and attitudes towards prostate cancer screening amongst men in Oshana Region*.

Namibia, C. A. (n.d.). *Cancer Registry*. Retrieved from Cancer Association of Namibia (W030): www.can.org.na/?page_id=493

Namibia, C. A. (2019). *Company Profile and Fact Sheet*. Cancer Association of Namibia.

Nasri, F., & Mtibaa, A. (2017). Smart Mobile Healthcare System based on WBSN and 5G. *International Journal of Advanced Computer Science and Applications*, 8(10), 147–156. DOI: 10.14569/IJACSA.2017.081020

Nastjuk, I., Trang, S., Grummeck-Braamt, J. V., Adam, M. T., & Tarafdar, M. (2024). Integrating and synthesising technostress research: A meta-analysis on technostress creators, outcomes, and IS usage contexts. *European Journal of Information Systems*, 33(3), 361–382. DOI: 10.1080/0960085X.2022.2154712

National Cancer Institute. (2021). *Cancer cost and care*. Retrieved from https://www.cancer.gov/about-cancer/treatment/costs

Nayak, J., Naik, B., Dinesh, P., Vakula, K., Dash, P. B., & Pelusi, D. (2022). Significance of deep learning for Covid-19: State-of-the-art review. *Research on Biomedical Engineering*, 38(1), 243–266. DOI: 10.1007/s42600-021-00135-6

Naylor, M., Ridout, B., & Campbell, A. (2020). A scoping review identifying the need for quality research on the use of virtual reality in workplace settings for stress management. *Cyberpsychology, Behavior, and Social Networking*, 23(8), 506–518. DOI: 10.1089/cyber.2019.0287 PMID: 32486836

Nduka, A., Samual, J., Elango, S., Divakaran, S., & Umar, U., & SenthilPrabha, R. (2019). Internet of Things Based Remote Health Monitoring System Using Arduino. *2019 Third International Conference on I-SMAC (IoT in Social, Mobile, Analytics and Cloud) (I-SMAC)*, 572–576. DOI: 10.1109/I-SMAC47947.2019.9032438

Nedungadi, P., Jayakumar, A., & Raman, R. (2017). Personalized Health Monitoring System for Managing Well-Being in Rural Areas. *Journal of Medical Systems*, 42(1), 22. DOI: 10.1007/s10916-017-0854-9 PMID: 29242996

Neiman, A. B., Ruppar, T., Ho, M., Garber, L., Weidle, P. J., Hong, Y., George, M. G., & Thorpe, P. G. (2018). CDC Grand Rounds: Improving medication adherence for chronic disease management — Innovations and opportunities. *American Journal of Transplantation*, 18(2), 514–517. DOI: 10.1111/ajt.14649 PMID: 29381269

Neto, M. M., Coutinho, E. F., Moreira, L. O., de Souza, J. N., & Agoulmine, N. (2018). A Proposal for Monitoring People of Health Risk Group Using IoT Technologies. *2018 IEEE 20th International Conference on E-Health Networking, Applications and Services (Healthcom)*, 1–6. DOI: 10.1109/HealthCom.2018.8531196

Newspaper, T. N. (2016). *Fighting cancer in Namibia*.

Nghitanwa Emma Maano*, H. T. (2019). Awareness and perception of women of reproductive age (15-49) regarding breast cancer at Okuryangava clinic, Namibia.

Nguyen, H. D., Chitturi, S., & Maple-Brown, L. J. (2016). Management of diabetes in Indigenous communities: Lessons from the Australian Aboriginal population. *Internal Medicine Journal*, 46(11), 1252–1259. https://doi.org/https://dx.doi.org/10.1111/imj.13123. DOI: 10.1111/imj.13123 PMID: 27130346

NIH. (2001, July 31). *PA-01-124: Patient-Centered Care: Customizing Care to Meet Patients' Needs*. https://grants.nih.gov/grants/guide/pa-files/PA-01-124.html

Nijhawan, R., & Bhatia, S. (2023). Edge-AI tools and techniques for healthcare. In Vyas, S., Upadhyaya, A., Bhargava, D., & Shukla, V. (Eds.), *Edge-AI in Healthcare Trends and Future Perspectives* (p. 14). CRC Press. DOI: 10.1201/9781003244592-2

Nijland, N., van Gemert-Pijnen, J., Kelders, S. M., & Seydel, E. R. 2009. "Evaluation of an Internet-Based Application for Supporting Self-Care of Patients with Diabetes Mellitus Type 2," in *eTELEMED*. DOI: 10.1109/eTELEMED.2009.33

Nilashi, M., Ibrahim, O., Ahmadi, H., Shahmoradi, L., & Farahmand, M. (2018). A hybrid intelligent system for the prediction of Parkinson's disease progression using machine learning techniques. *Biocybernetics and Biomedical Engineering*, 38(1), 1–15. DOI: 10.1016/j.bbe.2017.09.002

Nittas, V., Zecca, C., Kamm, C., Kuhle, J., Chan, A., & Wyl, V. (2023). Digital health for chronic disease management: An exploratory method to investigating technology adoption potential. *PLoS One*, 18(4), e0284477. Advance online publication. DOI: 10.1371/journal.pone.0284477 PMID: 37053272

Nugraha, B., Ekasurya, I., Osman, G., & Alaydrus, M. (2017). Analysis of Power Consumption Efficiency on Various IoT and Cloud-Based Wireless Health Monitoring Systems: A Survey. *International Journal of Information Technology and Computer Science*, 9(5), 31–39. DOI: 10.5815/ijitcs.2017.05.05

Nunnally, J. C. (1978). *Psychometric Theory* (2nd ed.). McGraw-Hill.

Nwosu, A. C., Sturgeon, B., McGlinchey, T., Goodwin, C. D., Behera, A., Mason, S., Stanley, S., & Payne, T. R. (2019). Robotic technology for palliative and supportive care: Strengths, weaknesses, opportunities and threats. *Palliative Medicine*, 33(8), 1106–1113. DOI: 10.1177/0269216319857628 PMID: 31250734

Nyasulu, T. (2016). Smart under-five health care system. *2016 IST-Africa Week Conference*, 1–8. DOI: 10.1109/ISTAFRICA.2016.7530674

Obayya, M., Alhebri, A., Maashi, M., Salama, S., Mustafa, A., Hilal, A., Alsaid, M. I., & Alneil, A. A. (2023). Henry Gas Solubility Optimization Algorithm based Feature Extraction in Dermoscopic Images Analysis of Skin Cancer. *Cancers (Basel)*, 15(7). Advance online publication. DOI: 10.3390/cancers15072146 PMID: 37046806

Obermeyer, Z., Powers, B., Vogeli, C., & Mullainathan, S. (2019). Dissecting racial bias in an algorithm used to manage the health of populations. *Science*, 366(6464), 447–453. DOI: 10.1126/science.aax2342 PMID: 31649194

Observatory, G. (2011). *mHealth: New horizons for health through mobile technologies*. Switzerland: World Health Organization.

Office for National Statistics. Living longer: how our population is changing and why it matters. Overview of population ageing in the UK and some implications for the economy, public services, society and the individual. Office for National Statistics. https://www.ons.gov.uk/peoplepopulationandcommunity/birthsdeathsandmarriages/ageing/articles/livinglongerhowourpopulationischangingandwhyitmatters/2018-08 -13. Census 2021. Accessed 26 October 2022.

Olde Keizer, R. A., van Velsen, L., Moncharmont, M., Riche, B., Ammour, N., Del Signore, S., Zia, G., Hermens, H., & N'Dja, A. (2019). Using socially assistive robots for monitoring and preventing frailty among older adults: A study on usability and user experience challenges. *Health and Technology*, 9(4), 595–605. DOI: 10.1007/s12553-019-00320-9

Omar, E., Garaix, T., Augusto, V., & Xie, X. (2015). A stochastic optimization model for shift scheduling in emergency departments. *Health Care Management Science*, 18(3), 289–302. DOI: 10.1007/s10729-014-9300-4 PMID: 25270574

Onakpojeruo, E., Al-Turjman, F., Mustapha, M., Altrjman, C., & Ozsahin, D. (2022). Emerging AI and cloud computing paradigms applied to healthcare. International Conference on Forthcoming Networks and Sustainability (p. 2022.2557). Cyprus: IET. DOI: 10.1049/icp.2022.2557

Onasanya, A., Lakkis, S., & Elshakankiri, M. (2019). Implementing IoT/WSN based smart Saskatchewan Healthcare System. *Wireless Networks*, 1(7), 3999–4020. Advance online publication. DOI: 10.1007/s11276-018-01931-2

Oncology, A. S. (n.d.). *Cancer.Net Mobile*. Retrieved from Cancer.Net: https://www.cancer.net/navigating-cancer-care/managing-your-care/cancernet-mobile

Ong, S. K., Zhao, M. Y., & Nee, A. Y. C. (2023). Augmented Reality-Assisted Healthcare Exercising Systems. In Springer Handbook of Augmented Reality, pp. 743-763. DOI: 10.1007/978-3-030-67822-7_30

Organization, W. H. (2010, January). *Cancer Fact Sheet*. Retrieved from World Health Organization: www.who.int/cancer/fact-sheet/

Organization, W. H. (2014). *Namibia Cancer Profile*. World Health Organization.

Oriwoh, E., & Conrad, M. (2015). *'Things' in the Internet of Things: Towards a Definition*. 5.

Ostchega, Y., Fryar, C. D., Nwankwo, T., & Nguyen, D. T. (2020). Hypertension prevalence among adults aged 18 and over: United States, 2017–2018, NCHS, National Health and Nutrition Examination Survey, 2017–2018: https://stacks.cdc.gov/view/cdc/87559

Ostertagová, E. (2012, December). Modelling using polynomial regression. *Procedia Engineering*, 48, 500–506. DOI: 10.1016/j.proeng.2012.09.545

Ozturk, O., Begen, M. A., & Zaric, G. S. (2014). A branch and bound based heuristic for makespan minimization of washing operations in hospital sterilization services. *European Journal of Operational Research*, 239(1), 214–226. DOI: 10.1016/j.ejor.2014.05.014

Paas, F., Renkl, A., & Sweller, J. (2003). Cognitive Load Theory and instructional design: Recent developments. *Educational Psychologist*, 38(1), 1–4. DOI: 10.1207/S15326985EP3801_1

Pace, P., Aloi, G., Caliciuri, G., Gravina, R., Savaglio, C., Fortino, G., Ibanez-Sanchez, G., Fides-Valero, A., Bayo-Monton, J., Uberti, M., Corona, M., Bernini, L., Gulino, M., Costa, A., De Luca, I., & Mortara, M. (2019). INTER-Health: An Interoperable IoT Solution for Active and Assisted Living Healthcare Services. *2019 IEEE 5th World Forum on Internet of Things (WF-IoT)*, 81–86. DOI: 10.1109/WF-IoT.2019.8767332

Page, M. J., McKenzie, J. E., Bossuyt, P. M., Boutron, I., Hoffmann, T. C., Mulrow, C. D., Shamseer, L., Tetzlaff, J. M., Akl, E. A., Brennan, S. E., Chou, R., Glanville, J., Grimshaw, J. M., Hróbjartsson, A., Lalu, M. M., Li, T., Loder, E. W., Mayo-Wilson, E., McDonald, S., & Moher, D. (2021). The PRISMA 2020 statement: An updated guideline for reporting systematic reviews. *BMJ (Clinical Research Ed.)*, 372(71), n71. Advance online publication. DOI: 10.1136/bmj.n71 PMID: 33782057

Pal, T., Saha, R., Sen, S., Saif, S., & Biswas, S. (2022). Architecture for Smart Healthcare: Cloud Versus Edge. In S. Biswas, C. Chowdhury, B. Acharya, & C. Liu, Internet of Things Based Smart Healthcare-Intelligent and Secure Solutions Applying Machine Learning Techniques (pp. 23-48). Singapore: Springer Singapore. DOI: 10.1007/978-981-19-1408-9_2

Pal, A., Rath, H. K., Shailendra, S., & Bhattacharyya, A. (2018). *IoT Standardization: The Road Ahead. Internet of Things - Technology*. Applications and Standardization., DOI: 10.5772/intechopen.75137

Panagioti, M., Richardson, G., Murray, E., Rogers, A., Kennedy, A., Newman, S., Small, N., & Bower, P. (2014). *Reducing Care Utilisation through Self-management Interventions (RECURSIVE): A systematic review and meta-analysis*. NIHR Journals Library. https://www.ncbi.nlm.nih.gov/books/NBK263888/

Pantalone, K. M., Hobbs, T. M., Wells, B. J., Kong, S. X., Kattan, M. W., Bouchard, J., Yu, C., Sakurada, B., Milinovich, A., Weng, W., Bauman, J. M., & Zimmerman, R. S. (2015). Clinical characteristics, complications, comorbidities and treatment patterns among patients with type 2 diabetes mellitus in a large integrated health system. *BMJ Open Diabetes Research & Care*, 3(1), e000093. DOI: 10.1136/bmjdrc-2015-000093 PMID: 26217493

Panthakkan, A., Anzar, S. M., Jamal, S., & Mansoor, W. (2022). Concatenated Xception-ResNet50 — A novel hybrid approach for accurate skin cancer prediction. *Computers in Biology and Medicine*, 150, 106170. Advance online publication. DOI: 10.1016/j.compbiomed.2022.106170 PMID: 37859280

Papadopoulos, I., Koulouglioti, C., Lazzarino, R., & Ali, S. (2020). Enablers and barriers to the implementation of socially assistive humanoid robots in health and social care: A systematic review. *BMJ Open*, 2020(1), 10. DOI: 10.1136/bmjopen-2019-033096 PMID: 31924639

Papadopoulos, P., Soflano, M., Chaudy, Y., Adejo, W., & Connolly, T. M. (2022). A systematic review of technologies and standards used in the development of rule-based clinical decision support systems. *Health and Technology*, 12(4), 713–727. DOI: 10.1007/s12553-022-00672-9

Parliament, U. K. Parliamentary Office of Science & Technology (POST). Robotics in Social Care. 2018 (12 December). Available from: https://post.parliament.uk/research-briefings/post-pn-0591

Parviainen, J., & Pirhonen, J. (2017). Vulnerable bodies in human–robot interactions: Embodiment as ethical issue in robot care for the elderly.

Patangia, B., Sankruthyayana, R. G., Sathiyaseelan, A., & Balasundaram, S. (2021). How could Mindfulness Help? A Perspective on the Applications of Mindfulness in Enhancing Tomorrow's Workplace. *i-Manager's. Journal of Management*, 16(3), 52.

Patel, V., Moosa, S., Sundaram, S., Langer, L., MacMillan, T. E., Cavalcanti, R., Cram, P., Gunaratne, K., Bayley, M., & Wu, R. (2022). Perceptions of patients and nurses regarding the use of wearables in inpatient settings: A mixed methods study. *Informatics for Health & Social Care*, 47(4), 444–452. DOI: 10.1080/17538157.2022.2042304

Pătrașcu, A. 2014. "Document Management Processes and Use Case Scenarios Elaboration.," *Economic Insights - Trends & Challenges* (66:3), pp. 91–98.

Pazvakawambwa, L., & Embela, S. P. (2017). Prevalence, trends and risk factors of Breast Cancer Mortality in Namibia: 200-2015. Retrieved from https://repository .unam.edu.na/server/api/core/bitstreams/fcc5998a-c36f-454f-ba31-285d6d79513a/ content

Peak, J., Barrett, H., Halloran, J., & Szczepura, A. (2019). All for one and one for all? Can communities in care homes support ageing in place? National Seminar, Possibilities of DDRI in Senior People's Care in Japan, (Poster).

Pearce, J., Mann, M. K., Jones, C., Van Buschbach, S., Olff, M., & Bisson, J. I. (2012). The most effective way of delivering a Train-the-Trainers program: A systematic review. *The Journal of Continuing Education in the Health Professions*, 32(3), 215–226. DOI: 10.1002/chp.21148 PMID: 23173243

Peeranuch LeSeure, S. C. (2015). The Experience of Caregivers Living with Cancer Patients: A Systematic Review and Meta-Synthesis. *Journal of Personalized Medicine*, 5(4), 406–439. DOI: 10.3390/jpm5040406 PMID: 26610573

Pegoraro, V., Bidoli, C., Dal Mas, F., Bert, F., Cobianchi, L., Zantedeschi, M., Campostrini, S., Migliore, F., & Boriani, G. (2023). Cardiology in a digital age: opportunities and challenges for e-health: a literature review. *Journal of Clinical Medicine*, 12(13), 4278. DOI: 10.3390/jcm12134278 PMID: 37445312

Pekmezaris, R., Williams, M. S., Pascarelli, B., Finuf, K. D., Harris, Y. T., Myers, A. K., Taylor, T., Kline, M., Patel, V. H., Murray, L. M., McFarlane, S. I., Pappas, K., Lesser, M. L., Makaryus, A. N., Martinez, S., Kozikowski, A., Polo, J., Guzman, J., Zeltser, R., & Granville, D. (2020). Adapting a home telemonitoring intervention for underserved Hispanic/Latino patients with type 2 diabetes: An acceptability and feasibility study [Article]. *BMC Medical Informatics and Decision Making*, 20(1), 324. Advance online publication. DOI: 10.1186/s12911-020-01346-0 PMID: 33287815

Peng, Y., & Nagata, M. H. (2020). An empirical overview of nonlinearity and overfitting in machine learning using COVID-19 data. *Chaos, Solitons, and Fractals*, 139, 110055. Advance online publication. DOI: 10.1016/j.chaos.2020.110055 PMID: 32834608

Perego, P., Scagnoli, M., & Sironi, R. (2021). *Co-design the acceptability of wearables in the healthcare field*. 21–32.

Petersen, R. C. (2016). Mild cognitive impairment. *CONTINUUM: Lifelong Learning in Neurology*, 22(2 Dementia), 404-418.

Petersen, R. C., Lopez, O., & Armstrong, M. J.. (2018). Practice guideline update summary: Mild cognitive impairment: Report of the Guideline Development, Dissemination, and Implementation Subcommittee of the American Academy of Neurology. *Neurology*, 90(3), 126–135. DOI: 10.1212/WNL.0000000000004826

Pham, M., Mengistu, Y., Do, H., & Sheng, W. (2018). Delivering home healthcare through a Cloud-based Smart Home Environment (CoSHE). *Future Generation Computer Systems*, 81, 129–140. DOI: 10.1016/j.future.2017.10.040

Piasek, J., & Wieczorowska-Tobis, K. (2018, July). Acceptance and long-term use of a social robot by elderly users in a domestic environment. In 2018 11th international conference on human system interaction (HSI) (pp. 478-482). IEEE. DOI: 10.1109/HSI.2018.8431348

Pickering, T. G. (2001). Mental stress as a causal factor in the development of hypertension and cardiovascular disease. *Current Hypertension Reports*, 3(3), 249–254. DOI: 10.1007/s11906-001-0047-1 PMID: 11353576

Pierleoni, P., Belli, A., Bazgir, O., Maurizi, L., Paniccia, M., & Palma, L. (2019). A Smart Inertial System for 24h Monitoring and Classification of Tremor and Freezing of Gait in Parkinson's Disease. *IEEE Sensors Journal*, 19(23), 11612–11623. DOI: 10.1109/JSEN.2019.2932584

Pino, M., Boulay, M., Jouen, F., & Rigaud, A. S. (2015). "Are we ready for robots that care for us?" Attitudes and opinions of older adults toward socially assistive robots. *Frontiers in Aging Neuroscience*, 7, 141. DOI: 10.3389/fnagi.2015.00141 PMID: 26257646

Piwek, L., Ellis, D. A., Andrews, S., & Joinson, A. (2016). The Rise of Consumer Health Wearables: Promises and Barriers. *PLoS Medicine*, 13(2), e1001953. Advance online publication. DOI: 10.1371/journal.pmed.1001953 PMID: 26836780

Plaza, A. M., Díaz, J., & Pérez, J. (2018). Software architectures for health care cyber-physical systems: A systematic literature review. *Journal of Software (Malden, MA)*, 30(7), e1930. DOI: 10.1002/smr.1930

Pol, M., Van Nes, F., Van Hartingsveldt, M., Buurman, B., De Rooij, S., & Kröse, B. (2016). Older people's perspectives regarding the use of sensor monitoring in their home. *The Gerontologist*, 56(3), 485–493. DOI: 10.1093/geront/gnu104 PMID: 25384761

Popov, V., Kudryavtseva, E., Katiyar, N., Shishkin, A., Stepanov, S., & Goel, S. (2022). Industry 4.0 and Digitalisation in Healthcare. *Materials (Basel)*, 15(6), 2140. Advance online publication. DOI: 10.3390/ma15062140 PMID: 35329592

Possik, J., Asgary, A., Solis, A. O., Zacharewicz, G., Shafiee, M. A., Najafabadi, M. M., Nadri, N., Guimaraes, A., Iranfar, H., & Ma, P.. (2021). An agent-based modeling and virtual reality application using distributed simulation: Case of a covid-19 intensive care unit. *IEEE Transactions on Engineering Management*, 2022. Brittin J, Araz O.M., Ramirez-Nafarrate A, and Huang T.T. An agent-based simulation model for testing novel obesity interventions in school environment design. *IEEE Transactions on Engineering Management*.

Prasad, V., Bhavsar, M., & Tanwar, S. (2019). Influence of Montoring: Fog and Edge Computing. Scalable Computing: Practice and Experience. DOI: 10.12694/scpe.v20i2.1533

Prev., A. P. (2011). RESEARCH METHODOLOGY a step-by-step guide for beginners. 1751–1763.

Price, W. N., & Cohen, I. G. (2019). Privacy in the age of artificial intelligence. In *Artificial intelligence in health care* (pp. 39–55). Springer., DOI: 10.1007/978-3-030-12723-8_3

Prieto, K. (2022). Current forecast of COVID-19 in Mexico: A Bayesian and machine learning approaches. *PLoS ONE, 17*(1 January), 1–21. DOI: 10.1371/journal.pone.0259958

Prince, J., & De Vos, M. (2018, July). A deep learning framework for the remote detection of Parkinson's disease using smart-phone sensor data. In 2018 40th Annual International Conference of the IEEE Engineering in Medicine and Biology Society (EMBC) (pp. 3144-3147). IEEE.

Puri, A., Kim, B., Nguyen, O., Stolee, P., Tung, J., & Lee, J. (2017). User acceptance of wrist-worn activity trackers among community-dwelling older adults: Mixed method study. *JMIR mHealth and uHealth*, 5(11), e8211. DOI: 10.2196/mhealth.8211 PMID: 29141837

Puri, V., Kumar, R., Le, D. N., Jagdev, S. S., & Sachdeva, N. (2020). BioSenHealth 2.0-a low-cost, energy-efficient Internet of Things-based blood glucose monitoring system. In Balas, V. E., Solanki, V. K., & Kumar, R. (Eds.), *Emergence of Pharmaceutical Industry Growth with Industrial Iot Approach* (pp. 305–324). Academic Press LTD-Elsevier Science LTD., DOI: 10.1016/B978-0-12-819593-2.00011-X

Pustiek, M., Beristain, A., & Kos, A. (2015). Challenges in Wearable Devices Based Pervasive Wellbeing Monitoring. *2015 International Conference on Identification, Information, and Knowledge in the Internet of Things (IIKI)*, 236–243. DOI: 10.1109/IIKI.2015.58

Putri, A. M., Wijaya, K., Salomo, O. A., & Santoso Gunawan, A. A., & Anderies. (2022). A Review Paper: Accuracy of Machine Learning for Depression Detection in Social Media. *2022 IEEE International Conference on Communication, Networks and Satellite (COMNETSAT)*, 39–45. DOI: 10.1109/COMNETSAT56033.2022.9994553

Quintero, L. (2019). *Facilitating Technology-based Mental Health Interventions with Mobile Virtual Reality and Wearable Smartwatches* (Doctoral dissertation, Department of Computer and Systems Sciences, Stockholm University).

Quy, V., Hau, N., Anh, D., & Ngoc, L. (2022). Smart healthcare IoT applications based on fog computing: Architecture, applications and challenges. *Complex & Intelligent Systems*, 8(5), 3805–3815. DOI: 10.1007/s40747-021-00582-9 PMID: 34804767

Radovic, , ABadawy, , S. M. (2020). Technology use for adolescent health and wellness. *Pediatrics*, 145(Supplement_2), S186–S194.

Rahimi, I., Chen, F., & Gandomi, A. H. (2023). A review on COVID-19 forecasting models. *Neural Computing & Applications*, 35(33), 23671–23681. DOI: 10.1007/s00521-020-05626-8 PMID: 33564213

Rahman, Md. A., & Hossain, M. S. (2018). M-Therapy: A Multisensor Framework for in-Home Therapy Management: A Social Therapy of Things Perspective. *IEEE Internet of Things Journal, 5*(4, SI), 2548–2556. DOI: 10.1109/JIOT.2017.2776150

Rahmani, A. M., Gia, T. N., Negash, B., Anzanpour, A., Azimi, I., Jiang, M., & Liljeberg, P. (2018). Exploiting smart e-Health gateways at the edge of healthcare Internet-of-Things: A fog computing approach. *Future Generation Computer Systems*, 78, 641–658. DOI: 10.1016/j.future.2017.02.014

Rahman, M., & Hossain, M. S. (2019). A cloud-based virtual caregiver for elderly people in a cyber physical IoT system. *Cluster Computing*, 22(1), 2317–2330. DOI: 10.1007/s10586-018-1806-y

Rahman, M., Peeri, N. C., Shrestha, N., Zaki, R., Haque, U., & Hamid, S. H. A. (2020, June). S., Peeri, N. C., Shrestha, N., Zaki, R., Haque, U., & Hamid, S. H. A. (2020). Defending against the Novel Coronavirus (COVID-19) Outbreak: How Can the Internet of Things (IoT) help to save the World? *Health Policy and Technology*, 9(2), 136–138. Advance online publication. DOI: 10.1016/j.hlpt.2020.04.005 PMID: 32322475

Rahman, R. A., Omar, K., Mohd Noah, S. A., Danuri, M. S. N. M., & Al-Garadi, M. A. (2020). Application of Machine Learning Methods in Mental Health Detection: A Systematic Review. *IEEE Access : Practical Innovations, Open Solutions*, 8, 183952–183964. DOI: 10.1109/ACCESS.2020.3029154

Rajeshkumar, K., Ananth, C., & Mohananthini, N. (2023). Optimal Hybrid Image Encryption with Machine Learning Model for Blockchain-Assisted Secure Skin Lesion Diagnosis. *International Journal of Engineering Trends and Technology*, 71(6), 96–106. Advance online publication. DOI: 10.14445/22315381/IJETT-V71I6P211

Rajesh, P., Murugan, A., Muruganantham, B., & Ganesh Kumar, S. (2020). Lung Cancer Diagnosis and Treatment Using AI and Mobile Applications. *International Journal of Interactive Mobile Technologies*, 14(17), 189. Advance online publication. DOI: 10.3991/ijim.v14i17.16607

Raj, S. (2020). An Efficient IoT-Based Platform for Remote Real-Time Cardiac Activity Monitoring. *IEEE Transactions on Consumer Electronics*, 66(2), 106–114. DOI: 10.1109/TCE.2020.2981511

Rakibul, M., & Islam, B. B. (n.d.). Barriers to Cervical Cancer and Breast Cancer Screening Uptake in Low-Income and Middle-Income Countries. *Systematic Reviews*.

Raoof, S., & Durai, M. (2022). A Comprehensive Review on Smart Health Care: Applications, Paradigms, and Challenges with Case Studies. *Contrast Media & Molecular Imaging*, 18(1), 4822235. Advance online publication. DOI: 10.1155/2022/4822235

Raskar, R., Welch, G., & Fuchs, H. (1998). Spatially Augmented Reality, *First International Workshop on Augmented Reality*, San Francisco.

Rathore, M. M., Ahmad, A., Paul, A., Wan, J., & Zhang, D. (2016). Real-time Medical Emergency Response System: Exploiting IoT and Big Data for Public Health. *Journal of Medical Systems*, 40(12), 283. DOI: 10.1007/s10916-016-0647-6 PMID: 27796839

Rathore, P. S., & Sharma, B. K. (2022). Improving Healthcare Delivery System using Business Intelligence. *Journal of IoT in Social, Mobile, Analytics, and Cloud*, 4(1), 11–23. DOI: 10.36548/jismac.2022.1.002

Rath, S., Tripathy, A., & Tripathy, A. R. (2020). Prediction of new active cases of coronavirus disease (COVID-19) pandemic using multiple linear regression model. *Diabetes & Metabolic Syndrome*, 14(5), 1467–1474. DOI: 10.1016/j.dsx.2020.07.045 PMID: 32771920

Ray, J., Kumar, S., Pandey, S., & Akram, S. V. (2023, June). The Role of Augmented Reality and Virtual Reality in Shaping the Future of Health Psychology. In *2023 3rd International Conference on Pervasive Computing and Social Networking (ICPCSN)* (pp. 1604-1608). IEEE. DOI: 10.1109/ICPCSN58827.2023.00268

Ray, P. P. (2018). A survey on Internet of Things architectures. *Journal of King Saud University. Computer and Information Sciences*, 30(3), 291–319. DOI: 10.1016/j.jksuci.2016.10.003

Rebecca, L., & Siegel, K. D. (2020). Cancer Statistics 2020. *American Cancer Society*, 7-30.

Reeder, B., Chung, J., Joe, J., Lazar, A., Thompson, H. J., & Demiris, G. (2016). Understanding older adults' perceptions of in-home sensors using an obtrusiveness framework. In Foundations of Augmented Cognition: Neuroergonomics and Operational Neuroscience: 10th International Conference, AC 2016, Held as Part of HCI International 2016, Toronto, ON, Canada, July 17-22, 2016 [Springer International Publishing.]. *Proceedings*, 10(Part II), 351–360.

Reger, G. M. (Ed.). (2020). *Technology and mental health: a clinician's guide to improving outcomes*. Routledge. DOI: 10.4324/9780429020537

Rehman, H., Kamal, A. K., Sayani, S., Morris, P. B., Merchant, A. T., & Virani, S. S. (2017). Using mobile health (mHealth) technology in the management of diabetes mellitus, physical inactivity, and smoking. *Current Atherosclerosis Reports*, 19(4), 1–11. DOI: 10.1007/s11883-017-0650-5 PMID: 28243807

Rghioui, A., Lloret, J., Parra, L., Sendra, S., & Oumnad, A. (2019). Glucose Data Classification for Diabetic Patient Monitoring. In *Applied Sciences-Basel* (Vol. 9, Issue 20). MDPI. DOI: 10.3390/app9204459

Riazul Islam, S. M., Daehan Kwak, , Humaun Kabir, M., Hossain, M., & Kyung-Sup Kwak, . (2015). The Internet of Things for Health Care: A Comprehensive Survey. *IEEE Access : Practical Innovations, Open Solutions*, 3, 678–708. DOI: 10.1109/ACCESS.2015.2437951

Ricciardi, F., Rossignoli, C., & De Marco, M. (2013). Participatory networks for place safety and livability: organisational success factors. *International Journal of Networking and Virtual Organisations 4, 13* (1), 42-65.

Richir, S., Kadri, A., & Ribeyre, N. (2022). Virtual Reality and Augmented Reality to Fight Effectively against Pandemics. In *The Nature of Pandemics* (pp. 311–348). CRC Press. DOI: 10.4324/9781315170220-20

Richmond, L., Rajappan, K., Voth, E., Rangavajhala, V., Earley, M. J., Thomas, G., Harris, S., Sporton, S. C., & Schilling, R. J. (2008). Validation of computed tomography image integration into the EnSite NavX mapping system to perform catheter ablation of atrial fibrillation. *Journal of Cardiovascular Electrophysiology*, 19(8), 821–827. DOI: 10.1111/j.1540-8167.2008.01127.x

Roberts, C. K., & Barnard, R. J. (2005). Effects of exercise and diet on chronic disease. *Journal of Applied Physiology*, 98(1), 3–30. DOI: 10.1152/japplphysiol.00852.2004 PMID: 15591300

Roberts, L. D., Howell, J. A., & Seaman, K. (2017). Give me a customizable dashboard: Personalized learning analytics dashboards in higher education. *Technology. Knowledge and Learning*, 22(3), 317–333. DOI: 10.1007/s10758-017-9316-1

Robey, D. (1996). Research commentary: diversity in information systems research: threat, promise, and responsibility. *Information Systems Research*, (7:4), 400-408.

Rodriguez-Leyva, D., Weighell, W., Edel, A. L., LaVallee, R., Dibrov, E., Pinneker, R., Maddaford, T. G., Ramjiawan, B., Aliani, M., Guzman, R., & Pierce, G. N. (2013). Potent antihypertensive action of dietary flaxseed in hypertensive patients. *Hypertension*, 62(6), 1081–1089. DOI: 10.1161/HYPERTENSIONAHA.113.02094 PMID: 24126178

Ro, H., Park, Y. J., Byun, J. H., & Han, T. D. (2019). Display methods of projection augmented reality based on deep learning pose estimation, *Proceedings of ACM SIGGRAPH 2019*, ACM. DOI: 10.1145/3306214.3338608

Romero-Perales, E., Sainz-de-Baranda Andujar, C., & López-Ongil, C. (2023). Electronic Design for Wearables Devices Addressed from a Gender Perspective: Cross-Influences and a Methodological Proposal. *Sensors (Basel)*, 23(12), 5483. DOI: 10.3390/s23125483

Rosales, C. R., Magazine, M. J., & Rao, U. S. (2019). Dual sourcing and joint replenishment of hospital supplies. *IEEE Transactions on Engineering Management*, 67(3), 918–931. DOI: 10.1109/TEM.2019.2895242

Rose, K., Eldridge, S., & Chapin, L. (2015). *The Internet of Things: An Overview— Understanding the Issues and Challenges of a More Connected World*. Internet Society.

Rossi, A., Puppato, A., & Lanzetta, M. (2013). Heuristics for scheduling a two-stage hybrid flow shop with parallel batching machines: Application at a hospital sterilisation plant. *International Journal of Production Research*, 51(8), 2363–2376. DOI: 10.1080/00207543.2012.737942

Rossi, M. C., Nicolucci, A., Pellegrini, F., Bruttomesso, D., Di Bartolo, P., Marelli, G., & Miselli, V. (2017). Interactive diary for diabetes: A useful and easy-to-use new telemedicine system to support the decision-making process in Type 1 diabetes. *Diabetes Technology & Therapeutics*, 15(1), 18–24. DOI: 10.1089/dia.2012.0091 PMID: 27982707

Rössler, W. (2016). The stigma of mental disorders: A millennia-long history of social exclusion and prejudices. *EMBO Reports*, 17(9), 1250–1253. DOI: 10.15252/embr.201643041 PMID: 27470237

Rupprecht, P., Kueffner-Mccauley, and H., Schlund, S. (2020). Information provision utilizing a dynamic projection system in industrial site assembly, *Procedia CIRP* (93:1), pp. 1182-1187.

Russell, Hugo & Ayliffe's: Principles and Practice of Disinfection. (2013). (pp. 445–458). Preservation and Sterilization.

Rutala, W. A., & Weber, D. J. (2019). Guideline for disinfection and sterilization in healthcare facilities, 2008. update: May 2019.

Ryan, P. 2009. "Integrated Theory of Health Behavior Change: Background and Intervention Development," *Clin Nurse Spec* (23:3), pp. 161–172.

Ryan, P., and Sawin, K. J. 2009. "The Individual and Family Self-Management Theory: Background and Perspectives on Context, Process, and Outcomes," *Nursing Outlook* (57:4), pp. 217-225.e6. ().DOI: 10.1016/j.outlook.2008.10.004

Sääskilahti, K., Kangaskorte, R., Pieskä, S., Jauhiainen, J., & Luimula, M. (2012). Needs and user acceptance of older adults for mobile service robot. 2012 IEEE RO-MAN: The 21st IEEE International Symposium on Robots and Human Interactive Communication (pp. 559-564). Paris, France: IEEE. Paris, France: IEEE.

Sadoughi, F., Behmanesh, A., & Sayfouri, N. (2020). Internet of things in medicine: A systematic mapping study. *Journal of Biomedical Informatics*, 103, 103383. DOI: 10.1016/j.jbi.2020.103383 PMID: 32044417

Safia Naveed, S. (2023). Prediction of breast cancer through Random Forest. *Current Medical Imaging*, 19(10).

Saha, J., Saha, A. K., Chatterjee, A., Agrawal, S., Saha, A., Kar, A., & Saha, H. N. (2018). Advanced IOT based combined remote health monitoring, home automation and alarm system. *2018 IEEE 8th Annual Computing and Communication Workshop and Conference (CCWC)*, 602–606. DOI: 10.1109/CCWC.2018.8301659

Said, O., & Masud, M. (2013). *Towards Internet of Things: Survey and Future Vision*. 17.

Saju, B., Asha, V., Murali, S. C., Vinayaka, D., Kumar, V., & Nithya, B. (2022). ML based Prototype for Skin Cancer Detection. In *Proceedings of the 2022 3rd International Conference on Communication, Computing and Industry 4.0, C2I4 2022*. Retrieved from https://doi.org/DOI: 10.1109/C2I456876.2022.10051378

Sakar, B. E., Serbes, G., & Sakar, C. O. (2017). Analyzing the effectiveness of vocal features in early telediagnosis of Parkinson's disease. *PLoS One*, 12(8), e0182428. DOI: 10.1371/journal.pone.0182428 PMID: 28792979

Sakthi, A. S., Inbamani, A., Elango, R., Niveda, S., Preethi, M., Rajalakshmi, R., & Veerasamy, V. (2022). Healthcare Solutions Using Wearable Devices. In *Smart and Secure Internet of Healthcare Things* (pp. 1–16). CRC Press. DOI: 10.1201/9781003239895-1

Salas-Zárate, R., Alor-Hernández, G., Salas-Zárate, M. del P., Paredes-Valverde, M. A., Bustos-López, M., & Sánchez-Cervantes, J. L. (2022). Detecting Depression Signs on Social Media: A Systematic Literature Review. *Health Care*, 10(2), 2. Advance online publication. DOI: 10.3390/healthcare10020291 PMID: 35206905

Salmanpour, M. R., Shamsaei, M., Saberi, A., Setayeshi, S., Klyuzhin, I. S., Sossi, V., & Rahmim, A. (2019). Optimized machine learning methods for prediction of cognitive outcome in Parkinson's disease. *Computers in Biology and Medicine*, 111, 103347. DOI: 10.1016/j.compbiomed.2019.103347 PMID: 31284154

Sam Wambugu, C. V. (2014). mHealth for Health Information Systems in Low-and-Middle-Income Countries: Challenges and Opportunities in Data Quality, Privacy and Security. *MEASURE Evaluation*, 1-20.

Sanyaolu, A., Okorie, C., Qi, X., Locke, J., & Rehman, S. (2019). Childhood and adolescent obesity in the United States: a public health concern. *Global pediatric health*, 6, 2333794X19891305.

Schneider, M. J. (2020). *Introduction to public health*. Jones & Bartlett Learning.

Schulman-Green, D., Jaser, S., Martin, F., Alonzo, A., Grey, M., McCorkle, R., Redeker, N. S., Reynolds, N., and Whittemore, R. 2012. "Processes of Self-Management in Chronic Illness," *Journal of Nursing Scholarship* (44:2), pp. 136–144.

Science Council of Japan. (2020). *Clinical Medicine Committee/Health/Life Science Committee Joint Care Science Subcommittee in an Aging Society with a Declining Birthrate, Recommendation: Forming the Foundation of Care Science and Creating a Future Society*. Science Council of Japan. (in Japanese)

Sefcik, J. S., Johnson, M. J., Yim, M., Lau, T., Vivio, N., Mucchiani, C., & Cacchione, P. Z. (2018). Stakeholders' perceptions sought to inform the development of a low-cost mobile robot for older adults: A qualitative descriptive study. *Clinical Nursing Research*, 27(1), 61–80. DOI: 10.1177/1054773817730517 PMID: 28918654

Segall, R. S., & Sankarasubbu, V. (2022). Survey of Recent Applications of Artificial Intelligence for Detection and Analysis of COVID-19 and Other Infectious Diseases. *International Journal of Artificial Intelligence and Machine Learning*, 12(2), 1–30. Advance online publication. DOI: 10.4018/IJAIML.313574

Sehulster, L. M. (2004). Prion inactivation and medical instrument reprocessing: Challenges facing healthcare facilities. *Infection Control and Hospital Epidemiology*, 25(4), 276–279. DOI: 10.1086/502391 PMID: 15108722

Seidel, D., Richardson, K., Crilly, N., Matthews, F. E., Clarkson, P. J., & Brayne, C. (2010). Design for independent living: Activity demands and capabilities of older people. *Ageing and Society*, 30(7), 1239–1255. DOI: 10.1017/S0144686X10000310

Self Care Forum. (2020). *What do we mean by self care and why is it good for people?* https://www.selfcareforum.org/about-us/what-do-we-mean-by-self-care -and-why-is-good-for-people/

Senbekov, M., Saliev, T., Bukeyeva, Z., Almabayeva, A., Zhanaliyeva, M., Aitenova, N., Toishibekov, Y., & Fakhradiyev, I. (2020). The recent progress and applications of digital technologies in healthcare: A review. *International Journal of Telemedicine and Applications*, 2020, 2020. DOI: 10.1155/2020/8830200 PMID: 33343657

Seneviratne, S., Hu, Y., Nguyen, T., Lan, G., Khalifa, S., Thilakarathna, K., Hassan, M., & Seneviratne, A. (2017). A Survey of Wearable Devices and Challenges. *IEEE Communications Surveys Tutorials, 19*(4), 2573–2620. *IEEE Communications Surveys and Tutorials*. Advance online publication. DOI: 10.1109/COMST.2017.2731979

Seng, K., Ang, L., & Ngharamike, E. (2022). Artificial intelligence Internet of Things: A new paradigm of distributed sensor networks. *International Journal of Distributed Sensor Networks*, 18(3). Advance online publication. DOI: 10.1177/15501477211062835

Sethi, P., & Sarangi, S. R. (2017). Internet of Things: Architectures, Protocols, and Applications. *Journal of Electrical and Computer Engineering*, 2017, 1–25. DOI: 10.1155/2017/9324035

Sewal, P., & Singh, H. (2022). A Machine Learning Approach for Predicting Execution Statistics of Spark Application. *PDGC 2022 - 2022 7th International Conference on Parallel, Distributed and Grid Computing*, 331–336. DOI: 10.1109/PDGC56933.2022.10053356

Sewal, P., & Singh, H. (2023). Analyzing distributed Spark MLlib regression algorithms for accuracy, execution efficiency and scalability using best subset selection approach. *Multimedia Tools and Applications*, 0123456789(15), 44047–44066. Advance online publication. DOI: 10.1007/s11042-023-17330-5

Sewal, P., & Singh, H. (2024). Performance Comparison of Apache Spark and Hadoop for machine learning based iterative GBTR on HIGGS and Covid-19 datasets. *Scalable Computing: Practice and Experience*, 25(3), 1373–1386. DOI: 10.12694/scpe.v25i3.2687

Shafik, W. (2024b). Data-Driven Future Trends and Innovation in Telemedicine. In *Improving Security, Privacy, and Connectivity Among Telemedicine Platforms* (pp. 93-118). IGI Global. https://doi.org/DOI: 10.4018/979-8-3693-2141-6.ch005

Shafik, W. (2024d). IoMT Future Trends and Challenges: Emerging Technologies, Policy Implications, and Research Questions. *Lightweight Digital Trust Architectures in the Internet of Medical Things* (IoMT), 348-370. https://doi.org/DOI: 10.4018/979-8-3693-2109-6.ch019

Shafik, W. (2024e). IoT-Enabled Secure and Intelligent Smart Healthcare: Beyond 5G in Enabling Smart Cities. In *Secure and Intelligent IoT-Enabled Smart Cities* (pp. 308-333). IGI Global. https://doi.org/DOI: 10.4018/979-8-3693-2373-1.ch015

Shafik, W., Hidayatullah, A. F., Kalinaki, K., & Aslam, M. M. (2024a). Artificial Intelligence (AI)-Assisted Computer Vision (CV) in Healthcare Systems. In *Computer Vision and AI-Integrated IoT Technologies in the Medical Ecosystem* (pp. 17-36). CRC Press. https://doi.org/DOI: 10.1201/9781003429609-2

Shafik, W., Tufail, A., Liyanage, C. D. S., & Apong, R. A. A. H. M. (2024b). Medical Robotics and AI-Assisted Diagnostics Challenges for Smart Sustainable Healthcare. In *AI-Driven Innovations in Digital Healthcare: Emerging Trends, Challenges, and Applications* (pp. 304-323). IGI Global. https://doi.org/DOI: 10.4018/979-8-3693-3218-4.ch016

Shafik, W. (2023). *Artificial intelligence and Blockchain technology enabling cybersecurity in telehealth systems. Artificial Intelligence and Blockchain Technology in Modern Telehealth Systems* (Vol. 1). IET., DOI: 10.1049/PBHE061E_ch11

Shafik, W. (2024a). Artificial Intelligence and the Medical Tourism. In *Examining Tourist Behaviors and Community Involvement in Destination Rejuvenation* (pp. 207–233). IGI Global., DOI: 10.4018/979-8-3693-6819-0.ch016

Shafik, W. (2024c). Digital healthcare systems in a federated learning perspective. In *Federated Learning for Digital Healthcare Systems* (pp. 1–35). Academic Press., DOI: 10.1016/B978-0-443-13897-3.00001-1

Shafik, W. (2024f). Science of Emotional Intelligence. In *Enhancing and Predicting Digital Consumer Behavior with AI* (pp. 284–310). IGI Global., DOI: 10.4018/979-8-3693-4453-8.ch015

Shafik, W. (2024g). *The Future of Healthcare: AIoMT—Redefining Healthcare with Advanced Artificial Intelligence and Machine Learning Techniques. Artificial Intelligence and Machine Learning in Drug Design and Development.* Wiley., DOI: 10.1002/9781394234196.ch19

Shafik, W. (2024h). Toward a More Ethical Future of Artificial Intelligence and Data Science. In *The Ethical Frontier of AI and Data Analysis* (pp. 362–388). IGI Global., DOI: 10.4018/979-8-3693-2964-1.ch022

Shankar, K., Perumal, E., & Gupta, D. (2021). *Artificial Intelligence for the Internet of Health Things.* CRC Press., DOI: 10.1201/9781003159094

Sharma, A., Harrington, R. A., McClellan, M. B., Turakhia, M. P., Eapen, Z. J., Steinhubl, S., Mault, J. R., Majmudar, M. D., Roessig, L., Chandross, K. J., Green, E. M., Patel, B., Hamer, A., Olgin, J., Rumsfeld, J. S., Roe, M. T., & Peterson, E. D. (2018). Using digital health technology to better generate evidence and deliver evidence-based care. *Journal of the American College of Cardiology*, 71(23), 2680–2690. DOI: 10.1016/j.jacc.2018.03.523 PMID: 29880129

Sharma, A., & Singh, B. (2022). Measuring Impact of E-commerce on Small Scale Business: A Systematic Review. *Journal of Corporate Governance and International Business Law*, 5(1).

Shastry, K. A., & Sanjay, H. A. (2022). Cancer diagnosis using artificial intelligence: A review. *Artificial Intelligence Review*, 55(4), 2641–2673. Advance online publication. DOI: 10.1007/s10462-021-10074-4

Shaw, F. E., Asomugha, C. N., Conway, P. H., & Rein, A. S. (2024). The Patient Protection and Affordable Care Act: Opportunities for prevention and public health. *Lancet*, 384(9937), 75–82. DOI: 10.1016/S0140-6736(14)60259-2 PMID: 24993913

Shinde, G. R., Kalamkar, A. B., Mahalle, P. N., Dey, N., Chaki, J., & Hassanien, A. E. (2020). Forecasting Models for Coronavirus Disease (COVID-19): A Survey of the State-of-the-Art. *SN Computer Science*, 1(4), 197. Advance online publication. DOI: 10.1007/s42979-020-00209-9 PMID: 33063048

Shiomi, M., Iio, T., Kamei, K., Sharma, C., & Hagita, N. (2015). Effectiveness of social behaviors for autonomous wheelchair robot to support elderly people in Japan. *PLoS One*, 10(5), e0128031. DOI: 10.1371/journal.pone.0128031 PMID: 25993038

Shore, L., de Eyto, A., & O'Sullivan, L. (2022). Technology acceptance and perceptions of robotic assistive devices by older adults–implications for exoskeleton design. *Disability and Rehabilitation. Assistive Technology*, 17(7), 782–790. DOI: 10.1080/17483107.2020.1817988 PMID: 32988251

Shore, L., Power, V., De Eyto, A., & O'Sullivan, L. W. (2018). Technology acceptance and user-centred design of assistive exoskeletons for older adults: A commentary. *Robotics (Basel, Switzerland)*, 7(1), 3. DOI: 10.3390/robotics7010003

Shrivastava, P., Shukla, A., Vepakomma, P., Bhansali, N., & Verma, K. (2017). A survey of nature-inspired algorithms for feature selection to identify Parkinson's disease. *Computer Methods and Programs in Biomedicine*, 139, 171–179. DOI: 10.1016/j.cmpb.2016.07.029 PMID: 28187888

Siervo, M., Lara, J., Chowdhury, S., Ashor, A., Oggioni, C., & Mathers, J. C. (2015). Effects of the Dietary Approach to Stop Hypertension (DASH) diet on cardiovascular risk factors: A systematic review and meta-analysis. *British Journal of Nutrition*, 113(1), 1–15. DOI: 10.1017/S0007114514003341 PMID: 25430608

Silvello, A. (2017). IoT and Connected Insurance Reshaping The Health Insurance Industry. A Customer-centric "From Cure To Care" Approach. *ICST Transactions on Ambient Systems*, 4(15), 153462. DOI: 10.4108/eai.8-12-2017.153462

Simango, D., Mushiri, T., Yahya, A., & Nyanduwa, L. (2023). Brain tumor detection and classification based on machine learning systems. In *AIP Conference Proceedings* (Vol. 2581). Retrieved from https://doi.org/DOI: 10.1063/5.0126334

Simons, L. P. A. (2020a). Health 2050: Bioinformatics for Rapid Self-Repair; A Design Analysis for Future Quantified Self, pp. 247-261, *33rd Bled eConference*. June 28-29, Bled, Slovenia, Proceedings retrieval from www.bledconference.org. ISBN-13: 978-961-286-362-3, DOI: https://doi.org/DOI: 10.18690/978-961-286-362-3.17

Simons, L. P. A., & Hampe, J. F. (2010). Service Experience Design for Healthy Living Support; Comparing an In-House with an eHealth Solution. The *23rd Bled eConference*, pp. 423-440. Accessed 2010 from www.bledconference.org

Simons, L. P. A., Foerster, F., Bruck, P. A., Motiwalla, L., & Jonker, C. M. (2014b). Microlearning mApp to Improve Long Term Health Behaviours: Design and Test of Multi-Channel Service Mix. Paper presented at the 27th Bled eConference. Bled, Slovenia, Proceedings. Retrieval from www.bledconference.org and https://aisel .aisnet.org/bled2014/4

Simons, L. P. A., Gerritsen, B., Wielaard, B., & Neerincx, M. A. (2022a). Health Self-Management Support with Microlearning to Improve Hypertension, pp. 511-524, *35th Bled eConference*. June 26-29, Bled, Slovenia, Proceedings retrieval from www.bledconference.org. ISBN-13: 978-961-286-616-7, DOI: DOI: 10.18690/um/ fov.4.2022

Simons, L. P. A., Neerincx, M. A., & Jonker, C. M. (2021). Health Literature Hybrid AI for Health Improvement; A Design Analysis for Diabetes & Hypertension, pp. 184-197, *34th Bled eConference*. June 27-30, Bled, Slovenia, Proceedings retrieval from www.bledconference.org. ISBN-13: 978-961-286-385-9, DOI: https://doi.org/ DOI: 10.18690/978-961-286-385-9

Simons, L. P. A., van den Heuvel, A. C., & Jonker, C. M. (2018). eHealth WhatsApp Group for Social Support; Preliminary Results, pp. 225-237, *presented at the 31st Bled eConference*. Bled, Slovenia, Proceedings retrieval from www.bledconference .org. ISBN-13: 978-961-286-170-4, DOI: https://doi.org/DOI: 10.18690/978-961- 286-170-4

Simons, L. P., Pijl, H., Verhoef, J., Lamb, H. J., ... (2016). Intensive Lifestyle (e) Support to Reverse Diabetes-2. In *Bled eConference* (p. 24), accessed Dec 20, 2016 www.bledconference.org

Simons, LPA, Gerritsen, B, Wielaard, B, Neerincx MA (2023). Hypertension Self-Management Success in 2 weeks; 3 Pilot Studies, pp.19-34, *36th Bled eConference*. June 25-28, Bled, Slovenia, Proceedings. ISBN-13: 978-961-286-751-5, DOI: DOI: 10.18690/um.feri.6.2023

Simons, LPA, Murukannaiah, PK, Neerincx, MA (2024). Designing and Evaluating an LLM-based Health AI Research Assistant for Hypertension Self-Management; Using Health Claims Metadata Criteria, pp.283-298, *37th Bled eConference*. June 9-12, Bled, Slovenia, Proceedings. ISBN-13: 978-961-286-871-0, DOI: DOI: 10.18690/um.fov.4.2024

Simons, L. P. A., Foerster, F., Bruck, P. A., Motiwalla, L., & Jonker, C. M. (2015). Microlearning mApp Raises Health Competence: Hybrid Service Design. *Health and Technology*, 5(1), 35–43. DOI: 10.1007/s12553-015-0095-1 PMID: 26097799

Simons, L. P. A., Hafkamp, M. P. J., Bodegom, D., Dumaij, A., & Jonker, C. M. (2017). Improving Employee Health; Lessons from an RCT. *Int. J. Networking and Virtual Organisations*, 17(4), 341–353. DOI: 10.1504/IJNVO.2017.088485

Simons, L. P. A., Hampe, J. F., & Guldemond, N. A. (2013). Designing Healthy Living Support: Mobile applications added to hybrid (e)Coach Solution. *Health and Technology*, 3(1), 85–95. DOI: 10.1007/s12553-013-0052-9

Simons, L. P. A., Hampe, J. F., & Guldemond, N. A. (2014). ICT supported healthy lifestyle interventions: Design Lessons. *Electronic Markets*, 24(3), 179–192. DOI: 10.1007/s12525-014-0157-7

Simons, L. P. A., Neerincx, M. A., & Jonker, C. M. (2022c). Is Google Making us Smart? Health Self-Management for High Performance Employees & Organisations. *International Journal of Networking and Virtual Organisations*, 27(3), 200–216. DOI: 10.1504/IJNVO.2022.128454

Simons, L. P. A., Pijl, M., Verhoef, J., Lamb, H. J., van Ommen, B., Gerritsen, B., Bizino, M. B., Snel, M., Feenstra, R., & Jonker, C. M. (2022b). e-Health Diabetes; 50 Weeks Evaluation. *International Journal of Biomedical Engineering and Technology*, 38(1), 81–98. DOI: 10.1504/IJBET.2022.120864

Simons, L. P. A., van den Heuvel, A. C., & Jonker, C. M. (2020b). eHealth WhatsApp for social support: Design lessons. *International Journal of Networking and Virtual Organisations*, 23(2), 112–127. DOI: 10.1504/IJNVO.2020.108857

Simons, L. P. A., van den Heuvel, W. A., & Jonker, C. M. (2019). WhatsApp Peer Coaching Lessons for eHealth. In *Handbook of Research on Optimizing Healthcare Management Techniques* (pp. 16–32). IGI Global.

Singh, B. (2023). Blockchain Technology in Renovating Healthcare: Legal and Future Perspectives. In *Revolutionizing Healthcare Through Artificial Intelligence and Internet of Things Applications* (pp. 177-186). IGI Global.

Singh, B., & Kaunert, C. (2024). Future of Digital Marketing: Hyper-Personalized Customer Dynamic Experience with AI-Based Predictive Models. *Revolutionizing the AI-Digital Landscape: A Guide to Sustainable Emerging Technologies for Marketing Professionals*, 189.

Singh, B., & Kaunert, C. (2024). Salvaging Responsible Consumption and Production of Food in the Hospitality Industry: Harnessing Machine Learning and Deep Learning for Zero Food Waste. In *Sustainable Disposal Methods of Food Wastes in Hospitality Operations* (pp. 176-192). IGI Global.

Singh, B., Jain, V., Kaunert, C., & Vig, K. (2024). Shaping Highly Intelligent Internet of Things (IoT) and Wireless Sensors for Smart Cities. In *Secure and Intelligent IoT-Enabled Smart Cities* (pp. 117-140). IGI Global.

Singh, B., Vig, K., & Kaunert, C. (2024). Modernizing Healthcare: Application of Augmented Reality and Virtual Reality in Clinical Practice and Medical Education. In Modern Technology in Healthcare and Medical Education: Blockchain, IoT, AR, and VR (pp. 1-21). IGI Global.

Singhal, A., Singh, P., Lall, B., & Joshi, S. D. (2020). Modeling and prediction of COVID-19 pandemic using Gaussian mixture model. *Chaos, Solitons, and Fractals*, 138, 110023. DOI: 10.1016/j.chaos.2020.110023 PMID: 32565627

Singh, B. (2022). Relevance of Agriculture-Nutrition Linkage for Human Healthcare: A Conceptual Legal Framework of Implication and Pathways. *Justice and Law Bulletin*, 1(1), 44–49.

Singh, B. (2022). Understanding Legal Frameworks Concerning Transgender Healthcare in the Age of Dynamism. *Electronic Journal Of Social And Strategic Studies*, 3(1), 56–65. DOI: 10.47362/EJSSS.2022.3104

Singh, B. (2023). Federated Learning for Envision Future Trajectory Smart Transport System for Climate Preservation and Smart Green Planet: Insights into Global Governance and SDG-9 (Industry, Innovation and Infrastructure). *National Journal of Environmental Law*, 6(2), 6–17.

Singh, B. (2023). Unleashing Alternative Dispute Resolution (ADR) in Resolving Complex Legal-Technical Issues Arising in Cyberspace Lensing E-Commerce and Intellectual Property: Proliferation of E-Commerce Digital Economy. *Revista Brasileira de Alternative Dispute Resolution-Brazilian Journal of Alternative Dispute Resolution-RBADR*, 5(10), 81–105. DOI: 10.52028/rbadr.v5i10.ART04.Ind

Singh, B. (2024). Biosensors in Intelligent Healthcare and Integration of Internet of Medical Things (IoMT) for Treatment and Diagnosis. *Indian Journal of Health and Medical Law*, 7(1), 1–7.

Singh, B. (2024). Evolutionary Global Neuroscience for Cognition and Brain Health: Strengthening Innovation in Brain Science. In Prabhakar, P. (Ed.), *Biomedical Research Developments for Improved Healthcare* (pp. 246–272). IGI Global., DOI: 10.4018/979-8-3693-1922-2.ch012

Singh, B. (2024). Featuring Consumer Choices of Consumable Products for Health Benefits: Evolving Issues from Tort and Product Liabilities. *Journal of Law of Torts and Consumer Protection Law*, 7(1), 53–56.

Singh, B. (2024). Green Infrastructure in Real Estate Landscapes: Pillars of Sustainable Development and Vision for Tomorrow. *National Journal of Real Estate Law*, 7(1), 4–8.

Singh, B. (2024). Legal Dynamics Lensing Metaverse Crafted for Videogame Industry and E-Sports: Phenomenological Exploration Catalyst Complexity and Future. *Journal of Intellectual Property Rights Law*, 7(1), 8–14.

Singh, B. (2024). Lensing Legal Dynamics for Examining Responsibility and Deliberation of Generative AI-Tethered Technological Privacy Concerns: Infringements and Use of Personal Data by Nefarious Actors. In Ara, A., & Ara, A. (Eds.), *Exploring the Ethical Implications of Generative AI* (pp. 146–167). IGI Global., DOI: 10.4018/979-8-3693-1565-1.ch009

Singh, B. (2024). Transformative Wave of IoMT, EHRs, RPM Technologies to Revolutionize Public Health. *Indian Journal of Health and Medical Law*, 7(2), 22–26.

Singh, B., Dutta, P. K., & Kaunert, C. (2024). Replenish Artificial Intelligence in Renewable Energy for Sustainable Development: Lensing SDG 7 Affordable and Clean Energy and SDG 13 Climate Actions With Legal-Financial Advisory. In Derbali, A. (Ed.), *Social and Ethical Implications of AI in Finance for Sustainability* (pp. 198–227). IGI Global., DOI: 10.4018/979-8-3693-2881-1.ch009

Singh, B., Jain, V., Kaunert, C., Dutta, P. K., & Singh, G. (2024). Privacy Matters: Espousing Blockchain and Artificial Intelligence (AI) for Consumer Data Protection on E-Commerce Platforms in Ethical Marketing. In Saluja, S., Nayyar, V., Rojhe, K., & Sharma, S. (Eds.), *Ethical Marketing Through Data Governance Standards and Effective Technology* (pp. 167–184). IGI Global., DOI: 10.4018/979-8-3693-2215-4.ch015

Singh, B., & Kaunert, C. (2024). Aroma of Highly Smart Internet of Medical Things (IoMT) and Lightweight Edge Trust Expansion Medical Care Facilities for Electronic Healthcare Systems: Fortified-Chain Architecture for Remote Patient Monitoring and Privacy Protection Beyond Imagination. In Hassan, A., Bhattacharya, P., Tikadar, S., Dutta, P., & Sagayam, M. (Eds.), *Lightweight Digital Trust Architectures in the Internet of Medical Things (IoMT)* (pp. 196–212). IGI Global., DOI: 10.4018/979-8-3693-2109-6.ch011

Singh, B., & Kaunert, C. (2024). Augmented Reality and Virtual Reality Modules for Mindfulness: Boosting Emotional Intelligence and Mental Wellness. In Hiran, K., Doshi, R., & Patel, M. (Eds.), *Applications of Virtual and Augmented Reality for Health and Wellbeing* (pp. 111–128). IGI Global., DOI: 10.4018/979-8-3693-1123-3.ch007

Singh, B., & Kaunert, C. (2024). Computational Thinking for Innovative Solutions and Problem-Solving Techniques: Transforming Conventional Education to Futuristic Interdisciplinary Higher Education. In Fonkam, M., & Vajjhala, N. (Eds.), *Revolutionizing Curricula Through Computational Thinking, Logic, and Problem Solving* (pp. 60–82). IGI Global., DOI: 10.4018/979-8-3693-1974-1.ch004

Singh, B., & Kaunert, C. (2024). Future of Digital Marketing: Hyper-Personalized Customer Dynamic Experience with AI-Based Predictive Models. In *Revolutionizing the AI-Digital Landscape* (pp. 189–203). Productivity Press. DOI: 10.4324/9781032688305-14

Singh, B., & Kaunert, C. (2024). Harnessing Sustainable Agriculture Through Climate-Smart Technologies: Artificial Intelligence for Climate Preservation and Futuristic Trends. In Kannan, H., Rodriguez, R., Paprika, Z., & Ade-Ibijola, A. (Eds.), *Exploring Ethical Dimensions of Environmental Sustainability and Use of AI* (pp. 214–239). IGI Global., DOI: 10.4018/979-8-3693-0892-9.ch011

Singh, B., & Kaunert, C. (2024). Integration of Cutting-Edge Technologies such as Internet of Things (IoT) and 5G in Health Monitoring Systems: A Comprehensive Legal Analysis and Futuristic Outcomes. *GLS Law Journal*, 6(1), 13–20. DOI: 10.69974/glslawjournal.v6i1.123

Singh, B., & Kaunert, C. (2024). Revealing Green Finance Mobilization: Harnessing FinTech and Blockchain Innovations to Surmount Barriers and Foster New Investment Avenues. In Jafar, S., Rodriguez, R., Kannan, H., Akhtar, S., & Plugmann, P. (Eds.), *Harnessing Blockchain-Digital Twin Fusion for Sustainable Investments* (pp. 265–286). IGI Global., DOI: 10.4018/979-8-3693-1878-2.ch011

Singh, B., & Kaunert, C. (2024). Salvaging Responsible Consumption and Production of Food in the Hospitality Industry: Harnessing Machine Learning and Deep Learning for Zero Food Waste. In Singh, A., Tyagi, P., & Garg, A. (Eds.), *Sustainable Disposal Methods of Food Wastes in Hospitality Operations* (pp. 176–192). IGI Global., DOI: 10.4018/979-8-3693-2181-2.ch012

Singh, B., Kaunert, C., & Vig, K. (2024). Reinventing Influence of Artificial Intelligence (AI) on Digital Consumer Lensing Transforming Consumer Recommendation Model: Exploring Stimulus Artificial Intelligence on Consumer Shopping Decisions. In Musiolik, T., Rodriguez, R., & Kannan, H. (Eds.), *AI Impacts in Digital Consumer Behavior* (pp. 141–169). IGI Global., DOI: 10.4018/979-8-3693-1918-5.ch006

Singh, C., Mallesha, M., Vijayaragavan, M., Sureshbabu, J., & Alsekait, D. (2022). IoT BASED SECURED HEALTHCARE USING 6G TECHNOLOGY AND DEEP LEARNING TECHNIQUES. *Journal of Pharmaceutical Negative Results*, ●●●, 462–472. DOI: 10.47750/pnr.2022.13.S09.053

Singh, H., & Bawa, S. (2016). IGSIM : An Integrated Architecture for High Performance Spatial Data Analysis. [IJCSIS]. *International Journal of Computer Science and Information Security*, 14(11), 302–309.

Singh, H., & Bawa, S. (2017). A mapreduce-based efficient H-bucket PMR quadtree spatial index. *Computer Systems Science and Engineering*, 32(5), 405–415.

Singh, H., & Bawa, S. (2019). An improved integrated Grid and MapReduce-Hadoop architecture for spatial data: Hilbert TGS R-Tree-based IGSIM. *Concurrency and Computation*, 31(17), e5202. https://doi.org/https://doi.org/10.1002/cpe.5202. DOI: 10.1002/cpe.5202

Singh, H., & Bawa, S. (2022). Predicting COVID-19 statistics using machine learning regression model: Li-MuLi-Poly. *Multimedia Systems*, 28(1), 113–120. DOI: 10.1007/s00530-021-00798-2 PMID: 33976474

Singh, H., Kaushik, S., Talyan, S., & Dwivedi, K. (2022). Skin Cancer Detection Using Deep Learning techniques. *International Journal for Research in Applied Science and Engineering Technology*, 10(5). Advance online publication. DOI: 10.22214/ijraset.2024.62662

Singh, R., Mathiassen, L., Stachura, M. E., & Astapova, E. V. (2011). Dynamic capabilities in home health: IT-enabled transformation of post-acute care. *Journal of the Association for Information Systems*, 12(2), 2. DOI: 10.17705/1jais.00257

Singh, S., Chowdhary, S. K., Rawat, S., & Acharya, B. M. (2023). 5G Revolution Transforming the Delivery in Healthcare. In Swarnkar, T., Patnaik, S., Mitra, P., Misra, S., & Mishra, M. (Eds.), *Ambient Intelligence in Health Care* (pp. 179–188). Springer Nature., DOI: 10.1007/978-981-19-6068-0_17

Sivaparthipan, C. B., Muthu, B. A., Manogaran, G., Maram, B., Sundarasekar, R., Krishnamoorthy, S., & Chandran, K. (2019). Innovative and efficient method of robotics for helping the Parkinson's disease patient using IoT in big data analytics. *Transactions on Emerging Telecommunications Technologies*, ●●●, e3838.

Smarr, C. A., Mitzner, T. L., Beer, J. M., Prakash, A., Chen, T. L., Kemp, C. C., & Rogers, W. A. (2014). Domestic robots for older adults: Attitudes, preferences, and potential. *International Journal of Social Robotics*, 6(2), 229–247. DOI: 10.1007/s12369-013-0220-0 PMID: 25152779

Smarr, C. A., Prakash, A., Beer, J. M., Mitzner, T. L., Kemp, C. C., & Rogers, W. A. (2012, September). Older adults' preferences for and acceptance of robot assistance for everyday living tasks. []. Sage CA: Los Angeles, CA: Sage Publications.]. *Proceedings of the Human Factors and Ergonomics Society Annual Meeting*, 56(1), 153–157. DOI: 10.1177/1071181312561009 PMID: 25284971

Smith, B., & Magnani, J. W. (2019). New technologies, new disparities: The intersection of electronic health and digital health literacy. *International Journal of Cardiology*, 292, 280–282. DOI: 10.1016/j.ijcard.2019.05.066 PMID: 31171391

Smuck, M., Odonkor, C. A., Wilt, J. K., Schmidt, N., & Swiernik, M. A. (2021). The emerging clinical role of wearables: Factors for successful implementation in healthcare. *NPJ Digital Medicine*, 4(1), 1–8. DOI: 10.1038/s41746-021-00418-3

Soares, L., Leal, T., Faria, A. L., Aguiar, A., & Carvalho, C. (2023). Cardiovascular disease: A review. *Biomedical Journal of Scientific & Technical Research, 51*(3).

Sodhro, A. H., & Shah, M. A. (2017). Role of 5G in medical health. *2017 International Conference on Innovations in Electrical Engineering and Computational Technologies (ICIEECT)*, 1–5. DOI: 10.1109/ICIEECT.2017.7916586

Softbank Robotics. "NAO the humanoid and programmable robot" (2020). Available: https://www.softbankrobotics.com/emea/en/nao

Softbank Robotics. "Pepper the humanoid and programmable robot" (2020). Available: https://www.softbankrobotics.com/emea/en/pepper

Solanas, A., Patsakis, C., Conti, M., Vlachos, I., Ramos, V., Falcone, F., Postolache, O., Perez-martinez, P., Pietro, R., Perrea, D., & Martinez-Balleste, A. (2014). Smart health: A context-aware health paradigm within smart cities. *IEEE Communications Magazine*, 52(8), 1558–1896. DOI: 10.1109/MCOM.2014.6871673

Sommerville, I. (2011). *Software Engineering* (9th ed.). Pearson Education Inc.

Sood, S. K., & Mahajan, I. (2017). Wearable IoT sensor based healthcare system for identifying and controlling chikungunya virus. *Computers in Industry*, 91, 33–44. DOI: 10.1016/j.compind.2017.05.006 PMID: 32287550

Sood, S. K., & Mahajan, I. (2019). IoT-Fog-Based Healthcare Framework to Identify and Control Hypertension Attack. *IEEE Internet of Things Journal*, 6(2), 1920–1927. DOI: 10.1109/JIOT.2018.2871630

Souza, D. J., Barbosa Baptista, M. H., dos Santos Gomides, D., & Emilia Pace, A. (2017). Adherence to diabetes mellitus care at three levels of health care. *Anna Nery School Journal of Nursing / Escola Anna Nery Revista de Enfermagem, 21*(4), 1-9. https://doi.org/DOI: 10.1590/2177-9465-EAN-2017-0045

Srinidhi, N. N., Kumar, S. D., & Venugopal, K. R. (2019). Network optimizations in the internet of things: A review. *Eng. Sci. Technol. Int. J.*, 22(1), 1–21. DOI: 10.1016/j.jestch.2018.09.003

Srivastav, S., Allam, K., & Mustyala, A. (2023). Software Automation Enhancement through the Implementation of DevOps. *International Journal of Research Publication and Reviews*, 4(6), 2050–2054. DOI: 10.55248/gengpi.4.623.45947

Staff, M. C. (2018, June 26). *Stress management*. Retrieved from Mayo Clinic: www.mayoclinic.org/healthy-lifestyle/stress-management/in-depth/support-groups/art-20044655

Starr, J. (2008). *The coaching manual: the definitive guide to the process, principles and skills of personal coaching*. Prentice Hall.

Stavropoulos, T. G., Papastergiou, A., Mpaltadoros, L., Nikolopoulos, S., & Kompatsiaris, I. (2020). IoT Wearable Sensors and Devices in Elderly Care: A Literature Review. *Sensors (Basel)*, 20(10), 2826. DOI: 10.3390/s20102826 PMID: 32429331

Steele, R., Lo, A., Secombe, C., & Wong, Y. K. (2009). Elderly persons' perception and acceptance of using wireless sensor networks to assist healthcare. *International Journal of Medical Informatics*, 78(12), 788–801. DOI: 10.1016/j.ijmedinf.2009.08.001 PMID: 19717335

Steffen, J. H., Gaskin, J. E., Meservy, T. O., Jenkins, J. L., & Wolman, I. (2019). Framework of affordances for virtual reality and augmented reality. *Journal of Management Information Systems*, 36(3), 683–729. DOI: 10.1080/07421222.2019.1628877

Stowell, F., & Mingers, J. (1997). *Information Systems: An Emerging Discipline?* McGraw-Hill Education.

Stradford, L., Curtis, J. R., Zueger, P., Xie, F., Curtis, D., Gavigan, K., Clinton, C., Venkatachalam, S., Rivera, E., & Nowell, W. B. (2024). Wearable activity tracker study exploring rheumatoid arthritis patients' disease activity using patient-reported outcome measures, clinical measures, and biometric sensor data (the wear study). *Contemporary Clinical Trials Communications*, 38, 101272. DOI: 10.1016/j.conctc.2024.101272 PMID: 38444876

Straub, D., Boudreau, M. C., & Gefen, D. (2004). Validation guidelines for IS positivist research. *Communications of the Association for Information systems*, (13:1), 24.

Stuck, R. E., & Rogers, W. A. (2018). Older adults' perceptions of supporting factors of trust in a robot care provider. *Journal of Robotics*, 2018(1), 6519713. DOI: 10.1155/2018/6519713

Subhedar, M., Jadhav, V., Tekade, S., & Prajapati, M. (2018). A Real Time Healthcare Monitoring System Based on Open Source IoT and ANFIS. *2018 Second International Conference on Intelligent Computing and Control Systems (ICICCS)*, 281–286. DOI: 10.1109/ICCONS.2018.8663037

Subramanian, G., & Sreekantan Thampy, A. (2021). Implementation of Blockchain Consortium to Prioritize Diabetes Patients' Healthcare in Pandemic Situations [Article]. *IEEE Access : Practical Innovations, Open Solutions*, 9, 162459–162475. DOI: 10.1109/ACCESS.2021.3132302

Suhasini, V. K., Patil, P. B., Vijaykumar, K. N., Manjunatha, S. C., Sudha, T., Kumar, P., & Manjunath, T. C. (2022). Detection of Skin Cancer using Artificial Intelligence & Machine Learning Concepts. In *Proceedings of 4th International Conference on Cybernetics, Cognition and Machine Learning Applications, ICCCMLA 2022*. Retrieved from https://doi.org/DOI: 10.1109/ICCCMLA56841.2022.9989146

Suiçmez, Ç., Tolga Kahraman, H., Suiçmez, A., Yılmaz, C., & Balcı, F. (2023). Detection of melanoma with hybrid learning method by removing hair from dermoscopic images using image processing techniques and wavelet transform. *Biomedical Signal Processing and Control*, 84, 104729. Advance online publication. DOI: 10.1016/j.bspc.2023.104729

Sun, T. N. (2014). Breast cancer: Knowing is best. Windhoek.

Sun, J., Chen, X., Zhang, Z., Lai, S., Zhao, B., Liu, H., Wang, S., Huan, W., Zhao, R., Ng, M. T. A., & Zheng, Y. (2020). Forecasting the long-term trend of COVID-19 epidemic using a dynamic model. *Scientific Reports, 10*(1), 1–10. DOI: 10.1038/s41598-020-78084-w PMID: 33273592

Supernor, B. (2018). *Why the cost of cloud computing is dropping dramatically.* App Developer Magazine. https://appdevelopermagazine.com/why-the-cost-of-cloud-computing-is-dropping-dramatically/

Suraki, M. Y., & Suraki, M. Y. (2013). Technology therapy for obsessive-compulsive disorder based on Internet of Things. *2013 7th International Conference on Application of Information and Communication Technologies*, 1–4. DOI: 10.1109/ICAICT.2013.6722800

Suresh Babu, C. V., Akshayah, N. S., & Maclin Vinola, P. (2024). Artificial Intelligence in Healthcare: Assessing Impacts, Challenges, and Recommendations for Achieving Healthcare Independence. In Geada, N., & Jamil, G. (Eds.), *Perspectives on Artificial Intelligence in Times of Turbulence: Theoretical Background to Applications* (pp. 61–80). IGI Global., DOI: 10.4018/978-1-6684-9814-9.ch005

Susan, S., & Hendrick, E. C. (2010). Practical Model for Psychosocial Care. *Journal of Oncology Practice / American Society of Clinical Oncology*, •••, 34–36. PMID: 20539730

Swan, K. (2003). Learning effectiveness online: What the research tells us. *Elements of quality online education, practice and direction, 4*(1), 13-47.

Swan, M. (2012). Health 2050: The realization of personalized medicine through crowdsourcing, the quantified self, and the participatory biocitizen. *Journal of Personalized Medicine, 2*(3), 93–118. DOI: 10.3390/jpm2030093 PMID: 25562203

Swan, M. (2013). The quantified self: Fundamental disruption in big data science and biological discovery. *Big Data, 1*(2), 85–99. DOI: 10.1089/big.2012.0002 PMID: 27442063

Sweller, J. (1988). Cognitive load during problem solving: Effects on learning. *Cognitive Science, 12*(2), 257–285. DOI: 10.1207/s15516709cog1202_4

Sweller, J., Van Merriënboer, J. J., & Paas, F. G. (1998). Cognitive architecture and instructional design. *Educational Psychology Review, 10*(3), 251–296. DOI: 10.1023/A:1022193728205

Sylla, B. S. C. W. (2012). Cancer burden in Africa in 2030. *International Agency for Research on Cancer*, 1-2.

Szczepura, A., Collinson, M., Moody, L., Jing, Y., Ward, G., Bul, K., Arnab, S., Asbury, C., Russell, E., Gibbons, C., & Dashwood, R. (2018). PP89 Living Lab Concept: An Innovation Hub For Elderly Residential Care. *International Journal of Technology Assessment in Health Care*, 34(S1), 99–100. DOI: 10.1017/S0266462318002362

Tacken, M., Marcellini, F., Mollenkopf, H., Ruoppila, I., & Szeman, Z. (2005). Use and acceptance of new technology by older people. Findings of the international MOBILATE survey: 'Enhancing mobility in later life'. *Gerontechnology (Valkenswaard)*, 3(3), 126–137. DOI: 10.4017/gt.2005.03.03.002.00

Taghian, A., Abo-Zahhad, M., Sayed, M. S., & Abdel-Malek, A. (2021, December). Virtual, Augmented Reality, and Wearable Devices for Biomedical Applications: A Review. In *2021 9th International Japan-Africa Conference on Electronics, Communications, and Computations (JAC-ECC)* (pp. 93-98). IEEE.

Taimoor, N., & Rehman, S. (2022). Reliable and Resilient AI and IoT-Based Personalised Healthcare Services: A Survey [Article]. *IEEE Access: Practical Innovations, Open Solutions*, 10, 535–563. DOI: 10.1109/ACCESS.2021.3137364

Tai, W., Kalanithi, L., & Milstein, A. (2014). What can be achieved by redesigning stroke care for a value-based world? *Expert Review of Pharmacoeconomics & Outcomes Research*, 14(5), 585–587. DOI: 10.1586/14737167.2014.946013 PMID: 25095813

Takiddin, A., Schneider, J., Yang, Y., Abd-Alrazaq, A., & Househ, M. (2021). Artificial intelligence for skin cancer detection: Scoping review. *Journal of Medical Internet Research*, 23(11), e22934. Advance online publication. DOI: 10.2196/22934 PMID: 34821566

Tan, E. T., & Halim, Z. A. (2019). Health care Monitoring System and Analytics Based on Internet of Things Framework. In *IETE Journal of Research* (Vol. 65, Issue 5, pp. 653–660). Taylor & Francis LTD. DOI: 10.1080/03772063.2018.1447402

Tariq, M. U. (2024). Advanced wearable medical devices and their role in transformative remote health monitoring. In *Transformative Approaches to Patient Literacy and Healthcare Innovation* (pp. 308–326). IGI Global. DOI: 10.4018/979-8-3693-3661-8.ch015

Tavares, P., Costa, C.M., Rocha, L., Malaca, P., Costa, P., Moreira, A.P., Sousa, A., and Veiga, G. 2019. Collaborative Welding System using BIM for Robotic Reprogramming and Spatial Augmented Reality, *Automation in Construction* (106:1), pp. 1-12.

Taylor, K. (2015). How digital technology is transforming health and social care. *Deloitte Center for Health Solutions*, 2-37.

Taylor, J. P., Smith, N., Prato, L., Damant, J., Jasim, S., Toma, M., Hamashima, Y., McLeod, H., Towers, A.-M., Keemink, J., Nwolise, C., Giebel, C., & Fitzpatrick, R. (2023). Care planning interventions for care home residents: A scoping review. *Journal of Long-Term Care*. Advance online publication. DOI: 10.31389/jltc.223

Tene, T., Vique López, D. F., Valverde Aguirre, P. E., Orna Puente, L. M., & Vacacela Gomez, C. (2024). Virtual reality and augmented reality in medical education: An umbrella review. *Frontiers in Digital Health*, 6, 1365345. DOI: 10.3389/fdgth.2024.1365345

Than, N. N. (2023). *Journey to Wellbeing: Seeing Beyond the Mind's Eye Through Story in a Virtual Therapeutic Space* (Doctoral dissertation, New York University Tandon School of Engineering).

Thompson, A. H. (2021). A Holistic Approach to Employee Functioning: Assessing the Impact of a Virtual-Reality Mindfulness Intervention at Work.

Thomson, R. G., Eccles, M. P., Steen, I. N., Greenaway, J., Stobbart, L., Murtagh, M. J., & May, C. R. (2007). A patient decision aid to support shared decision-making on anti-thrombotic treatment of patients with atrial fibrillation: Randomised controlled trial. *BMJ Quality & Safety*, 16(3), 216–223. DOI: 10.1136/qshc.2006.018481 PMID: 17545350

Tian, S. W., Yu, A. Y., Vogel, D., & Kwok, R. C. W. (2011). The impact of online social networking on learning: A social integration perspective. *International Journal of Networking and Virtual Organisations*, 8(3-4), 264–280. DOI: 10.1504/IJNVO.2011.039999

Tian, S., Yang, W., Grange, J., Wang, P., Huang, W., & Ye, Z. (2019). Smart healthcare: Making medical care more intelligent. *Global Health Journal (Amsterdam, Netherlands)*, 62-65(3), 62–65. Advance online publication. DOI: 10.1016/j.glohj.2019.07.001

Tobias, C. R., Downes, A., Eddens, S., & Ruiz, J. (2012). Building blocks for peer success: Lessons learned from a train-the-trainer program. *AIDS Patient Care and STDs*, 26(1), 53–59. DOI: 10.1089/apc.2011.0224 PMID: 22103430

Toh, X., Tan, H., Liang, H., & Tan, H. (2016). Elderly medication adherence monitoring with the Internet of Things. *2016 IEEE International Conference on Pervasive Computing and Communication Workshops (PerCom Workshops)*, 1–6. DOI: 10.1109/PERCOMW.2016.7457133

Tomlin, A., & Asimakopoulou, K. (2014). Supporting behaviour change in older people with type 2 diabetes. *British Journal of Community Nursing*, 19(1), 22–27. http://ez.library.latrobe.edu.au/login?url=https://search.ebscohost.com/login.aspx ?direct=true&db=cul&AN=103994423&login.asp&site=ehost-live&scope=site. DOI: 10.12968/bjcn.2014.19.1.22 PMID: 24800323

Touati, F., & Tabish, R. (2013). u-Healthcare system: State-of-the-art review and challenges. *Journal of Medical Systems*, 37(3), 9949. DOI: 10.1007/s10916-013-9949-0 PMID: 23640734

Traeger, M. L., Strohkorb Sebo, S., Jung, M., Scassellati, B., & Christakis, N. A. (2020). Vulnerable robots positively shape human conversational dynamics in a human–robot team. *Proceedings of the National Academy of Sciences of the United States of America*, 117(12), 6370–6375. DOI: 10.1073/pnas.1910402117 PMID: 32152118

Trainum, K., Tunis, R., Xie, B., & Hauser, E. (2023). Robots in Assisted Living Facilities: Scoping Review. *JMIR Aging*, 6, e42652. DOI: 10.2196/42652 PMID: 36877560

Trawley, S., Baptista, S., Browne, J. L., Pouwer, F., & Speight, J. (2016). The use of mobile applications among adults with type 1 and type 2 diabetes: Results from a national survey. *Journal of Diabetes Science and Technology*, 10(6), 1335–1343. DOI: 10.1177/1932296816666503 PMID: 27301981

Triono, T., Darmayanti, R., Saputra, N. D., Afifah, A., & Makwana, G. (2023). Open Journal System: Assistance and training in submitting scientific journals to be well-indexed in Google Scholar. *Jurnal Inovasi dan Pengembangan Hasil Pengabdian Masyarakat, 1*(2), 106-114.

Tsanas, A., Little, M. A., McSharry, P. E., & Ramig, L. O. (2010, March). Enhanced classical dysphonia measures and sparse regression for telemonitoring of Parkinson's disease progression. In *2010 IEEE International Conference on Acoustics, Speech and Signal Processing* (pp. 594-597). IEEE.

Tschandl, P., Rosendahl, C., & Kittler, H. (2020). The state of the art in dermatoscopy and skin cancer detection. *Dermatology (Basel, Switzerland)*, 236(1), 4–11. DOI: 10.1159/000506973

Tschofenig, H., Arkko, J., Thaler, D., & McPherson, D. (2015). *Architectural considerations in smart object networking. RFC 7452.* http://hjp.at/doc/rfc/rfc7452.html

Tsoi, K., & Wong, M. (2021). Digital health for chronic disease management. In Fong, B., & Wong, M. (Eds.), *The Routledge Handbook of Public Health and the Community* (p. 12). Routledge., DOI: 10.4324/9781003119111-24-28

Tuli, S., Tuli, S., Wander, G., Wander, P., Gill, S., Dustdar, S., & Rana, O. (2019). Next generation technologies for smart healthcare: Challenges, vision, model, trends and future directions. *Internet Technology Letters*, 15. Advance online publication. DOI: 10.1002/itl2.145

Tun, S. Y. Y., Madanian, S., & Mirza, F. (2020). Internet of things (IoT) applications for elderly care: A reflective review. *Aging Clinical and Experimental Research*. Advance online publication. DOI: 10.1007/s40520-020-01545-9 PMID: 32277435

Twohig, P. A., Rivington, J. R., Gunzler, D., Daprano, J., & Margolius, D. (2019). Clinician dashboard views and improvement in preventative health outcome measures: A retrospective analysis. *BMC Health Services Research*, 19(1), 475. https://doi.org/https://dx.doi.org/10.1186/s12913-019-4327-3. DOI: 10.1186/s12913-019-4327-3 PMID: 31296211

Ullah, M., Hamayun, S., Wahab, A., Khan, S. U., Rehman, M. U., Haq, Z. U., Rehman, K. U., Ullah, A., Mehreen, A., Awan, U. A., Qayum, M., & Naeem, M. (2023). Smart technologies used as smart tools in the management of cardiovascular disease and their future perspective. *Current Problems in Cardiology*, 48(11), 101922. DOI: 10.1016/j.cpcardiol.2023.101922 PMID: 37437703

United Nations. (2022). *World Population Prospects 2022*. Department of Economic and Social Affairs, Population Division.

Upadhyay, S., Kumar, M., Upadhyay, A., Verma, S., Kavita, M., Khurma, R., & Castillo, P. (2023). Challenges and Limitation Analysis of an IoT-Dependent System for Deployment in Smart Healthcare Using Communication Standards Features. Sensors, 11. doi:https://www.mdpi.com/1424-8220/23/11/5155

Usta, Y. Y. (2012). Importance of Social Support in Cancer Patients. *Asian Pacific Journal of Cancer Prevention*, 13(8), 3569–3572. DOI: 10.7314/APJCP.2012.13.8.3569 PMID: 23098436

Uva, A. E., Gattullo, M., Manghisi, V. M., Spagnulo, D., Cascella, G. L., & Fiorentino, M. (2018). Evaluating the effectiveness of spatial augmented reality in smart manufacturing: A solution for manual working stations. *International Journal of Advanced Manufacturing Technology*, 94(1-4), 509–521. DOI: 10.1007/s00170-017-0846-4

Vaishnavi, V., & Kuechler, W. 2004. Design Research in Information Systems. Last updated August 16, 2009 from http://desrist.org/design-research-in-information -systems

Van Belle, G. (2011). *Statistical Rules of Thumb*. John Wiley & Sons.

Van Den Haak, M., De Jong, M., & Jan Schellens, P. (2003). Retrospective vs. concurrent think-aloud protocols: Testing the usability of an online library catalogue. *Behaviour & Information Technology*, 22(5), 339–351. DOI: 10.1080/0044929031000

van Kleef, E., Robotham, J. V., Jit, M., Deeny, S. R., & Edmunds, W. J. (2013). Modelling the transmission of healthcare associated infections: A systematic review. *BMC Infectious Diseases*, 13(1), 1–13. DOI: 10.1186/1471-2334-13-294 PMID: 23809195

Vansimaeys, C., Benamar, L., & Balagué, C. (2021). Digital health and management of chronic disease: A multimodal technologies typology. *The International Journal of Health Planning and Management*, 36(4), 1107–1125. DOI: 10.1002/hpm.3161 PMID: 33786849

Varonen, H., Kortteisto, T., & Kaila, M.EBMeDS Study Group. (2008). What may help or hinder the implementation of computerized decision support systems (CDSSs): A focus group study with physicians. *Family Practice*, 25(3), 162–167. DOI: 10.1093/fampra/cmn020 PMID: 18504253

Vasconcelos, M. J. M., Moreira, D., Alves, P., Graça, R., Franco, R., & Rosado, L. (2022). Improving Teledermatology Referral with Edge-AI: Mobile App to Foster Skin Lesion Imaging Standardization. In *Communications in Computer and Information Science* (Vol. 1710 CCIS). Retrieved from https://doi.org/DOI: 10.1007/978-3-031-20664-1_9

Vavilis, S., Petković, M., & Zannone, N. (2012). Impact of ICT on Home Healthcare. In M. D. Hercheui, D. Whitehouse, W. McIver, & J. Phahlamohlaka (Eds.), *ICT Critical Infrastructures and Society* (pp. 111–122). Springer. DOI: 10.1007/978-3-642-33332-3_11

Venkatesh, V., Brown, S. A., & Bala, H. (2013). Bridging the qualitative-quantitative divide: Guidelines for conducting mixed methods research in information systems. *Management Information Systems Quarterly*, 37(1), 21–54. DOI: 10.25300/MISQ/2013/37.1.02

Venkatesh, V., Morris, M. G., Davis, G. B., & Davis, F. D. (2003). User acceptance of information technology: Toward a unified view. *Management Information Systems Quarterly*, 27(3), 425–478. DOI: 10.2307/30036540

Verma, R., Akhai, S., & Wadhwa, A. S. (2024). Use of Smart Materials in Physiotherapy. In *Revolutionizing Healthcare Treatment With Sensor Technology* (pp. 300–319). IGI Global. DOI: 10.4018/979-8-3693-2762-3.ch019

Vertucci, R., D'Onofrio, S., Ricciardi, S., & De Nino, M. (2023). History of Augmented Reality, In: Nee, A.Y.C., Ong, S.K. (eds) *Springer Handbook of Augmented Reality*. Springer Handbooks. Springer, Cham. DOI: 10.1007/978-3-030-67822-7_2

Vesselkov, A., Hämmäinen, H., & Töyli, J. (2018). Technology and value network evolution in telehealth [Article]. *Technological Forecasting and Social Change*, 134, 207–222. DOI: 10.1016/j.techfore.2018.06.011

Vijayakumar, V., Malathi, D., Subramaniyaswamy, V., Saravanan, P., & Logesh, R. (2019). Fog computing-based intelligent healthcare system for the detection and prevention of mosquito-borne diseases. In *Computers in Human Behavior* (Vol. 100, pp. 275–285). Pergamon-Elsevier Science LTD., DOI: 10.1016/j.chb.2018.12.009

Vlaanderen, F. P., Tanke, M. A., Bloem, B. R., Faber, M. J., Eijkenaar, F., Schut, F. T., & Jeurissen, P. P. T. (2019). Design and effects of outcome-based payment models in healthcare: A systematic review. *The European Journal of Health Economics*, 20(2), 217–232. DOI: 10.1007/s10198-018-0989-8 PMID: 29974285

Volland, J., Fugener, A., Schoenfelder, J., & Brunner, J. O. (2017). Material logistics in hospitals: A literature review. *Omega*, 69, 82–101. DOI: 10.1016/j.omega.2016.08.004

Von Arnim, C. A. F., Bartsch, T., Jacobs, A. H., Holbrook, J., Bergmann, P., Zieschang, T., Polidori, M. C., & Dodel, R. (2019). Diagnosis and treatment of cognitive impairment. *Zeitschrift für Gerontologie und Geriatrie*, 52(4), 309–315. DOI: 10.1007/s00391-019-01560-0

Vorraber, W., Gasser, J., Webb, H., Neubacher, D., & Url, P. (2020). Assessing augmented reality in production: Remote-assisted maintenance with HoloLens. *Procedia CIRP*, 88, 139–144. DOI: 10.1016/j.procir.2020.05.025

Vukicevic, S., Stamenkovic, Z., Murugesan, S., Bogdanovic, Z., & Radenkovic, B. (2016). A New Telerehabilitation System Based on Internet of Things. *FACTA Universitatis-Series Electronics and Energetics*, 29(3), 395–405. DOI: 10.2298/FUEE1603395V

Vuong, A. M., Ory, M. G., Begaye, D., & Forjuoh, S. N. (2012). Factors Affecting Acceptability and Usability of Technological Approaches to Diabetes Self-Management: A Case Study. *Diabetes Technology & Therapeutics*, 14(12), 12. DOI: 10.1089/dia.2012.0139 PMID: 23013155

Vyas, S., & Bhargava, D. (2021). *Smart Health Systems - Emerging Trends*. Springer Singapore., DOI: 10.1007/978-981-16-4201-2

Vyas, S., Upadhyaya, A., Bhargava, D., & Shukla, V. (2023). *Edge-AI in Healthcare-Trends and Future Perspectives*. CRC Press., DOI: 10.1201/9781003244592

Wan, K., & Alagar, V. (2015, August). Context-aware, knowledge-intensive, and patient-centric Mobile Health Care Model. In *2015 12th International Conference on Fuzzy Systems and Knowledge Discovery (FSKD)* (pp. 2253-2260). IEEE. DOI: 10.1109/FSKD.2015.7382303

Wang, H., Dauwed, M., Khan, I., Sani, N., Omar, H., Amano, H., & Mostafa, S. (2023). MEC-IoT-Healthcare: Analysis and Prospects. *Computers, Materials & Continua*, 32. Advance online publication. DOI: 10.32604/cmc.2022.030958

Wang, W., Tang, J., & Wei, F. (2020). Updated understanding of the outbreak of 2019 novel coronavirus (2019-nCoV) in Wuhan, China. *Journal of Medical Virology*, 92(4), 441–447. DOI: 10.1002/jmv.25689 PMID: 31994742

Wang, X., Han, Y., Leung, V., Niyato, D., Yan, X., & Chen, X. (2021). *Edge AI - Convergence of Edge Computing and Artificial Intelligence*. Springer Singapore., DOI: 10.1007/978-981-15-6186-3

Wan, J., Al-awlaqi, M. A. A. H., Li, M., O'Grady, M., Gu, X., Wang, J., & Cao, N. (2018). Wearable IoT enabled real-time health monitoring system. *EURASIP Journal on Wireless Communications and Networking*. Advance online publication. DOI: 10.1186/s13638-018-1308-x

Webber, L., Divajeva, D., Marsh, T., McPherson, K., Brown, M., Galea, G., & Breda, J. (2014). The future burden of obesity-related diseases in the 53 WHO European-Region countries and the impact of effective interventions: A modelling study. *BMJ Open*, 4(7), e004787. DOI: 10.1136/bmjopen-2014-004787 PMID: 25063459

Wegerich, A., Dzaack, J., & Rötting, M. (2010). Optimizing Virtual Superimpositions: User–centered Design for a UAR Supported Smart Home System. IFAC Proceedings Volumes, 43(13), 71-76.

Welcome to Know Cancer. (n.d.). Retrieved from Know Cancer: https://www.knowcancer.com/

Whelan, S., Murphy, K., Barrett, E., Krusche, C., Santorelli, A., & Casey, D. (2018). Factors affecting the acceptability of social robots by older adults including people with dementia or cognitive impairment: A literature review. *International Journal of Social Robotics*, 10(5), 643–668. DOI: 10.1007/s12369-018-0471-x

White Baker, E., Eden, R., & Xue, Y. (2023). Health Information Systems Research: Opportunities to Further Advance the Field. *Communications of the Association for Information Systems*, 53(1), 984–1002. DOI: 10.17705/1CAIS.05342

Whiten, A., & van de Waal, E. (2018). The pervasive role of social learning in primate lifetime development. *Behavioral Ecology and Sociobiology*, 72(80), 1–16. DOI: 10.1007/s00265-018-2489-3 PMID: 29755181

Whitmore, A., Agarwal, A., & Da Xu, L. (2015). The Internet of Things—A survey of topics and trends. *Information Systems Frontiers*, 17(2), 261–274. DOI: 10.1007/s10796-014-9489-2

Wickramasinghe, N., & Goldberg, S. (2010). Transforming online communities into support environments for chronic disease management through cell phones and social networks. *International journal of Networking and Virtual Organisations*, 7(6), 581-591.

Wikipedia. T. free encyclopedia. (n.d.). *Covid-19 pandemic lockdown in India.* Https://En.Wikipedia.Org/Wiki/COVID-19_pandemic_lockdown_in_India#Unlock_1.0_(1%E2%80%9330_June)

Wilson, A. D., & Benko, H. (2010, October). Combining multiple depth cameras and projectors for interactions on, above and between surfaces. In *Proceedings of the 23nd annual ACM symposium on User interface software and technology*, 273-282. DOI: 10.1145/1866029.1866073

Wohlin, C., Runeson, P., Höst, M., Ohlsson, M. C., Regnell, B., & Wesslén, A. (2012). *Experimentation in software engineering* (Vol. 236). Springer. DOI: 10.1007/978-3-642-29044-2

Wojahn, R. D., Foeger, N. C., Gelberman, R. H., & Calfee, R. P. (2014). Long-term outcomes following a single corticosteroid injection for trigger finger. [Comment in: J Bone Joint Surg Am. 2014 Nov 19;96(22) [:e191 PMID: 25410519] [. *The Journal of Bone and Joint Surgery. American Volume*, 96(22), 1849–1854. https://www.ncbi.nlm.nih.gov/pubmed/25410519. DOI: 10.2106/JBJS.N.00004 PMID: 25410501

Wongkoblap, A., Vadillo, M. A., & Curcin, V. (2017). Researching Mental Health Disorders in the Era of Social Media: Systematic Review. *Journal of Medical Internet Research*, 19(6), e7215. DOI: 10.2196/jmir.7215 PMID: 28663166

World Health Organization. (2022). Noncommunicable diseases: progress monitor 2022. Genevra: WHO. Retrieved from https://iris.who.int/handle/10665/353048

World Health Organization. (2023). Global report on diabetes. Retrieved from https://www.who.int/news-room/fact-sheets/detail/diabetes

World Health Organization. (2024). World health statistics 2024. Retrieved from https://www.who.int/data/gho/publications/world-health-statistics

Worldometer. (2022). Https://Www.Worldometers.Info/Coronavirus/Country/India/

Wortman, C. B. (1984, May). Social Support and the Cancer Patient: Conceptual and Methodologic Issues. *Cancer,* 53(S10), 2339–2360. DOI: 10.1002/cncr.1984.53. s10.2339 PMID: 6367944

Wu, H.-T., & Tsai, C.-W. (2018). A home security system for seniors based on the beacon technology. *Concurrency and Computation-Practice & Experience, 30*(15, SI). DOI: 10.1002/cpe.4496

Wu, M., Lu, T.-J., Ling, F.-Y., Sun, J., & Du, H.-Y. (2010). Research on the architecture of Internet of Things. *2010 3rd International Conference on Advanced Computer Theory and Engineering(ICACTE), 5*, V5-484-V5-487. DOI: 10.1109/ICACTE.2010.5579493

Wu, A. Y., & Munteanu, C. (2018, April). Understanding older users' acceptance of wearable interfaces for sensor-based fall risk assessment. In *Proceedings of the 2018 CHI conference on human factors in computing systems* (pp. 1-13). DOI: 10.1145/3173574.3173693

Wu, J., Chang, L., & Yu, G. (2021). Effective Data Decision-Making and Transmission System Based on Mobile Health for Chronic Disease Management in the Elderly. *IEEE Systems Journal,* 15(4), 5537–5548. DOI: 10.1109/JSYST.2020.3024816

Würfel, D., Lutz, R., & Diehl, S. (2016). Grounded Requirements Engineering: An Approach to Use Case Driven Requirements Engineering. *Journal of Systems and Software,* 117, 645–657. DOI: 10.1016/j.jss.2015.10.024

Wu, T., Wu, F., Qiu, C., Redoute, J., & Yuce, M. R. (2020). A Rigid-Flex Wearable Health Monitoring Sensor Patch for IoT-Connected Healthcare Applications. *IEEE Internet of Things Journal,* 7(8), 1–1. DOI: 10.1109/JIOT.2020.2977164

Wu, Y. H., Wrobel, J., Cornuet, M., Kerhervé, H., Domene, S., & Rigaud, A. S. (2014). Acceptance of an assistive robot in older adults: A mixed-method study of human–robot interaction over a 1-month period in the Living Lab setting. *Clinical Interventions in Aging,* ●●●, 801–811. DOI: 10.2147/CIA.S56435 PMID: 24855349

Yacchirema, D., Sarabia-Jacome, D., Palau, C. E., & Esteve, M. (2018a). A Smart System for Sleep Monitoring by Integrating IoT With Big Data Analytics. *IEEE Access : Practical Innovations, Open Solutions,* 6, 35988–36001. DOI: 10.1109/ACCESS.2018.2849822

Yacchirema, D., Sarabia-Jacome, D., Palau, C. E., & Esteve, M. (2018b). System for monitoring and supporting the treatment of sleep apnea using IoT and big data. *Pervasive and Mobile Computing*, 50, 25–40. DOI: 10.1016/j.pmcj.2018.07.007

Yadav, P., Steinbach, M., Kumar, V., & Simon, G. (2018). Mining electronic health records (EHRs) A survey. *ACM Computing Surveys*, 50(6), 1–40. DOI: 10.1145/3127881

Yang, G., Deng, J., Pang, G., Zhang, H., Li, J., Deng, B., Pang, Z., Xu, J., Jiang, M., Liljeberg, P., Xie, H., & Yang, H. (2018). An IoT-Enabled Stroke Rehabilitation System Based on Smart Wearable Armband and Machine Learning. *IEEE Journal of Translational Engineering in Health and Medicine, 6*, 1–10. *IEEE Journal of Translational Engineering in Health and Medicine*. Advance online publication. DOI: 10.1109/JTEHM.2018.2822681 PMID: 29805919

Yang, G., Xie, L., Mantysalo, M., Zhou, X., Pang, Z., Xu, L. D., Kao-Walter, S., Chen, Q., & Zheng, L.-R. (2014). A Health-IoT Platform Based on the Integration of Intelligent Packaging, Unobtrusive Bio-Sensor, and Intelligent Medicine Box. *IEEE Transactions on Industrial Informatics*, 10(4), 2180–2191. DOI: 10.1109/TII.2014.2307795

Yang, P., Bi, G., Qi, J., Wang, X., Yang, Y., & Xu, L. (2021). Multimodal wearable intelligence for dementia care in healthcare 4.0: A survey. *Information Systems Frontiers*, ●●●, 1–18. DOI: 10.1007/s10796-021-10163-3

Yang, Q., Mamun, A. A., Hayat, N., Jingzu, G., Hoque, M. E., & Salameh, A. A. (2022). Modeling the Intention and Adoption of Wearable Fitness Devices: A Study Using SEM-PLS Analysis. *Frontiers in Public Health*, 10, 918989. Advance online publication. DOI: 10.3389/fpubh.2022.918989

Yang, Y., Park, Y. J., Ro, H., Chae, S., & Han, T. D. (2018). *CARe-bot: Portable Projection-based AR Robot for Elderly, Companion of HRI 2018*. ACM. DOI: 10.1145/3173386.3177528

Yin, C., Chen, J., Miao, X., Jiang, H., & Chen, D. (2021). Device-free human activity recognition with low-resolution infrared array sensor using long short-term memory neural network. *Sensors (Basel)*, 21(10), 3551. DOI: 10.3390/s21103551 PMID: 34065183

Yoo, Y., Henfridsson, O., and Lyytinen, K. 2010. "The New Organizing Logic of Digital Innovation: An Agenda for Information Systems Research," *Information Systems Research* (21:4), pp. 724–735.

Yu, W., Liang, F., He, X., Hatcher, W., Lu, C., Lin, J., & Yang, X. (2017). A Survey on the Edge Computing for the Internet of Things. *IEEE Access, PP*, 1–1. DOI: 10.1109/ACCESS.2017.2778504

Yudistira, N., Sumitro, S. B., Nahas, A., & Riama, N. F. (2021). Learning where to look for COVID-19 growth: Multivariate analysis of COVID-19 cases over time using explainable convolution–LSTM. *Applied Soft Computing*, 109, 107469. DOI: 10.1016/j.asoc.2021.107469 PMID: 33994895

Yu, J., Lam, C. L., & Lee, T. M. (2017). White matter microstructural abnormalities in amnestic mild cognitive impairment: A meta-analysis of whole-brain and ROI-based studies. *Neuroscience and Biobehavioral Reviews*, 83, 405–416. DOI: 10.1016/j.neubiorev.2017.10.026

Yu, S., Chai, Y., Chen, H., Brown, R. A., Sherman, S. J., & Nunamaker, J. F.Jr. (2021). Fall detection with wearable sensors: A hierarchical attention-based convolutional neural network approach. *Journal of Management Information Systems*, 38(4), 1095–1121. DOI: 10.1080/07421222.2021.1990617

Zenkoukai: Social Welfare Corporation & Zenkoukai Research Institute. https://zenkou-lab.co.jp/

Zhang, X. M., & Zhang, N. (2011). An Open, Secure and Flexible Platform Based on Internet of Things and Cloud Computing for Ambient Aiding Living and Telemedicine. *2011 International Conference on Computer and Management (CAMAN)*, 1–4. DOI: 10.1109/CAMAN.2011.5778905

Zhou, B., Perel, P., Mensah, G. A., & Ezzati, M. (2021). Global epidemiology, health burden and effective interventions for elevated blood pressure and hypertension. *Nature Reviews. Cardiology*, 18(11), 785–802. DOI: 10.1038/s41569-021-00559-8 PMID: 34050340

Zhou, J., Lee, I., Thomas, B., Menassa, R., Farrant, A., & Sansome, A. (2012). In-situ support for automotive manufacturing using spatial augmented reality. *The International Journal of Virtual Reality: a Multimedia Publication for Professionals*, 11(1), 33–41. DOI: 10.20870/IJVR.2012.11.1.2835

Zhou, T., Wang, Y., Yan, L., & Tan, Y. (2023). Spoiled for choice? Personalized recommendation for healthcare decisions: A multiarmed bandit approach. *Information Systems Research*, 34(4), 1493–1512. DOI: 10.1287/isre.2022.1191

Zhu, H., Samtani, S., Chen, H., & Nunamaker, J. F.Jr. (2020). Human identification for activities of daily living: A deep transfer learning approach. *Journal of Management Information Systems*, 37(2), 457–483. DOI: 10.1080/07421222.2020.1759961

Zhu, T., Kuang, L., Daniels, J., Herrero, P., Li, K., & Georgiou, P. (2023). IoMT-Enabled Real-Time Blood Glucose Prediction With Deep Learning and Edge Computing [Article]. *IEEE Internet of Things Journal*, 10(5), 3706–3719. DOI: 10.1109/JIOT.2022.3143375

About the Contributors

Nilmini Wickramasinghe Currently, Professor Wickramasinghe is the inaugural Optus Chair and Professor of Digital Health at La Trobe University . She holds or has held honorary research professor positions at Epworth HealthCare, Peter MacCallum Cancer Centre, Northern Health and Murdoch Children's Research Institute. After completing 5 degrees at the University of Melbourne, she was awarded a full scholarship to complete PhD studies at Case Western Reserve University, Cleveland, OH, USA and later she was sponsored to complete executive education at Harvard Business School, Harvard University, Cambridge, MA, USA in Value-based HealthCare. For over 20 years, Professor Wickramasinghe has been actively, researching and teaching within the health informatics/digital health domain in US, Germany and Australia with a particular focus on designing, developing and deploying suitable models, strategies and techniques grounded in various management principles to facilitate the implementation and adoption of technology solutions to effect superior, value-based patient centric care delivery. Professor Wickramasinghe collaborates with leading scholars at various premier healthcare organizations and universities throughout Australasia, US and Europe and is well published with more than 400 referred scholarly articles, more than 15 books, numerous book chapters, an encyclopaedia and a well established funded research track record securing over \$25M in funding from grants in US, Australia, Germany and China as a chief investigator. She holds a patent around analytics solution for managing healthcare data and is the editor-in-chief of Intl J Networking and Virtual Organisations by InderScience as well as series editor of the Springer book series Healthcare Delivery in the Information Age and the CRC Routledge book series Analytics and AI for Healthcare. In 2020 she was awarded the prestigious Alexander von Humboldt award for outstanding contribution to Digital Health, the first time this honour has been bestowed to someone in the discipline of Digital Health

***

Shalom Akhai has established himself as a prominent figure in the field of engineering, leveraging over 17 years of academic, research, and technical experience to make significant contributions. With a robust portfolio of over 50 publications in prestigious journals and conferences, Dr. Akhai demonstrates a commitment to advancing knowledge through scholarly work. Additionally, he has authored/co-authored several technical textbooks, further solidifying his expertise and dedication to education in the field. Beyond academia, Dr. Akhai's impact extends to real-world applications through the establishment of IGNIS Technical Solutions, a consultancy firm to translate his knowledge into real-world applications. His skills have resulted in the successful development of over 50 patents+, underscoring his innovative approach and influence in shaping the engineering landscape. Moreover, Dr. Akhai's involvement in professional societies, notably as a member of the Indian Society of Heating Ventilation and Air Conditioning Engineers (ISHRAE) Chandigarh Chapter, reflects his commitment to fostering collaboration and knowledge exchange within the society. As an influential figure, Dr. Akhai continues to drive progress and innovation, leaving an indelible mark on the field of engineering landscape.

C.V. Suresh Babu is a pioneer in content development. A true entrepreneur, he founded Anniyappa Publications, a company that is highly active in publishing books related to Computer Science and Management. Dr. C.V. Suresh Babu has also ventured into SB Institute, a center for knowledge transfer. He holds a Ph.D. in Engineering Education from the National Institute of Technical Teachers Training & Research in Chennai, along with seven master's degrees in various disciplines such as Engineering, Computer Applications, Management, Commerce, Economics, Psychology, Law, and Education. Additionally, he has UGC-NET/SET qualifications in the fields of Computer Science, Management, Commerce, and Education. Currently, Dr. C.V. Suresh Babu is a Professor in the Department of Information Technology at the School of Computing Science, Hindustan Institute of Technology and Science (Hindustan University) in Padur, Chennai, Tamil Nadu, India. For more information, you can visit his personal blog at https://sites.google .com/view/cvsureshbabu/.

Doris Behrens is a professor of Healthcare Management and Head of the Department for Economy and Health at the University of Krems in Austria. Additionally, Doris serves the NHS Wales as Wellbeing Analytics Lead, following years of previous employment as principal mathematician and epidemiologist. In these roles, she was part of a team jointly based at Cardiff University and Aneurin Bevan University Health Board that used Operations Research techniques to increase the efficiency and effectiveness of the healthcare system. Doris' work typically sits at the interface of mathematics, operations research, economics and management.

It covers projects such as (cost-)effective pathway design for diabetes, forecasting A&E attendances for planning and increasing patient safety by enabling clinical staff to improve their systems. Doris has a PhD in Technical Sciences from the Vienna University of Technology, focusing on Operations Research and Biomathematics.

Dinesh Chander has presently been working as a Professor and Head Department of Computer Applications at Panipat Institute of Engineering & Technology. He has more than 20 years of teaching experience. He has published more than 20 papers in reputed journals/conferences. His areas of interest are MANET, Data Science, and Machine Learning.

William Alberto Cruz Castañeda AI Researcher. Experience in Biomedical Engineering and Computer Science. Research topics include ubiquitous computing, the internet of things, wearable devices, ubiquitous health, machine learning, multi-criteria decision-analysis, healthcare technology management, home care, chronic disease management, and digital assistive technologies. It includes the design, development, and implementation of large-scale computational solutions that empower the acquisition, processing, transmission, and management of heterogeneous data.

Thomas Davies has earned his BSc degree at the School of Mathematics at Cardiff University, UK. His final year undergraduate project covered the problem of improving staffing at a Hospital Sterilization and Decontamination Unit (HSDU).

Upasna Deep is an Intensive Care Unit Consultant Assistant Professor at the prestigious Christian Medical College and Hospital Ludhiana, where she has been serving for the last 5 years. Her experience also includes tenures at institution Frances Newton Mission Hospital at Firozpur, Punjab (2 years). Holding post graduate degree MD and Diplomat National Board in Anaesthesiology, Dr. Upasna has consistently demonstrated exceptional expertise in intensive care and anaesthesiology. Alongside her extensive hospital experience, she is actively engaged in research projects and has several publications to her credit, contributing significantly to advancements in her field.

Omar El-Gayar, Ph.D. is a Professor of Information Systems at Dakota State University. Dr. El-Gayar has extensive administrative experience at the college and university levels as the Dean of the College of Information Technology at United Arab Emirates University (UAEU) and the Founding Dean of Graduate Studies and Research at Dakota State University. His research interests include analytics, business intelligence, and decision support with applications in domains such as healthcare, environmental management, and security planning and management.

His interdisciplinary educational background and training include information technology, computer science, economics, and operations research. Dr. El-Gayar's industry experience includes working as an analyst, modeler, and programmer. His numerous publications have appeared in various fields related to information technology. Dr. El-Gayar serves as a peer and program evaluator for accrediting agencies such as the Higher Learning Commission and ABET, a panelist for the National Science Foundation, and a peer-reviewer for numerous journals and conferences. He is a member of a number of professional organizations such as the Association for Information Systems (AIS) and the Association for Computing Machinery (ACM).

Sherif El-Gayar M.D. completed a B.S. in Biology at the South Dakota State University where he assisted research on antibiotic resistance and the SPRTN gene. For postgraduate, he trained at the Mayo Clinic Alix School of Medicine where he authored a publication analyzing patient emergency department complaints and assisted research in adolescent alcohol withdrawal. He is currently practicing as a psychiatry resident in Las Vegas and is assisting research in psychiatric and medical comorbidities and undergoing a QI project involving data-assisted psychopharmacology education.

Tracey England is a senior post-doctoral research fellow with approximately 30 years of developing mathematical models and simulations, typically in healthcare related areas. Her areas of interest focus on discrete event simulation and system dynamics. She has spent approximately 20 years in academia in Russell Group Universities as well as 6 years in an embedded healthcare modelling team in the NHS. Her current research involves developing a system dynamics model for frailty incidence and progression in the older population which she is now adapting into a workforce model.

G.Bhuvaneswar I received the B.E degree in Computer Science & Engineering from Bharathidasan University, M.E degree in Computer Science & Engineering from Anna University, Ph.D degree in Computer Science & Engineering at Anna University. She is having more than 20 years of experience in Academics, Research & Development and Administration. She is currently working as a Professor in Computer Science and Engineering Department at Saveetha Engineering College. She is having two Patents and one Copyright on various topics. She has published more than 15 Research papers in Scopus / SCI / WoS Journals and more than 20 Research papers presented in different National and International level Conferences. Her area of interests includes Image Processing, Computer Vision, Data mining, Artificial Intelligence and Machine Learning.

G.Manikandan received the B.E degree in Computer Science & Engineering from Madras University, M.E degree in Computer Science & Engineering from Sathyabama University, Post Graduate Diploma in Geo Spatial Information Technology from Periyar Maniammai University, the M.B.A degree in HR from Tamil Nadu Open University, Ph.D degree in Computer Science & Engineering at Sathyabama University. He is having more than 24 years of Valuable in depth and extensive experience in Academics, Research & Development and Administration. He is Currently working as a Professor in the department of Artificial Intelligence and Data Science Department at R.M.K Engineering College. He completed the Post-doctoral Research in the topic of "Enhanced AI Based machine learning model for an accurate segmentation and classification method", under the guidance of Dr. Bui Thanh Hung, Artificial Intelligence Laboratory, Faculty of Information Technology, Industrial University of Ho Chi Minh City VIETNAM. He is having more than seven pattern and one Copyright on different topics. He has published more than 36 Research papers in Scopus / SCI / WoS Journals and more than 32 Research papers presented in different National and International level Conferences. His area of interests includes Data mining, Spatial Databases, Geographic information System and intelligent Transportation Systems, Artificial Intelligence and Machine Learning.

G Revathy is working in SASTRA Deemed University. She has 15 years of teaching experience. She has published around 30 international journals and authored 10 books

Daniel Gartner is a Professor of Operational Research at Cardiff University, School of Mathematics. His research has been recognized by awards such as the OR Society's Lyn Thomas Impact Medal. Besides his researcher-in-residence appointment with NHS Wales, Daniel serves as an editor-in-chief for the OR Society's journal Health Systems.

Sumana Haldar is a dynamic and driven individual with a keen interest in technology and healthcare innovation. With both undergraduate and graduate degrees in Information Technology, Sumana has cultivated a deep understanding of software engineering principles and their application in real-world settings. Currently working as a Senior Software Engineer at Canon Medical Informatics, Sumana plays a pivotal role in developing advanced software solutions for medical imaging. In addition to her professional pursuits, Sumana is pursuing a doctorate program in Information Systems with a specialization in Healthcare from Dakota State University. This academic pursuit reflects his commitment to advancing the intersection of technology and healthcare. At the core of Sumana's academic and research interests lies a deep-seated passion for mental health advocacy. She is particularly interested in exploring the potential of Artificial Intelligence (AI) in the mental health domain and is dedicated to utilizing AI-driven technologies to promote mental well-being and create a healthier society.

V Hashiyana is a Namibian national. He obtained his Doctorate in Computer Engineering from Saint -Petersburg State University of Information Technologies, Mechanics and Optics (Russia). Currently he is a Senior Lecturer at Computing, Mathematical and Statistical Science Department at University of Namibia. His area of research are Wireless technologies, Computer Networks and IT Security, Next -generation Computing, Artificial Intelligence and Educational Technologies

Yanguo Jing is the Dean of the Faculty of Business, Computing and Digital Industries, Leeds Trinity University. He is a Professor of Artificial Intelligence. Prior joining LTU, Professor Jing was a Professor in Artificial Intelligence and an Associate Dean in Coventry University, having held senior leadership roles in all three faculties – namely the Faculty of Business and Law, the Faculty of Engineering, Environment and Computing and the Faculty of Arts and Humanities.

M. Robinson Joel received the Doctorate Ph.D degree in Computer and Information Technology from the Manonmaniam Sundaranar University, Tirunelveli in March 2019. He completed his M.Tech and MCA from the same university year 2008 and 2002 respectively. He is currently working as an Associate Professor in the Department of Information Technology, at Kings Engineering College, Chennai. He has 16 years of teaching experience.

Yordanka Karayaneva is a Lecturer in Computer Science at the School of Computing, Engineering and Digital Technologies at Teesside University. She completed her PhD at Coventry University with a thesis title "Machine Learning for Human Activity Recognition Using Non-Intrusive Sensors" in 2021. Previously, she obtained a BSc in Computer Science at Coventry University in 2017. Dr Yordanka Karayaneva has published articles in both high-impact journals and conferences. Her main research interests are in the field of machine learning, signal processing and human activity recognition.

Christian Kaunert is Professor of International Security at Dublin City University, Ireland. He is also Professor of Policing and Security, as well as Director of the International Centre for Policing and Security at the University of South Wales. In addition, he is Jean Monnet Chair, Director of the Jean Monnet Centre of Excellence and Director of the Jean Monnet Network on EU Counter-Terrorism (www.eucter.net).

Ekta Mala is a renowned clinical microbiologist at the Alchemist Hospitals Multi-Specialty Hospital in Panchkula, where she has been serving for over 2 years. Her extensive experience also includes tenures at prestigious institutions such as Christian Medical College, Ludhiana (3 years), and Mission Hospital, Ferozpur, Punjab (2 years). Holding a postgraduate degree in Microbiology, Dr. Mala has consistently demonstrated exceptional expertise in clinical Microbiology. Alongside her extensive hospital experience, she is actively engaged in research projects and has several publications to her credit, contributing significantly to advancements in her field.

Shaveta Mala is a renowned ICU Specialist and Medical Officer at the Government Multi-Specialty Hospital in Chandigarh, where she has been serving for over 10 years. Her extensive experience also includes tenures at prestigious institutions such as Christian Medical College, Ludhiana (4 years), Philadelphia Hospital, Ambala, Haryana (2 years), and Mission Hospital, Ferozpur, Punjab (2 years). Holding a postgraduate degree in Anesthesia, Dr. Mala has consistently demonstrated exceptional expertise in intensive care and anesthesiology. Alongside her extensive hospital experience, she is actively engaged in research projects and has several publications to her credit, contributing significantly to advancements in her field.

James Mutuku is a Lecturer at the Department of Computing, Mathematical & Statistical Sciences under the Faculty of Agriculture, Engineering and Natural Sciences, University of Namibia. His main areas of Research are ICT4D, AI, IT Security, Next-generation Computing, and Educational Technologies.

Nevine Nawar is a Lecturer at the Department of Public Health, School of Medicine, Alexandria University, Egypt. Her research interests emphasize preventive strategies that recognize and address risk factors as key to health promotion and disease prevention. Dr. Nawar taught courses in nutrition, child and maternity health, health education, rural health, health care delivery systems, and communicable diseases. She has engaged in funded research including a World Health Organization funded survey to identify microbial causes for diarrhea among preschool children living in rural communities in Egypt. She was also part of a community-based surveys to recognize health problems in urban Alexandrian communities. Dr. Nawar holds a medical degree and a Master's in Public Health from Alexandria University. She obtained her Ph.D. in Public Health also from Alexandria University through a joint-supervision with Harvard University (channel system).

Mark A. Neerincx is a Professor in Human-Centered Computing and Principal Scientist at TNO Human-Machine Teaming. He focuses on the socio-cognitive engineering of ePartners in health and safety, which enhance the social, cognitive and affective processes in human-agent teams.

Hari Singh is PhD, M.Tech and B.Engg. (Honors) in Computer Science & Engineering. He has been presently working as a faculty in Computer Science & Engineering Department at Jaypee University of Information Technology, Solan, Himachal Pradesh, India. He has a teaching experience of 21+ years that includes a significant administrative and research experience. His areas of interest are Distributed and Parallel Computing, Grid Computing, Cloud Computing, Machine Learning and Deep Learning, Programming and logic development. He has many awards, honors and recognitions to his credit. He has delivered several invited/ expert talks on recent research topics at renowned institutes and universities. He has published several research papers/book chapters in SCI/Scopus indexed/ peer-reviewed International Journals, edited books and National/International Conferences. He has also worked as editor of proceedings of various International/ National Conferences. He has attended/participated and organized several Conferences/Seminars/Workshops. He has/has been supervised/supervising several M.Tech/PhD scholars.

Ruban S Associate professor and Head of the department of software technology, St Aloysius Deemed to be university, Mangalore. With a teaching and research experience of 22 years in post graduate department, he has received various external funded research projects and has many Scopus Index publications. His areas of interest include Clinical Machine Learning, Big Data Analytics, Artificial Intelligence in Healthcare and Design Thinking. He has been to Sophia University, Japan as a Visiting Associate Faculty to the Science and Technology department recently.

Piyush Sewal is an Assistant Professor in the Yogananda School of AI, Computers, and Data Science (YSAICDS) at Shoolini University, Solan. He is currently pursuing his PhD in the Department of Computer Science & Engineering and Information Technology at Jaypee University of Information Technology. Mr. Sewal holds a Master's degree in Computer Applications from the Department of Computer Science at Himachal Pradesh University. With over 12 years of professional experience, he has a diverse background in teaching and training. He has delivered numerous talks and training sessions as a resource person at various government, semi-government, and private organizations. His areas of expertise include distributed data processing, data analytics, artificial intelligence, and machine learning.

Wasswa Shafik (Member, IEEE) received a Bachelor of Science degree in information technology engineering with a minor in mathematics from Ndejje University, Kampala, Uganda, a Master of Engineering degree in information technology engineering (MIT) from Yazd University, Iran, and a Ph.D. degree in computer science with the School of Digital Science, Universiti Brunei Darussalam, Brunei Darussalam. He is also the Founder and a Principal Investigator of the Dig Connectivity Research Laboratory (DCRLab) after serving as a Research Associate at Network Interconnectivity Research Laboratory, Yazd University. Prior to this, he worked as a Community Data Analyst at Population Services International (PSI-Uganda), Community Data Officer at Programme for Accessible Health Communication (PACE-Uganda), Research Assistant at the Socio-Economic Data Centre (SEDC-Uganda), Prime Minister's Office, Kampala, Uganda, an Assistant Data Officer at TechnoServe, Kampala, IT Support at Thurayya Islam Media, Uganda, and Asmaah Charity Organization. He has 70+ publications in renowned journals and conferences. His research interests include AI, smart agriculture, health computing and ecological informatics.

Sara Sharifzadeh completed her PhD study in Computer Science at Technical University of Denmark, in 2015, with an external research period at Waterloo University, Canada. Upon Completion of her PhD, she started her new career as Research Associate in Data Science at Loughborough University. In 2018, she joined Coventry University as a Lecturer. She has joined Swansea University as senior lecturer in 2021. During her study and research career, Dr Sharifzadeh was involved in several industrial research projects funded by EPSRC and Danish Council for Strategic Research and industrial partners. Her main areas of research include machine learning, artificial intelligence, multivariate data analysis with application in spectral signal/image analysis, digital health e.g. human activity recognition, satellite image analysis and analysis of 3D point cloud data acquired from robot-mounted laser scanner sensors. She has supervised several PhD and Msc projects on these research topics. She is a reviewer of several high impact international journals and member of IEEE.

Luuk P.A. Simons is a Senior Fellow in the field of persuasive technology, hybrid eHealth systems, self-management support, lifestyle medicine and high impact health coaching.

Bhupinder Singh working as Professor at Sharda University, India. Also, Honorary Professor in University of South Wales UK and Santo Tomas University Tunja, Colombia. His areas of publications as Smart Healthcare, Medicines, fuzzy logics, artificial intelligence, robotics, machine learning, deep learning, federated learning, IoT, PV Glasses, metaverse and many more. He has 3 books, 139 paper publications, 163 paper presentations in international/national conferences and seminars, participated in more than 40 workshops/FDP's/QIP's, 25 courses from international universities of repute, organized more than 59 events with international and national academicians and industry people's, editor-in-chief and co-editor in journals, developed new courses. He has given talks at international universities, resource person in international conferences such as in Nanyang Technological University Singapore, Tashkent State University of Law Uzbekistan; KIMEP University Kazakhstan, All'ah meh Tabatabi University Iran, the Iranian Association of International Criminal law, Iran and Hague Center for International Law and Investment, The Netherlands, Northumbria University Newcastle UK,

Ala Szczepura is Professor of Health Technology Assessment in the Research Centre for Healthcare and Communities, and Visiting Professor at University Hospitals Coventry and Warwickshire Trust. Originally a scientist, she has over thirty years' experien of interdisciplinary health services research with specific interests in: health and care technology assessment; re-design and assessment of services; and addressing population diversity for cost-effective care.

Bo Tan is an Associate Professor at Tampere Wireless Research Centre, Tampere University, Finland. He received his PhD from the Institute for Digital Communications (IDCOM), the University of Edinburgh, UK, in Nov 2013. He conducted multiple postdoctoral research projects at the University College London and the University of Bristol, UK, contributing to radar design and applications in security and healthcare. From 2017 to 2018, he was a lecturer at Coventry University, UK. Since 2019, he has been an assistant professor and then promoted to associate professor at Tampere University. His research interests include radio signal processing for sensing and connectivity, mobile networks, distributed machine learning for intelligent machines, and healthcare. He is the PI and coordinator of multiple research projects funded by the Academy of Finland, Business Finland, and Horizon Europe. He is currently the vice chair of the IEEE Finland AP/ED/ MTT Chapter, editor of IEEE Wireless Communications Letters, and reviewer of multiple IEEE/ACM/IET journals, as well as organizer and TPC member of multiple international conferences.

Arulkumar V P received his B.E Degree in Computer Science and Engineering from Anna University in 2010 and M.E. Computer Science and Engineering in Karpagam Academy of Higher Education in 2013. He is currently pursuing Ph.D in IoT, and Machine Learning at Karpagam Academy of Higher Education. He is currently an Assistant Professor, Department of IT, Karpagam Institute of

Technology. His main research interest includes IoT, AI-ML, Wireless Sensor Network and Cloud Computing.

Nilmini Wickramasinghe, PhD, MBA, is the Professor and Optus chair of Digital Health at La Trobe University within the School of Computing, Engineering and Mathematical Sciences. She also holds honorary research professor positions at the Peter MacCallum Cancer Centre, MCRI, Epworth HealthCare and Northern Health. After completing 5 degrees at the University of Melbourne, she completed PhD studies at Case Western Reserve University, and later executive education at Harvard Business School, USA in Value-based HealthCare. For over 25 years, she has been actively, researching and teaching within the health informatics/ digital health domain with over 350 scholarly publications, a patent, 25 books, numerous posters and book chapters and a very successful grant funding portfolio. In 2020, she was awarded the prestigious Alexander von Humboldt award for her outstanding contribution to digital health. Professor Wickramasinghe is the editor in chief of International Journal Networking and Virtual Organisations, published by InderScience. In addition, she is the editor of two book series in digital health 1) Healthcare Delivery in the Information Age, published by Springer 2) Analytics and AI for healthcare Delivery, published by CRC Routledge.

Bas Wielaard is a health coach and lifestyle expert specialised in cardiac and metabolic health, diet and self-management support.

Index

A

ageing population 4, 19, 24

AI Algorithms 107, 110, 126, 133, 135, 167, 171, 187, 188, 195, 197, 198, 199, 200, 201, 202, 225, 226, 285, 286

Artificial Intelligence 57, 71, 101, 102, 115, 117, 118, 121, 122, 123, 124, 125, 126, 127, 128, 129, 130, 131, 133, 134, 135, 136, 137, 139, 141, 142, 143, 144, 145, 167, 184, 185, 189, 190, 191, 192, 193, 200, 228, 229, 232, 254, 285, 342, 345, 373, 379, 380, 381, 387, 393, 397, 402, 404, 414, 449, 484, 489, 498

Augmented Reality 56, 58, 95, 106, 139, 140, 141, 144, 145, 409, 410, 412, 414, 437, 438, 439, 440, 441, 442, 443, 444

B

Breast Cancer 172, 176, 189, 191, 439, 445, 446, 447, 448, 449, 450, 452, 453, 454, 458, 461, 462, 463, 464, 465, 468, 469, 470, 471, 473, 474, 475, 476, 477, 478, 479

C

Cancer Association 446, 477, 479

Cardiovascular Risk Factors 277, 379, 382, 390, 395, 397

Caregivers 9, 25, 27, 55, 56, 60, 88, 100, 293, 388, 446, 448, 449, 450, 451, 453, 465, 466, 467, 468, 470, 473, 474, 478, 479

Chronic Diseases 56, 57, 73, 101, 102, 104, 132, 249, 341, 342, 343, 344, 346, 347, 349, 350, 351, 352, 358, 360, 395, 488, 491, 496

Clinical Decision Support Systems (CDSS) 105, 187, 231, 232, 233, 234, 235, 236, 237, 238, 239, 240, 241, 242, 243, 244, 245, 246, 247, 248, 249, 251, 253, 254, 255

Cognitive Adoption 410, 411, 412, 430, 431, 434, 438

Comparative Analysis 409, 411, 412, 417, 418, 420, 421, 423, 424, 434

Covid-19 61, 72, 81, 151, 160, 191, 303, 304, 305, 306, 307, 308, 309, 310, 314, 315, 320, 333, 335, 336, 337, 338, 339, 393, 396, 402, 405, 413, 481, 483, 484, 485, 486, 487, 489, 490, 491, 492, 493, 494, 496, 498

D

Decision Tree 172, 173, 174, 303, 306, 310, 312, 313, 318, 320, 323, 335, 368

Deep learning 4, 70, 100, 103, 117, 118, 135, 144, 145, 186, 189, 190, 192, 197, 198, 200, 201, 207, 212, 213, 221, 226, 228, 236, 254, 288, 290, 292, 293, 301, 305, 307, 308, 336, 337, 368, 372, 373, 374, 377, 416, 442, 500

Design Principles 341, 342, 343, 344, 346, 347, 349, 351, 353, 355, 358, 379, 387

Design Science 441

Diabetes Management 250, 251, 347, 351, 353, 359, 481, 483, 484, 485, 486, 487, 488, 489, 490, 491, 492, 493, 494, 495, 497

Diabetes Mellitus 255, 361, 398, 481, 482, 484, 488, 489, 491, 494, 495, 498

Digital Health Interventions 380, 382, 481, 484, 485, 486, 488, 491, 493, 494

Digital Health Technologies 118, 379, 380, 381, 382, 383, 384, 385, 386, 387, 388, 389, 390, 391, 411, 412, 430, 431, 434, 438, 481, 484, 486, 491, 494

Digital Technology 347, 394, 478

E

eHealth 69, 72, 94, 257, 259, 278, 279, 387, 496

Electronic Health Record (EHR) 232, 254

employee health 278

Z

Milton Keynes UK
Ingram Content Group UK Ltd.
UKHW012104151124
451073UK00027B/302

9 798369 352373